BSAVA Manual of Canine and Feline Nephrology and Urology
third edition

T0203239

Editors:

Jonathan Elliott
MA VetMB PhD CertSAC DipECVPT FHEA MRCVS
Comparative Biomedical Sciences,
The Royal Veterinary College,
Royal College Street, London NW1 0TU, UK

Gregory F. Grauer
DVM MS DipACVIM (Small Animal Internal Medicine)
College of Veterinary Medicine,
Kansas State University,
Manhattan, KS 66506, USA

Jodi L. Westropp
DVM PhD DipACVIM
UC Davis School of Veterinary Medicine,
One Shields Avenue, Davis, CA 95616, USA

Published by:

British Small Animal Veterinary Association
Woodrow House, 1 Telford Way,
Waterwells Business Park, Quedgeley,
Gloucester GL2 2AB

A Company Limited by Guarantee in England
Registered Company No. 2837793
Registered as a Charity

ISBN 978 1 905319 94 7

The publishers, editors and contributors cannot take responsibility for information provided on
dosages and methods of application of drugs mentioned or referred to in this publication.
Details of this kind must be verified in each case by individual users from up to date literature
published by the manufacturers or suppliers of those drugs. Veterinary surgeons are reminded
that in each case they must follow all appropriate national legislation and regulations (for
example, in the United Kingdom, the prescribing cascade) from time to time in force.

Printed by Cambrian Printers, Aberystwyth, UK
Printed on ECF paper made from sustainable forests

3700PUBS17

Titles in the BSAVA Manuals series

For further information on these and all BSAVA publications, please visit our website: **www.bsava.com**

Contents

Contributors

Larry Adams
DVM PhD
Department of Veterinary Clinical Sciences,
Purdue University, 625 Harrison Street,
West Lafayette, IN 47907, USA

Rick Alleman
DVM PhD DipACBVP DipACVP
Lighthouse Veterinary Consultants,
13337 NW 172nd Avenue, Alachua, FL 32615, USA

Clarke Atkins
DVM DipACVIM
Department of Clinical Sciences,
College of Veterinary Medicine, North Carolina
State University, 1060 William Moore Drive,
Raleigh, NC 27607, USA

Joe Bartges
DVM PhD DipACVIM DipACVN
Department of Small Animal Medicine and Surgery,
College of Veterinary Medicine, The University of
Georgia, Athens, GA 30602, USA

Allyson Berent
DVM DipACVIM
Animal Medical Center,
510 East 62nd Street, New York, NY 10065, USA

Cathy Brown
VMD PhD DipACVP
Department of Pathology,
College of Veterinary Medicine, The University of
Georgia, Athens, GA 30602, USA

Scott A. Brown
VMD PhD DipACVIM (Small Animal Internal Medicine)
Departments of Physiology & Pharmacology and
Small Animal Medicine & Surgery, College of
Veterinary Medicine, The University of Georgia,
Athens, GA 30602, USA

Tony Buffington
DVM PhD DipACVN
California, USA

Julie Byron
DVM MS DipACVIM
Department of Veterinary Clinical Sciences,
College of Veterinary Medicine, The Ohio State
University, 601 Vernon L. Tharp Street, Columbus,
OH 43210, USA

Dennis J. Chew
DVM DipACVIM
Department of Veterinary Clinical Sciences,
College of Veterinary Medicine, The Ohio State
University, 601 Vernon L. Tharp Street,
Columbus, OH 43210, USA

Amanda E. Coleman
DVM DipACVIM (Cardiology)
Department of Small Animal Medicine and Surgery,
College of Veterinary Medicine, The University of
Georgia, Athens, GA 30602, USA

Larry D. Cowgill
DVM PhD DipACVIM
UC Davis School of Veterinary Medicine,
One Shields Avenue, Davis, CA 95616, USA

William T. N. Culp
VMD DipACVS
UC Davis School of Veterinary Medicine,
One Shields Avenue, Davis, CA 95616, USA

Autumn P. Davidson
DVM MS DipACVIM
UC Davis School of Veterinary Medicine,
One Shields Avenue, Davis, CA 95616, USA

Jonathan Elliott
MA VetMB PhD CertSAC DipECVPT FHEA MRCVS
Comparative Biomedical Sciences,
The Royal Veterinary College, Royal College Street,
London NW1 0TU, UK

Natalie Finch
BVSc PhD DipECVIM-CA MRCVS
School of Clinical Sciences and School of Veterinary
Sciences, University of Bristol, Whitson Street,
Bristol BS1 3NY, UK

Julie R. Fischer
DVM DipACVIM (Small Animal Internal Medicine)
Veterinary Specialty Hospital,
10435 Sorrento Valley Road, San Diego, CA 92121, USA

Rebecca Geddes
MA VetMB GPCert(FelP) PhD MRCVS
Queen Mother Hospital for Animals,
The Royal Veterinary College, Hawkshead Lane,
North Mymms, Hatfield AL9 7TA, UK

Alexander J. German
BVSc(Hons) PhD CertSAM DipECVIM-CA MRCVS
Institute of Veterinary Science,
University of Liverpool, Leahurst Campus,
Chester High Road, Neston CH64 7TE, UK

Gregory F. Grauer
DVM MS DipACVIM (Small Animal Internal Medicine)
College of Veterinary Medicine,
Kansas State University, Manhattan, KS 66506, USA

Sarah Crilly Guess
DVM MS
Columbia River Veterinary Specialists,
6607 NE 84th Street, Suite 109, Vancouver,
WA 98665, Canada

Reidun Heiene
DVM PhD MRCVS
Oslo, Norway

Rosanne Jepson
BVSc MVetMed PhD DipACVIM DipECVIM MRCVS
Queen Mother Hospital for Animals,
The Royal Veterinary College, Hawkshead Lane,
North Mymms, Hatfield AL9 7TA, UK

India F. Lane
DVM MS EdD DipACVIM (Small Animal Internal Medicine)
Academic Affairs and Student Success,
The University of Tennessee, 823 Andy Holt Tower,
Knoxville, TN 37996, USA

Cathy Langston
DVM DipACVIM
Department of Veterinary Clinical Sciences,
College of Veterinary Medicine, The Ohio State
University, 601 Vernon L. Tharp Street, Columbus,
OH 43210, USA

Meryl P. Littman
VMD DipACVIM
School of Veterinary Medicine,
University of Pennsylvania, 3900 Delancey Street,
PA 19104, USA

Jody Lulich
DVM PhD DipACVIM
Department of Veterinary Clinical Sciences,
College of Veterinary Medicine, University of Minnesota,
1352 Boyd Avenue, St Paul, MN 55108, USA

Philipp D. Mayhew
BVM&S DipACVS
UC Davis School of Veterinary Medicine,
One Shields Avenue, Davis, CA 95616, USA

Shelly Olin
DVM, DipACVIM (Small Animal Internal Medicine)
Veterinary Medical Center,
The University of Tennessee, 2407 River Drive,
Knoxville, TN 37996, USA

Mark A. Oyama
DVM MSCE DipACVIM
Department of Clinical Studies, School of Veterinary
Medicine and Ryan Veterinary Hospital, University of
Pennsylvania, 3900 Spruce Street, PA 19104, USA

Carrie A. Palm
DVM DipACVIM
UC Davis School of Veterinary Medicine,
One Shields Avenue, Davis, CA 95616, USA

Ludovic Pelligand
DocMedVet CertVA DipECVAA DipECVPT PhD MRCVS
Queen Mother Hospital for Animals,
The Royal Veterinary College, Hawkshead Lane,
North Mymms, Hatfield AL9 7TA, UK

Kathryn L. Phillips
DVM
Department of Molecular Biomedical Sciences,
College of Veterinary Medicine, North Carolina State
University, Raleigh, NC 27607, USA

Rachel E. Pollard
DVM PhD DipACVR
UC Davis School of Veterinary Medicine,
One Shields Avenue, Davis, CA 95616, USA

David J. Polzin
DVM PhD DipACVIM (Small Animal Internal Medicine)
Department of Veterinary Clinical Sciences,
College of Veterinary Medicine, University of Minnesota,
1352 Boyd Avenue, St Paul, MN 55108, USA

Sheri Ross
DVM PhD DipACVIM
UC Veterinary Medical Center - San Diego,
10435 Sorrento Valley Road, Suite 101,
San Diego, CA 92121, USA

Xavier Roura
DVM PhD DipECVIM-CA
Hospital Clinic Veterinari,
Universitat Autònoma de Barcelona,
08193 Bellaterra (Cerdanyola del Vallès), Spain

Gilad Segev
DipECVIM-CA (Internal Medicine)
Koret School of Veterinary Medicine,
The Hebrew University of Jerusalem,
PO Box 12, Rehovot 76100, Israel

Harriet Syme
BSc BVetMed PhD FHEA DipACVIM DipECVIM MRCVS
Small Animal Medicine and Surgery Group,
The Royal Veterinary College, Hawkshead Lane,
North Mymms, Hatfield AL9 7TA, UK

Mary Thompson
BVSc(Hons) PhD DipACVIM MANZCVS
School of Veterinary and Life Sciences,
College of Veterinary Medicine,
South Street Campus, 90 South Street,
Murdoch 6150, Western Australia, Australia

Shelly L. Vaden
DVM PhD DipACVIM
Department of Clinical Sciences,
College of Veterinary Medicine,
North Carolina State University, 1060 William Moore
Drive, Raleigh, NC 27607, USA

Heather L. Wamsley
BS DVM PhD DipACVP (Clinical)
ANTECH Diagnostics, Tampa, FL 32614, USA

A. David J. Watson
BVSc PhD FAAVPT MACVSc DipECVPT FRCVS
Sydney, Australia

Jodi L. Westropp
DVM PhD DipACVIM
UC Davis School of Veterinary Medicine,
One Shields Avenue, Davis, CA 95616, USA

Tim Williams
MA VetMB PhD FRCPath DipECVCP MRCVS
Department of Veterinary Medicine,
University of Cambridge, Madingley Road,
Cambridge CB3 0ES, UK

Foreword

This is the third edition of the *BSAVA Manual of Canine and Feline Nephrology and Urology*, and it has been a full decade since the publication of the previous edition. Readers will, therefore, soon discover that whilst the arrangement and layout of the manual are similar, this is a radically different book to the previous edition, reflecting the enormous advances in this field over the last 10 years.

Chapters on imaging and diagnostic techniques are interspersed between chapters describing clinical presentations and others covering clinical syndromes. The manual has been designed as a practical and usable guide for busy practitioners and one that, I am sure, will find everyday use in small animal practice.

The editors, Jonathan Elliott, Gregory Grauer and Jodi Westropp, have put together a world class team of authors, and the quality of the *BSAVA Manual of Canine and Feline Nephrology and Urology* is provided by the breadth and depth of knowledge of both the authors and editors, and their ability to effectively communicate this knowledge to the reader. I would like to congratulate the editors and authors on producing this new edition that, I am sure, will prove to be as useful and enduring as its predecessors. On behalf of practitioners, thank you!

John Chitty
BVetMed CertZooMed MRCVS
BSAVA President 2017–2018

Preface

It is 10 years since the publication of the second edition of the *BSAVA Manual of Canine and Feline Nephrology and Urology*. For this third edition, a new scientific editor has joined the editorial team, bringing deeper insight into lower urinary tract disorders in particular. New technologies are clearly influencing our ability to understand, diagnose and treat urinary tract disorders in dogs and cats, and are reflected in the additions made to this new edition.

The third edition follows the successful format of the first two manuals with sections on presenting problems, diagnostic and therapeutic techniques, and management of specific problems. A series of new chapters has been added explaining how other systemic diseases (or drug treatments) affect the kidney, influencing diagnostic tests or contributing to kidney damage. We hope these will aid practitioners in considering the kidney when tackling cardiovascular and endocrine disorders and when treating osteoarthritis.

A fresh look has been taken at many of the tried and tested chapters by inviting new authors to provide their perspectives on these familiar topics. The number of clinical experts from Europe and the United States who are actively publishing original clinical research papers in nephrology and urology has grown in recent years, so we have had no difficulty in identifying new truly international experts as authors.

There are some exciting new developments in urinary diseases included in this new edition. For example, rapid advances in molecular genetics mean that the genomic basis of many more inherited diseases of the urinary tract are now known with genetic tests available. The International Renal Interest Society's (IRIS) grading system for acute kidney injury (AKI) is a novel framework for veterinary medicine that should enable practitioners to pick up cases of AKI early and so manage these more successfully, particularly if the field of urinary biomarkers advances over the next 10 years, as it has the potential to do. Early diagnostics for chronic kidney disease (CKD) are also under development, including symmetric dimethylarginine (SDMA) which was launched commercially in 2015. Experience of using this marker alongside creatinine is in its infancy – time will tell what SDMA beings, but the initial data look promising. The discovery of the role of FGF-23 in mineral and bone disorders associated with CKD and its prognostic value in the CKD patient is an exciting advance in knowledge, the application of which will become apparent in the next decade.

The work of the WSAVA Renal Pathology Group has made significant advances in our knowledge of canine glomerular disease pathology and this stimulated a series of consensus papers written by groups of experts coordinated by IRIS reviewing the evidence-base treatment of glomerular disease in dogs. These recommendations are summarized in the manual. In future years we expect further research to provide the evidence on which to use biopsy results to further define the most appropriate approach to treatment.

Diagnosing and managing various lower urinary tract disorders in companion animals has evolved immensely over the past 10 years, particularly with the advances in minimally invasive procedures. For example, the use of laser ablation for the correction of ectopic ureters in dogs has meant far fewer surgical procedures for this anomaly. Minimally invasive stone removal was one of the highlights discussed in the ACVIM Consensus Statement for Recommendations on the Treatment and Prevention on Uroliths in Dogs and Cats in 2016, and many of these recommendations are discussed in the manual, including voiding urohydropropulsion, holmium:YAG laser lithotripsy and percutaneous cystolithotomy. With the advent of ureteral stents and subcutaneous ureteral bypass procedures, we now have alternative and often better ways to manage obstructive kidney disease in cats and dogs, and details are provided in this new edition. The most recent medical management strategies for urolithiasis prevention are also provided in a dedicated chapter. Finally, this edition provides a comprehensive overview as well as various updates on other aspects of lower urinary tract disorders, which make these sections a valuable resource for students and practitioners, as well as various veterinary specialists.

Editing a manual of this size is a hugely enjoyable if time-consuming task as one learns so much in the process. This task has been made as easy as it could be by the efficient editorial team at BSAVA, who have supported us so effectively throughout the process. We hope the end result will be a useful addition to your practice library.

Jonathan Elliott, Gregory F. Grauer and Jodi L. Westropp
June 2017

Chapter 1

Stranguria and haematuria

Mary Thompson and A. David J. Watson

Stranguria and haematuria can occur concurrently in dogs and cats but may be seen separately as signs of disease.

- **Stranguria** is defined as difficulty in micturition.
- **Haematuria** denotes the presence of blood in the urine.

Stranguric animals usually adopt the typical urinating posture but show obvious effort or difficulty while attempting to pass urine and may appear distressed. If urine is passed, the flow may be weak, attenuated or intermittent. If little or no urine is passed, either because the bladder is nearly empty or the excretory pathway is obstructed, stranguria may continue for some time, with the animal shifting position repeatedly between attempts.

Whether occurring separately or together, these signs are often associated with two other abnormalities:

- **Dysuria** suggests pain upon urination, which can be difficult to ascertain in some animals
- **Pollakiuria** is defined as the abnormally frequent passage of small amounts of urine.

When pollakiuria is present, a small volume of urine is passed each time the animal urinates. This pattern must be distinguished from **polyuria**, which refers to an increase in daily urine volume. With polyuria, the animal will also urinate more frequently than usual, but a large volume is passed each time, and the urine is usually dilute (low specific gravity).

Stranguria generally results from disorders of the lower urinary tract (bladder or urethra), the genital tract (prostate or vagina) or both. Haematuria can be more difficult to localize because bleeding may occur anywhere in the urinary tract, from the kidneys to the urethral meatus, as well as from the prostate, penis or prepuce in the male, and from the uterus, vagina or vulva in the female. When haematuria and stranguria occur together, lower urinary tract disease or a genital lesion is most likely to be present.

Stranguria – defining the problem

If stranguria is *suspected* on the basis of the history provided by the owners, it is important to *confirm* that this is indeed the problem with key questions to distinguish stranguria from other problems that may confuse owners such as polyuria/polydipsia (PU/PD), dyschezia (difficulty in defecating), urinary incontinence, and behavioural causes of inappropriate urination. It is also important to note the bladder size of the patient, because an animal that presents with stranguria and a large bladder may have a urethral obstruction, which may constitute a medical emergency.

- Animals with PU/PD should pass large volumes when urinating, and drinking is increased (see Chapter 2).
- An animal with urinary incontinence caused by urethral sphincter mechanism incompetence may void small amounts of urine frequently but would not typically appear to be in pain and, by definition, is not aware that urine is being passed.
- A pet urinating in inappropriate places or at unusual times might be described as 'incontinent' by the owner when the problem could be attributed to stranguria and pollakiuria.
- Behavioural urination typically occurs in locations outside of what is considered normal/acceptable.

Confirmation may require the veterinary surgeon (veterinarian) or nurse/technician to observe the animal's behaviour during the process of urination and this can be extremely useful. The importance of spending the time in taking a thorough history from the owner also cannot be overemphasized in terms of confirming the true nature of the problem or problems (some animals will present with more than one of the above clinical signs) (Figure 1.1).

Once the clinician is comfortable that stranguria is the problem, they can use the information gained on the frequency of urination, volume passed, and location of urination to gain further insight into potential causes of stranguria and other signs that may be present.

- Is the volume of urine passed small or large?
- What is the frequency of urination?
- Is the animal urinating in inappropriate places?
- Is there excessive straining or apparent discomfort?
- Is the stream interrupted, attenuated or weak?
- Is the urine cloudy, discoloured or malodorous?
- Is the animal licking its penis or vulva?
- Does the animal appear aware that urine is being passed?
- What is the drinking behaviour of the animal?
- How long have the signs been apparent?
- Have there been any previous episodes?
- Has there been any previous treatment? If so, how did the animal respond?

1.1 Important history questions to ask about a patient with suspected or confirmed stranguria.

Two distinct processes have the potential to cause stranguria:

- Non-obstructive stranguria (small bladder):
  - Diseases of the lower urinary or genital tract that result in mucosal irritation or inflammation
  - Mucosal inflammation can cause pain and urgency to urinate
- Obstructive stranguria (large bladder):
  - Conditions that produce obstruction or narrowing of the urethra or bladder neck:
    - Mechanical obstruction caused by urethral calculi or plugs, neoplasia and prostatic diseases (e.g. benign prostatic hypertrophy or prostatic neoplasia)
    - 'Functional' obstructions can also occur when increased urethral pressure results (e.g. urethral dyssynergia) (see Chapter 30).

A combination of history findings and careful clinical examination of the urinary tract will usually allow the clinician to distinguish between the two processes (Figure 1.2).

The prevalence of different stranguric disorders differs between dogs and cats:

- In dogs, the two most common causes of stranguria are bacterial infections of the lower urinary tract (bacterial cystitis/urethritis) and urinary calculi
- In cats under 10 years of age, the main causes of stranguria (often accompanied by pollakiuria and other lower urinary tract signs) are idiopathic cystitis (obstructive or non-obstructive) and urolithiasis.

However, various other conditions cause stranguria in both species (especially in dogs) and care is warranted before excluding them as possible diagnoses. Potential causes of stranguria in dogs and cats are listed in Figure 1.3.

Process	Frequency of urination	Volume of urination	Bladder size	Systemically unwell
Non-obstructive stranguria	Increased	Decreased	Small	Unlikely
Obstructive stranguria	Increased	Decreased to none	Large	Unlikely

1.2 Clinical features of obstructive and non-obstructive stranguria.

Urinary bladder

- Bacterial cystitis
- Cystic calculi
- Idiopathic cystitis in cats
- Neoplasia – transitional cell carcinoma most common (rare in cats)
- Polypoid cystitis

Urinary bladder and urethra

- Detrusor–urethral dyssynergia (male dogs)

Urethra

- Calculi
- Plugs (cats)
- Stricture
- Bacterial urethritis
- Rupture
- Neoplasia
- Proliferative urethritis

1.3 Sites and processes potentially involved in dogs and cats with stranguria. (continues) ▶

Prostate (conditions rare in cats)

- Benign hyperplasia
- Bacterial prostatitis
- Prostatic abscess
- Carcinoma or other neoplasia of the prostate
- Paraprostatic cysts

Penis, prepuce, vagina (tumours of external genitalia rarely present as dysuria; bloody discharge or visible mass noted more often)

- Transmissible venereal tumour in dogs (mainly in regions with many feral or stray dogs and unregulated breeding)
- Squamous cell carcinoma
- Neoplasia (mast cell tumour, leiomyoma)
- Fibroma
- Vaginitis

Other

- Perineal hernia

1.3 (continued) Sites and processes potentially involved in dogs and cats with stranguria.

Haematuria and other causes of red, brown or black urine (pigmenturia)

As is the case with stranguria, pollakiuria and dysuria, the key to a successful diagnostic investigation of haematuria (both gross and microscopic) lies to a good extent in confirming that this is the correct assignation of the problem. When an animal passes discoloured urine, there are several possibilities as to the cause, and a logical approach to identifying the problem correctly is necessary in order to formulate a diagnostic plan. Prior to undertaking a diagnostic investigation for haematuria, these other causes of discoloured urine must be considered and eliminated as possibilities. For a complete description on the interpretation of urinalysis, see Chapter 6.

Causes of pigmenturia other than gross haematuria

Red, brown or black urine without the presence of intact red blood cells (RBCs) is an uncommon finding in dogs and cats. The most likely cause is haemoglobinuria, but myoglobinuria or chemicals are also potential causes. Important points to note in the diagnostic work-up (Figure 1.4) are:

- Turbidity: samples with gross haematuria are turbid, whereas those due to other causes of pigmenturia are not, unless an additional factor causing turbidity is present
- Test strip results: the common tests for haematuria react positively to haemoglobin and myoglobin but negatively if pigmenturia is caused by a drug or dye
- After centrifugation: the supernatant remains equally discoloured with other causes of pigmenturia, whereas with gross haematuria it becomes less discoloured, or even normal in colour, as RBCs are spun out (Figure 1.5).

Diagnostic procedure

Test urine for occult blood with a dipstick:

- Positive: haematuria (gross or microscopic), haemoglobinuria or myoglobinuria.
- Negative: drugs or dyes the likely cause.

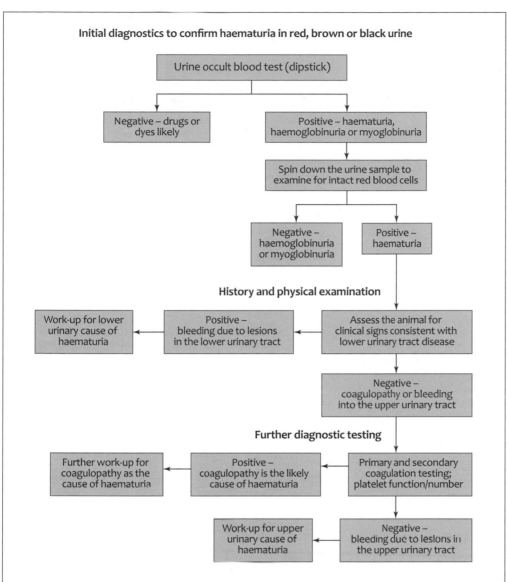

1.4 Diagnostic approach to haematuria (confirmation and work-up).

Initial diagnostics to confirm haematuria in red, brown or black urine

Urine occult blood test (dipstick)

- Negative – drugs or dyes likely
- Positive – haematuria, haemoglobinuria or myoglobinuria

Spin down the urine sample to examine for intact red blood cells

- Negative – haemoglobinuria or myoglobinuria
- Positive – haematuria

History and physical examination

Work-up for lower urinary cause of haematuria ← Positive – bleeding due to lesions in the lower urinary tract ← Assess the animal for clinical signs consistent with lower urinary tract disease

Negative – coagulopathy or bleeding into the upper urinary tract

Further diagnostic testing

Further work-up for coagulopathy as the cause of haematuria ← Positive – coagulopathy is the likely cause of haematuria ← Primary and secondary coagulation testing; platelet function/number

Work-up for upper urinary cause of haematuria ← Negative – bleeding due to lesions in the upper urinary tract

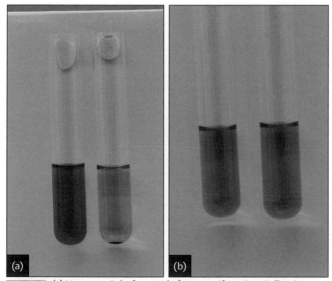

1.5 (a) Haematuria before and after centrifugation. Following centrifugation the urine is no longer turbid, the pigment has largely dissipated and there is a red sediment pellet. (b) Haemoglobinuria before and after centrifugation. The prespin sample is similar in appearance to the haematuric urine in (a) but is less turbid. The urine remains pink following centrifugation and there is no visible sediment.

In rare cases, red, pink, red-brown, red-orange or orange urine that tests negatively for haem pigments may indicate the presence of bromsulphthalein or phenol-sulphthalein (in alkaline urine), or porphyrins, Congo red, phenazopyridine, phenothiazine, or (in humans) various other drugs and chemicals (Bartges, 2005).

Centrifuge the urine sample to examine for intact RBCs:

- Supernatant clear with pellet of RBCs present: haematuria (gross or microscopic) (see Figure 1.5a).
- Supernatant pigmented with absence of RBCs in pellet: haemoglobinuria or myoglobinuria (see Figure 1.5b).

Haemoglobinuria

Haemoglobinuria gives urine a pink to red colour, although this may darken over time with oxidation. Two processes can cause haemoglobinuria (Figure 1.6).

- Intravascular lysis of RBCs. Many processes (e.g. primary or secondary immune-mediated disease, infectious, toxic, chemical) cause RBCs to lyse within blood vessels. The lysed cells release haemoglobin into the plasma, where it forms a complex with haptoglobin. Once the binding capacity of haptoglobin

Cause of haemoglobinuria	Suggestive clinical findings
Intravascular haemolysis	• Haemoglobinuria without RBC ghosts or lysed RBCs in urine sediment • Haemoglobinaemia (pinkish or red plasma) • Suggestive changes in RBCs (spherocytes, Heinz bodies, *Babesia* spp., *Mycoplasma haemofelis*) • Regenerative anaemia (allow 4–5 days for bone marrow response to appear) • Exposure to a known haemolytic drug, chemical or toxin • Inherited intrinsic erythrocyte defect known to cause haemolysis in that breed
Lysis of RBCs within urine	• Haemoglobinuria with RBC ghosts in urine sediment • Hypotonic and/or alkaline urine • Normal plasma colour • Absence of regenerative anaemia • Delayed processing of urine specimen

1.6 Causes of haemoglobinuria and suggestive clinical findings.

is saturated, free haemoglobin appears in the plasma. The plasma becomes visibly pink if the concentrations of free haemoglobin, bound haemoglobin and various derivatives exceed a certain level. Some of the free haemoglobin cleared from the plasma by glomerular filtration is taken up by renal tubular cells and metabolized to bilirubin. Haemoglobin appears in urine once this tubular uptake mechanism becomes saturated.
• Lysis of RBCs within the urinary excretory pathway. When urine is hypotonic (urine specific gravity <1.008), many RBCs may lyse within the excretory pathway. Urine alkalinity (pH >7) also contributes to lysis, both *in vivo* and *in vitro*. In these circumstances, RBCs in the urine sediment appear as faint colourless circles ('ghost cells') or become invisible because of lysis.

Myoglobinuria

Myoglobinuria is rarely detected in dogs and cats, but is possible whenever extensive destruction of muscle fibres releases substantial amounts of myoglobin into the plasma. One such condition is 'exertional rhabdomyolysis' (also known as 'tying up' or 'cramping') in unfit racing Greyhounds. Other potential causes are toxic, traumatic, infectious or ischaemic myopathies.

When myoglobinuria is present:

• Active muscle necrosis should be apparent: look for swelling or atrophy of muscles, pain and/or weakness, increased plasma creatine kinase (CK) activity
• Plasma colour is not altered: myoglobin released from myocytes is rapidly eliminated in urine because it does not bind to plasma protein and the renal threshold for myoglobin is low
• Differentiation between myoglobinuria and haemoglobinuria is usually based on plasma colour and the other pointers mentioned previously, but a myoglobin solubility test can be performed if required.

The patient with haematuria or other causes of pigmenturia

It is important to remember that haematuria and other causes of pigmenturia can result from systemic disorders as well as from urogenital abnormalities, and both possibilities should be covered when obtaining the history and performing the physical examination. The aspects discussed below should be explored.

Causes of pigmenturia other than gross haematuria

Urine discoloration in these cases is present throughout urination, as with total haematuria. There are several possibilities to explore.

• Haemoglobinuria:
  • In the breed presented, is there an inherited erythrocyte defect causing intravascular haemolysis?
  • Has there been exposure to a haemolysin (e.g. drug, chemical, onions)?
  • Are there systemic signs suggesting anaemia and/or jaundice?
  • During the physical examination, look for evidence of anaemia and jaundice, and for enlargement of liver, spleen and lymph nodes.
• Myoglobinuria: check history and physical findings for evidence of myopathy.
• Other pigmenturias: enquire about exposure to unusual drugs or chemicals.

Gross haematuria

When haematuria is sufficient to be apparent to the naked eye, the urine has a brownish to red (occasionally blackish) colour and turbid appearance. This is known as gross or macroscopic haematuria. Sometimes small blood clots may be present. For haematuria to be detected visually, at least 0.5 ml of whole blood must be present per litre of urine, corresponding to about 2500 RBCs per microlitre, and >150 RBCs per high-power field (hpf) in urine sediment. Figure 1.7 lists the reference ranges for RBCs in urine sediment samples.

Sample type	Red blood cells per high-power field
Voided	0–8
Catheterized	0–5
Cystocentesis	0–5

1.7 Suggested reference values for red blood cells (RBCs) in urine sediment, although it is not uncommon for urine obtained by cystocentesis to contain up to 15–20 RBCs per high-power field.

Gross haematuria does not always appear consistently throughout urination. By noting when it does occur, i.e. the pattern of haematuria, it may be possible to identify potential bleeding sites, as indicated in Figure 1.8. Potential origins and causes of haematuria in dogs and cats are presented in Figure 1.9.

Haematuria can arise from blood loss within the renal parenchyma or, more often, from discontinuity of endothelial or epithelial barriers anywhere in the urine collecting system, from the renal pelvis to the external urethral orifice. It can also occur with disorders affecting genital or accessory sex organs and with coagulation disorders.

Occult haematuria

Haematuria that is present but not visible to the naked eye is known as occult or microscopic haematuria. Urine from healthy dogs and cats can contain some RBCs without this being clinically relevant. Occult haematuria is identified if urine contains >5 RBCs/hpf but is not visibly pink. Interpretation is difficult if catheterization or cystocentesis causes overt trauma.

The various conditions that cause gross haematuria can also cause occult haematuria if present in less severe forms. Occult haematuria often accompanies pollakiuria, dysuria and/or stranguria caused by idiopathic cystitis in cats, and bacterial cystitis or urinary calculi in dogs and cats.

Observation	Possible origin of haemorrhage
Initial haematuria (at beginning of voiding)	• Lower urinary tract (bladder neck, urethra, vagina, vulva, penis, prepuce) • Genital tract (proestrus, metritis, pyometra, prostate, genital neoplasia)
Terminal haematuria (at end of voiding)	• Upper urinary tract (bladder, ureters, kidneys; intermittent bleeding allowing RBCs to settle in bladder, to be expelled with final bladder contents) or lesion of the ventrolateral aspect of the urinary bladder
Total haematuria (throughout voiding)	• Upper urinary tract (bladder, ureters, kidneys; bleeding frequent to continuous, or intermittent but mixing occurring because animal is physically active) • Diffuse bladder disease • Severe prostatic or proximal urethral lesion (blood refluxing into bladder) • Coagulopathies
Bloody fluid dripping from penis or vulva independent of urination	• Bleeding distal to urethral sphincter (prostate, urethra, penis, uterus, vagina, vulva)

1.8 Observed patterns of haematuria and possible origins.

Origin	Possible cause	Clinical/historical features
Coagulation abnormality	Platelet or clotting factor disorders	Bleeding from other sites; breed or family history suggesting inherited defect; access to anticoagulant rodenticide; snake envenomation; strenuous exercise; disseminated intravascular coagulation (DIC) secondary to systemic disease
Renal	Blunt trauma; idiopathic renal haematuria; renal infarction; renal cysts; renal pelvic haematoma; urinary calculi; telangiectasia (Welsh Corgi); glomerulonephritis; passive congestion; neoplasia; *Dioctophyma renale*, *Dirofilaria immitis* microfilaraemia	Haematuria (gross or microscopic) may occur throughout urination (total haematuria); possibly haemoglobinuria if RBCs lyse in hypotonic urine
Bladder, ureters, urethra	Calculi; bacterial infection; feline idiopathic cystitis; trauma; neoplasia; cyclophosphamide therapy; *Capillaria plica*; polypoid cystitis; proliferative urethritis	Haematuria (gross or microscopic) may occur at beginning or end of urination (sometimes throughout, see Figure 1.8); dysuria may be concurrent
Genital tract	Prostatic disease; oestrus; subinvolution of placental sites; neoplasia; infection; trauma	Haematuria (gross or microscopic) at beginning of voiding or independent of urination

1.9 Origin, causes and clinical features of haematuria.

Diagnostic approach to stranguria and haematuria

As with all clinical problems, a detailed history, including a full dietary history, and thorough physical examination, including body and muscle condition scoring, are the cornerstones of diagnosis in patients with stranguria, haematuria or both of these signs. Although this discussion will centre on the urinary tract, all body systems and the general health of the patient should be evaluated, to ensure that any contributing factors or systemic consequences are detected. Once basic data have been collected by means of history taking and physical examination, these findings should be assessed carefully, enabling tentative decisions to be made about the nature of the problem, the probable differential diagnoses, and the diagnostic and therapeutic measures required.

History and physical examination
The stranguric patient without haematuria

As outlined above, stranguria usually results from disorders of the lower urinary tract (bladder or urethra), genital tract (prostate or vagina) or both.

Physical examination:
Assessment of urethral patency: As urinary obstruction can be life-threatening, urethral patency should be ascertained from the history and physical examination during the first phase of the investigation. This is especially important if the clinical signs suggest uraemia (e.g. depression, anorexia, vomiting). Observing the animal attempting to urinate provides the ideal opportunity to verify urethral patency and confirm the owner's account

of events. When the bladder is distended and urine is not passed, urethral blockage should be suspected and catheterization attempted. This will often require initial decompressive cystocentesis, which allows for stabilization of the animal in conjunction with intravenous fluid therapy and pain relief, sedation for diagnostic imaging, and general anaesthesia for urethral catheterization in cats. The decompressive cystocentesis also allows collection of a urine sample suitable for urinalysis and culture. Serum biochemistry should be evaluated for the presence or absence of azotaemia and electrolyte disturbances at the same time, and blood gas analysis considered if available.

- If catheterization is easy, this suggests that the cause may be functional urethral obstruction from detrusor–urethral dyssynergia, wherein sphincter muscle relaxation and detrusor muscle contraction are uncoordinated (see Chapters 3 and 30). However, a mechanical obstruction cannot be excluded because small urethral plugs can be dislodged and catheters can be passed easily around some mass lesions and urethroliths. Contrast urography or cystoscopy may be considered.
- If catheterization is difficult or impossible, cystocentesis is highly recommended to reduce intravesicular pressure and facilitate catheterization. In the case of obstructive urolithiasis, a further option is retrograde urohydropropulsion (see Chapter 20).

Bladder palpation: Palpation of the urinary bladder is very important in stranguric animals, but must be done carefully because a tightly distended bladder can rupture under pressure. It is advisable to palpate the bladder again after emptying, to improve the chances of feeling intraluminal or intramural masses. Findings and interpretation of bladder palpation are summarized in Figure 1.10.

Finding	Interpretation
Small bladder, thickened wall, gentle palpation readily elicits voiding	Bladder inflammation
Large bladder, flaccid feel, gentle palpation readily expels urine	Bladder atony or lower motor neuron disease
Large bladder, tense wall, urine not easily expressed (exercise caution)	Urinary tract obstruction or increased outflow resistance
Irregular, hard masses within lumen, possibly with a grating feeling (easier to appreciate if bladder empty of urine)	Cystic calculi or mineralized mass

1.10 Abnormal findings on bladder palpation and their interpretation.

Digital rectal palpation: Ideally, this should be performed in all stranguric dogs. Rectal examination can be considered in sedated cats if clinically indicated. Structures that may be evaluated include:

- Prostate gland
- Trigone of the bladder
- Pelvic urethra
- Vagina and cervix
- Masses in the caudal abdominal or pelvic region.

Palpation of the prostate and trigone area can often be assisted by pressing upwards and backwards on the caudal abdomen with the other hand at the same time.

Examination of perineum and external genitalia: Inspection and palpation are advisable in both sexes.

- Males: palpate the perineum and urethra. A soft fluctuant perineal swelling could indicate perineal herniation (which sometimes causes stranguria and/or dysuria) or urine accumulation following urethral obstruction and rupture. Extrude the penis and examine both the penis and inside the prepuce for masses, inflammation, haemorrhage, trauma or discharge. In cats with urethral obstruction, the penis may be partly extruded and reddened, and a plug may be visible protruding from the urethral meatus.
- Females: examine the vulva for swelling, masses, inflammation or discharge and assess for proestrus or oestrus. Consider digital vaginal palpation to identify masses or strictures and abnormalities of the urethral papilla.

The haematuric patient

If haematuria is determined to be present, the clinician needs to distinguish between systemic disorders such as coagulopathies and disorders localized to the urinary tract, which may or may not result in signs of lower urinary tract disease (LUTD) (see Figure 1.4).

- Clinical signs of LUTD absent: coagulopathy or bleeding into the upper urinary tract is most likely.
- Clinical signs of LUTD present: bleeding due to lesions in the lower urinary tract (for example infectious, inflammatory, neoplastic or traumatic causes) is most likely.

Important questions to ask during history taking of haematuric patients:

- Enquire as to the presence of clinical signs of LUTD.
- Has bleeding been noticed from any other sites? (Consider the possibility of a breed or familial haemostatic defect.)

- Ask about trauma, exposure to anticoagulant rodenticides and systemic signs suggesting anaemia.
- Find out whether there is a consistent pattern to the urine discoloration that may suggest its origin (see Figure 1.3).

Physical examination:

- Look for haemorrhage at other sites, including the abdomen, thorax, subcutis, skin and mucosae (especially mouth, axillae, groin and inside pinnae and other mucosal surfaces).
- Examine faeces grossly for blood.
- Palpate the kidneys and assess for size, symmetry and discomfort.
- Perform digital rectal palpation, assessing structures as suggested for stranguric patients.
- Examine the external genitalia.

The stranguric patient with haematuria or haemoglobinuria

Stranguria accompanied by haematuria (gross or microscopic) or haemoglobinuria is most likely to be caused by lesions in the lower urinary tract (bladder or urethra) and/or the genital tract (prostate or vagina). Accordingly, the approach to the history and physical examination in these patients should cover all aspects mentioned separately for stranguric patients and for patients with reddish urine.

Making an assessment and planning the investigation and treatment

The assessment of individual patients will naturally depend on the findings from the history and physical examination. Once a tentative diagnosis or list of diagnostic possibilities is established, this should lead to logical plans for further investigation and treatment. In patients with urinary tract obstruction and uraemia, establishing urethral patency and instituting appropriate therapy may well take precedence over investigations to establish a definitive diagnosis.

In many, but not all, patients with stranguria and/or haematuria, diagnostic aids will be required to confirm the tentative diagnosis or to decide among several diagnostic possibilities. Available options include:

- Urinalysis, either routine or specialized, depending on the case (see Chapter 6)
- Assessment for alterations to platelet number and/or prothrombin time (PT) and activated partial thromboplastin time (aPTT) (primary and secondary coagulation problems)
- Assessment of renal function if renal disease and failure seem likely (see Chapter 10)
- Diagnostic imaging studies, especially to assess the involvement of the kidneys, urinary bladder and prostate, or to detect urinary tract rupture: for example, ultrasonography for patients with suspected renal haematuria, urolithiasis or prostatic disease; double-contrast cystography for suspected bladder wall disease; positive-contrast retrograde urethrography for suspected urethral lesions and/or prostatic disease (see Chapter 7)
- Haematological and blood biochemical tests to evaluate underlying causes of dysuria/haematuria and possible systemic consequences.

Figure 1.11 lists various diagnostic aids that may be used when investigating patients with dysuria/haematuria, together with comments on indications for their use and interpretation of findings. Aspects of treatment for various urinary and prostatic diseases are presented later in this Manual.

Test and indication	Finding	Interpretation and action
Haematology (not useful in most cases)	Inflammatory leucogram	Compatible with inflammation but typically not useful in lower urinary disorders Origin: renal, prostatic or elsewhere?
	'Stress' leucogram	Suggests severe illness, glucocorticoid therapy or hyperadrenocorticism
	Anaemia with microcytosis	Suggestive for iron deficiency anaemia
	Anaemia	Suggestive for pronounced haematuria
Blood biochemical tests (to assess azotaemia and metabolic effects if uraemia suspected or to detect disorders predisposing to urinary infection or calculus formation)	Increased concentrations of creatinine, urea, phosphate in fasting sample (see Chapter 10)	Azotaemia present – post-renal (urinary obstruction or rupture), renal or pre-renal? Check hydration status, urinary specific gravity and other findings
	Changes compatible with hyperadrenocorticism, kidney disease, diabetes mellitus	May predispose to bacterial cystitis or pyelonephritis
	Hypercalcaemia or evidence of hepatopathy	May predispose to urolith formation
Coagulation tests (to investigate a bleeding disorder as the cause of haematuria)	Severely decreased platelet numbers and/or increased coagulation times (PT/aPTT)	Coagulopathy is the likely cause of haematuria
Prostatic fluid examination (see Chapter 25) – advisable if any prostatic disease other than uncomplicated benign prostatic hypertrophy is suspected	Leucocytes and bacteria	Prostatitis or prostatic abscess
	Epithelial cell clumps with abnormal appearance	Neoplasia, hyperplasia, squamous metaplasia or reactive change Further prostatic sampling may be necessary (see Chapter 25)
Diagnostic imaging (see Chapter 7)	Findings depend on disorder present and techniques used (plain and contrast radiography, ultrasonography)	See Chapter 7
Endoscopy (see Chapter 8) (recommended if dysuria or haematuria remains unexplained following preliminary diagnostics)	Mucosal lesions in bladder, urethra or vagina Uroliths in urethra, bladder, ureters and/or kidneys Localization of origin of haemorrhage	Inflammatory or neoplastic changes, strictures Biopsy and culture are usually performed Uroliths may be collected, analysed and bacterial culture performed Ureteroscopy may be helpful in the case of renal haematuria Vessel cauterization may be possible if a renal vascular malformation is detected

1.11 Use of ancillary diagnostic aids in patients with dysuria and/or haematuria.

References and further reading

Bartges JW (2005) Discolored urine. In: *Textbook of Veterinary Internal Medicine, 6th edn*, ed. SJ Ettinger and EC Feldman, pp.112–114. Elsevier Saunders, St Louis

Chew DJ and DiBartola SP (1998) Normal urinalysis reference ranges of the dog and cat. In: *Interpretation of Canine and Feline Urinalysis*, p. 65. Ralston Purina, Wilmington

Grauer GF (2003) Clinical manifestations of urinary disorders. In: *Small Animal Internal Medicine, 3rd edn*, ed. RW Nelson and GC Couto, pp.568–583. Mosby, St Louis

Osborne CA and Finco DR (1995) *Canine and Feline Nephrology and Urology.* Williams and Wilkins, Baltimore

Osborne CA and Stevens JB (1999) *Urinalysis: a Clinical Guide to Compassionate Patient Care.* Veterinary Learning Systems, Trenton

Chapter 2

Polyuria and polydipsia

Rosanne Jepson

Polyuria (PU) is defined as the production of increased volumes of urine whilst polydipsia (PD) is defined as an increase in drinking. Although patients may appear to present with either PU or PD, by the nature of the physiology of water balance, these signs usually occur together. The pathophysiology underlying PU/PD in different conditions may vary, but PU/PD can be considered broadly in two categories. Most commonly, conditions cause an alteration in urine production that results in polyuria, so that the patient drinks excessively to compensate for this fluid loss. Alternatively, and much less commonly, a primary polydipsia results in a secondary increase in urination.

PU/PD can be a frustrating presentation for clients trying to cope in particular with the increased volume of urine produced by their pet. A logical approach is therefore required for the investigation of any patient presenting with PU/PD to ensure that an expedient diagnosis is made and, where possible, appropriate treatment started. In order to understand the pathophysiology of PU/PD it is important to understand the physiological mechanisms which control thirst, urine production and urine concentrating mechanisms.

Physiology of water balance and thirst

Thirst and urine production are controlled by complex physiology involving the central nervous system (hypothalamus, posterior pituitary gland and thirst centre), plasma volume, plasma osmolality and the kidneys. In health, ingested water (from food and drinking water) and water produced through metabolism are balanced by insensible losses from the respiratory tract and skin, and sensible losses via faeces and urine (Barrett et al., 2010). Insensible losses may vary with environmental and patient factors, e.g. environmental temperature, humidity, hyperthermia, pyrexia and exercise. However, a minimum volume of urine must be produced on a daily basis to facilitate excretion of waste products. Provided there is free access to water and the patient is able to drink, the insensible losses will be met and homeostatic mechanisms involving the kidney and urine concentrating ability will be sufficient to maintain fluid balance.

Plasma volume and osmolality (plasma solute concentration) are tightly regulated, with osmolality being determined principally by plasma sodium concentration

and being the main determinant of secretion of arginine vasopressin (AVP), also called antidiuretic hormone (ADH). A review of the physiology of urine concentration is provided in Figure 2.1. In the presence of AVP and an osmotic gradient, water moves from the tubular fluid in the distal tubule and collecting duct into the renal interstitium. AVP also increases urea transport in the inner medullary collecting duct and recycling such that urea contributes significantly to the hypertonicity of the medullary interstitium under conditions where plasma AVP concentrations are high. Tubular fluid increases in osmolality as water is conserved and more concentrated urine is produced. An absence of AVP (central diabetes insipidus, CDI) or an inability of the distal tubule or collecting duct to respond to AVP (nephrogenic diabetes insipidus, NDI) results in failure to conserve water. In this scenario, the hypotonic fluid passing from the earlier portions of the loop of Henle into the distal tubule and collecting duct remain hypotonic and large volumes of dilute urine are produced, resulting in PU.

Decreases in plasma volume and increased osmolality sensed at the hypothalamus also mediate an increase in thirst, although the threshold is higher than for AVP secretion. The two mechanisms can be independently stimulated such that a decrease in circulating volume (e.g. from haemorrhage) can stimulate thirst without a change in plasma osmolality.

Cats and dogs may also demonstrate a degree of habitual drinking, where increased water intake is associated with eating (prandial drinking). This habitual water intake ensures that water consumption is typically in excess of insensible losses and the minimum urine volume required for solute excretion. Studies have demonstrated that increased frequency of feeding increases water intake and, although this is considered a learned or habitual response, it may reflect changes in plasma osmolality associated with eating. Other psychological factors that may influence thirst include dry pharyngeal mucous membranes and pain.

Pathophysiology of polyuria and polydipsia

Four main pathophysiological mechanisms can result in an increase in thirst and/or urination (Nelson, 2014). These may occur alone or in combination.

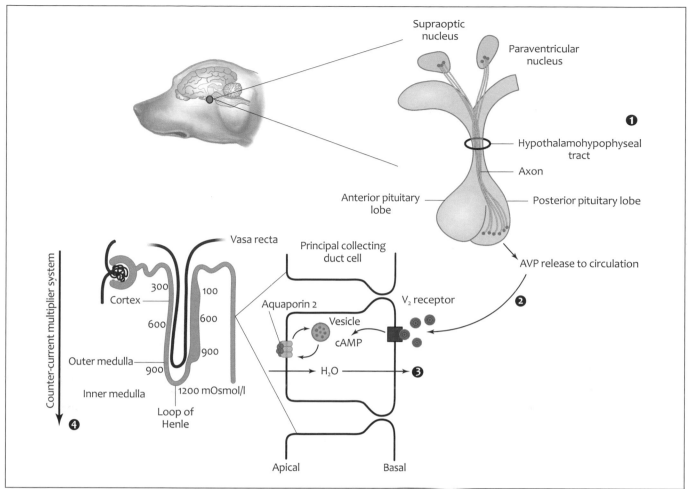

2.1 Arginine vasopressin production and action in the kidney. 1 = Antidiuretic hormone (ADH), otherwise known as arginine vasopressin (AVP), is synthesized in the hypothalamus as a preprohormone and stored in vesicles within the posterior pituitary. Secretion of AVP from the posterior pituitary is stimulated by increasing plasma osmolality sensed by osmoreceptors in the hypothalamus or decreased total circulating plasma volume sensed by change in pressure within the atria, veins and the carotid sinus. 2 = Circulating AVP has its primary action in the kidney, more specifically in the distal tubule and the collecting ducts. Here AVP interacts with its receptor (V2) and via a cascade of events facilitates the transient insertion of water channels (aquaporin-2) which increases the permeability of these epithelial cells to water. By an independent pathway, AVP also regulates urea transport within the inner medullary collecting duct. AVP results in an increase in transepithelial transport of urea, important for maintenance of the urea gradient. 3 = The fluid in the distal tubule is dilute, allowing passive movement of water from the tubule to the hypertonic medullary interstitium along an osmotic gradient. 4 = Maintenance of the osmotic gradient is dependent on the counter-current multiplier system between the loop of Henle and the vasa recta blood supply, which concentrates solutes (urea and sodium) within the medullary interstitium. cAMP = cyclic adenosine monophosphate.

Lack of vasopressin production

Lack of AVP production by the hypothalamus results in CDI. Without AVP, the epithelial cells in the distal tubule and collecting ducts fail to express aquaporin-2, the transmembrane channel required for water reabsorption. Water therefore remains within the distal tubule and collecting duct, the tubular fluid remains hypotonic and an increased volume of hypotonic urine is produced. In order to maintain fluid balance, water intake increases (increased thirst is driven by increased plasma osmolality) and individuals therefore demonstrate primary polyuria with a secondary polydipsia (Figure 2.2).

- Congenital central diabetes insipidus
- Acquired central diabetes insipidus:
  - Hypothalamic/pituitary neoplasia (primary/metastatic)
  - Post-transsphenoidal surgery for hyperadrenocorticism/acromegaly
  - Trauma, particularly associated with skull fracture
  - Idiopathic
  - Vascular

2.2 Conditions causing central diabetes insipidus.

Inability of distal tubular and collecting duct epithelial cells to respond to vasopressin

Inability to respond to AVP at the level of the distal tubule and collecting duct epithelial cells is referred to as NDI and can either be congenital or secondary.

Congenital nephrogenic diabetes insipidus

This occurs when a mutation is present in the AVP receptor gene, resulting in either reduced insertion of the AVP receptor in the plasma membrane or an inability of AVP to bind to the receptor. This will result in a secondary failure of recycling and insertion of aquaporin-2. Alternatively, mutations have been described in the gene encoding aquaporin-2 such that, although AVP signalling is intact, recycling and insertion of aquaporin-2 are reduced. In both scenarios, reduced insertion of aquaporin-2 results in lack of water movement from the tubular filtrate to the interstitium, hypotonic tubular filtrate, and production of large volumes of dilute urine. Patients therefore demonstrate primary polyuria with a compensatory polydipsia (Figure 2.3).

- Congenital nephrogenic diabetes insipidus
- Secondary nephrogenic diabetes insipidus:
  - Reduced response to arginine vasopressin:
    - Hyperadrenocorticism
    - Hypercalcaemia
    - Endotoxin formation (pyelonephritis/pyometra)
  - Loss of osmotic gradient:
    - Hypoadrenocorticism
    - Hepatic failure
    - Hypokalaemia
    - Chronic kidney disease
    - Diuretic therapy

2.3 Conditions causing nephrogenic diabetes insipidus.

Secondary nephrogenic diabetes insipidus

Secondary NDI is brought about by reduced response to AVP at the distal tubule or collecting duct epithelial cells, or an inability of the kidney to maintain the osmotic gradient between tubular fluid and the medullary interstitium. Many factors (e.g. hypercalcaemia, corticosteroids and endotoxins) are known to interfere with the AVP response, thus limiting the recycling and insertion of aquaporins. This reduces water movement from the tubular filtrate to the medullary interstitium, despite the presence of an adequate concentration gradient. Conversely, other conditions may result in loss of the hypertonicity present in the medullary interstitium. In this scenario, despite adequate availability of aquaporin-2, the loss of concentration gradient means that water movement is reduced, tubular fluid remains hypotonic and large volumes of urine are produced with a compensatory increase in thirst to maintain water balance (see Figure 2.3).

Osmotic diuresis

A minimum volume of water must be excreted with waste solutes by the kidney. Increased concentration of solutes within the tubular filtrate results in an increased requirement for water excretion by the kidney; this results in primary polyuria with a compensatory increase in thirst (Figure 2.4).

- Diabetes mellitus
- Administration of the following medications:
  - Diuretics
  - Mannitol
  - Sodium chloride intravenous fluid therapy
- Postobstructive diuresis
- Primary renal glucosuria/Fanconi syndrome

2.4 Conditions resulting in osmotic diuresis.

Primary polydipsia

Primary polydipsia is uncommon in companion animals and refers to an increase in thirst which occurs without physiological stimulus. In dogs, behavioural alteration resulting in increased drinking has been referred to as psychogenic polydipsia (Figure 2.5).

- Primary 'psychogenic' polydipsia
- Hyperthyroidism
- Hepatic encephalopathy
- Gastrointestinal disease

2.5 Conditions resulting in a primary polydipsia.

Pathophysiology and diagnosis of conditions resulting in polyuria and polydipsia

A large number of conditions can lead to polyuria and polydipsia, but differential diagnoses can often be narrowed down on the basis of an assessment of signalment, history, physical examination (Figure 2.6) and a minimum diagnostic database (Figures 2.7 and 2.8). Conditions resulting in PU/PD in the dog and cat are listed in Figure 2.9.

Assessment	Findings and causes
Mentation/ neurological examination	• **Abnormal mentation/neurological examination:** Primary or metastatic neoplasia affecting pituitary/hypothalamus, hepatic encephalopathy • **Hyperactivity:** Primary polydipsia, hyperthyroidism
Ocular examination	• **Icteric sclera:** Primary hepatic disease • **Cataract formation:** Diabetes mellitus • **Congested sclera/conjunctival hyperaemia:** Polycythaemia • **Hyphaema/tortuous retinal vessels/focal bullous detachment:** Systemic hypertension (acute kidney injury, chronic kidney disease, hyperthyroidism, hyperadrenocorticism, polycythaemia, phaeochromocytoma) • **Corneal lipidosis:** Diabetes mellitus, hyperadrenocorticism • **Scleral haemorrhage:** *Angiostrongylus vasorum*[a] • **Blindness:** Pituitary/hypothalamic neoplasia, hepatic encephalopathy • **Papillary oedema:** Pituitary neoplasia
Oral mucous membrane appearance	• **Icteric:** Primary hepatic disease • **Hyperaemic/congested:** Polycythaemia, hypoadrenocorticoid crisis[a], sepsis/systemic inflammatory response syndrome (pyelonephritis/pyometra) • **Pale:** chronic kidney disease, hypoadrenocorticism[a], anaemia of chronic disease/neoplasia
Oral examination	• **Lingual ulceration:** Severe azotaemia (chronic kidney disease, acute kidney injury, pyelonephritis) • **Halitosis:** Severe azotaemia (chronic kidney disease, acute kidney injury, pyelonephritis) • **Widened interdental spaces/enlarged facial features:** Acromegaly
Cervical palpation	• **Thyroid goitre:** Hyperthyroidism • **Parathyroid nodule:** Hyperparathyroidism[a] (may be appreciated in the cat, not usually palpable in dogs)
Dermatological manifestations	• **Skin thinning, alopecia, pigmentation change, comedones, calcinosis cutis:** Hyperadrenocorticism • **Fragile skin/skin tears:** Hyperadrenocorticism (cats)
Thoracic auscultation	• **Tachypnoea:** Pulmonary metastatic disease[a], primary pulmonary neoplasia[a], mediastinal mass[a], pleural effusion associated with neoplasia, pulmonary granulomatous disease[a] • **Panting:** Hyperadrenocorticism • **Dull/muffled lung sounds:** Mediastinal mass (lymphoma)[a] • **Cough:** Angiostrongylosis[a], metastatic disease[a], primary pulmonary neoplasia[a], granulomatous pulmonary disease[a] • **Tachycardia:** Hyperthyroidism, phaeochromocytoma, sepsis (pyelonephritis/pyometra) • **Bradycardia:** Hypoadrenocorticism[a]

2.6 Physical examination findings which may indicate the underlying aetiology for polyuria and polydipsia. [a] Indicates that hypercalcaemia may be either the main or one of several mechanisms driving polyuria/polydipsia. (continues) ▶

Assessment	Findings and causes
Renal palpation	• **Enlarged/painful kidneys:** Acute kidney injury, pyelonephritis, renal lymphoma • **Small irregular kidneys:** Chronic kidney disease
Abdominal palpation	• **Hepatomegaly:** Acute hepatic disease, hyper-adrenocorticism, diabetes mellitus, hepatic neoplasia[a] • **Microhepatica:** End-stage liver disease (cirrhosis), portosystemic shunt • **Enlarged uterus:** Pyometra • **Lymphadenopathy:** Lymphoma[a], metastatic neoplastic disease[a]
Lymph-adenomegaly	• **Lymphoma**[a] • **Granulomatous disease**[a]: Fungal disease, sterile neutrophilic/granulomatous lymphadenitis
Rectal examination	• **Rectal mass:** Anal sac adenocarcinoma[a] • **Sublumbar lymph node enlargement:** Metastasis from anal sac adenocarcinoma[a], lymphoma[a]
Vaginal examination	• **Vaginal discharge:** Pyometra (open)
Change in body condition	• **Poor body condition:** Diabetes mellitus, hepatic disease, chronic kidney disease, neoplastic disease[a], hyperthyroidism (cats) • **Abdominal enlargement:** Hyperadrenocorticism
Small stature/poor growth	• **Portovascular anomaly** • **Congenital renal disease**

2.6 (continued) Physical examination findings which may indicate the underlying aetiology for polyuria and polydipsia.
[a] Indicates that hypercalcaemia may be either the main or one of several mechanisms driving polyuria/polydipsia.

• Packed cell volume/total solids and/or complete blood count
• Serum biochemical profile
• Total thyroxine concentration (cat)
• Urinalysis:
  ◦ Specific gravity
  ◦ Dipstick assessment
  ◦ Sediment examination
  ◦ Culture

2.8 Minimum diagnostic database for the patient with polyuria and polydipsia.

Assessment of the signalment of the patient may allow prioritization of the likely underlying cause for PU/PD. For example, pyometra is more likely to be identified in the middle-aged to older entire bitch, hyperadrenocorticism and neoplasia in older dogs, whilst in patients less than 1 year of age consideration should be given to congenital or familial conditions. Certain conditions may also have breed predispositions; for example, Fanconi syndrome in the Basenji or primary hyperparathyroidism in the Keeshound.

Historical information regarding the clinical presentation is fundamental to ensuring that the primary presentation is indeed PU/PD and that this presentation is differentiated from other clinical signs relating to the urinary tract such as urinary incontinence, pollakiuria (increased frequency of urination), stranguria (difficulty in urination) and dysuria (pain during urination). However, these clinical present-ations and PU/PD may not always be mutually exclusive.

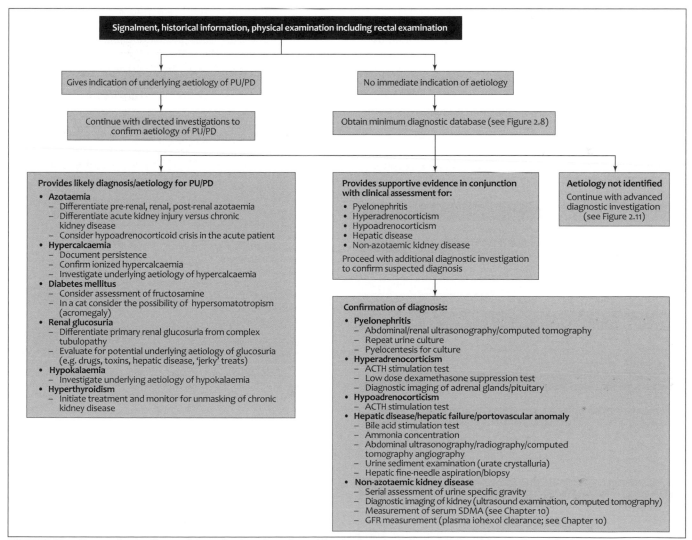

2.7 Flow diagram for the diagnostic investigation of a patient with polyuria and polydipsia. ACTH = adrenocorticotrophic hormone; GFR = glomerular filtration rate; PD = polydipsia; PU = polyuria; SDMA = symmetric dimethylarginine.

Incidence	Canine conditions	Feline conditions
Common	• Chronic kidney disease[a] • Hyperadrenocorticism[c] • Diabetes mellitus[c]; juvenile diabetes mellitus[b] • Hypercalcaemia (dependent on aetiology)[a] • Pyometra[c] • Iatrogenic (diet/diuretic/fluid/drug administration)[a] • Hepatic disease[c]; portovascular anomaly[b]	• Chronic kidney disease[c] • Diabetes mellitus[c] • Hyperthyroidism[c] • Postobstructive diuresis[a] • Iatrogenic (fluid/diuretic/drug administration)[a]
Uncommon	• Pyelonephritis[a] • Hypoadrenocorticism[a] • Postobstructive diuresis[a] • Acute kidney injury (polyuric recovery phase)[a]	• Primary hyperaldosteronism (Conn's syndrome)[c] • Hypersomatotropism (acromegaly with diabetes mellitus)[c] • Hepatic disease[c] • Pyelonephritis[a] • Acute kidney injury (polyuric recovery phase)[a]
Rare	• Primary 'psychogenic' polydipsia[a] • Central diabetes insipidus: acquired[a]; congenital[b] • Primary nephrogenic diabetes insipidus (congenital)[b] • Hyperviscosity syndrome/polycythaemia[a] • Primary renal glycosuria/Fanconi syndrome: acquired[a]; in Basenjis (typically 3–4 years of age at onset of glycosuria)[b] • Hypokalaemia[a] • Primary hyperaldosteronism/deoxycorticosterone production[c]	• Central diabetes insipidus: acquired[c]; congenital[b] • Hypercalcaemia[a] • Hyperadrenocorticism (with diabetes mellitus)[c] • Hypoadrenocorticism[a] • Congenital nephrogenic diabetes insipidus is not reported in the cat

2.9 Conditions resulting in polyuria and polydipsia in the dog and cat. [a] Patients can be any age at presentation. [b] Patients are young at presentation. [c] Patients are middle-aged to older at presentation.

Further information regarding the presentation of patients with lower urinary tract disease and urinary incontinence can be found in Chapters 1 and 3.

Before embarking on lengthy and expensive investigations, if there is any doubt regarding the presence of PU/PD an attempt should be made to quantify water intake. In the dog polydipsia is defined as water intake >100 ml/kg/24h. However, this criterion should not be considered absolute because astute owners may appreciate more subtle changes in thirst, which should still be considered abnormal if they are persistent. Indeed, water intake of >60–100 ml/kg/day may be abnormal, particularly if there is a documented recent increase in water consumption. A clear criterion for polydipsia is not reported for the cat, although it is widely accepted that water intake is lower than the dog. It is uncommon for urine output to be quantified owing to the requirement for hospitalization and catheterization for accurate assessment.

Fluid administration
• Subcutaneous or intravenous fluid administration
Diuretics
• Loop diuretics (e.g. furosemide) • Thiazide diuretics (e.g. hydrochlorothiazide) • Aldosterone antagonists (e.g. spironolactone) • Osmotic diuretics (e.g. mannitol)
Corticosteroids
• Oral, intramuscular, intravenous, topical corticosteroids • Fludrocortisone (combined mineralocorticoid and glucocorticoid supplementation)
Antiepileptic medication
• Phenobarbital
Dietary modification
• Increased frequency of feeding • Dry diet • Sodium supplemented diets • Dietary indiscretion
Environmental factors
• Exercise • Ambient temperature/humidity • Hyperthermia

2.10 Iatrogenic causes of polyuria and polydipsia.

Careful assessment of a patient's history is also important to exclude the many iatrogenic causes of PU/PD (Figure 2.10). Many conditions that result in PU/PD are systemic, involving multiple body systems. Therefore, historical information and careful physical examination may reveal key information (see Figure 2.6), which together with the presence of PU/PD narrows the likely differential diagnoses and can focus the diagnostic investigation. For many conditions, after initial assessment of the signalment, history, patient and minimum diagnostic database, further diagnostic procedures are required in order to confirm or investigate the suspected diagnosis (Figure 2.11).

• **Diagnostic imaging**
  ○ Abdominal ultrasonography/radiography/computed tomography
  ○ Thoracic radiography/ultrasonography/computed tomography
  ○ Spinal/long bone radiography/computed tomography
• **Adrenal gland function testing**
  ○ Urine cortisol to creatinine ratio
  ○ ACTH stimulation test
  ○ Low dose dexamethasone suppression test
• **Liver function testing**
  ○ Bile acid stimulation
  ○ Ammonia concentration
• **Repeat urine culture**
• **Serial assessment of USG**
  ○ Consider performing with change of environment (e.g. hospitalization for patients where suspicion for primary polydipsia)
• **Pyelocentesis (culture)**
• **Antibiotic trial therapy**
  ○ Should only be performed with index of suspicion for occult pyelonephritis
• **GFR measurement**
  ○ Iohexol clearance

2.11 Advanced diagnostic database. ACTH = adrenocorticotrophic hormone; GFR = glomerular filtration rate; USG = urine specific gravity.

Kidney disease

Chronic kidney disease (CKD) is one of the most common conditions in both dogs and cats that results in PU/PD. In acute kidney injury (AKI), oliguria (reduced urine production) or anuria (no urine production) are more often identified, although in the reparative phases of AKI extreme polyuria can ensue.

CKD is most often the result of tubulointerstitial nephritis. Nephrons are lost and replaced with inflammatory and fibrous tissue. Adaptive mechanisms that occur when the total nephron number is reduced lead to hyperfiltration in the remaining functioning nephrons in order to try and maintain the glomerular filtration rate (GFR; see Chapter 23). Increased solute load and tubular flow rates within the remaining nephrons lead to reduced water reabsorption within the distal tubules and collecting ducts. A simultaneous inability to maintain the counter-current mechanism, and therefore a reduction in the osmotic gradient between the tubular filtrate and medullary interstitium, also impairs water reabsorption, with the consequence of polyuria and an associated compensatory polydipsia to maintain hydration.

Key diagnostic information

CKD can typically be diagnosed on the basis of signalment, compatible history, clinical signs and physical examination, in conjunction with persistent azotaemia and inappropriate urine concentrating ability (see Chapters 10 and 12). Cats with CKD due to tubulointerstitial nephritis are typically older (>9 years) at the time of presentation. However, CKD should remain a differential diagnosis for any age of patient presenting with PU/PD, and in younger patients renal dysplasia or congenital renal conditions should be considered. For a diagnosis of CKD, clinical signs will usually have been present for >2–3 months. Renal azotaemia must be differentiated from pre-renal and post-renal azotaemia.

Isosthenuria (urine specific gravity (USG) 1.008–1.015) is not a requirement for the diagnosis of CKD although it may be identified, perhaps more commonly in the dog. Indeed the presence of isosthenuric urine, particularly in the cat, should prompt the clinician to consider whether conditions in addition to CKD could be contributing to PU/PD (e.g. concurrent pyelonephritis; see below). In addition, patients that present with hyposthenuric urine (USG <1.008) are unlikely to have a diagnosis of CKD, at least not alone, because tubular function and active transportation of solutes out of the tubular filtrate in excess of water are required for the production of hyposthenuric urine, which is not possible with significant loss of functioning nephrons.

Diagnostic imaging may be useful in the diagnosis of CKD (see Chapter 7). On ultrasound examination the kidneys typically appear small and irregular. They may also show evidence of loss of corticomedullary differentiation, mild pyelectasia and mineralization. The presence of a nonregenerative anaemia, weight loss, reduced body condition, hypokalaemia, hyperphosphataemia with renal secondary hyperparathyroidism and elevated carbamylated haemoglobin may also increase suspicion for chronic disease.

Much effort is being devoted to diagnosing CKD at an earlier stage in the course of disease (see Chapter 10). The International Renal Interest Society (IRIS) staging system (see Chapter 12) accommodates the situation that a patient can be diagnosed with non-azotaemic CKD (IRIS Stage 1 and non-azotaemic IRIS Stage 2). Such patients may demonstrate persistently poor urine concentrating ability despite remaining non-azotaemic. In this scenario, other methods to assess GFR should be considered (see Chapter 10). Additional information regarding the likelihood of CKD may be ascertained from serial documentation of poor or declining urine concentrating ability, ultrasound examination of the kidneys and the presence of persistent renal proteinuria (see Chapter 5). Assessment of GFR may be useful for non-azotaemic patients where there is an index of suspicion for reduced renal function and CKD (see Chapter 10).

Pyelonephritis

Pyelonephritis refers to inflammation of the renal pelvis and parenchyma, most often due to a bacterial infection, and it may cause PU/PD by several mechanisms. First, the presence of an inflammatory process within the interstitium may interfere with the maintenance of the medullary osmotic gradient through altered expression of urea transporters and aquaporins (water channels). Second, Gram-negative bacteria (e.g. *Escherichia coli*) produce endotoxins (e.g. lipopolysaccharide) that interfere with the action of AVP on the AVP receptors in the distal tubule and collecting duct epithelium, resulting in secondary NDI. In addition, chronic damage to renal parenchyma caused by pyelonephritis may result in loss of nephrons and PU/PD by the mechanisms described above for CKD.

Pyelonephritis may be acute or chronic in onset. It is most often the result of ascending infections, although haematogenous spread is also possible. Given the superior concentrating ability of the feline kidney, which results in more hostile urine, pyelonephritis is less common in this species than in the dog, especially without another predisposing condition such as CKD, glucosuria or congenital renal abnormalities.

Key diagnostic information

The diagnosis of pyelonephritis can be challenging. PU/PD can be severe in patients with pyelonephritis. However, patients with pyelonephritis may also show clinical signs relating to lower urinary tract infection such as haematuria, pollakiuria, stranguria or dysuria, if infection is not restricted to the upper urinary tract. Patients with acute pyelonephritis will often demonstrate systemic signs such as pyrexia and lethargy, which may be combined with a left-shifted inflammatory leucogram. In such patients there may be evidence of renal/lumbar/spinal pain and unilateral or bilateral renomegaly on abdominal palpation. While it is usual for patients with pyelonephritis to present with azotaemia, this is not always the case.

Ultrasound examination of the kidneys is likely to be more informative than radiography. It can reveal renomegaly, changes in echogenicity of the renal parenchyma, pyelectasia and dilatation of the proximal ureter (see Chapter 7). Ultrasonography of the urinary tract may also allow identification of predisposing factors for urinary tract infections (e.g. urolithiasis, structural abnormalities, nephroliths). Radiographs may confirm the presence of renomegaly, and intravenous excretory urography may indicate poor contrast enhancement of the kidney with dilatation and/or incomplete filling of the renal pelvis (see Chapter 7).

The presentation of patients with chronic pyelonephritis can be more insidious, with the degree of PU/PD varying in severity. Patients with chronic pyelonephritis may not always demonstrate pyrexia, or pyrexia may wax and wane, and a left-shifted inflammatory leucogram is not consistent. Particularly in feline patients with mild CKD, where isosthenuric urine (USG 1.008–1.015) is identified and appears discordant with the magnitude of azotaemia, a secondary pyelonephritis should be considered. The same may be true for the dog, although is potentially a less consistent phenomenon.

Chronic pyelonephritis may be suspected on the basis of ultrasound examination of the kidneys (see Chapter 7) combined in some instances with a more rapid than anticipated deterioration in renal function. However, the degree of pyelectasia must be interpreted with caution as mild renal pelvis dilatation can also be attributed to intravenous fluid therapy and CKD alone.

In both acute and chronic pyelonephritis, pyelocentesis with ultrasound guidance resulting in a positive culture from urine obtained from the renal pelvis gives a definitive diagnosis. Culture of renal aspirates or biopsy samples would also provide a definitive diagnosis but is rarely performed. However, pyelocentesis should be considered a specialized procedure, and more often a presumed diagnosis of acute or chronic pyelonephritis is made on the basis of compatible clinical signs, ultrasonographic findings, urinalysis and positive anaerobic bacterial urine culture performed on a cystocentesis sample. However, if the infection is predominantly affecting the renal parenchyma, urine obtained from the bladder may not have an active sediment and urine culture may be negative. In this scenario, if there is still a high index of suspicion for pyelonephritis based on clinical presentation and ultrasonographic changes, empirical antibacterial therapy, using an agent likely to have good activity against the probable causative organism, may be considered before pyelonephritis is excluded as a cause of PU/PD. Clinical improvement in PU/PD, and in renal parameters if azotaemia has been documented, would be anticipated if an occult pyelonephritis is present.

Pyometra

Pyometra is a common condition in older entire bitches and cardinal presenting signs can include PU/PD (Hagman, 2012). Ascending bacteria from the normal vaginal flora establish an infection in the progesterone-primed uterus. The most common bacterial organism (in over 70% of cases) is *E. coli*. As stated above, endotoxin produced by certain strains of bacteria such as *E. coli* can interfere with AVP–receptor interaction, resulting in a temporary secondary NDI.

Key diagnostic information

Entire bitches with pyometra typically present in dioestrus 2–12 weeks after their season, although infection of the uterine stump (stump pyometra) in neutered bitches is possible. The condition is most often seen in older bitches (mean 7 years; range 4 months to 18 years). In bitches with open pyometra, a mucoid to purulent discharge may be present at the vulva, although in patients with a closed cervix this may not be appreciated. Other typical presenting signs can include lethargy, pyrexia, inappetence, abdominal discomfort, vomiting and diarrhoea. Patients may present with clinical signs compatible with systemic inflammatory response syndrome, and on abdominal palpation an enlarged uterus may be palpable.

Diagnosis is based on historical information of an entire bitch with compatible clinical signs and physical examination. Patients invariably demonstrate a left-shifted inflammatory leucogram although overwhelming demand may result in neutropenia. Azotaemia may be documented in bitches with pyometra and can be either pre-renal or renal in origin. Proteinuria may also be identified, which has been ascribed to immune-mediated glomerulonephritis although conclusive evidence for this from comparison with age-matched control dogs is not available. Abdominal ultrasound examination and/or radiography typically reveals a fluid-filled enlarged uterus. PU/PD is anticipated to resolve after ovariohysterectomy. Pyometra is rare in cats.

Hyperthyroidism

PU/PD is reported in up to 75% of cats with hyperthyroidism. The exact pathogenesis of PU/PD in hyperthyroidism is uncertain but psychogenic polydipsia and heat intolerance may be factors. The sensation of thirst may occur at a lower plasma osmolality in hyperthyroidism compared with the euthyroid state. However, experimental studies in rodents suggest that PU/PD may also be contributed to by an alteration in renal haemodynamics, which may lead to increased solute excretion, a non-osmotic related suppression of AVP production and down-regulation of aquaporins (Syme, 2007).

Key diagnostic information

Hyperthyroidism should be considered as a differential diagnosis for PU/PD in all cats over the age of 7 years. A diagnosis of hyperthyroidism is suspected on the basis of compatible history and clinical signs, including polyphagia with weight loss, intermittent vomiting and diarrhoea, hyperactivity and behavioural changes (Peterson, 2013). On physical examination, poor body condition, tachycardia, heart murmur and gallop rhythm and a unilateral or bilateral thyroid goitre may be noted. Increased alanine aminotransferase (ALT) activity is a common biochemical abnormality but definitive diagnosis of hyperthyroidism is usually achieved with measurement of serum/plasma total thyroxine (tT4) concentration. For those patients where there is a high clinical index of suspicion for hyperthyroidism but where tT4 does not confirm the diagnosis, additional diagnostics including repeat measurement of tT4 in 4–8 weeks, or assessment of free T4 by equilibrium dialysis may be required. Additional diagnostics that may be considered in such cases include assessment of serum thyroid-stimulating hormone (TSH) concentration, tri-iodothyronine (T3) suppression testing or, less commonly, a thyrotropin-releasing hormone (TRH) stimulation test and thyroid scintigraphy.

Both hyperthyroidism and CKD are common in older cats and therefore may occur concurrently (Vaske *et al.*, 2015). The relationship between hyperthyroidism and renal function is discussed further in Chapter 17. The increase in GFR associated with the hyperthyroid state and variable urine concentrating ability means that renal function cannot be adequately assessed until the hyperthyroidism has been treated and a euthyroid state achieved.

Hyperadrenocorticism

Hyperadrenocorticism is a common condition in the middle-aged to older dog (>6 years) and PU/PD is reported in approximately 80–85% of dogs with this condition (see Chapter 19). In hyperadrenocorticism, high circulating concentrations of glucocorticoids result in interference with the action of AVP at the AVP receptor in the distal tubule and collecting duct, resulting in a secondary NDI. In addition, increased cortisol concentrations may have an effect on the set point and relative release of AVP, resulting in a secondary CDI. For this reason, many dogs with hyperadrenocorticism will show at least a partial response to exogenous administration of desmopressin acetate (DDAVP), making it important to exclude hyperadrenocorticism before performing either a water deprivation test or a desmopressin trial. Cortisol may also have a direct impact on GFR, increasing diuresis. CDI due to direct compression of the posterior pituitary or hypothalamus by an anterior pituitary mass (pituitary macroadenoma) could theoretically modulate thirst and result in PU/PD although this is considered rare. Exogenous steroid administration, and ensuing iatrogenic hyperadrenocorticism, is a common cause of the development of PU/PD in the dog (see Figure 2.10).

Hyperadrenocorticism is a rare condition in the cat and PU/PD is not typically reported as a presenting sign unless the patient has concurrent diabetes mellitus. Cats, unlike dogs, do not typically develop PU/PD in response to exogenous steroid administration. The presence of PU/PD in cats receiving corticosteroids should always raise concern for the onset of diabetes mellitus.

Key diagnostic information

A diagnosis of hyperadrenocorticism should be suspected on the basis of historical information, clinical signs and physical examination findings. The median age for diagnosis of hyperadrenocorticism is 11 years, with over 75% of dogs being >9 years (Behrend et al., 2013). Hyperadrenocorticism is therefore an unlikely diagnosis in young dogs, and other differential diagnoses should be considered in such patients. Typical clinical signs in the dog include PU/PD, polyphagia, panting, change in appearance (e.g. pot-bellied with muscle wastage), skin thinning and changes in haircoat (see Figure 2.6). On biochemical assessment approximately 90–95% of dogs will have increased alkaline phosphatase (ALP) activity, therefore hyperadrenocorticism should be considered an unlikely diagnosis if ALP activity is normal. Dogs with hyperadrenocorticism typically demonstrate reduced urine concentrating ability, with USG <1.020 in over 80% of cases. However, many affected dogs will be able to concentrate their urine to >1.025–1.030. This phenomenon may be appreciated when dogs have a change in environment, for example during hospitalization.

A number of diagnostic tests are available although no test has 100% sensitivity and specificity and therefore false-negative and -positive results are possible. It is important that diagnostic testing is only performed when there is a clinical suspicion of hyperadrenocorticism. Diagnostic tests that are commonly performed to confirm a diagnosis of hyperadrenocorticism include an adreno-corticotrophic hormone (ACTH) stimulation test and/or a low dose dexamethasone suppression test. The urine cortisol to creatinine ratio (UCCR) has a high sensitivity and is therefore a useful test when the index of suspicion for hyperadrenocorticism is low and exclusion of this condition is required. However, the specificity of the UCCR diagnostic test is low and therefore a positive test result should not be used to confirm a diagnosis of hyperadrenocorticism because of the high possibility of false-positive results. Urine samples for UCCR assessment should be collected in a home environment, avoiding any potentially stressful episodes such as visiting the veterinary clinic.

Hyperadrenocorticism is a rare condition in cats. It is most often considered as a differential diagnosis in cats with diabetes mellitus and particularly those where diabetic control has been poor. However, PU/PD has been reported rarely as a primary presenting clinical sign in cats with hyperadrenocorticism in the absence of diabetes mellitus. Other typical clinical signs include polyphagia, thin, fragile or torn skin, curled ear-tips, weight loss, failure of hair regrowth, lethargy and abdominal enlargement. In contrast to dogs, <10% of cats with hyperadrenocorticism are reported to have an elevation in ALP activity, although around 30% may have increased ALT activity and hypercholesterolaemia. Diagnostic testing, similar to that described above for dogs, can be used to confirm a diagnosis of hyperadrenocorticism in cats.

Hypoadrenocorticism

Hypoadrenocorticism is a condition where loss of 85–90% of adrenocortical cells results in clinical signs relating to glucocorticoid and mineralocorticoid deficiency. Hypoadrenocorticism is an uncommon cause of PU/PD, with only approximately 20% of dogs showing evidence of PU/PD as part of their initial presentation (see Chapter 19). Rarely, dogs may present with isolated glucocorticoid deficiency although a proportion of such dogs go on to develop mineralocorticoid deficiency. Polyuria in patients with hypoadrenocorticism results from hyponatraemia secondary to mineralocorticoid deficiency, which results in loss of the osmotic gradient required between the tubular filtrate and the tubulointerstitium for water reabsorption and is therefore a form of secondary NDI. Approximately 30% of dogs with hypoadrenocorticism also demonstrate hypercalcaemia, which may be a contributing factor in the development of polyuria and polydipsia in these dogs (Schenck and Chew, 2013; Van Lanen and Sande, 2014).

Key diagnostic information

Patients with hypoadrenocorticism often present with vague clinical signs including variable appetite, lethargy, weight loss, vomiting/diarrhoea, weakness, waxing and waning disease course, shaking/shivering and collapse. The mean age at diagnosis is 4–5 years although diagnosis is possible at a wide range of ages. Bitches are predisposed, and over-represented breeds include the Great Dane, poodles and West Highland White Terrier. Pertinent physical examination findings can include depression, lethargy, weakness and bradycardia (see Figure 2.6). Patients presenting in a hypoadrenocorticoid crisis will have clinical signs of shock including hypovolaemia, dehydration, poor peripheral pulses, hypothermia, melaena and/or haematochezia. Serum biochemistry may reveal the presence of key electrolyte abnormalities, hyperkalaemia and hyponatraemia, in addition to mild hypercalcaemia and hypoglycaemia. On complete blood count the absence of a stress leucogram and the presence of eosinophilia and lymphocytosis should be noted.

The diagnosis of hypoadrenocorticism can be confirmed by performing an ACTH stimulation test, to which the patient with hypoadrenocorticism will demonstrate no response. An atypical form of hypoadrenocorticism is identified in some dogs, where the typical electrolyte abnormalities (hyperkalaemia and hyponatraemia) are not identified. These dogs may only have deficiency in glucocorticoids but recent studies support the notion that, even without typical electrolyte abnormalities, many dogs do demonstrate mineralocorticoid deficiency when aldosterone concentrations are assessed pre- and post-administration of ACTH (Baumstark et al., 2014).

Patients that present in a hypoadrenocorticoid crisis must be differentiated from patients with AKI. During a hypoadrenocorticoid crisis, hypovolaemia and dehydration attributable to diuresis, gastrointestinal fluid losses and reduced fluid intake can result in hypotension and hypoperfusion of the kidneys and a pre-renal azotaemia. Gastrointestinal bleeding may further increase plasma urea concentrations. In patients with normal renal function, pre-renal azotaemia should be accompanied by an increase in USG, typically >1.030 in the dog. However, loss of the osmotic gradient due to hyponatraemia occurring in hypoadrenocorticism prevents adequate urine concentrating ability. As a result, some dogs with hypoadrenocorticism may present with a pre-renal azotaemia in conjunction with USG of 1.008–1.020 which, without due care, can be mistaken for AKI.

Diabetes mellitus

Diabetes mellitus with persistent hyperglycaemia results in glucosuria and an osmotic diuresis (see Chapter 19). Glucose is a low molecular weight molecule, which is freely filtered at the glomerulus. In health, >99% of filtered glucose should be reabsorbed in the proximal tubule such that the glucose concentration of the tubular filtrate in the remaining nephron is low. The plasma glucose concentration at which glucosuria is first identified is referred to as the renal threshold, which is approximately 9–12 mmol/l (~180–200 mg/100 ml) in dogs and 11–16 mmol/l (~290 mg/100 ml) in cats. When plasma glucose values exceed the tubular transport maximum for glucose reabsorption, glucose remains in the tubular filtrate and an osmotic diuresis ensues.

Key diagnostic information

The diagnosis of diabetes mellitus in dogs can be made on the basis of the combination of glucosuria with a persistently elevated blood glucose concentration and compatible physical examination findings (see Figure 2.6), with clinical signs including weight loss despite an increased appetite/polyphagia and lethargy. In cats, the presence of stress hyperglycaemia may make the initial diagnosis of diabetes mellitus more challenging. Stress-related hyperglycaemia which exceeds the tubular maximum for glucose reabsorption in the kidney can result in glucosuria. However, the short-term increase in blood glucose means that, in this scenario, clinical PU/PD should not be appreciated. A diagnosis of diabetes mellitus in the cat should therefore always be made in association with compatible clinical signs, documentation of persistent hyperglycaemia and glucosuria, with the latter sample potentially obtained in a less stressful home environment. In dogs, and particularly in cats, assessment of fructosamine concentration or glycosylated haemoglobin may give additional information about the persistence of hyperglycaemia.

Primary renal glycosuria

In human patients, primary renal glycosuria results from either a congenital abnormality in the glucose transporters within the proximal tubule membrane or an abnormality in transtubular glucose movement. Primary renal glycosuria results in polyuria through osmotic diuresis with compensatory polydipsia, although some patients may be asymptomatic at the time of diagnosis. Complex tubular disorders are also reported where glycosuria with euglycaemia may be identified in addition to variable alteration in electrolyte (sodium, potassium, phosphate, calcium and bicarbonate) and amino acid reabsorption. In both congenital and acquired complex tubulopathies, polyuria results from osmotic diuresis, although AVP-resistant polyuria may also be present.

Key diagnostic information

Primary renal glycosuria is uncommon but has been reported in Scottish Terriers and as a familial condition in Norwegian Elkhounds. Patients demonstrate persistent glucosuria in the face of euglycaemia. Fructosamine concentrations may aid in documenting normoglycaemia. In addition, patients with glucosuria are predisposed to secondary bacterial and fungal urinary tract infections, and clinical signs therefore may relate to these secondary conditions in addition to PU/PD.

Complex tubulopathies can be identified on the basis of urinalysis and venous blood gas analysis to assess for evidence of renal tubular acidosis, and by performing renal clearance studies to identify reabsorptive defects in electrolytes and amino acids. Fanconi syndrome is the complex tubulopathy that is most commonly reported in veterinary medicine. In the Basenji, Fanconi syndrome is presumed to be familial, although the onset of clinical signs frequently does not occur until adulthood with dogs typically being 3–4 years of age when glycosuria and PU/PD are first appreciated.

Acquired renal glycosuria, or Fanconi-like syndromes, can be identified secondary to any condition that results in damage to tubular cells or generally disrupts normal tubular reabsorptive mechanisms. Renal glycosuria and Fanconi-like syndromes have been reported in association with acute kidney injury, a number of drugs and toxins including heavy metals (e.g. lead, copper, mercury), ethylene glycol, certain antibiotics (e.g. aminoglycosides, tetracyclines) and chemotherapeutic agents (e.g. cisplatin, carboplatin), and also with infections such as pyelonephritis and leptospirosis (Tangeman and Littman, 2013). Certain antibiotics (such as ciprofloxacin when using the glucose oxidase test reagent (Drysdale et al., 1988; Rees and Boothe, 2004), penicillin and cephalosporin antibiotics when using copper sulphate-based reagents (Rotblatt and Koda-Kimble, 1987; Rees and Boothe, 2004)) may also give false-positive results on a urine glucose dipstick test, due to their sugar-reducing properties. More recently, acquired tubulopathies have also been reported in Labrador Retrievers with copper hepatopathy (Langlois et al., 2013), and in patients with malignancies (e.g. multiple myeloma), primary hypoparathyroidism and with feeding of jerky treats (Thompson et al., 2013). The toxic component in the last scenario remains unknown.

Hypercalcaemia

Hypercalcaemia is a common cause of PU/PD in the dog, but it is a rare cause in the cat. Calcium sensing receptors (CaSR) are identified on the serosal side of the collecting duct epithelium. Activation of the CaSR in this region by high circulating concentrations of calcium down-regulates aquaporin-2 expression, resulting in a secondary NDI, and PU with a compensatory PD (Khanna, 2006). In addition, persistent hypercalcaemia and interaction with the CaSR in the thick ascending limb may modulate activity of the $Na^+K^+2Cl^-$ channels, affecting the kidney's ability to maintain an osmotic gradient between the tubular fluid and medullary interstitium (Hebert et al., 1997).

Key diagnostic information

A number of different underlying disease conditions can result in hypercalcaemia, with the severity of clinical signs associated with the magnitude of the hypercalcaemia (Figure 2.12). Hypercalcaemia is often first identified on the basis of a serum biochemical profile, where total calcium is usually reported. Total calcium reflects the combined quantification of protein-bound and ionized (free) calcium and can therefore be influenced, in particular, by albumin concentrations. Where possible, total hypercalcaemia should be confirmed by assessment of ionized calcium concentration, ideally repeated on at least two occasions to document persistence. Reported adjustment factors for total calcium to estimate ionized calcium have been shown to be inaccurate and should not be used (Schenck and Chew, 2005; 2010). Unless immediate in-house assessment

Incidence	Causes
Common	• Neoplasia (lymphoma, anal sac adenocarcinoma, nasal adenocarcinoma, pancreatic adenocarcinoma, pulmonary carcinoma, mammary carcinoma, multiple myeloma, squamous cell carcinoma, thyroid adenocarcinoma) • Chronic kidney disease • *Angiostrongylus vasorum* infection • Hypoadrenocorticism • Idiopathic (cat)
Uncommon	• Primary hyperparathyroidism • Nutritional secondary hyperparathyroidism • Acute kidney injury
Rare	• Vitamin D toxicosis • Granulomatous disease (*Angiostrongylus vasorum*, immune-mediated, histoplasmosis, blastomycosis)
Miscellaneous	• Spurious/laboratory error • Haemoconcentration

2.12 Causes of hypercalcaemia.

of ionized calcium is available, careful sample handling is required to ensure that serum is not exposed to air, which may significantly increase pH and falsely decrease ionized calcium concentrations. Studies show that correctly handled serum samples can be stored for up to 72 hours for ionized calcium assessment, at room temperature or at 4°C (Schenck *et al.*, 1995).

The initial clinical presentation, history, physical examination and routine biochemistry are important in differentiating the underlying aetiology of a patient's hypercalcaemia. For example, identification of underlying neoplasia should be prioritized in the older or systemically unwell patient and the history may provide important information regarding potential access to vitamin D sources (e.g. psoriasis cream, rodenticides, vitamin D supplements). Physical examination findings, e.g. peripheral lymphadenopathy or a mass on rectal examination, may provide immediate insight into the possibility of lymphoma or anal sac adenocarcinoma, respectively (see Figure 2.6).

Additional diagnostics, including abdominal (metastatic disease or primary neoplasia) and thoracic (mediastinal mass/metastatic disease) imaging combined with fine-needle aspiration and/or biopsy may be useful when evaluating for underlying neoplasia, and spinal/long bone radiography or computed tomography may be required for identification of lytic lesions (multiple myeloma/bone metastasis). If there is a high index of suspicion for neoplasia, which cannot otherwise be identified, parathyroid hormone related peptide (PTHrp) may be assessed.

For key diagnostic information relating to the diagnosis of acute and chronic kidney disease and hypoadrenocorticism, readers are directed to the relevant section in this chapter. However, secondary effects of persistent hypercalcaemia can include renal mineralization and therefore caution must be exercised when a patient presents with concurrent azotaemia, hypercalcaemia and hyperphosphataemia in order to ascertain whether these biochemical abnormalities are due to primary renal disease, hypoadrenocorticoid crisis or the secondary consequence of hypercalcaemia.

Primary hyperparathyroidism (PHPTH) is an uncommon condition resulting from adenomatous proliferation of chief cells in the parathyroid gland. The condition usually affects just one parathyroid gland, although more than one gland may be affected. PHPTH is most often diagnosed in middle-aged to older dogs (median age 11 years, range 4–17 years) and the Keeshond is over-represented.

Although PU/PD may be recognized, the identification of hypercalcaemia is serendipitous in many patients with PHPTH when routine biochemistry is performed for an alternative reason, e.g. pre-anaesthetic screening. Mild clinical signs including PU/PD, weakness, reduced appetite, muscle wastage, muscle tremors and reduced activity may be identified with PHPTH. However, many clients only recognize these changes after parathyroidectomy has been performed and PTH and calcium concentrations have normalized, suggesting that the hypercalcaemia is insidious in onset and chronic.

Approximately 25% of dogs with PHPTH present with urolithiasis; this means that clinical signs relating to the lower urinary tract (e.g. stranguria, pollakiuria, dysuria) may also trigger diagnostic investigation.

Physical examination of patients with PHPTH is typically unremarkable and the enlarged parathyroid gland cannot usually be palpated but may be readily visualized with ultrasonography and compared with the contralateral glands. In general, if a patient is systemically unwell on presentation, an alternative diagnosis or second condition in addition to PHPTH should be considered as an explanation for hypercalcaemia. Serum biochemistry in patients with PHPTH will reveal the presence of variable total hypercalcaemia and low normal or low serum phosphorus concentrations. A diagnosis of PHPTH can be confirmed by the presence of normal or elevated parathyroid hormone concentrations in the face of hypercalcaemia, where physiologically the parathyroid hormone concentrations should be suppressed.

Hepatic disease

Hepatic disease can result in PU/PD through a number of mechanisms. Urea is one of the main solutes required for the maintenance of the osmolality of the medullary interstitium and the counter-current multiplier system (see above). Reduced synthesis of urea with decreased hepatic function can lead to failure in the maintenance of the osmotic gradient, reduced water reabsorption from the tubular filtrate and therefore PU. However, the build-up of hepatic toxins in hepatic encephalopathy may have a direct central effect at the hypothalamus, resulting in a form of primary PD. In certain hepatic diseases, e.g. copper hepatopathy in Labrador Retrievers, primary renal glycosuria has been reported, which results in osmotic diuresis and PU.

Key diagnostic information

Hepatic disease is usually suspected on the basis of historical and physical examination findings and routine biochemistry. Dogs of any age may be affected by hepatic disease ranging from congenital portovascular anomalies detected early in life, through to chronic hepatopathies presenting in middle to older age. Numerous breed predispositions have been identified for different hepatic conditions and readers are directed to comprehensive medicine texts for further information on specific hepatic conditions (e.g. Ettinger and Feldman, 2010). Historical and physical examination findings can be non-specific, e.g. lethargy, reduced appetite, vomiting, diarrhoea and weight loss, or may more directly raise concern regarding hepatic function, e.g. icterus, small or large liver on abdominal palpation or the presence of ascites. In the young dog or cat, poor growth, neurological signs particularly associated with feeding, seizures and hypersalivation may increase suspicion of a portovascular anomaly.

On serum biochemistry, elevated liver enzyme activities (ALT, ALP, gamma-glutamyltransferase) indicate liver pathology or hepatic stress, but do not reflect liver function. Reduction in urea, hypocholesterolaemia, hypoalbuminaemia and low glucose concentrations can be used in conjunction with a bile acid stimulation test and blood ammonia concentration to give information about hepatic function. Further information on hepatic disease may be gained from diagnostic imaging, including abdominal radiographs, ultrasound examination and computed tomography. In the patient with a suspected portovascular anomaly, abdominal ultrasound examination and/or computed tomography angiography not only may allow identification of the anomalous vessel but may also indicate microhepatica, renomegaly and the presence of urate uroliths. Hepatic fine-needle aspiration and/or biopsy is usually required for a definitive diagnosis of most acute or chronic hepatopathies.

Central diabetes insipidus

CDI results from lack of production of AVP by the hypothalamus and/or posterior pituitary, which in turn prevents adequate concentration of urine and results in a primary PU. In human medicine, a number of different underlying aetiologies have been reported including familial conditions, vascular disease, autoimmune disease, trauma and benign or malignant neoplasia affecting the hypothalamopituitary system. However, in over 50% of human patients the condition is idiopathic.

CDI is a rare condition in dogs and cats, although both partial and complete CDI have been reported in dogs. In complete CDI, patients exhibit a complete lack of AVP production despite rising plasma osmolality, whereas in patients with partial CDI the production of AVP in response to osmolality appears blunted, with inadequate AVP production for a given plasma osmolality. In both scenarios, reduced or absent AVP means lack of interaction between vasopressin and its receptor in the distal tubule and collecting ducts. As a result, reduced insertion of aquaporin-2 for water reabsorption leads to production of large volumes of dilute urine.

Key diagnostic information

CDI has been reported as an idiopathic disease in young dogs and may occur as part of panhypopituitarism syndrome. However, in middle-aged to older dogs the most common aetiology is pituitary neoplasia (macroadenoma), although craniopharyngioma, meningioma, lymphoma and metastatic disease have also been reported. CDI may also occur secondary to traumatic brain injury, frequently associated with skull fracture, and in this scenario CDI may be a permanent phenomenon although regrowth of neurons may afford some clinical improvement with time. A more common cause of CDI in recent years is in association with transsphenoidal surgery for hyperadrenocorticism or acromegaly; this again may be transient with spontaneous recovery, or permanent if there is degeneration of the hypothalamic neurons.

Clinical signs in patients with CDI include an extreme PU with compensatory and near incessant PD, which may be insidious or acute in onset depending on the underlying aetiology. For those patients where neoplasia underlies the CDI, other associated neurological signs may be present and in such patients the emphasis in diagnostic investigation should be to perform a full neurological assessment and to assess the pituitary/hypothalamic region with either computed tomography or magnetic resonance imaging.

Diagnostic investigation for CDI is infrequently performed in veterinary practice because this is a rare condition; it should only be performed after exclusion of other more common causes of PU/PD (see Figure 2.9). A normal dog or cat is able to produce concentrated urine and osmolality can reach >2300 mOsm/kg, with normal plasma osmolality ranging between 280 and 310 mOsm/kg (Nelson, 2014). Patients with severe CDI typically have USG values that are persistently <1.008 (urine osmolality <310 mOsm/kg); although, in milder or partial forms of CDI, USG may be higher with urine osmolality up to 600 mOsm/kg. Serum biochemistry in patients with CDI is typically unremarkable, although patients may have a tendency towards hypernatraemia or a sodium concentration at the top end of the laboratory reference interval. Spot plasma osmolality may be elevated; however, this is not always the case and plasma osmolality in dogs with CDI has been reported to range between 281 and 339 mOsm/kg (Nelson, 2014). Elevated plasma osmolality/sodium concentrations may be of particular concern if patients with CDI have their water intake inadvertently restricted, when failure to keep up with large excretory water losses can result in rapid-onset hypernatraemia (plasma sodium >160 mmol/l), hypertonic encephalopathy and clinical signs of stupor, ataxia and obtundation.

Differentiation of CDI from primary PD and NDI can be achieved by performing a water deprivation test, often in conjunction with a desmopressin trial (DDAVP: 1-deamino, 9-D-arginine vasopressin), which is referred to as a modified water deprivation test (Figures 2.13 and 2.14). However, a water deprivation test is not without considerable risk to the patient and should be considered a specialized procedure requiring hospitalization and careful monitoring to be performed safely and correctly. A water deprivation test should never be performed in a patient that is azotaemic or already dehydrated.

In normal dogs in a clinical setting, if a water deprivation test were to be performed, the expectation would be that urine osmolality would typically reach >1100 mOsm/kg and USG >1.030 after 5% dehydration within a period of 20–40 hours. During a water deprivation test, patients with CDI will continue to produce dilute urine (typically USG <1.008) and will not be able to concentrate their urine to above their plasma osmolality, typically <310 mOsm/kg. Dehydration will ensue typically over a period of 3–10 hours with evidence of reduction in bodyweight, development of hypernatraemia and increase in plasma osmolality. However, with administration of desmopressin, patients with complete CDI will demonstrate a >50% increase in urine osmolality. During water deprivation in patients with partial CDI, urine osmolality may increase to >300 mOsm/kg with a concomitant minimal increase in USG, typically to 1.008–1.020 (see Figure 2.14). However, patients with partial CDI will also subsequently show a response to desmopressin administration, but the response is usually incomplete and increases in urine osmolality of only >15% but <50% are anticipated. These findings in complete and partial CDI are in contrast to patients with congenital NDI who demonstrate low urine osmolality (<310 mOsm/kg), normal to increased spot plasma osmolality, but who show no alteration in urine osmolality with 5% dehydration and no response to administration of desmopressin (see Figure 2.14), with urine osmolality remaining <310 mOsm/kg and USG <1.006–1.012. This is also in contrast to the patient with psychogenic polydipsia, where a normal to low result (e.g. <280 mOsm/kg) is expected on a spot plasma osmolality test.

Careful review of signalment, historical and physical data to ensure that all conditions other than central diabetes insipidus, nephrogenic diabetes insipidus and primary polydipsia have been excluded

Yes:
- Consider serial USG assessment at home or in a new environment (e.g. during hospitalization) for patients with suspected primary polydipsia
- Consider desmopressin trial (see Figure 2.15)
- Consider requirements for water deprivation test and seek specialist advice if necessary

No:
Proceed with further diagnostic investigations (see Figure 2.7)

Prior to water deprivation test:
- Consider gradual water restriction (see Figure 2.16)
- Ensure no clinical signs of dehydration or azotaemia – if present **DO NOT PERFORM WDT**
- Withhold food for 12 hours

Water deprivation phase:
- Begin early in the morning
- Empty the bladder and ideally place urinary catheter to enable complete bladder emptying throughout test
- Assess and record USG and if possible osmolality
- Obtain and record accurate weight of patient
- Obtain blood sample for plasma creatinine, sodium and osmolality, and record
- Continuously:
  - Monitor the patient for signs of depression/lethargy/behavioural change
- Every 1–2 hours:
  - Assess the patient for clinical signs of dehydration
  - Empty bladder/urine bag – measure and record USG and urine osmolality
  - Record weight of patient (ensure the same scales are used on each occasion)
  - Obtain sample for plasma creatinine, sodium and osmolality, and record

Water deprivation test end points:
The WDT should be ended when one or more of the following is noted:
- Azotaemia and/or hypernatraemia
- Patient becomes depressed/lethargic/obtunded/shows behavioural changes
- Urine specific gravity exceeds 1.030
- Patient loses 5% of bodyweight

On stopping the WDT obtain samples for:
- USG, urine osmolality, plasma osmolality, plasma creatinine and sodium concentrations

Response to exogenous vasopressin:
- Administer desmopressin (0.5 IU/kg i.m. once; maximal dose 5 IU/animal; subcutaneous administration is not recommended owing to variable absorption) or desmopressin acetate (intranasal solution: 4 drops placed in conjunctival sac; injectable solution: 1–4 µg/dog i.v. once)
- Continue restriction of water and food
- Continuously:
  - Evaluate mentation and monitor for depression
- Every 30 minutes for 2 hours (every 1–2 hours for up to 8–12 hours if desmopressin acetate is used):
  - Empty bladder/urine bag
  - Measure and record USG and urine osmolality
  - Obtain sample for assessment of plasma creatinine, sodium and osmolality

Continuation of monitoring beyond 2 hours may be required for some patients. However, extreme caution is required if the patient is becoming dehydrated. See Figure 2.14 for anticipated response to water deprivation testing

2.13 Modified water deprivation test (WDT). USG = urine specific gravity.

Patient	Starting urine osmolality and urine specific gravity	Random plasma osmolality with free access to water	Time to test endpoint	Maximal urine osmolality and urine specific gravity after 5% dehydration	Urine osmolality and urine specific gravity response to vasopressin
Normal dog	160–2500 mOsm/kg 1.006–1.040	280–300 pOsm	Up to 40 hours	>1100 mOsm/kg >1.030	–
Complete central diabetes insipidus	<310 mOsm/kg <1.006–1.012	Normal to ↑	Mean 4 hours Range 3–10 hours	<310 mOsm/kg <1.006–1.012	>50% ↑mOsm/kg >1.025
Partial central diabetes insipidus	<310 mOsm/kg <1.006–1.012	Normal to ↑	Mean 8 hours Range 3–10 hours	>310 mOsm/kg 1.008–1.020	15–50% ↑mOsm/kg >1.025
Nephrogenic diabetes insipidus	<310 mOsm/kg <1.006–1.012	Normal to ↑	Mean 5 hours Range 3–10 hours	<310 mOsm/kg <1.006–1.012	<300 mOsm/kg <1.006–1.012
Primary polydipsia	<150–1100 mOsm/kg 1.002–1.020	Normal to ↓	Mean 13 hours Up to 24 hours	>1100 mOsm/kg >1.030	–

2.14 Anticipated response to modified water deprivation testing.

USG can be monitored instead of urine osmolality during a water deprivation test, but the results can be more difficult to interpret. Patients who demonstrate no change in USG with water deprivation but an increase in USG to >1.030 with administration of desmopressin can be considered to have complete CDI, whereas an increase in USG to between 1.012 and 1.025 supports partial CDI.

Whereas complete CDI and severe NDI may be relatively easily distinguished with a water deprivation test, there must be caution in interpreting the results of a modified water deprivation test that appear to be compatible with partial CDI, for a number of reasons. Many disease conditions which result in a secondary NDI can give similar results, with only a slight or lack of increase in urine osmolality and USG in response to water deprivation, and a slight increase in both parameters after administration of desmopressin. This is at least partly due to medullary washout and highlights the importance of ensuring that all the more common causes of PU/PD have been excluded before rare conditions such as CDI are considered. Differentiating partial CDI from primary PD on a water deprivation test can also be difficult if medullary washout prevents the patient with primary PD from adequately concentrating their urine and increasing urine osmolality during the water deprivation phase. In addition, some patients with partial CDI appear to show an enhanced response to the small amount of AVP they secrete on maximal osmotic stimulation. In this scenario, their maximal response to AVP is achieved during the water deprivation phase and no further increase in urine osmolality or change in USG is appreciated during administration of a synthetic vasopressin analogue.

Other reported diagnostic tests for the differentiation of CDI include measurement of AVP during osmotic stimulation (saline diuresis), direct assessment of plasma osmolality without requirement for water restriction and an isolated desmopressin trial (Figure 2.15). Assessment of plasma osmolality without water restriction may increase

suspicion of CDI providing other, more common, differential diagnoses have been excluded. Given that congenital NDI is extremely rare, if all other causes of secondary NDI have been excluded, CDI is the more likely diagnosis.

Some clinicians prefer to perform a desmopressin trial (see Figure 2.15) rather than a modified water deprivation test. In patients with CDI, provision of exogenous AVP should facilitate an increase in urine osmolality and USG. However, the apparent speed of this response will be partially dependent on the presence of an osmotic gradient between the tubular fluid and medullary interstitium. For patients with CDI, sufficient time must therefore be allowed (usually 5–7 days) for medullary washout to correct, before a full response to desmopressin will be appreciated. Caution is required when undertaking a desmopressin trial to ensure that all other potential causes of PU/PD have been excluded because patients with secondary NDI of many aetiologies will show a partial response to administration of exogenous desmopressin, giving a false-positive interpretation of this test.

Nephrogenic diabetes insipidus

Congenital NDI results from a lack of response to AVP by the kidney. In human medicine, this condition is most often the result of an X-linked mutation in the arginine vasopressin receptor gene (*AVPR2*) or a mutation in aquaporin-2 gene (*AQP2*), affecting water reabsorption from the tubule. Congenital NDI is extremely rare in dogs, with only a few case reports in the veterinary literature, and has never been reported in cats. A familial form of NDI has been reported in Huskies in which a mutation resulted in reduced affinity of the AVP receptor for AVP. A large number of causes of secondary NDI have been discussed in this chapter (see Figure 2.3) and it is important that these are excluded before primary NDI is considered as a differential diagnosis.

Key diagnostic information

Patients with congenital NDI present at a young age (<2 years) with extreme polyuria and compensatory polydipsia. As with CDI, routine biochemistry is usually unremarkable apart from a tendency towards hypernatraemia or a sodium concentration at the upper end of the reference interval. Similar to patients with CDI, those with congenital NDI may demonstrate a normal to increased spot plasma osmolality, with values in the literature reported to range between 283 and 340 mOsm/kg (Nelson, 2014). Patients with congenital NDI are unable to modify urinary osmolality in response to water deprivation, resulting in 5% dehydration and an increase in plasma osmolality whilst urine osmolality remains <290–310 mOsm/kg (see Figure 2.14). Such patients will consistently show USG values <1.012 throughout a water deprivation test. In contrast to patients with CDI, dogs with congenital NDI will show no response to subsequent administration of desmopressin. However, given the extreme rarity of this condition, if the results of a modified water deprivation test are compatible with NDI, it is advisable to review all previous diagnostic investigations to ensure that all causes of secondary NDI, which are much more common, have been excluded (see Figure 2.7).

Primary (psychogenic) polydipsia

Primary PD is an uncommon condition where excessive thirst drives a secondary PU. It is considered more common in highly strung or hyperactive young dogs and may reflect a behavioural response to lack of environmental

---

Owner monitors water intake at home over two 24-hour periods with free water access. Serial urine specific gravity (USG) assessment performed

↓

Synthetic desmopressin administered (0.05–0.2 mg/dog orally q8h; 1–4 drops of intranasal solution applied to conjunctival sac q12h) for 5–7 days

↓

Days 5–7: Owner monitors water intake at home over one 24-hour period. Serial USG/urine osmolality assessment period

↓

CDI suspected when:
- Dramatic reduction in water intake on days 5–7 *versus* day 1
- Increase in USG >1.030 or >50% increase in urine osmolality

Congenital NDI: Dogs will show no response
Secondary NDI: Dogs may show partial response, in particular with hyperadrenocorticism
Primary polydipsia: Dogs may show partial response

2.15 Schedule for performing a desmopressin trial. CDI = central diabetes insipidus; NDI = nephrogenic diabetes insipidus.

stimulation. A component of primary PD may underpin the PU/PD which is identified in cats with hyperthyroidism. Lesions within the hypothalamus and thirst centre may also rarely lead to primary PD.

Key diagnostic information

Dogs with primary PD are typically young and may have a history of a lack of environmental stimulation, or an environmental change such as rehoming. Traditionally, a water deprivation test has been used for diagnosis of primary PD. In a water deprivation test, dogs with primary PD should have adequate capacity to concentrate their urine and increase urine osmolality before dehydration occurs. However, an individual's ability to do this may be impaired by medullary washout, which can lead to equivocal results. Some clinicians support a period of gradual water restriction prior to a water deprivation test (Figure 2.16) to accommodate this, but it is strongly advocated that such an approach should only ever be undertaken in a hospital environment with careful 24-hour monitoring.

Given the concern regarding the risks associated with a water deprivation test, if primary PD is suspected, sequential assessment of USG measurements, both at home when the dog is active and after a change in environment (e.g. during a period of hospitalization), can be a useful and safer alternative. If USG >1.025 can be documented, then CDI can be excluded and, providing there are no other clinical or biochemical abnormalities, a diagnosis of primary PD is likely and will preclude the requirement for further diagnostic testing.

For patients with long-term medullary washout, gradual water restriction may be beneficial prior to performing a water deprivation test.

1. Monitor unrestricted water intake in a hospitalized environment over 24 hours with serial USG monitoring.
2. Over 2–5 days **gradually** restrict water intake to 100 ml/kg/24h by providing water in divided amounts throughout the day. Careful monitoring of bodyweight, serial USG, plasma sodium and creatinine, and patient demeanour should be performed throughout this period in a hospitalized environment.
3. If USG >1.025 or azotaemia develops do not proceed to water deprivation test.

2.16 Gradual water restriction prior to water deprivation test. USG = urine specific gravity.

References and further reading

Barrett KE, Barman SM, Boitano S and Brooks HL (2010) *Ganong's Review of Medical Physiology*. McGraw Hill Medical, New York

Bartges JW (2012) Chronic kidney disease in dogs and cats. *Veterinary Clinics of North America: Small Animal Practice* **42**, 669–692

Baumstark ME, Sieber-Ruckstuhl NS, Muller C *et al.* (2014) Evaluation of aldosterone concentrations in dogs with hypoadrenocorticism. *Journal of Veterinary Internal Medicine* **28**, 154–159

Behrend EN, Kooistra HS, Nelson R, Reusch CE and Scott-Moncrieff JC (2013) Diagnosis of spontaneous canine hyperadrenocorticism: 2012 ACVIM Consensus Statement (Small Animal). *Journal of Veterinary Internal Medicine* **27**, 1292–1304

Boag AK, Murphy KE and Connolly DJ (2005) Hypercalcaemia associated with *Angiostrongylus vasorum* in three dogs. *Journal of Small Animal Practice* **46**, 79–84

Brown SA, Atkins CE, Bagley R *et al.* (2007) Guidelines for the identification, evaluation and management of systemic hypertension in dogs and cats. *Journal of Veterinary Internal Medicine* **21**, 542–558

Drysdale L, Gilbert L, Thomson A *et al.* (1988) Pseudoglycosuria and ciprofloxacin. *The Lancet* **332**, 961

Ettinger SJ and Feldman EC (2010) *Textbook of Veterinary Internal Medicine*. Saunders, St Louis, Missouri

Hagman R (2012) Clinical and molecular characteristics of pyometra in female dogs. *Reproduction in Domestic Animals* **47**, 323–325

Hebert SC, Brown EM and Harris HW (1997 Role of the Ca^{2+}-sensing receptor in divalent mineral ion homeostasis. *Journal of Experimental Biology* **200**, 295–302

Khanna A (2006) Acquired nephrogenic diabetes insipidus. *Seminars in Nephrology* **26**, 244–248

Langlois DK, Smedley RC, Schall WD and Kruger JM (2013) Acquired proximal renal tubular dysfunction in 9 Labrador Retrievers with copper-associated hepatitis (2006–2012). *Journal of Veterinary Internal Medicine* **27**, 491–499

Nelson RW (2014) Water metabolism and diabetes insipidus. In: *Canine and Feline Endocrinology 2nd edn*, ed. EC Feldman *et al.*, pp. 1–36. Elsevier Health Sciences, St Louis, Missouri

Peterson ME (2013) More than just T4: Diagnostic testing for hyperthyroidism in cats. *Journal of Feline Medicine and Surgery* **15**, 765–777

Pressler BM (2013) Clinical approach to advanced renal function testing in dogs and cats. *Veterinary Clinics of North America: Small Animal Practice* **43**, 1193–1208

Rees CA and Boothe DM (2004) Evaluation of the effect of cephalexin and enrofloxacin on clinical laboratory measurements of urine glucose in dogs. *Journal of the American Veterinary Medical Association* **224**, 1455–1458

Rotblatt MD and Koda-Kimble MA (1987) Review of drug interference with urine glucose tests. *Diabetes Care* **10**, 103–110

Schenck PA and Chew DJ (2005) Prediction of serum ionized calcium concentration by use of serum total calcium concentration in dogs. *American Journal of Veterinary Research* **66**, 1330–1336

Schenck PA and Chew DJ (2010) Prediction of serum ionized calcium concentration by serum total calcium measurement in cats. *Canadian Journal of Veterinary Research* **74**, 209–213

Schenck PA and Chew DJ (2013) Hypercalcemia in dogs. In: *Clinical Endocrinology of Companion Animals*, ed. J Rand *et al.* pp. 356–373. John Wiley & Sons Ltd, Ames, Iowa

Schenck PA, Chew DJ and Brooks CL (1995) Effects of storage on serum ionized calcium and pH values in clinically normal dogs. *American Journal of Veterinary Research* **56**, 304–307

Syme HM (2007) Cardiovascular and renal manifestations of hyperthyroidism. *Veterinary Clinics of North America: Small Animal Practice* **37**, 723–743

Tangeman LE and Littman MP (2013) Clinicopathologic and atypical features of naturally occurring leptospirosis in dogs: 51 cases (2000–2010). *Journal of the American Veterinary Medical Association* **243**, 1316–1322

Thompson MF, Fleeman LM, Kessell AE, Steenhard LA and Foster SF (2013) Acquired proximal renal tubulopathy in dogs exposed to a common dried chicken treat: retrospective study of 108 cases (2007–2009). *Australian Veterinary Journal* **91**, 368–373

Van Lanen K and Sande A (2014) Canine hypoadrenocorticism: pathogenesis, diagnosis and treatment. *Topics in Companion Animal Medicine* **29**, 88–95

Vaske HH, Schermerhorn T and Grauer GF (2015) Effects of feline hyperthyroidism on kidney function: a review. *Journal of Feline Medicine and Surgery* **18(2)**, 55–59

Useful websites

www.research.vet.upenn.edu/InstructionsforSampleSubmission/SampleCollectionShipping/MetabolicFanconiCystinuria/tabid/7607/Default.aspx

Case example 1: Polydipsia and muscle weakness in a Domestic Shorthaired Cat

SIGNALMENT

A 13-year-old male neutered Domestic Shorthaired Cat.

HISTORY

PD and gradual muscle weakness reported over the past 2–3 months but without any other notable clinical signs. Urination unmonitored because the cat did not use a litter tray.

PHYSICAL EXAMINATION

Physical examination revealed mild generalized muscle wastage and borderline small kidneys on abdominal palpation. No thyroid goitre palpable.

INITIAL INVESTIGATION

- Haematology: unremarkable.
- Biochemistry: moderate hypokalaemia (2.5 mmol/l; reference interval (RI) 3.5–5.5 mmol/l).
- Total thyroxine: 23 nmol/l (RI 10–60 nmol/l).
- Urinalysis: specific gravity 1.020, otherwise unremarkable; urine protein to creatinine ratio 0.18.
- Urine culture: negative.
- Non-invasive blood pressure (Doppler technique): average systolic blood pressure (SBP) 190 mmHg.
- Fundic examination: unremarkable.

FURTHER DIAGNOSTIC INVESTIGATIONS

- Repeat biochemistry: persistent moderate hypokalaemia (2.8 mmol/l).
- Repeat urinalysis: specific gravity 1.018, otherwise unremarkable.
- Repeat SBP: confirmed systemic hypertension (SBP 210 mmHg).
- Fundic examination remained within normal limits.
- Abdominal ultrasound examination revealed a right-sided adrenal mass. Both kidneys were slightly small with an irregular contour.
- Plasma aldosterone concentration: 1573 pmol/l (RI 150–430 pmol/l).

OUTCOME

Primary hyperaldosteronism was confirmed on the basis of persistent hypokalaemia, an adrenal mass lesion and elevated aldosterone concentrations. Plasma renin activity was low, supporting primary aldosterone production. The cat was started on spironolactone 3 mg/kg orally q24h, potassium supplementation 2 mEq orally q12h and amlodipine besylate 0.625 mg/cat orally q24h. Potassium concentrations normalized with this therapy after 4 weeks. SBP returned to the American College of Veterinary Internal Medicine (ACVIM) Hypertension Consensus Guidelines mild risk category for target organ damage (Brown *et al.*, 2007) (SBP 150–160 mmHg).

The polydipsia did not change with medical therapy instituted for hyperaldosteronism despite normalization of potassium concentrations. Surgical resection of the adrenal mass was discussed but declined. Based on persistent poor urine concentrating ability and the changes in renal size and architecture present on the initial ultrasound examination, non-azotaemic chronic kidney disease was suspected (non-azotaemic IRIS Stage 2). Continued monitoring of renal function was recommended and at re-examination after 5 months the cat had developed mild azotaemia (plasma creatinine 201 μmol/l; RI 84–177 μmol/l) IRIS Stage 2 (140–250 μmol/l) with inappropriately dilute urine (USG 1.022).

In this patient, the initial polydipsia was most likely to be compensatory for primary polyuria brought about by non-azotaemic CKD. CKD should be considered as a continuum with some cats demonstrating gradual loss of urine concentrating ability prior to the onset of azotaemia. Poor muscle condition may also have a direct impact on creatinine concentrations, falsely reducing creatinine concentration when body condition is reduced. In this non-azotaemic patient assessment of GFR by iohexol clearance or assessment of symmetric dimethylarginine (see Chapter 10) could have been considered.

In this cat, the presence of hypokalaemia may, at least initially, also have contributed to the polyuria. Hypokalaemia affects the function of the $Na^+K^+2Cl^-$ co-transporters within the thick ascending limb of the loop of Henle and also the Na^+ and K^+ channels in the collecting ducts. Reduced function of these channels decreases sodium reabsorption, and sodium is a driving solute for water retention within the tubules. In addition, hypokalaemia has a direct impact on reducing expression of the AVP receptor. Hypokalaemia may therefore, via both methods, have contributed to secondary nephrogenic diabetes insipidus.

Case example 2: Polydispia and polyuria in a Labrador Retriever with a cough

SIGNALMENT

An 8-month-old neutered Labrador Retriever bitch.

HISTORY

Mild polyuria and polydipsia noted over the past month with mild lethargy and an intermittent harsh cough of the same duration. Fully vaccinated and no known toxin exposure or travel history.

PHYSICAL EXAMINATION

Physical examination revealed slightly harsh lung sounds bilaterally on thoracic auscultation but was otherwise unremarkable.

INITIAL INVESTIGATION

- 24-hour water quantification: 86 ml/kg/24h.
- Haematology: mild eosinophilia (2.3×10^9/l; RI $0.0–1.3 \times 10^9$/l), neutrophilia (13.6×10^9/l; RI $3–11.5 \times 10^9$/l) and lymphopenia (0.6×10^9/l; RI $1–4.8 \times 10^9$/l).
- Biochemistry: mild increase in ALP activity (310 IU/l; RI 19–285 IU/l), mild hyperphosphataemia (2.3 mmol/l; RI 0.8–2.0 mmol/l) and mild total hypercalcaemia (2.91 mmol/l; RI 2.1–2.7 mmol/l).
- Urinalysis: specific gravity 1.017; otherwise unremarkable.
- Urine culture: negative.

FURTHER DIAGNOSTIC INVESTIGATIONS

- Ionized calcium: 1.58 mmol/l (RI 1.13–1.33 mmol/l).
- Thoracic radiographs: right lateral and dorsoventral views were obtained and revealed a peripheral alveolar–insterstitial pattern.
- Faecal smear and Baermann faecal flotation: positive for *Angiostrongylus vasorum*.

OUTCOME

Total water quantification in the home environment did not exceed 100 ml/kg/24h. However, the owners were concerned that there had been a change in drinking and urination habits, which warranted further investigation in conjunction with clinical signs of lethargy and coughing. In this patient, the biochemical profile revealed a total hypercalcaemia, which was confirmed with assessment of free calcium. Considering differential diagnoses for hypercalcaemia, the age of the patient meant that neoplasia was considered unlikely. Azotaemia was not identified, excluding azotaemic chronic kidney disease. Hyperphosphataemia, which could have been renal in origin, was likely to be age-related in this patient. Non-azotaemic CKD remained a possible differential diagnosis, particularly if congenital or dysplastic renal disease was present. Abdominal ultrasound examination would have been required to provide further information about renal architecture. Lack of typical electrolyte abnormalities (i.e. hyponatraemia and hyperkalaemia) made hypoadrenocorticism unlikely, combined with the young age of onset. There was no history of vitamin D intoxication. Although elevation in ALP activity was identified, hyperadrenocorticism was excluded on the basis of signalment and was attributed to the young age.

The history of a chronic cough prompted thoracic radiographs, which revealed a typical peripheral distribution of an alveolar–interstitial pattern suggestive of *A. vasorum* infection. A faecal smear and Baermann flotation confirmed this diagnosis. The mild peripheral eosinophilia was most likely due to the parasite burden.

Angiostrongylosis is known to lead to formation of pulmonary granulomas and there were radiographic changes supportive of *A. vasorum* infection in this patient. In human medicine, granulomatous disease can result in increased production of calcitriol (1,25-dihydroxycholecalciferol) by activated macrophages, resulting in an increase in calcium concentration (Boag *et al.*, 2005). Hypercalcaemia secondary to *A. vasorum* infection was identified as the underlying cause of PU/PD. Hypercalcaemia can result in alteration in the interaction between AVP and the AVP receptor on the distal tubule and collecting duct epithelial cells, and therefore result in a secondary nephrogenic diabetes insipidus and clinical signs of PU/PD.

While granulomatous disease is an uncommon differential diagnosis for hypercalcaemia in patients that have not travelled outside the UK, *A. vasorum* should always be considered. The dog was treated with fenbendazole (50 mg/kg for 10 days) and was continued on monthly anthelmintic (moxidectin/imidacloprid) spot-on therapy. PU/PD and the cough resolved.

Chapter 3

Urinary incontinence and urine retention

Julie R. Fischer and India F. Lane

Normal micturition consists of a urine storage phase during which the bladder slowly fills and relaxes while the urethra remains closed, and a urine voiding phase during which the bladder contracts and urine is expelled through a relaxed urethra. The bladder remains in the storage phase the vast majority of the time. Appropriate urine storage and voiding depend on the intricate and coordinated interaction of the nervous system, urinary bladder and urethra. Urine storage disorders usually manifest clinically as urinary incontinence, whilst urine voiding disorders usually manifest as urine retention. Successful management of incontinence and urine retention depends foremost on accurate description of the problem and localization of the disorder, augmented by a clear understanding of the associated neurophysiology.

Lower urinary tract anatomy

The key anatomical components of the lower urinary tract include the bladder, the ureterovesicular junction (UVJ), the trigone and the urethra (Figure 3.1).

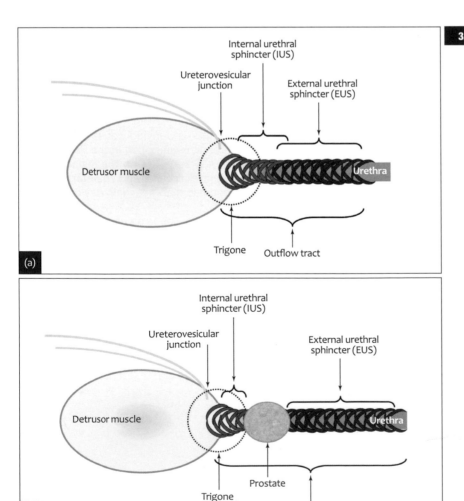

3.1 Basic anatomy of the (a) female and (b) male lower urinary tract.

BSAVA Manual of Canine and Feline Nephrology and Urology, third edition. Edited by Jonathan Elliott, Gregory F. Grauer and Jodi L. Westropp. ©BSAVA 2017

Urinary bladder

The bladder consists of a rounded body for receiving and storing urine, and a funnel-shaped neck through which urine is expelled. The bladder wall has four layers (from the outer surface to the lumen): serosa, smooth muscle and extracellular matrix, lamina propria and urothelium (mucosal layer). The smooth muscle cells of the detrusor are oriented in a seemingly random fashion in small functional fascicular units, although in the trigone the fascicles organize into three layers. The individual myocytes fuse with one another at specialized connexin-based gap junctions, resulting in low-resistance electrical pathways across cells. This permits the propagation of action potentials from one myocyte to the next, enabling simultaneous contraction of the entire detrusor muscle. Smooth muscle generally contracts at a slower velocity than striated muscle, and during the process of bladder contraction the detrusor extracellular matrix serves as a tension-generating scaffold, helping maintain a steady tension over a wide range of muscle fibre lengths. In states of over-distension, however, the fascicles become positioned in more of a tangential orientation to the lumen, rather than an encompassing one, and the detrusor loses some mechanical advantage for increasing intravesical pressure.

The lamina propria (or submucosa) is strongly fibro-elastic and contains fibroblasts, mast cells, myofibroblasts (also called interstitial cells), nerve endings (sensory, afferent and efferent), collagen and elastin fibres, and some smooth muscle fascicles. It is replete with blood and lymphatic vessels. This layer also acts as a protective barrier between the detrusor and irritating substances (e.g. noxious solutes dissolved in urine) that may damage and penetrate the urothelium.

The innermost layer, the urothelium, functions as a barrier that protects the bladder wall from components of urine. The urothelium is a transitional-type epithelium, comprising a basal cell layer, an intermediate layer and a flattened superficial layer. The cells of the superficial layer are also known as umbrella cells and have modifications that decrease permeability to improve barrier function; the cell membranes have specialized lipids and are uroplakin-rich to reduce permeability to small substances (e.g. water, urea, protons), the lateral margins are sealed to each other by claudin- and occludin-rich tight junctions, and the luminal membranes are covered by a glycosaminoglycan layer that may provide antibacterial and anti-adherence properties. In addition to functioning as a barrier, the urothelium is becoming increasingly understood and appreciated as a responsive structure with sensory and signalling properties that allow communication with local nerves and muscle tissue.

Urothelial cells express receptors for bradykinins and neurotrophins, as well as cholinergic (both nicotinic and muscarinic), adrenergic, purinergic and transient-receptor-potential vanilloid receptors, and have the capacity for release of neurotransmitters and other signalling molecules (e.g. nitric oxide, adenosine triphosphate (ATP), acetylcholine, prostaglandins, substance P, neurotrophins) that influence the sensitivity and reactivity of suburothelial afferents. The dense nexus of sensory nerves in the sub-epithelium has terminal projections into the urothelium, and thus it is thought that urothelial cells (as well as myofibroblasts in the lamina propria) actually play an autocrine/paracrine role in urinary sensory mechanisms.

Bladder compliance is a measure of resistance to filling and reflects the capacity to maintain appropriately low wall tension and intravesical pressure during the filling process.

Compliance is measured by calculating the change in bladder volume divided by the change in intravesical pressure (expressed as ml/cmH$_2$0). The bladder maintains appropriate compliance throughout filling by reorientation of detrusor fibres to run parallel to the bladder lumen, elongation of individual smooth muscle cells, thinning of the lamina propria and flattening of the urothelium, which occur in response to volume-generated increases in tension, the so called 'relaxation compliance phase' of bladder filling. Compliance depends on bladder wall viscoelasticity and varies based on a number of factors, including congenital anomalies (e.g. hypoplastic bladder), modulation of neurological stimulation (e.g. lower motor neuron lesion causing decreased cholinergic input), neuromuscular wall changes (e.g. atony due to chronic overdistension) and changes in wall collagen content and type (e.g. with fibrosis due to severe, chronic inflammatory bladder disease).

Ureterovesicular junction

The ureters travel obliquely through the caudodorsal bladder wall and terminate in slit-like openings at the cranial margin of the trigone, a triangular region of smooth mucosa at the dorsal bladder neck. The ureteral muscle is chiefly circular, but inner and outer smooth muscle 'coats' of longitudinal fascicles become more prominent at the UVJ. Fascicles extend from the detrusor to form part of the outer ureteral muscle coat, whilst the inner longitudinal fascicles extend to merge with the smooth muscle of the trigone, which also has a fascicular layer oriented in a somewhat longitudinal fashion. The longitudinal orientation of these fascicles facilitates opening of the bladder outlet during detrusor contraction. The ureters do not have specific anatomical valves, *per se*, but rather the oblique nature of ureteral transit through the wall combined with luminal pressure and tension during bladder filling keep the distal ureter closed, precluding the reflux of urine into the upper urinary tract.

Urethra

Traditionally, the urethral smooth muscle is referred to as the internal urethral sphincter (IUS) and the urethral striated muscle is termed the external urethral sphincter (EUS). In male dogs and cats, the IUS and EUS are separated by the prostatic region, and in females they are more merging than discrete anatomical structures, but in both sexes discussion of them as individual entities aids understanding of their mechanistic interactions. Continence is maintained by the normal structure and function of the bladder neck; the smooth and striated musculature, mucosa, submucosal elastic fibres and stratum spongiosum of the urethra; and regional fibromuscular tissues. Collectively, this is called the urethral sphincter mechanism (or the 'closure mechanism'). These structures are also collectively referred to as the 'outflow tract' or 'outlet' (see Figure 3.1).

The urethral mucosa is thinner than the bladder mucosa. The proximal urethra is lined with 2–3 layers of transitional epithelial cells, which become stratified cuboidal cells in the mid-urethra and then stratified squamous cells in the distal/terminal urethra. In the closed urethra, mucosal enfolding plays a significant role in static passive generation of outlet resistance.

Females

The urethra of female dogs and cats is structurally similar, with approximately two-thirds consisting of circularly-oriented smooth muscle that arises from the circular smooth muscle of the bladder neck. This circular smooth muscle begins to blend with striated muscle in the mid-urethra in dogs and a bit further caudally in cats. The caudal third of the urethra consists entirely of encircling striated muscle (longer and thicker in the dog than in the cat) that extends caudally to the vestibular floor, opening at the urethral tubercle in the dog and as a groove in the cat. The striated muscle encircles both the urethra and vagina at the caudal-most extent, anchoring the urethra to the vagina.

Males

The male urethra is divided into four segments: pre-prostatic, prostatic, post-prostatic and penile. The pre-prostatic segment of the urethra in cats consists chiefly of circular smooth muscle and extends to the prostate gland located at the midpoint of the pelvic urethral segment. The prostate lies on the dorsal urethral surface and the dorsal sub-mucosa contains the ductus deferens and prostatic duct openings. The prostatic urethral wall contains little muscle tissue. The post-prostatic urethra consists of encircling striated muscle extending to the root of the penis and covering the bulbourethral glands that lie there.

In dogs, urethral smooth muscle is confined primarily to the bladder neck. The prostate is situated just caudal to the trigone and encircles the urethra. Although the smooth muscle fibres cover the proximal portion of the prostate, they do not extend into the prostatic urethra, which plays no role in maintaining continence. The thick, encircling striated muscle coat of the post-prostatic urethra covers the caudal surface of the prostate and extends to cover the bulbospongiosus at the ischial arch. No significant smooth muscle is present in the post-prostatic urethra.

Neurophysiology of micturition

Nervous control of the micturition cycle involves the brainstem and cerebral cortex of the central nervous system (CNS), as well as both the autonomic (involuntary) and somatic (voluntary) arms of the peripheral nervous system. Normal urine storage and voiding requires intricate interaction amongst all components.

Innervation of the bladder and urethra

The bladder and urethra are innervated by three sets of nerves: thoracolumbar sympathetic (arising from spinal segments L1–L4 in the dog and L2–L5 in the cat), sacral parasympathetic (arising from spinal segments S1–S3) and somatic (arising from spinal segments S1–S3). Sympathetic and parasympathetic preganglionic neurons are located in the lumbar and sacral intermediate grey matter, respectively. Parasympathetic axons travel via the lumbosacral plexus and pelvic nerves to the paired pelvic plexuses, while sympathetic axons travel through lumbar splanchnic nerves, where most synapse at the caudal mesenteric ganglion, and then continue through the hypogastric nerves to the pelvic plexuses.

The pelvic plexuses are bilateral nervous meshworks, where autonomic ganglia housing both sympathetic and (chiefly) parasympathetic postganglionic neurons are located. The mesh of nerves from the pelvic plexuses extend into the caudal portion of the bladder wall, where they adopt a tortuous course as they spread cranially so that bladder distension does not result in excessive nerve stretching. The nervous plexus is thickest in the bladder neck and progressively less dense as nerves extend towards the apex, ending around the equatorial region. These neurons elaborate non-myelinated axons, with varicosities containing synaptic vesicles along the terminal branches. Distinct neuromuscular junctions are not present; rather the synaptic vesicles 'spill' neurotransmitters within diffusion proximity of myocyte receptors, inducing excitatory (causing myocyte contraction) or inhibitory (causing myocyte relaxation) junction potentials. Somatic innervation of the striated muscle of the EUS involves the motor nuclei in the ventral horn of the sacral spinal cord. Axons travel through the lumbosacral plexus and the pudendal nerve.

Urine storage

The urine storage phase of micturition occurs chiefly under sympathetic (adrenergic) nervous control (Figure 3.2) and is aided by the intrinsic structural and anatomical properties of the bladder and urethra (see above). Sympathetic postganglionic neurons release noradrenaline (norepinephrine) which binds to detrusor beta adrenoceptors (primarily beta-3 in dogs and likely beta-1 or -2 in cats). This permits smooth muscle relaxation via a second messenger system: beta-3 adrenoceptors are linked to G proteins (guanine nucleotide-binding proteins that act as intracellular molecular switches) which decrease levels of cyclic adenosine monophosphate (cAMP), resulting in increased K^+ efflux and decreased Ca^{2+} influx. This results in myocyte hyperpolarization and inhibition of contraction, and allows bladder filling under low pressure. Noradrenaline also binds to alpha-1 (in dogs, chiefly alpha-1A; alpha-1 adrenoceptor subtypes remain unelucidated in the feline urinary tract)

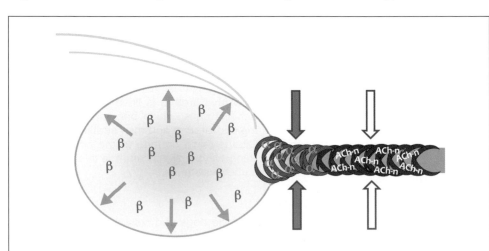

3.2 The urine storage phase of micturition. Sympathetic input to the beta (β) adrenoceptors in the bladder stimulates detrusor muscle relaxation; sympathetic input to the alpha (α) adrenoceptors in the IUS stimulates smooth muscle contraction. Voluntary input to the nicotinic cholinergic receptors (Ach-n) in the EUS stimulates striated muscle contraction. During the storage phase, outlet resistance must exceed intravesicular pressure to maintain continence.

adrenoceptors in the bladder neck and urethral smooth muscle (the IUS). This induces smooth muscle contraction via a second messenger system: alpha-1 adrenoceptors are linked to G proteins that generate inositol triphosphate, driving the sarcoplasmic reticulum to release Ca^{2+}, which then initiates smooth muscle contraction, closing the bladder outlet and maintaining continence. Sympathetic input also modulates and minimizes parasympathetic-mediated contraction of the detrusor muscle.

As bladder filling progresses, sensory information from the detrusor stretch receptors (slowly adapting mechano-receptors) is passed to higher centres via the myelinated ($A\delta$) axons (filling sensation, urge to void) of the pelvic nerves (in dogs; in cats both pelvic and hypogastric nerves are involved) to the sacral cord, and then through the ventral portion of the lateral funiculus to the pontine micturition centre and to the periaqueductal grey matter of the mid-brain, as well as the hypothalamus and thalamus. The pontine continence centre (located lateral to the micturition centre) sends axons through the dorsal portion of the lateral funiculus, and then through the hypogastric nerve to activate the EUS and pelvic diaphragm. The full bladder (in quadrupeds) tends to be drawn cranially into the abdomen by gravity, which increases tension in the urethral wall, providing additional outlet closure strength.

Voluntary input to the striated urethral musculature (the EUS) is supplied via the pudendal nerve (Figure 3.3) to temporarily maintain continence when tonic closure provided by the IUS is breached (e.g. reflex closure during coughing or sneezing, temporary voluntary overriding of the urge to void and midstream stoppage of flow). During the storage phase, the stimulation of urine flow into the urethra and/or conscious input from cortical centres causes the pudendal nerve to release acetylcholine, stimulating nicotinic cholinergic receptors in the EUS. Acetylcholine-induced opening of non-selective cation channels on striated myocytes permits the influx of Na^+ and efflux of K^+, causing rapid EUS (as well as muscles of the anal canal and root of the penis) contraction, providing swift additional closure of the outlet.

The pelvic and hypogastric nerves also contain unmyelinated (C) axons, which are insensitive to physiological distension/contraction conditions (thus are termed 'silent' C-fibres) and respond primarily to chemical irritation, cooling or other noxious stimuli. Sensation carried via these fibres may play a role in conditions such as interstitial cystitis in women and idiopathic cystitis in cats.

Urine voiding

The urine voiding phase of micturition is chiefly under parasympathetic control via release of acetylcholine. Voiding may be initiated when the forebrain receives sufficient notice of increasing bladder wall tension. The sensation of stretch is transmitted via afferent pelvic nerves associated with detrusor mechanoreceptors. Degree of fullness, environmental factors and other inputs are processed to determine whether voiding is situationally appropriate; voiding is then either initiated or inhibited. If the decision not to void is made, the continence centre of the pons causes EUS contraction and tonic contraction of the IUS is maintained, along with ongoing beta adrenoceptor-mediated detrusor relaxation.

If voiding is elected, the pontine activity switches to favour micturition; sympathetic and somatic input to the outlet is actively inhibited, permitting IUS and EUS relaxation, respectively. Simultaneously, acetylcholine release by the pelvic nerve stimulates M3 muscarinic cholinergic receptors in the detrusor, causing sustained contraction and raising of intravesicular pressure, pulling the neck of the bladder open. Mammalian studies involving complete blockage of cholinergic receptors show that non-adrenergic and non-cholinergic (NANC) neurotransmission (most likely representing ATP acting on purinergic receptors) also plays a role in detrusor contraction. When intravesical pressure exceeds outlet closure pressure, voiding occurs (Figure 3.4). As the bladder empties, intravesical pressure and wall tension (and thus signalling from detrusor mechanoreceptors) decline. Complete bladder emptying is facilitated by input from the brain, which helps to maintain detrusor contraction as long as required. After voiding is complete, the system is 'reset' for the filling stage to begin again.

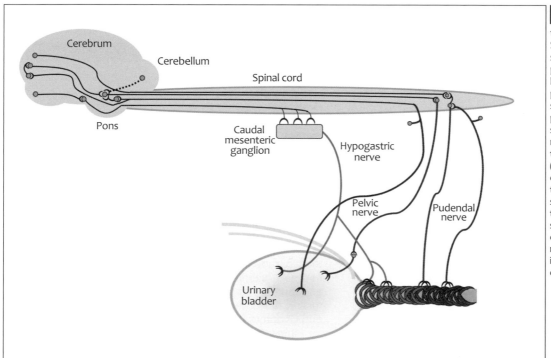

3.3 Central nervous system input to the lower urinary tract. Sympathetic input is supplied to the bladder and proximal urethra via the hypogastric nerve (green); parasympathetic input is supplied via the afferent pelvic nerve (red) and sensation of stretch is relayed to higher centres via the efferent pelvic nerve (blue). The afferent (red) and efferent (blue) branches of the pudendal nerve relay somatic input to and from the external urethral sphincter. Voiding is coordinated in the pontine micturition centre, with input from cerebrocortical centres.

Cerebrum
Cerebellum
Spinal cord
Pons
Caudal mesenteric ganglion
Hypogastric nerve
Pelvic nerve
Pudendal nerve
Urinary bladder

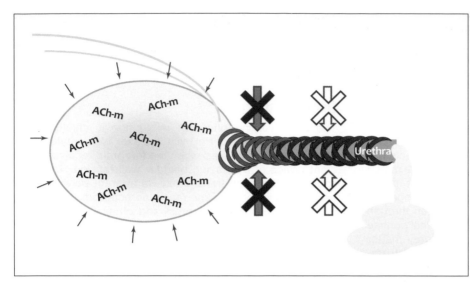

3.4 The urine voiding phase of micturition. Parasympathetic stimulation of muscarinic cholinergic receptors (Ach-m) causes contraction of the detrusor muscle. Parasympathetic inhibition of sympathetic input to the IUS (**X**) and voluntary inhibition of EUS contraction (☒) cause passive relaxation of the outflow tract and intravesicular pressure to exceed outlet pressure, permitting urine voiding.

Urinary incontinence

Continence requires that the ureters open solely into the bladder, bladder capacity and compliance permit low pressure filling, urethral closure pressure exceeds intravesical pressure, and bladder sensation be modulated appropriately by higher CNS centres. Urinary incontinence (hereafter simply incontinence) is defined as the involuntary leakage of urine through the urethra. Thus, diagnosis of this disorder first requires differentiation of unconscious leakage from behaviourally inappropriate urination and dysuria/pollakiuria (i.e. conscious inappropriate voiding). Incontinence is most common in bitches, but is also clinically recognized in male dogs and cats. Incontinence is usually due to failure of urine storage during filling and, in some patients, particularly in animals with congenital disorders, multiple mechanisms may be contributory. Causes of incontinence (Figures 3.5 and 3.6) are traditionally described as neurogenic or non-neurogenic in nature.

Neurogenic and functional
• Urethral sphincter mechanism incompetence
• Detrusor instability (overactive bladder)
• Pelvic nerve or pelvic plexus trauma
• Lumbosacral disease
• Intervertebral disc disease
• Lumbosacral stenosis
• Neoplasia
• Sacral malformation (Manx cats)
• Feline leukaemia virus-associated
• Generalized peripheral lower motor neuron disease
• Dysautonomia

Non-neurogenic
• Urethral hypoplasia
• Lower urinary tract inflammation
• Bacterial cystitis
• Sterile cystitis
• Urolithiasis
• Ectopic ureter
• Partial outflow obstruction (overflow incontinence)
• Uroliths
• Neoplasia
• Polyps
• Patent urachus
• Vestibulovaginal stenosis/septum causing urine pooling/spilling
• Primary detrusor atony with overflow

3.5 Causes of urinary incontinence in dogs and cats.

Adult female dogs
• Urethral sphincter mechanism incompetence
• Detrusor instability (bladder storage dysfunction)
• Vaginal pooling
• Vulvar conformation or positioning abnormality
• Lower urinary tract inflammation
• Neurogenic disorders
• Partial outflow obstruction (e.g. urethroliths, trigonal carcinoma)

Adult male dogs
• Prostatic disease
• Urethral sphincter mechanism incompetence
• Detrusor instability
• Neurogenic disorders
• Partial outflow obstruction (e.g. urethroliths, prostatic carcinoma)

Juvenile dogs
• Ectopic ureter
• Urethral or bladder hypoplasia
• Congenital urethral sphincter mechanism incompetence
• Vaginal or vulvar anomalies
• Intersex disorder
• Patent urachus

Cats
• Feline leukaemia virus-associated
• Urethral sphincter mechanism incompetence
• Overflow
• Neurogenic disorders
• Urethral anomalies

3.6 Common causes of urinary incontinence by signalment.

Urine retention disorders can ultimately result in a paradoxical incontinence, also termed overflow incontinence. This occurs when bladder overdistension eventually results in urine leakage. As the primary causative problem is voiding failure, and storage failure is an end result of that, paradoxical incontinence is most accurately classified as a voiding disorder rather than a storage disorder and must be approached and managed as such by determining the underlying cause of urine retention (see below and Chapters 9 and 30).

Figure 3.7 provides a summary of characteristics and useful diagnostics associated with common causes of incontinence.

Disorder	Characteristics	Diagnostic tests
Acquired urethral sphincter mechanism incompetence (reproductive hormone-responsive or 'spay' incontinence)	Medium to large-breed adult dogs (usually female) Prior ovariohysterectomy Intermittent urine leakage Resting urinary incontinence Otherwise normal	Response to treatment Urethral pressure profilometry
Urinary bladder storage dysfunction (detrusor instability, urge incontinence, overactive bladder)	Intermittent urinary incontinence Pollakiuria May appear behavioural or voluntary May be associated with excitement or activity	Response to treatment Cystometrography Cystourethrography
Ectopic ureter	Affected since birth Often continuous urine leakage	Urethrocystoscopy Contrast radiography, computed tomography Vaginourethrography Surgical exploration
Congenital urethral incompetence or hypoplasia	Severe or continuous urine leakage Juvenile animal Wide or short urethra in some cases Ectopic ureter not demonstrated	Urethrocystoscopy Cystourethrography Urethral pressure profile
Vaginal abnormality or urine pooling	Urine leakage at rest or when rising Urine leakage following voiding Recurrent or persistent vaginitis Vestibulovaginal stenosis/septum on digital examination	Assessment of vulvar conformation Digital vaginal examination and vaginoscopy Vaginourethrography
Prostatic disease (male dogs)	Intact or neutered Other signs of prostatic disease or concurrent dysuria Hindlimb weakness or stiff, stilted gait	Abdominal radiography Ultrasonography Contrast urethrography Prostatic brushing, aspiration or biopsy
Feline leukaemia virus (FeLV)-associated urinary incontinence (cats)	Intermittent urine leakage Anisocoria	FeLV test Neurological examination Urodynamic assessment

3.7 Characteristics of common disorders causing urinary incontinence.

Neurogenic incontinence

Neurogenic incontinence usually refers to sacral spinal cord level disorders (or less frequently involves spinal nerves bilaterally). Clinical signs associated with sacral cord lesions are characteristically lower motor neuron (LMN) in nature. With these disorders, end organs have the potential to function normally, but signal generation or transduction fails at some point between the CNS and the bladder and/or urethra.

Lesions of the sacral or sacrocaudal spinal cord interfere with normal function of the pudendal nerve, disrupting the local reflex arc and causing loss of normal EUS function, resulting in eventual involuntary leakage of urine when the bladder becomes distended (LMN bladder). Usually these animals also have loss of normal detrusor contractile function and cannot voluntarily urinate. Any cause of increased abdominal pressure or intravesical pressure (e.g. coughing, abdominal compression, manual bladder compression) may cause urine expression. In these dogs, urinary incontinence is rarely the sole overt neurological abnormality on physical examination; decreased anal tone and perineal reflexes and/or deficits of motor function of the pelvic limbs are usually also present. For these dogs, treatment of the incontinence and prognosis for resolution or clinical control depend primarily on diagnosis and management of the underlying cause.

Non-neurogenic incontinence

Non-neurogenic incontinence is associated with anatomical and functional disorders of the urinary tract. In these disorders, generation and conduction of neural impulses are intact throughout their course from the CNS to the end organs, but the bladder and/or urethra have a decreased ability to sense the input, respond to the input, or both.

Urethral sphincter mechanism incompetence

Urethral sphincter mechanism incompetence (USMI) is the most common cause of incontinence in dogs. USMI is most often an acquired disorder in medium to large-breed neutered bitches, but has been occasionally reported in cats and male dogs, and can be congenital. Animals with USMI should have normal and complete bladder emptying, and measurement or approximation of post-voiding residual urine volume is an important part of the initial assessment to rule out disorders of retention and consequent overflow incontinence. USMI involves decreased strength and responsiveness of the entire sphincter mechanism (urethral musculature and vasculature, urothelium, fibroelastic supportive tissue). Many different factors may affect the development and degree of USMI in a given patient.

Overactive bladder

An overactive bladder (urge incontinence, detrusor hyperreflexia, detrusor instability) is less common than USMI and manifests as intermittent incontinence, often associated with activity or excitement (rather than with recumbency, as is typical of USMI). It is sometimes difficult to discriminate an overactive bladder from pollakiuria or even inappropriate urination, since the sensation of detrusor contraction will often trigger dogs to assume a urination position. An overactive bladder is seen both as a sole disorder and in conjunction with USMI in dogs. This disorder is chiefly treated with antimuscarinic agents (e.g. oxybutynin, dicyclomine, flavoxate) or tricyclic antidepressants (e.g. imipramine), which increase bladder capacity and decrease detrusor spasticity.

Ectopic ureter

Ureteral ectopia results from dysembryogenesis of the metanephric ducts. It is defined as ureteral termination distal to the trigone, and other anatomical or functional abnormalities (e.g. reduced bladder capacity, USMI, hypoplastic urethra) often occur concurrently. Animals with ectopic ureters usually have continuous urine leakage from birth, but episodic leakage can be seen as well. Surgical or cystoscopic-guided correction is required for clinical improvement. Thorough preoperative evaluation of the urinary tract is recommended to determine the prognosis with surgical correction and to predict the need for postoperative medical management. For further information on the pathophysiology, diagnosis and management of ureteral ectopia, the reader is referred to Chapter 30.

Prostatic disease

Incontinent males should be screened for prostatic disease, particularly neoplasia and bacterial prostatitis (especially if entire), via rectal palpation, urine/prostatic fluid analysis, ultrasonography and (potentially) prostatic aspiration or biopsy. An easily palpable prostate or prostatic marginal irregularity found in a neutered dog (especially if the animal was neutered before adulthood) should markedly raise suspicion for prostatic neoplasia (see Chapter 25).

Cats

Urinary incontinence is rare in cats and may occur due to congenital anatomical anomalies (ureteral ectopia, urethral and/or vaginal hypoplasia, bladder hypoplasia), neurological injury or malformation, viral disease (specifically feline leukaemia), and congenital or acquired urethral incompetence. Juvenile cats should be screened for ectopic ureters and vaginourethral abnormalities; adults should be tested for feline leukaemia virus. Alpha adrenergic agonists may improve non-neurogenic urethral incompetence and a recent report (Pisu and Veronesi, 2014) suggests leuprolide or deslorelin could be effective. Medical and surgical aspects of management specific to cats are found in Chapter 30.

Diagnostic approach

The diagnostic approach to urinary incontinence is designed to:

- Verify the disorder is primarily of urine storage
- Rule out infectious, polyuric, pollakiuric or behavioural disorders
- Identify a neurological or anatomical lesion if present.

A detailed diagnostic approach to incontinence is presented in Chapter 9.

Treatment

Management options for patients with urinary incontinence are discussed in Chapter 30. Figure 3.8 summarizes the pharmacological agents that can be used in the treatment of urinary incontinence. Suggestions for the management of relapsing or refractory incontinence are given in Figure 3.9.

Drug class	Dosage	Mechanism of action	Contraindications or comments	Side effects
Alpha-1 agonists				
Phenylpropanolamine	1–2 mg/kg orally q8–24h (12.5–7.5 mg total dose per dog)	Sympathomimetic; causes noradrenaline (norepinephrine) release and alpha/beta adrenergic stimulation	Glaucoma; prostatic hypertrophy; hyperthyroidism; hypertension; diabetes mellitus	Restlessness; irritability; hypertension; anorexia; tachycardia
Oestrogen analogues				
Estriol	2.0 mg/dog orally q24h for 7–14 days, then reduce daily dose by 0.5 mg/week to minimum effective dose, then try q48h	Increases sensitivity of alpha-1 urethral smooth muscle receptors to noradrenaline; other mechanisms may play a role	Male dogs; cats; entire females; pregnant/lactating females Use with caution in liver disease, with glucocorticoids or with known immune-mediated disease	Gastrointestinal upset; decreased appetite; swollen vulva; vulvovaginitis; mammary hyperplasia; behavioural changes
Diethylstilbestrol	0.1–1.0 mg/dog orally q24h for 5–7 days, then weekly or prn			As per estriol Blood dyscrasias (rare)
Testosterone analogues				
Testosterone cypionate	2.2 mg/kg i.m. every 4 weeks	Precise mechanism of incontinence management unknown	Hypersensitivity; renal, cardiac or hepatic dysfunction Controlled Drug – Schedule 3	Perianal adenomas; perineal hernias; prostatic disorders; behavioural changes
Antimuscarinic agents				
Imipramine	5–15 mg/dog (total dose) orally q12h	Tricyclic antidepressant; anxiolytic; alpha antagonist; antihistamine; analgesic; anticholinergic; mast cell stabilizer	Bladder atony; urine retention Many drug interactions: concurrent administration of selective serotonin reuptake inhibitors, monoamine oxidase inhibitors or tramadol may cause serotonin syndrome May decrease seizure threshold	Dry mouth; constipation; tachycardia; hyperexcitability; tremors; myelosuppression

3.8 Formulary of agents useful in the management of urinary incontinence. (continues) ▶

Drug class	Dosage	Mechanism of action	Contraindications or comments	Side effects
Antimuscarinic agents continued				
Oxybutynin	0.2 mg/kg orally q8–12h or 1.25–5 mg/dog orally q8–12h	Antimuscarinic with some selectivity for the urinary system and antispasmodic	Urine retention; ileus; glaucoma; cardiac disease; hyperthyroidism	Diarrhoea; constipation; urinary retention; hypersalivation; sedation
Dicyclomine	5–10 mg/dog (total dose) orally q6–8h	Urinary antimuscarinic		
Gonadotrophin-releasing hormone (GnRH) agents				
Leuprolide (depot)	11.25 mg/dog s.c. every 3 months[a]	Precise mechanism of incontinence management unknown	Pregnancy	None documented
Deslorelin (depot)	5–10 mg/dog s.c. every 6 months[a]			
Buserelin (depot)	6.3 mg/dog s.c. every 2 months[a]			

3.8 (continued) Formulary of agents useful in the management of urinary incontinence. [a] Extrapolated from human doses.

Cause or complicating factor	Possible solution(s)
Inadequate dosage or frequency of medication	Increase dosage within recommended range Increase frequency of sympathomimetic (up to q8h) or oestrogen (up to q48h) as tolerated
Inappropriate medication	Consider change from oestrogen to sympathomimetic administration Consider addition of oestrogen to sympathomimetic administration
Desensitization or intolerance	Withdraw sympathomimetic treatment for 1–2 weeks and restart at a frequency of q24h
Poor owner compliance	Consider switch to long-acting sympathomimetic or to oestrogens to improve compliance
Underlying urinary tract infection	Monitor for infection and treat appropriately
Underlying polyuria	Evaluate for common, treatable polyuric disorders (e.g. hyperadrenocorticism, diabetes mellitus)
Mixed disorder of micturition	Consider addition of or trial treatment with anticholinergic agent
Underlying anatomical abnormality	Investigate anatomy with contrast radiography Consider surgical management of ectopic ureter, pelvic bladder or vaginal/vulvar abnormality
Underlying neurological lesion	Investigate for subtle lumbosacral disorder with neurological examination and imaging studies
Behavioural component or senility	Consider treatments for behavioural disorders or cognitive dysfunction
Refractory urethral incompetence	Consider combinations of medications or surgical treatment to enhance medical management Consider trial gonadotrophin-releasing hormone (GnRH) analogues or duloxetine Consider urethral bulking agents

3.9 Potential causes and possible solutions for refractory or relapsing urinary incontinence.

Urine retention

Urine retention occurs due to a failure of the urine voiding phase of micturition (voiding dysfunction). For normal and complete voiding to occur, intravesical pressure must rise quickly and exceed outlet pressure until the bladder is empty. Urine retention is caused by either failure of detrusor contraction or by inappropriately high outlet resistance during voiding (or both) (Figure 3.10). Failure of detrusor contraction can be either neurogenic or non-neurogenic in origin, as can increased outlet resistance.

In contrast with patients presented for incontinence, the clinical signs associated with voiding disorders commonly include stranguria and dysuria. The patient with urinary retention may make frequent attempts to void, with little or no success, or, particularly with animals who have chronic retention, may make little or no voiding effort. Determination of the aetiology of urine retention should be aggressively pursued, since early identification and correction of the underlying cause greatly improves the prognosis for functional recovery. Management strategies may include urinary catheterization to facilitate bladder emptying or surgical procedures to correct or bypass the obstruction. Pharmacological manipulation of outlet resistance and detrusor function (less commonly) is often used, either in conjunction with other procedures or as a sole therapy for certain disorders.

Neurogenic urine retention

In a similar fashion to incontinence, neurogenic retention disorders usually involve a spinal cord lesion, but can also occur secondary to bilateral nerve injury or generalized ganglionic disruption. Most cases have evidence of other neurological deficits on physical examination.

Lower motor neuron disorders

Disruption of sacral spinal cord segments S1–S3, or of the pelvic nerves or pelvic plexuses, results in LMN signs of decreased detrusor tone or complete atony and sphincter hypo- or areflexia. Patients with LMN disorders usually lack perineal reflexes and have distended bladders that are easily expressed. Overflow incontinence is often seen when the bladder is full, and in many of these patients the urinary problem is initially misidentified as a primary storage disorder rather than as a voiding disorder. LMN

Disorder	Characteristics	Diagnostic tests
Neurogenic causes		
Sacral spinal cord lesions (lower motor neuron)	Distended, flaccid urinary bladder Bladder easily expressed Depressed genitoanal reflexes Lumbosacral pain Possible overflow incontinence	Neurological examination Myelography, epidurography, computed tomography, magnetic resonance imaging
Suprasacral spinal cord lesions (upper motor neuron)	Distended, firm urinary bladder Bladder not easily expressed Incomplete voiding possible Gait and proprioceptive deficits	Neurological examination Myelography, epidurography, computed tomography, magnetic resonance imaging
Detrusor–urethral dyssynergia	Distended, firm urinary bladder Bladder not easily expressed Incomplete voiding possible; stream may be initiated but cannot be maintained Patient is otherwise normal Chronic management usually required	Observation Measurement of residual urine volume Urethral pressure profilometry ± cystometrography Response to alpha antagonists
Neurogenic detrusor atony	Distended bladder Bladder easily expressed Weak or absent urine stream Caused by dysautonomia, damage to hypogastric nerve	Observation Measurement of residual urine volume Response to treatment Cystometrography
Non-neurogenic causes		
Mechanical urethral obstruction	Difficult urethral catheterization Dysuria and stranguria ± haematuria Caused by uroliths, neoplasia, blood clots, urethral plugs (cats)	Urethral catheterization Radiography, contrast cystourethrography Cystourethroscopy Ultrasonography
Functional urinary obstruction	Distended bladder, difficult to express Easy urethral catheterization Voiding may be initiated then interrupted Usually male dogs and cats Idiopathic or caused by urethral irritation or previous obstruction Rarely and transiently occurs following abdominal, pelvic or pelvic limb surgery	Exclusion of mechanical or neurogenic causes Response to treatment with alpha antagonists Resolution over time Urethral pressure profile can be considered
Neurogenic detrusor atony	Distended bladder Weak or absent urine stream Caused by acute or chronic overdistension from any cause of obstruction, muscle weakness or drugs	Observation Measurement of residual urine volume Response to treatment Cystometrography
Medication (e.g. opioids, anticholinergics/antispasmodics, tricyclic antidepressants, calcium channel blockers)	Easy urethral catheterization Variable presentation otherwise	Medication history Exclusion of mechanical or functional obstruction Response to withdrawal of medication

3.10 Characteristics of common disorders causing urine retention.

disorders that can cause urine retention include cauda equina syndrome, sacral fracture, sacroiliac luxation, intervertebral disc disease, sacrococcygeal separation or fracture ('tail-pull' injury) and neoplasia.

Treatment for complete neurogenic detrusor atony and sphincter areflexia is generally unsuccessful, unless the underlying cause can be corrected (e.g. intervertebral disc disease or reparable fracture). Parasympathomimetic agents such as bethanechol (a muscarinic receptor agonist) are thought by some to help increase the strength of detrusor contraction if partial function is present, but clinical evidence of efficacy is not strong. Muscarinic receptor agonists agents are ineffective if pelvic nerve input to the detrusor is disrupted. Patients can be managed at home with scrupulous bladder and nursing hygiene, including manual bladder expression or, in male dogs, clean intermittent catheterization, ideally 3–4 times daily, and careful cleaning to prevent urine scald. Urine cultures can be monitored if clinically indicated because recurrent bacteriuria is common in patients with urine retention. Treating urinary tract infections (UTIs) may be appropriate initially; however, if infection persists or recurs in spite of appropriate therapy, then the decision whether or not to continue treatment should be made on an individual patient basis, taking into account factors such as bacterial characteristics (e.g. species, susceptibility, virulence), clinical signs and comorbidities.

Upper motor neuron disorders

Upper motor neuron (UMN) signs result from suprasacral injuries, meaning spinal cord damage between the sacral cord segments and the forebrain, but usually referring to lesions of the T3–L3 cord segments. Lesions occurring in this region disrupt normal modulating inhibitory signals to the hypogastric and pudendal nerves, causing reflex detrusor contraction with concurrent uninhibited urethral sphincter contraction. Patients with UMN disorders usually have overt paresis or paralysis of the hindlimbs with proprioceptive and nociceptive deficits, and cannot void voluntarily. Intervertebral disc disease and spinal trauma are the most common causes of UMN lesions in companion animals.

On examination, the bladder is large, turgid and challenging or impossible to safely express early in the disease course. Aggressive attempts at manual expression risk bladder rupture and should be avoided initially. In male dogs, regular, intermittent, aseptic urethral catheterization is preferred to expression in order to reduce the risk of detrusor trauma and the reflux of urine into the upper tract, and to ensure complete emptying. Unfortunately, this is not usually an option for cats and female dogs, and in these patients use of alpha-1 adrenergic antagonists (e.g. prazosin, tamsulosin, terazosin, alfuzosin) to relax the IUS and skeletal muscle relaxants (e.g. diazepam, dantrolene, baclofen, methocarbamol, acepromazine) to decrease EUS tone may be helpful. Some of the alpha-1 antagonists may also effect a decrease in EUS tone by interfering with overall central sympathetic output. Phenoxybenzamine, a non-selective alpha-1/alpha-2 antagonist, has historically been used for IUS relaxation, but the advent of selective alpha-1 (prazosin) and even uroselective alpha-1 (tamsulosin) agents permits greater clinical efficacy with decreased risk of adverse effects. Unless the newer, more selective agents are unavailable, there is no longer a strong clinical rationale for the use of phenoxybenzamine as a urethral relaxant. Most of the skeletal muscle relaxants available also cause some degree of sedation.

After days to weeks, recovery of local spinal reflexes may allow for resumption of some voiding activity. At that point, involuntary bladder emptying initiated when threshold capacity is reached, termed an automatic or reflex bladder, frequently develops. When automatic bladder activity occurs, safe manual expression is much easier, since stimulation of detrusor contraction now should result in sphincter relaxation and partial to complete automatic emptying. Alpha adrenergic blockade is still usually helpful in maximizing emptying in these patients. As with LMN disorders, patients should be monitored routinely for bacteriuria/clinical UTIs and treated when deemed clinically appropriate. Verification of adequate emptying and maintenance of good skin hygiene is critical for ongoing health, particularly if the patient remains recumbent.

Detrusor–urethral dyssynergia

A dyssynergic state results when initiation of detrusor contraction stimulates (or simply fails to inhibit) simultaneous contraction of the urethral musculature (either the IUS or the EUS), causing the bladder to contract against inappropriately increased outlet resistance. Detrusor–urethral dyssynergia (DUD) is thought to result from a nervous system defect (usually central), although in veterinary medicine the exact lesion often is not or cannot be determined. DUD can be caused by injury to the reticulospinal tract or Onuf's nucleus in the sacral cord, or by a lesion cranial to the caudal mesenteric ganglion, or it can be considered idiopathic. Regardless of specific lesion, the clinical signs associated with DUD likely result from disruption of normal inhibitory signalling to the hypogastric and pudendal nerves. Animals with idiopathic DUD usually have a normal neurological examination, in contrast with animals that have UMN lesions, although patients with both types of disease characteristically have large, firm bladders on physical examination. The diagnosis and management of DUD are discussed in detail in Chapter 30.

Dysautonomia

Dysautonomia is a rare generalized autonomic polyneuropathy that results in degeneration and functional loss of neuronal cell bodies of sympathetic and parasympathetic ganglia, intermediolateral spinal cord column and parasympathetic brainstem nuclei. Overflow incontinence due to bladder atony/distension and sphincter areflexia is often the clinical sign that prompts evaluation, but other signs of autonomic dysfunction (e.g. dilated, non-responsive pupils; relative bradycardia; xerostomia with dry/crusted nasal planum; nictitans prolapse; absent anal sphincter tone with faecal incontinence; vomiting; keratoconjunctivitis sicca; evidence of regurgitation and/or pneumonia) are often identified by owner questioning or found on examination. Any aged animal can be affected, although the median age of onset in affected dogs has been reported at 14 and 18 months, and clinical signs of autonomic dysfunction develop relatively rapidly (within 2 days in cats and within 2 weeks in dogs). The disorder appears strongly geographically clustered; most cases have been reported in cats in Great Britain and dogs in the Midwestern United States (particularly Missouri and Kansas), but it is seen sporadically in dogs and cats worldwide. Identified risks include a rural environment, wildlife/carrion consumption, outdoor lifestyle and access to livestock, their pastures and water sources. In dogs, most cases are reported between February and April.

Diagnosis is strongly suggested by physical examination and may be further supported by imaging findings, pupillary response to dilute pilocarpine, lack of intradermal histamine response, improved urination after subcutaneous bethanechol, unchanged heart rate after subcutaneous atropine, documentation of orthostatic hypotension and other tests. Definitive diagnosis relies on documentation of consistent histopathological lesions in the autonomic nervous system. Management is generally unrewarding if the gastrointestinal tract is affected (e.g. ileus, megaoesophagus), but may be possible with cholinergic agents and bladder expression or catheterization if signs are largely confined to the urinary tract. Prognosis is poor to grave, with a reported 70–90% mortality rate. Unfortunately, the aetiology, and thus methods for prevention, remains unknown, although geographical distribution and case clustering suggest involvement of toxic (including *Clostridium botulinum*), infectious and/or genetic factors.

Non-neurogenic urine retention

Non-neurogenic urine retention can occur secondary to mechanical, anatomical or functional disorders.

Mechanical outflow obstruction

Any intraluminal or extraluminal partial or complete obstruction of the outflow tract can disrupt normal voiding. The most common causes of mechanical obstruction include: urolithiasis; trigonal, prostatic or urethral neoplasia; severe proliferative urethritis or stricture; obstructive blood clot; extramurally-compressive non-urological neoplasia; and mucoid or crystalline urethral plugs (in cats). Treatment and prognosis depend on the cause, chronicity and potential for resolution of the underlying problem. The more chronic the obstruction, the more likely some degree of detrusor atony will result as well, and the likelihood of resolution of that atony component declines with increasing duration of obstruction.

Urethral functional obstruction

Functional urethral obstruction (increased outlet resistance not due to mechanical obstruction or neurological lesion) is thought to result from local irritation (e.g. urethral instrumentation, urethral stones) and possibly also from increased sympathetic stimulation of urethral musculature. It is thought sometimes to have a neurogenic component as well, but these hypotheses are all unproven. Increased sympathetic input from any cause (stress of hospitalization or illness, physical or psychological excitation) may increase IUS pressure, as well as EUS pressure with involvement of the higher brain centres, and inappropriately raise outlet resistance, restricting urine flow during voiding attempts. Functional obstruction may be difficult to distinguish definitively from DUD without actual urodynamic testing documenting high urethral pressure concomitant with simultaneous or induced detrusor contraction. The differentiation is usually clinical and based on known presence of urethral inflammation or irritation, or recent urethral obstruction or instrumentation, rather than definitive urodynamic diagnostics.

Obstruction due to urethral spasm seems to be a common occurrence in cats following relief of mechanical urethral obstruction. Management of urethral spasm includes treatment or prevention of bladder atony from overdistension, with indwelling catheterization if necessary, while decreasing IUS and/or EUS resistance. Anxiolytic therapy can help decrease stress and thus decrease sympathetic input to the lower urinary tract. Prognosis is variable, but usually good in situations involving acute urethral irritation (e.g. cats with urethral spasm post-obstruction) with sufficient time and patience.

Detrusor atony from overdistension

Any cause of persistent outlet obstruction can lead to bladder overdistension and consequent detrusor atony. Excessive stretch separates the detrusor muscular junctions, resulting in weak, uncoordinated or absent contraction. Animals with detrusor atony from overdistension may show stranguria, anuria or overflow incontinence and may have a large, full or flaccid bladder on physical examination. The bladder remains distended after voiding attempts, which are often partial or weak. Perineal reflexes are intact unless an LMN lesion is present, but the detrusor contraction is diminished or absent. For such patients, maintenance of an indwelling catheter for 72 hours up to 14 days is recommended to help re-establish tight junctions and permit return of detrusor function. If sustained indwelling catheterization is not feasible, frequent (3–4 times daily) intermittent aseptic catheterization is an acceptable alternative.

Although parasympathomimetic agents (e.g. bethanechol) may effectively help detrusor contraction (as pelvic nerve signalling is intact), they should not be administered without establishing a low resistance outflow conduit, either via indwelling catheterization, removal of the mechanical obstruction or pharmacological agents that relax the urethral outlet (in cases of functional obstruction or DUD). Urethral relaxants alone are usually not sufficient to assure reliable outflow patency, particularly in the initial stages of recovery from detrusor atony. Prognosis is dependent on cause and reversibility of obstruction, but is good for recovery of detrusor function in acute cases. Chronic detrusor atony resulting from any cause carries a guarded to poor prognosis for return to full function.

Diagnostic approach

The diagnostic approach to urine retention is designed to:

- Rule out neurogenically and mechanically obstructive disorders
- Assess urinary bladder contractile capacity and bladder outlet resistance
- Investigate possible underlying aetiologies for the primary disorder.

History and physical examination

As for most micturition disorders, history and physical examination provide the basis for localization of the problem and determination of diagnosis. Problem-specific historical questions related to urine retention are listed in Figure 3.11 and a comprehensive approach is provided in Chapter 9. Most animals with urine retention have a distended bladder that is readily palpable, and some patients have evidence of overflow incontinence. The bladder distension may or may not be painful; animals with chronic distension are often comfortable on palpation. Critical assessment of neurological status, particularly of the pelvic limb reflexes and reflexes testing the sacral arc (e.g. perineal, bulbospongiosus/vulvar), is specifically indicated.

Observation of voiding behaviour is an important part of the initial evaluation, especially (and more often easily) in male dogs, and begins with assessment of the patient's ability to initiate and maintain a strong urine stream. Mechanically obstructed patients typically strain and produce little to no urine. Functionally obstructed animals may initiate a stream that is quickly attenuated; this pattern may repeat several times in near-pulsatile fashion. Animals with bladder atony may slowly initiate a weak stream that often increases with manual abdominal compression. Some animals with chronic atony will not attempt to void at all. The bladder, as assessed by palpation, ultrasonography or catheterization, should be nearly empty following voiding, even in male dogs. If there is palpable distension following voiding, manual expression may be gently attempted. Inability to manually express a distended bladder indicates likely mechanical, neurogenic or functional outlet obstruction.

- How old was the patient when the problem began?
  - Was it related to neutering surgery?
- Have there been any previous medical problems?
- What is the estimated daily water consumption?
- Is there any history of prior urogenital disorders (e.g. urinary tract infections, urolithiasis, urethral obstructions)?
- Are there any systemic signs of illness, pain or weakness?
- Has there been any previous back surgery or trauma?
- Has there been any recent abdominal, pelvic or urogenital surgery or trauma?
- How frequent are voiding attempts?
- Is any urine passed during voiding attempts?

3.11 Problem-specific historical questions for patients with urine retention.

Catheterization

Catheterization of the urethra following voluntary voiding may allow assessment of outlet obstruction and permits quantification of residual urine volume. In healthy animals, resistance to the urethral catheter is normally encountered at the urethral flexure in male cats and at the distal os penis and pelvic brim/ischial arch in male dogs. Urethral catheters may pass smoothly by small uroliths and through or by some soft tissue lesions; thus, the ability to catheterize the urethra does not fully rule out mechanical obstruction. Use of the largest gauge soft catheter that will comfortably pass through the urethra increases the likelihood of detecting a small mechanical obstruction. Normal residual urine volume in dogs ranges from approximately 0.1–3.4 ml/kg bodyweight, but is usually <0.5 ml/kg. Serial measurement of residual urine volume can also be used to assess the response to therapy in animals with retention disorders.

Diagnostic imaging

Diagnostic imaging is usually required to positively identify and characterize, or rule out, mechanical obstruction. Plain radiography will demonstrate most mineralized obstructions >2–3 mm and thoracic radiographs are indicated if neoplasia is suspected or confirmed. Ultrasonography is a sensitive tool for detection of trigonal and proximal urethral lesions. Contrast urethrocystography helps delineate the location and extent of many obstructive lesions, as well as mineralized structures too small to easily detect on plain radiography. Urethrocystoscopy is often useful for visualization and/or biopsy of obstructing structures. Utility of scoping for biopsy may be limited in cats and small dogs. Urethroscopy has proven valuable for the detection of urethral lesions that are not readily visible on conventional imaging studies. Advanced imaging of the spinal cord (e.g. myelography/epidurography, computed tomography, magnetic resonance imaging) may be necessary to confirm and localize subtle neurological lesions. For additional information on various imaging modalities for the lower urinary tract, the reader is referred to Chapters 7 and 8.

Specialized urodynamic studies

Urethral pressure profilometry records a tracing of pressure measurements along the length of the outflow tract and urethra. In patients with urine retention, urethral pressure profilometry may help establish the presence and location of high pressure zones in animals with dyssynergic urination, functional urethral obstruction, stricture and other causes of incomplete emptying. Cystometrography measures the pressure within the bladder as it is filled with fluid or gas and helps assess bladder capacity and compliance, as well as detrusor overactivity or atony. On occasion, urethral pressure profilometry and cystometrography are combined with synchronized electromyographic recording of perineal muscle contractions. In patients with urine retention, cystometrography may be helpful in determining whether abnormal detrusor function is a component of the disease process. Indications, utility and methodology of urodynamic studies are discussed in greater detail in Chapter 9.

Treatment

A formulary of pharmacological agents commonly used for the management of urine retention is provided in Figure 3.12.

Drug class	Dosage	Mechanism of action	Contraindications or comments	Side effects
Urethral relaxants				
Acepromazine	Recommended starting dose: 0.02 mg/kg i.v. q12–24h, up to 1.1 mg/kg i.v. q12–24h (higher doses not generally needed or recommended) 0.55–2.2 mg/kg orally q12–24h	Neuroleptic skeletal muscle relaxant via postsynaptic dopamine receptor blockade in the central nervous system; smooth muscle relaxation via alpha antagonism; antiemetic and antispasmodic effects	Hypovolaemia; cardiac disease; general debilitation; sensitivity in giant breeds, Greyhounds and Boxers Reduce dose by 25% for *MDR1* heterozygotes and 30–50% for *MDR1* homozygotes	Hypotension; sedation; disinhibition of aggressive behaviour; hypothermia; possible interactions with many other medications
Baclofen	Dogs: 1–2 mg/kg or 5–10 mg/kg orally q8h; start with lower dose Cats: not recommended	GABA-derived skeletal muscle relaxant; decrease gamma efferent neuronal activity	Seizure disorders Discontinue gradually; hallucination and seizures reported in humans when stopped abruptly Narrow therapeutic index	Sedation; weakness; gastrointestinal upset; pruritus
Botulinum toxin type A as urethral injection	Dogs, cats: unknown Humans: 50–100 IU injection in saline every 1–6 months	Inhibition of acetylcholine release at neuromuscular junction	Hypersensitivity to toxin; infection at injection site	Spread of toxin effect (locally or systemically); hypersensitivity reaction
Dantrolene	Dogs: 1–5 mg/kg orally q8–12h Cats: 0.5–2.0 mg/kg orally q12h 1.0 mg/kg i.v.	Skeletal muscle relaxation via direct effects	Cardiac disease; hepatic dysfunction; pulmonary disease	Weakness; sedation; gastrointestinal upset; hepatotoxicity
Diazepam	Dogs: 2–10 mg/dog orally q8h Cats: 1–2.5 mg/cat orally q8h or prn	Skeletal muscle relaxation via central effects (benzodiazepine)	Pregnancy; hepatic disease	Sedation; paradoxical excitement; idiopathic hepatic necrosis (with oral use in cats only)
Phenoxybenzamine (considered obsolete for urinary indications if selective alpha-1 antagonists are available)	Dogs: 0.25 mg/kg orally q8–12h or 2.5–20 mg/dog orally q8–12h Cats: 1.25–7.5 mg/cat orally q8–12h	Urinary smooth muscle relaxation via non-specific alpha antagonism	Cardiac disease; hypovolaemia; glaucoma; renal failure; diabetes mellitus (type II)	Hypotension; tachycardia; gastrointestinal upset
Prazosin	Dogs: 1 mg/15 kg orally q8–12h Cats: 0.25–0.5 mg/cat orally q12–24h	Urinary smooth muscle relaxation via selective alpha-1 antagonism	Cardiac disease; renal failure; hypotension; hypovolaemia; *MDR1* mutation?	Hypotension; mild sedation; ptyalism
Tamsulosin	Dogs: 0.1–0.2 mg/10 kg orally q12–24h Cats: not recommended	Smooth muscle relaxation via uroselective alpha-1 antagonism	Hypersensitivity Do not crush or compound	Hypotension (uncommon unless overdosed)

3.12 Formulary of agents useful in the management of urine retention. GABA = gamma-aminobutyric acid; MDR = multi-drug resistance. (continues)

Drug class	Dosage	Mechanism of action	Contraindications or comments	Side effects
Detrusor stimulants				
Bethanechol	Dogs: 5–15 mg/dog orally q8–12h Cats: 1.25–7.5 mg/cat orally q8–12h	Stimulation of muscarinic receptors	Gastrointestinal or urinary obstruction	Ptyalism Vomiting Diarrhoea Possible abdominal pain
Cisapride	Dogs: 0.1–0.5 mg/dog orally q8–12h Cats: 2.5–5 mg/cat orally q8–12h	Prokinetic activity via acetylcholine release	Gastrointestinal obstruction Reduce dosage with liver disease	Diarrhoea Possible abdominal pain
Anxiolytic agents				
Alprazolam	Cats: 0.125–0.25 mg/cat orally q12h	Centrally acting anxiolytic benzodiazepine	May be a good alternative to diazepam if oral therapy is needed	Sedation; paradoxical excitement
Amitriptyline	Cats: 1–2 mg/kg/day orally or 2.5–10 mg/cat/day orally	Tricyclic antidepressant; anxiolytic; alpha antagonist; antihistamine; analgesic; anticholinergic; mast cell stabilizer	Bladder atony; urine retention Many drug interactions: concurrent administration of selective serotonin reuptake inhibitors, monoamine oxidase inhibitors or tramadol may cause serotonin syndrome	Sedation; neutropenia; thrombocytopenia; urine retention; weight gain
Acepromazine and diazepam are also anxiolytic agents; see above for information				

3.12 (continued) Formulary of agents useful in the management of urine retention. GABA = gamma-aminobutyric acid; MDR = multi-drug resistance.

References and further reading

Apodaca G (2004) The uroepithelium: not just a passive barrier. *Traffic* **5**, 117–128

Arnold S, Hubler M and Reichler I (2009) Urinary incontinence in spayed bitches: new insights into the pathophysiology and options for medical treatment. *Reproduction in Domestic Animals* **44(Suppl. 2)**, 190–192

Avelino A, Cruz F, Panicker JN *et al.* (2016) Basic principles. In: *Practical Functional Urology*, ed. J Heesakkers *et al.*, pp. 1–10. Springer International Publishing, Switzerland

Birder L, deGroat W, Mills I *et al.* (2010) Neural control of the lower urinary tract: peripheral and spinal mechanisms. *Neurourology and Urodynamics* **29(1)**, 128–139

Byron JK (2015) Micturition disorders. *Veterinary Clinics of North America: Small Animal Practice* **45**, 769–782

Clemens JQ (2010) Basic bladder neurophysiology. *Urologic Clinics of North America* **37(4)**, 487–494

Fowler CJ, Griffiths D and DeGroat WC (2008) The neural control of micturition. *Nature Reviews Neuroscience* **9(6)**, 453–466

Hamaide A (2014) Medical management of urinary incontinence and retention disorders. In: *Current Veterinary Therapy XV*, ed. JD Bonagura JD and DC Twedt, pp. 915–919. Saunders, Philadelphia

Hu HZ, Granger N and Jeffery ND (2016) Pathophysiology, clinical importance, and management of neurogenic lower urinary tract dysfunction caused by suprasacral spinal cord injury. *Journal of Veterinary Internal Medicine* **30**, 1575–1588

Labato MA and Acerno MJ (2010) Micturition disorders and urinary incontinence. In: *Textbook of Veterinary Internal Medicine, 7th edn*, ed. SJ Ettinger and E Feldman, pp. 160–164. Elsevier Saunders, St. Louis

Lane IF and Fischer JR (2003) Symposium: A diagnostic approach to micturition disorders; Treating urinary incontinence; and Medical treatment of voiding dysfunction in dogs and cats. *Veterinary Medicine* 49–74

Noël S, Claeys S and Hamaide A (2010) Acquired urinary incontinence in the bitch: update and perspectives from human medicine. Part 1: The bladder component, pathophysiology and medical treatment. Part 2: The urethral component, pathophysiology and medical treatment. Part 3: The urethral component and surgical treatment. *The Veterinary Journal* **186**, 10–31

Pisu MC and Veronesi MC (2014) Effectiveness of deslorelin acetate subcutaneolus implantation in a domestic queen with after spaying urinary incontinence. *Journal of Feline Medicine and Surgery* **16(4)**, 366–368

Reichler IM and Hubler M (2014) Urinary incontinence in the bitch: an update. *Reproduction in Domestic Animals* **49(Suppl. 2)**, 75–80

Stoffel JT (2016) Detrusor sphincter dyssynergia: a review of physiology, diagnosis and treatment strategies. *Translational Andrology and Urology* **5(1)**, 127–135

Chapter 4

Abnormal renal palpation

Alexander J. German

When renal disease is suspected, abdominal palpation is critical to the initial physical examination. Abdominal palpation will reveal changes in renal morphology (Figure 4.1) that accompany various pathological processes, but it is important to recognize that no direct information on renal function can be derived (see Chapter 10 for details on assessment of renal function).

• Increased size • Reduced size • Altered number • Altered shape • Altered consistency • Altered position • Pain	**4.1** Summary of abnormal findings on renal palpation.

The normal kidneys are bean-shaped organs that lie in a retroperitoneal position ventral to the sublumbar musculature. The right kidney lies cranial to the left. Anatomical relations of the right kidney are:

- Cranioventrally it is deeply recessed in the liver (renal notch)
- Medially and cranially are the right adrenal gland and vena cava
- Laterally are the last rib and abdominal wall.

The left kidney is positioned more caudally than the right. Anatomical relations of the left kidney are:

- Cranially is the spleen
- Medially are the left adrenal gland and aorta
- Laterally is the abdominal wall and ventrally the descending colon.

In dogs, the normal left kidney can be palpated in most animals, whilst the right kidney is only palpable in thin subjects. Relative to bodyweight, feline kidneys are larger than those of the dog; the normal left kidney and caudoventral surface of the right kidney are readily palpable in most cats. Kidneys are also more mobile in cats; both kidneys (but the left in particular) can be easily displaced from their normal positions on palpation.

When normal kidney morphology is altered it usually implies a pathological process, but some changes can be physiological. The main palpable abnormalities include enlargement (renomegaly), decreased size and abnormal shape, and changes can be unilateral or bilateral. Other abnormalities include altered number of kidneys (usually decreased, e.g. renal agenesis), abnormal position (e.g. renal ectopia), altered renal consistency and the presence of pain. Since a number of consequences can arise as a result of morphological abnormalities of the kidney (Figure 4.2), prognosis is variable.

Disorder	Azotaemia? Yes (Y) or no (N)	Unilateral (U) or bilateral (B)	Prognosis
Physiological: • Acromegaly • Nephrectomy • Portovascular anomalies	Y/N	 B U B	Variable
Acute pyelonephritis	Y/N	U or B	Guarded; can resolve with appropriate treatment
Perinephric pseudocysts	Y/N*	B>U	Good
Primary renal neoplasia	N	U unless cystadenocarcinoma	Guarded
Renal lymphoma	Y/N	B usually	Guarded short term; poor long term
Feline infectious peritonitis (FIP)	Y/N	B	Poor
Metastatic neoplasia	N	U/B	Poor
Disorder	**Renal failure? Yes (Y) or no (N)**	**Unilateral (U) or bilateral (B)**	**Prognosis**
Polycystic kidney disease	Y/N	B	Guarded to poor if multiple cysts and azotaemia develop
Hydronephrosis	Y/N	U/B	Guarded if unilateral; very poor if bilateral, unless obstruction can be relieved

4.2 Effects of selected diseases on kidney morphology. All of these diseases/disorders lead to renomegaly with the exception of chronic kidney disease (CKD) and selected congenital diseases, which give rise to small kidneys. *There is some evidence to suggest an association between perinephric pseudocysts and CKD although the reason for any such association has not been determined. (continues) ▶

Disorder	Renal failure? Yes (Y) or no (N)	Unilateral (U) or bilateral (B)	Prognosis
Congenital	See Chapter 14	U/B	See Chapter 14
Subcapsular haematoma	N	U	Good
Chronic kidney disease	Y	B	Guarded
Nephrolithiasis	N unless bilateral	U/B	Good unless bilateral
Trauma	N unless bilateral	U>B	Variable
Acute nephrosis	Y/N	B	Guarded; can resolve with appropriate treatment

4.2 (continued) Effects of selected diseases on kidney morphology. All of these diseases/disorders lead to renomegaly with the exception of chronic kidney disease (CKD) and selected congenital diseases, which give rise to small kidneys.

Abnormal findings on renal palpation

Increased size

Renomegaly may be physiological or pathological. Unilateral nephrectomy, congenital unilateral renal agenesis and other conditions that result in loss of function in one kidney induce compensatory physiological hypertrophy of the remaining kidney. Unilateral renomegaly is always a pathological finding if the opposite kidney is present and functional. Bilateral renomegaly usually implies renal pathology, although compensatory renal hypertrophy can be seen in animals with portovascular anomalies (PVA). Technically, renomegaly secondary to acromegaly is a physiological response to excess growth hormone and insulin-like growth factor-1 (IGF-1) production.

Several diseases that cause renomegaly occur more frequently in cats than in dogs. These include renal lymphoma, feline infectious peritonitis (FIP), idiopathic polycystic kidney disease (PCKD) and perinephric pseudocysts. Renal lymphoma occurs occasionally in dogs, PCKD is uncommon but is hereditary in certain breeds (West Highland White Terriers, English Bull Terriers), whilst a canine equivalent of FIP has not been reported. Other causes of renomegaly, such as hydronephrosis, acute pyelonephritis, some of the diseases leading to acute uraemia (e.g. nephrotoxicosis, renal ischaemia, obstructive uropathy), PVA, renal neoplasia, subcapsular haematomas and acromegaly, are less species-specific. In the dog, bilateral renomegaly is often accompanied by acute rather than chronic kidney disease, whereas in the cat, some of the diseases causing bilateral renomegaly can lead to chronic kidney disease.

Reduced size

Reduced renal size can occur in both dogs and cats, and usually suggests a chronic rather than acute cause. In contrast to renomegaly, small kidneys are usually abnormal whether unilateral or bilateral. Chronic kidney disease (see Chapters 10 and 23) is the most common cause, but other differential diagnoses are possible, including congenital diseases (dysplasia, familial nephropathies) and renal atrophy (e.g. as a long-term consequence of ureteral obstruction). The latter are usually unilateral rather than bilateral.

Altered number

Congenital diseases, although rare, are the most common reason for alterations in kidney number (Figure 4.3). Decreased number is seen with renal agenesis and fused (horseshoe) kidneys; increased renal number can be seen

Decreased number

Congenital:
- Renal agenesis
- Fused (horseshoe) kidneys

Acquired:
- Nephrectomy

Increased number

Congenital:
- Renal duplication

4.3 Causes of altered kidney number.

with renal duplication. Although many breeds can be affected, agenesis and duplication have been reported as familial diseases in Beagles and English Bull Terriers, respectively. Unilateral agenesis is also associated with Cavalier King Charles Spaniels, Dobermanns, Pekingese and Shetland Sheepdogs. Agenesis can be unilateral or bilateral, and is usually accompanied by ureteral aplasia. Not surprisingly, bilateral agenesis is invariably fatal and is a potential cause of fading puppy syndrome. The main acquired cause of decreased kidney number is prior nephrectomy. Renal duplication is the only, rare, abnormality that causes an increased number of kidneys, and this is usually an incidental finding.

Altered shape

Many of the diseases which alter the shape of the kidney (Figure 4.4) also lead to changes in size. Examples include renal dysplasia, congenital renal fusion (horseshoe kidney), perinephric pseudocysts, renal neoplasia, subcapsular haematomas and PCKD.

- Congenital
  - Renal fusion – horseshoe kidney
  - Renal dysplasia
- Perinephric pseudocysts
- Neoplasia
  - Primary renal neoplasia
  - Renal lymphoma
  - Metastatic neoplasia
- Polycystic kidney disease
- Chronic kidney disease (small and deformed)
- Hydronephrosis
  - Congenital
  - Acquired

4.4 Causes of altered renal shape.

Altered consistency

Palpable changes in consistency include kidneys that have a fluctuant feel, and those that are firmer than normal (Figure 4.5). The former is most often noted with perinephric

Kidney characteristic	Cause
Fluctuant	• Perinephric pseudocyst • Subcapsular haematoma • Cystic tumour • Hydronephrosis
Firm	• Neoplasia • Chronic kidney disease

4.5 Causes of altered renal consistency.

pseudocysts, subcapsular haematomas, cystic tumours and hydronephrosis; the latter is often detected with neoplasia (usually large, abnormally shaped, and/or asymmetrical) and chronic kidney disease (usually small, may be abnormally shaped).

Altered position

Causes of altered kidney position are listed in Figure 4.6. Renal ectopia is a congenital condition, which arises as a result of failure of normal embryonic ascent of the kidney. The condition is usually incidental, and the kidney can be identified either as a caudal abdominal, sublumbar or pelvic mass. Altered position can also accompany renomegaly (the enlarged kidney becomes displaced ventrally) and conditions which result in enlargement of an adjacent structure, e.g. hepatomegaly and adrenal gland tumours. In obese subjects, kidneys are displaced ventrally and often embedded within large amounts of fat. However, this finding is rarely documented on abdominal palpation.

• Renal ectopia
• Enlarged kidney
• Displaced kidney
• Enlargement of adjacent organs:
  • Adrenal gland tumour
  • Splenomegaly
  • Hepatomegaly
  • Alimentary tract disease
  • Sublumbar disease
• Obesity

4.6 Causes of altered kidney position.

Pain

Renal pain is most often seen with pyelonephritis, acute nephrosis, renal abscesses, neoplasia and in the early stage of hydronephrosis (Figure 4.7).

• Pyelonephritis
• Urolithiasis:
  • Renal calculi
  • Ureteric calculi causing obstruction
• Acute nephrosis
• Hydronephrosis
• Stretching of renal capsule:
  • Renal trauma (e.g. subcapsular haematoma)
  • Amyloidosis?
• Trauma
• Referred pain:
  • Spinal disease
  • Other abdominal disease
• Abscesses
• Neoplasia

4.7 Causes of kidney pain.

Diagnostic approach to abnormal renal morphology

As with diagnosis of a disease in any body system, a problem-oriented approach is recommended, taking into account information compiled from a minimum database of signalment, history, physical examination and a range of further diagnostic tests. Some diseases involve other body systems in addition to the renal system (e.g. lymphoma, FIP, PVA, metastatic neoplasia and acromegaly), whilst others are organ-specific (e.g. PCKD, hydronephrosis, perinephric pseudocysts, acute pyelonephritis and acute uraemia). From the minimum database, a problem list and set of differential diagnoses can be constructed. With subsequent diagnostic evaluations, the problem list is refined and the differential diagnoses are narrowed.

Signalment

Breed, gender and age predispositions are evident in some of the diseases that cause morphological renal abnormalities, allowing the clinician to prioritize the preliminary list of differential diagnoses. Examples of diseases where breed predispositions exist include PCKD (Persian cats, Figure 4.8; Cairn Terriers, West Highland White Terriers and English Bull Terriers), basement membrane disorders (Dobermanns, English Cocker Spaniels and Samoyeds) and amyloidosis (Beagles, English Foxhounds, Shar Peis

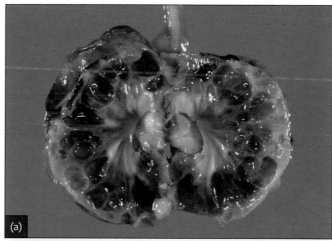

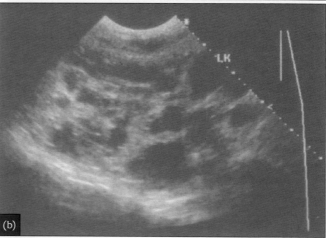

4.8 Polycystic kidney disease in a Persian cat. (a) The renal cortex is distorted with multiple fluid-filled cysts. (b) These cysts can readily be detected by ultrasonographic examination.
(Courtesy of the Feline Advisory Bureau)

and Abyssinian cats) (see Chapter 14). Diseases with a gender predisposition include acromegaly (male cats and neutered bitches) and the basement membrane disorder in male Samoyeds (X-linked recessive), whilst diseases with an age predisposition include congenital PVA (young animals) and most neoplastic diseases (older individuals). In contrast, German Shepherd Dogs have an inherited predisposition for nodular dermatofibrosis combined with renal cystadenocarcinomas (Lingaas *et al.*, 2003).

History

A full medical history should be obtained in all cases. Signs of disease in other body systems may be evident and, in some cases, concurrent acute or chronic kidney disease may be present (Figure 4.9). Further, there are some historical findings which, when present, may suggest the specific underlying cause. Cases of unilateral hydronephrosis and perinephric pseudocysts have simple histories of progressive abdominal enlargement, often with no systemic signs. In contrast, the history of acute pyelonephritis may be poorly defined, although pyrexia, anorexia, lethargy, dehydration and weight loss may be present. In severe cases there may be sublumbar pain and signs of systemic sepsis.

Physical examination

Physical examination provides the opportunity to evaluate the renal system indirectly (e.g. with abdominal palpation), and to assess the rest of the systemic health of the animal. Systematic abdominal palpation provides information on most aspects of renal morphology (size, shape and position), as well as providing evidence of other organ involvement. The following questions should be addressed:

- Are two kidneys palpable, and in their normal position? If not, is there evidence to suggest an alteration in kidney number or position?
- Are there alterations in renal size, e.g. either renomegaly or decreased size?
- Are the renal contours smooth or irregular?
- Are the abnormalities documented unilateral or bilateral?
- Are other abdominal masses present?
- Is there renal or sublumbar pain?
- Are there any other abnormalities present?

Other physical examination findings that may be relevant to the diagnosis are presented in Figure 4.9.

Historical and physical findings	Possible diagnostic implications
Signs of renal failure: buccal ulceration, uraemic breath, dehydration, poor concentrating ability and history of oliguria/polyuria (acute or decompensated chronic). Pallor and emaciation (additional findings which suggest a chronic problem)	• Acute nephrosis: ischaemic, toxic, infectious • Bilateral pyelonephritis • Bilateral hydronephrosis • Chronic kidney disease
Lymphadenopathy	• Lymphoma
Anterior uveitis and/or chorioretinitis	• FIP
Neurological/encephalopathic signs	• Renal encephalopathy • Portovascular anomaly • FIP • Lymphoma • (Acromegaly – pituitary problem)
Haematuria without dysuria	• Renal neoplasia • Pyelonephritis • Nephrolithiasis • Acute nephrosis? • Trauma • Telangiectasia
Dysuria and haematuria	• Nephrolithiasis: urinary calculi, renal or ureteral trauma • Pyelonephritis with lower urinary tract infection • Portovascular anomaly with ammonium biurate urolithiasis
Urinary calculi	• Hydronephrosis (renal calculi) • Portovascular anomaly with ammonium biurate urolithiasis
Urinary incontinence with urine scalding	• Congenital anatomical defect causing incontinence and hydronephrosis/pyelonephritis
Microhepatica	• Portovascular anomaly
Hepatomegaly	• Acute tubular nephrosis (leptospirosis) • Acromegaly and secondary diabetes mellitus • Amyloidosis in Siamese cats
Enlargement of the skull, mandible (prognathia inferior) and tongue in an adult animal	• Acromegaly
Enlargement/malformation of the mandibles in a young animal	• Osteodystrophy associated with chronic kidney disease
Signs of systemic sepsis: fever, depression, tachycardia, vomiting, petechiation	• Acute tubular nephrosis • Leptospirosis • Acute pyelonephritis • Sepsis
Skin nodules	• Renal cystadenocarcinoma • In German Shepherd Dogs, associated with dermatofibrosis

4.9 Significance of physical findings when associated with morphological abnormalities.

Further diagnostic tests

In some circumstances, altered renal morphology is physiological and an incidental finding (e.g. renomegaly associated with PVA, acromegaly and physiological hypertrophy of the remaining kidney after nephrectomy). However, in most cases it indicates a significant pathological process, which requires further diagnostic evaluation (see also Chapters 6 and 10). The initial approach is to collect baseline clinicopathological data:

- **Haematology**. Complete blood count and blood smear evaluation are recommended
- **Serum biochemical analysis**. A complete profile including electrolytes is recommended
- **Urinalysis**. This should include gross examination, dipstick, sediment examination and measurement of specific gravity by refractometer. Where sediment does not indicate the presence of inflammation, urine protein to creatinine ratio would be useful
- **Virology.** Serological tests for feline leukaemia virus (FeLV) antigen and anti-feline immunodeficiency virus (FIV) antibody should be performed in all cats, whilst coronavirus serology should also be considered.

In some cases, the above database is sufficient to obtain a definitive diagnosis. However, on occasion additional procedures may be warranted, including bacterial culture of urine, diagnostic imaging, tests of renal function, cytological examination and histopathological assessment of biopsy material. The routine measurement of blood pressure in animals where renal disorders are suspected is recommended (Chapter 15).

Bacterial culture of urine

Cystocentesis is the preferred method of urine collection if bacterial culture is required, and it is recommended that a laboratory is chosen which provides information on minimum inhibitory concentration (MIC) to assist in antimicrobial selection if appropriate (see Chapter 29). The presence of intracellular bacteria confirms that an active infection exists.

Diagnostic imaging

In cases of renomegaly, some form of diagnostic imaging is always recommended in order to characterize better the reason for renal enlargement (see Chapter 7). For cases presenting with small kidneys, diagnostic imaging is perhaps less likely to yield further information.

Survey radiographs of the abdomen and thorax are recommended, and orthogonal views of the abdomen should be taken if ultrasonography is not available. A complete ultrasonographic examination of the abdomen is indicated, paying particular attention to the kidneys. The ventrodorsal abdominal radiograph can be used to measure renal size, although this is greatly facilitated by the use of contrast radiography (see below). It is usual to compare renal length to the length of the second lumbar vertebral body in order to minimize the effects of magnification of the radiographic image. Size is better evaluated by ultrasonography, which avoids the problem of magnification, and ranges for normal renal size have been reported (Figure 4.10).

- Excretory urogram in the ventrodorsal view:
  - Dog: normal kidney length = 2.5–3.5 x L2 (length of second lumbar vertebra)
  - Cat: normal kidney length = 2.4–3.0 x L2
- Maximal sagittal dimension on ultrasonographic images:
  - In the dog, kidney length is directly proportional to bodyweight (Figure 4.10)
  - Cat = 38–44 mm.

Renal ultrasonography can also provide excellent detail of internal architecture, and many focal lesions, such as cysts, mass lesions, nephroliths, subcapsular fluid accumulation and renal pelvis dilatation, can be readily identified (Figures 4.11 and 4.12). Diffuse changes in echogenicity are also associated with certain diseases. Increased echogenicity may be seen in acute nephrosis and FIP, while lymphoma can increase or decrease echogenicity. Focal lesions are, thus, readily recognized. Ultrasonography can also facilitate fine-needle aspiration cytology and percutaneous collection of tissue core samples (see Chapters 7 and 13).

Weight range (kg)	Number of kidneys evaluated	Renal length (cm)		
		Range	*Mean*	*Standard deviation*
0–4	2	3.2–3.3	3.2	0.09
5–9	16	3.2–5.2	4.4	0.5
10–14	10	4.8–6.4	5.6	0.6
15–19	20	5–6.7	6	0.4
20–24	20	5.2–8	6.5	0.72
25–29	44	5.3–7.8	6.9	0.58
30–34	32	6.1–8.7	7.2	0.6
35–39	24	6.6–9.3	7.6	0.72
40–44	12	6.3–8.4	7.6	0.54
45–49	8	7.6–9.1	8.5	0.46
50–59	6	7.5–10.6	9.1	1.27
60–69	4	8.3–9.8	9	0.63
90–99	2	8.6–10.1	9.4	1.06

4.10 Relationship between kidney length and bodyweight in dogs.

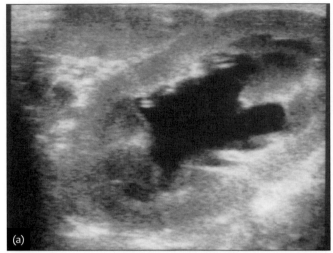

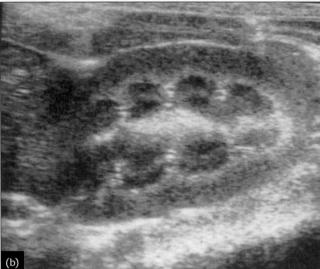

4.11 Ultrasonography demonstrating hydronephrosis.
Ultrasonograms of a 3-year-old female (recently neutered)
Chihuahua, presenting shortly after routine ovariohysterectomy.
(a) Longitudinal image of the left kidney shows the hyperechoic fat of
the renal pelvis markedly separated by anechoic fluid, consistent with
severe hydronephrosis. The outline of the kidney is expanded, the
normal architecture of the renal medulla is compressed, but the cortex is
relatively normal. (b) Longitudinal view of the right kidney in the same
dog showing normal renal architecture.
(Courtesy of Anna Newitt, University of Liverpool)

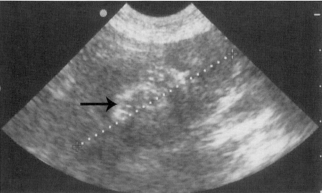

4.12 Ultrasonography demonstrating nephrolithiasis.
Ultrasongram of the left kidney of a 7-year-old male
Dalmatian, presenting with apparent sublumbar pain. Hyperechoic
shadowing regions are present in the renal pelvis (arrowed), consistent
with nephrolithiasis (probably urate given the breed).
(Courtesy of Anna Newitt and Alistair Freeman, University of Liverpool)

With the wider use of abdominal ultrasonography, the
indications for intravenous urography have declined (Figures
4.13 and 4.14). However, if ultrasonography is not available,
intravenous urography can be a useful method of providing
information on the size, shape, position and, to a lesser
extent, internal architecture of the kidney. Information can
also be gained regarding the size, integrity and course of
the ureters. Antegrade pyelography can be used to localize
the site of ureteral obstructions.

Advanced imaging techniques include excretory urography, renal scintigraphy, computed tomography (CT),
magnetic resonance imaging (MRI) and advanced ultrasonographic techniques. CT has become increasingly
available to veterinary surgeons (veterinarians) working in
practice, and the rapid acquisition of three-dimensional
information offers significant advantages in abdominal
imaging. CT may be used in combination with excretory
urography to increase the diagnostic information available. However, the cost of the technique and the high
radiation doses should be borne in mind by clinicians.
MRI is less often selected for abdominal imaging than CT
despite the exquisite soft tissue details; scan times are
longer than for CT and thus movement blur from respiration is a consideration.

Advanced ultrasonographic techniques may also be of
use. In human medicine, intrarenal blood flow impedance,
expressed as the renal resistive index (RRI) and obtained
by duplex Doppler ultrasonography, has been used to aid
in diagnosis and prognosis of renal failure (Rivers *et al.*,
1997). Increased RRI is seen in a variety of diseases,
including acute tubular necrosis and glomerulopathy, and

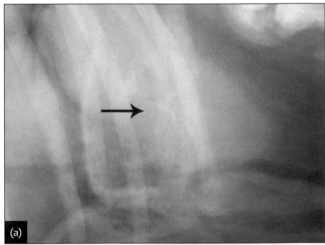

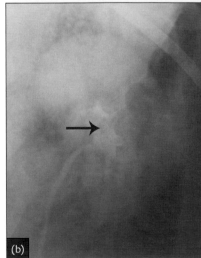

4.13 Excretory
urography
demonstrating
nephrolithiasis in a
7-year-old Dalmatian
presenting with apparent
sublumbar pain (same dog
as in Figure 4.12).
(a) Nephroliths (probably
urate) are evident on plain
lateral abdominal
radiography (arrowed).
(b) Filling defects can be
seen during subsequent
urography (arrowed).
(Courtesy of Anna Newitt and
Alistair Freeman, University of
Liverpool)

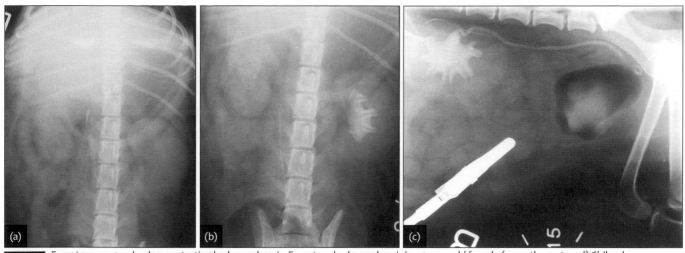

4.14 Excretory urography demonstrating hydronephrosis. Excretory hydronephrosis in a 3-year-old female (recently neutered) Chihuahua, presenting shortly after routine ovariohysterectomy (same dog as in Figure 4.11). There is evidence of (a) left-sided renomegaly, (b) dilatation of the left renal pelvis and (c) left ureter dilatation. The findings are suggestive of hydronephrosis secondary to iatrogenic ligation.
(Courtesy of Anna Newitt, University of Liverpool)

the RRI can return to normal upon successful treatment. Furthermore, after the administration of either mannitol or furosemide, RRI remains unchanged in non-obstructed kidneys but is increased in obstructed kidneys (Choi *et al.*, 2003). However, the diagnostic value of RRI in veterinary medicine has yet to be established. Contrast ultrasonography is a technique which offers the opportunity to evaluate renal perfusion in both focal and diffuse disease. Ultrasound shear wave elastography is an advanced technique, which is currently being explored in human and veterinary medicine; this technique assesses the elasticity of a tissue, and it is hoped that this may in future provide useful diagnostic information. However, at the time of publication, these advanced techniques are not widely used in a clinical setting. Further details of these advanced imaging techniques can be found in Chapter 7.

Tests of renal function

The initial database provides some information on renal function, e.g. serum creatinine and urine specific gravity. However, given the insensitivity of these methods, other techniques may be necessary in some cases. Examples of function tests include measurement of water intake, and assessment of glomerular filtration rate (GFR), all of which are covered in detail in Chapters 2 and 10.

Renal cytology

Fine-needle aspiration can be performed blind, if the kidney can be palpated and readily immobilized for the procedure. However, samples should ideally be taken under ultrasound guidance if at all possible; this enables appropriate sites to be chosen, renal vasculature to be avoided and specific lesions to be targeted. Cytology is potentially useful for assessing mass lesions; although, with neoplastic lesions such as lymphoma, cells often do not readily exfoliate, and samples usually have marked blood contamination.

Renal biopsy

Renal biopsy should only be considered when the information obtained is likely to alter the approach to management of a particular case (see Chapter 13), or when prognosis is deemed important for the owner. Biopsy is

more commonly indicated for assessment of renomegaly and changes in renal architecture, than for small kidneys, since the latter are almost invariably associated with end-stage disease, where the pathology is similar regardless of the initiating cause and so the information obtained does not inform management. Diseases such as lymphoma, other types of neoplasia, acute tubular nephrosis, FIP and familial nephropathy can all be diagnosed by renal biopsy (Figures 4.15 and 4.16).

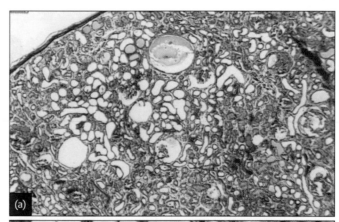

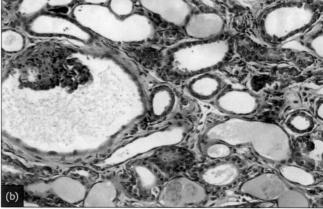

4.15 Histopathological images of renal parenchyma from an 11-month-old Cocker Spaniel bitch with familial nephropathy. The Bowman's spaces are dilated and empty; some contain components of vascular glomerular tufts and proteinaceous material. There is multifocal calcification of the Bowman's capsules, tubular basement membranes and glomerular basement membranes. (a) H&E stain; original magnification X100. (b) H&E stain; original magnification X400.

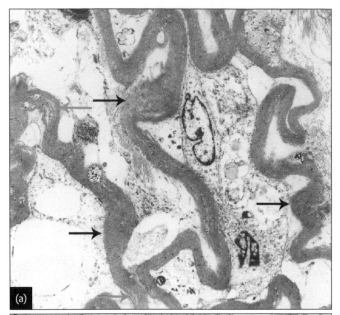

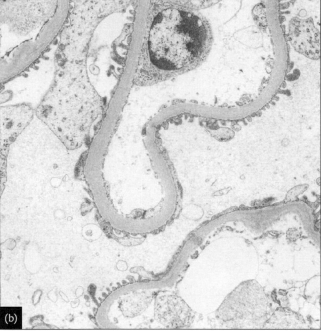

4.16 Transmission electron micrographs of glomeruli from (a) an 11-month-old Cocker Spaniel bitch with familial nephropathy and (b) a normal dog. In the affected dog, there is evidence of basement membrane thickening (red arrows) and splitting (green arrows). (Original magnification X5400).

Conditions causing abnormal renal morphology

Acute kidney injury

Acute kidney injury is defined as sudden, often catastrophic, failure of the kidney to meet the excretory, metabolic and endocrine demands of the body. The condition can arise secondary to disruptions to a number of renal functions, including haemodynamic, filtration, tubular and outflow tract disruptions. The proposed new grading of acute kidney injury is presented in Chapter 12 and the causes, consequences and management of acute kidney injury are discussed in Chapter 21. Affected kidneys are either normal or enlarged regardless of the cause of the acute uraemia unless a pre-existing chronic kidney disease is also evident. They often have a turgid feel to them and may be painful on palpation.

The mechanisms which underlie the renomegaly depend upon the underlying cause. In obstructive uropathy, the enlargement is due to dilatation of the renal pelvis and development of hydronephrosis (see below). In contrast, in cases of acute nephrosis (nephrotoxicosis, renal ischaemia, etc.) the enlargement is the result of the parenchymal damage associated with the insult, which leads to a pathogenetic process involving three stages (initiation, maintenance and recovery; see Chapter 21).

Amyloidosis

Amyloidosis involves the extracellular deposition of fibrils formed by polymerization of proteins with a beta-pleated sheet tertiary structure. Although several different types of protein have been recognized in human amyloidosis, fewer types are noted or reported in companion animals. The protein usually involved is amyloid A, which is produced from the polymerization of the N-terminal portion of serum amyloid A. Serum amyloid A is an acute phase protein predominantly synthesized in the liver. Therefore, amyloidosis is usually a sequel to a variety of chronic inflammatory disorders. Amyloid can be deposited in a number of organs, but the kidney is most often involved. Renal amyloidosis is more common in dogs than in cats and older animals are most often affected. The disease affects females more commonly than males. An increased incidence is reported in some breeds (e.g. Shar Pei, Beagle, English Foxhound, Walker Hound), and the disease is thought to be familial in most of the these cases. Although amyloidosis is uncommon in cats, certain breeds are reportedly predisposed, e.g. Abyssinian and Siamese.

In most breeds of dog, the glomerulus is the most common site of renal amyloid deposition, and hence the most common abnormality is proteinuria. However, in Shar Peis and Abyssinian cats, amyloid is predominantly deposited in the renal medulla and proteinuria is less commonly observed. Diagnosis requires renal biopsy and histopathological examination, where the amyloid can be readily identified if special staining procedures are employed, e.g. Congo red or Sirius red. Specific treatment options are limited because the beta-pleated sheet conformation is naturally resistant to breakdown. Suggested therapies have included colchicine (some success in Shar Peis) and dimethylsulfoxide. However, in most cases response is poor, especially after chronic kidney disease has developed.

Chronic kidney disease

Chronic kidney disease is the most common disorder involving the kidneys of dogs and cats, and is defined as the presence of functional or structural abnormalities of one or both kidneys (see Chapters 12 and 23). It is characterized by irreversible loss of functional nephrons, and leads ultimately to decreased renal function. In order to define that a particular patient has chronic kidney disease, either renal damage or reduced renal function (e.g. decreased GFR) must have been present for at least 3 months. Chronic kidney disease can be the result of a number of initiating causes, and in many patients the factor(s) responsible is not clear. Whatever the inciting insult and irrespective of where in the nephron it develops, the whole nephron eventually becomes involved, leading to destruction of the complete structure and replacement with non-functional connective tissue. Initially, any potential decrease in renal size resulting from such nephron loss is counteracted by compensatory hypertrophy of remaining (functional) nephrons. However, as nephron loss progresses, the overall kidney mass eventually declines and end-stage kidneys result. Therefore, in most cases of chronic kidney disease, the kidneys are small and this is a helpful finding in differentiating chronic from acute kidney disease. Nevertheless, some chronic kidney disease patients have kidneys that are of normal size or even enlarged (see above for examples).

Definitive diagnosis of chronic kidney disease theoretically involves renal biopsy, although this is seldom performed or indicated in most cases. Treatment is supportive and/or renoprotective (see Chapter 23), and prognosis depends upon duration, aetiology and rate of progression of the disease.

Congenital renal disease and familial nephropathies

The details of congenital and familial renal disorders are given in Chapter 14. Most of such disorders develop at a young age (e.g. less than 5 years), but some can arise in older individuals. Most of such diseases ultimately lead to chronic kidney disease, although the severity and rate of progression is variable. Therapeutic options are limited to conservative therapy only, and the prognosis is usually guarded to poor.

The key features of these conditions with regard to renal palpation are as follows:

- Amyloidosis – variable
- Tubular dysfunction – none?
- Basement membrane disorder – decreased size
- Glomerular disorders – decreased size
- Polycystic kidney disease – increased size ± altered shape
- Renal dysplasia – decreased size
- Unilateral renal agenesis – decreased number
- Cystadenocarcinoma – altered size and shape (occasionally normal)
- Telangiectasia -- none or altered size and shape
- Agenesis – decreased number
- Fusion (horseshoe kidney) – decreased number ± altered shape and position.

Hydronephrosis

Obstruction of urine flow causes a progressive dilatation of the renal pelvis (see Figures 4.11 and 4.14). In bilateral ureteric or urethral obstruction, the patient will die from acute post-renal failure before significant atrophy of renal parenchyma occurs; in cases of unilateral ureteric obstruction, compensation by the unobstructed kidney will allow the development of gross hydronephrosis. The renal pelvis progressively dilates causing pressure atrophy of the renal parenchyma and eventually the kidney becomes a distended, fibrous, fluid-filled sac. In the early stages, the distension of the renal capsule will induce signs of renal pain, but in many cases the first indication of hydronephrosis is progressive abdominal enlargement due to a large, unilateral, abdominal mass. Obstructive lesions may be congenital or acquired. Congenital obstructions can include ureteral atresia, stenosis, torsion and ureterocele. These abnormalities

may be seen in association with ectopic ureters. Acquired causes of obstruction can include neoplasms, blood clots, uroliths, trauma, inflammatory masses and inadvertent ureteral ligation.

As bilateral hydronephrosis presents with acute azotaemia, rapid diagnosis and urgent therapy are required if renal function is to be re-established. For unilateral cases, diagnosis is usually made by imaging, with ultrasonography providing the best information. Treatment depends upon the cause and duration of the condition. Unfortunately, most unilateral cases are not diagnosed until the condition is long-standing, and the only recourse is surgical resection of the affected kidney.

Infectious disorders

Feline infectious peritonitis

Renomegaly can be seen in the non-effusive form of FIP. Affected kidneys have multiple granulomas on the renal surface extending into the cortex and cytological aspirates have mixed lymphocytes, plasma cells, neutrophils and macrophages. Pathological change is usually also present in the liver, mesenteric lymph nodes, central nervous system and eyes. FIP should be suspected in patients presenting with enlarged irregular kidneys, ocular lesions and central nervous system signs.

Leptospirosis

Leptospirosis is a systemic infection which causes renal enlargement and acute uraemia in dogs. Several different forms are recognized, depending upon the infecting serovar, and can be peracute, subacute or chronic. Most animals affected by the peracute form die from the complications of systemic sepsis and disseminated intravascular coagulation, while subacute cases may develop renal enlargement, acute uraemia, hepatitis and jaundice.

Pyelonephritis

Pyelonephritis is interstitial inflammation of the kidney associated with bacterial infection. In acute cases, one or both kidneys may be enlarged. Chronic pyelonephritis causes structural damage, fibrosis and scarring and is associated with reduced renal size. Most cases in the dog are caused by ascending urinary tract infection, but the importance of ascending infection has not been fully established in the cat. Other possible mechanisms of infection include haematogenous spread or septic embolization in animals with bacteraemia or septicaemia, e.g. in cases of bacterial endocarditis, discospondylitis and pyometra. Pyelonephritis can also occur secondary to immunosuppression, e.g. hyperadrenocorticism.

Signs of acute pyelonephritis may be quite vague but include mild renomegaly, renal pain, fever, anorexia, dehydration, weight loss, polyuria, polydipsia and vomiting. Diagnosis is usually made from a combination of tests, including diagnostic imaging (especially ultrasonography) and laboratory findings (haematology, serum biochemistry, urinalysis and aerobic bacterial urine culture) (Figure 4.17). Ultrasonographic findings in acute pyelonephritis are variable (see Chapter 7). There may be:

- Dilatation of the renal pelvis
- A hyperechoic mucosal line within the renal pelvis
- Focal hypoechoic areas in the medulla
- Focal hyper- or hypoechoic cortical lesions.

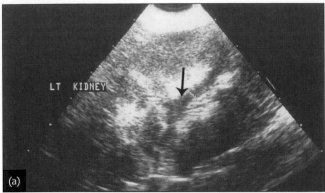

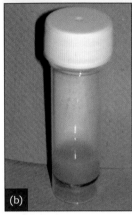

4.17 Pyelonephritis in a 9-year-old neutered Weimaraner bitch. (a) Ultrasonogram of the left kidney, demonstrating dilatation of the renal pelvis (arrowed) and poor corticomedullary definition. (b) Specimen of urine demonstrating gross turbidity.
(a, Courtesy of Annette Kerins, University of Liverpool)

Ultrasonography may also facilitate the collection of cytological specimens, by fine-needle aspiration, from the renal parenchyma or from a dilated renal pelvis.

Neutrophilic leucocytosis may be noted on haematological examination, whereas serum biochemical analysis may reveal azotaemia if excretory renal function is compromised. Urinalysis may demonstrate haematuria, pyuria, evidence of suboptimal concentrating ability (specific gravity usually within the hypersthenuric range, but not markedly concentrated, e.g. 1.015–1.025; often in the face of azotaemia) and a positive urine culture (see Chapter 6). The source of urinary tract infection may be difficult to localize, but the presence of white blood cell casts confirms the presence of inflammation in the upper urinary tract. Unfortunately, the absence of white cell casts does not rule out pyelonephritis. A definitive diagnosis can be made by renal biopsy, although this technique carries the risk of iatrogenic spread of infection within the abdomen and is rarely performed for this disease. Further, taking a biopsy of the cortex might miss the diagnosis since this region can be unaffected in pyelonephritis.

Perinephric pseudocysts

A small number of cats have been described with large fluid accumulations in fibrous pseudocysts surrounding one or both kidneys. The cysts are termed pseudocysts because they are not lined by epithelium and develop between the renal parenchyma and the renal capsule. The kidneys, which are enclosed within the cyst, are usually of normal size and fully functional. The pathogenesis is not understood, but trauma with subcapsular urine leakage has been suggested. Older entire male cats are most often affected and there are few clinical signs except progressive abdominal enlargement. The cyst fluid is a transudate and, after surgical resection and drainage of the cyst, there was no recurrence in cats followed up for 2 years.

Portovascular anomalies

Renomegaly is a relatively common finding in dogs and cats with congenital PVA. The increase in renal size is thought to be related to increased renal workload, to increased delivery of trophic factors to the kidneys and to increased renal blood flow. There is some evidence that exposure of renal cells to high ammonia concentrations causes hypertrophy; increased renal gluconeogenesis can also develop secondary to systemic hypoglycaemia and this can also cause hypertrophy. Renal enlargement can additionally occur secondary to increased GFR, which can be seen in animals with PVA. PVA are usually diagnosed with a combination of laboratory analyses (including dynamic bile acids) and diagnostic imaging (ultrasonography and portovenography).

Renal neoplasia

Tumours are important causes of unilateral renomegaly in the dog (Figure 4.18). Lymphoma is the most common renal neoplasm in the cat and is usually, but not invariably, bilateral (Figure 4.19). Other metastatic neoplasms, such as haemangiosarcoma, may also induce bilateral renomegaly. Primary renal malignancies, such as renal cell carcinoma and transitional cell carcinoma, are relatively rare in both species and vary in their behaviour. Some tumours are highly invasive locally and cause erosion of the renal artery and vein while others are quite static. Some metastasize early, whereas others are curable by excision. The presence of an irregular mass involving part or all of one kidney should always prompt careful evaluation for local and distant metastasis.

Renal lymphoma is relatively common in cats, and usually affects both kidneys, which may have an irregular outline (Figure 4.19). As a result, signs of renal insufficiency are common. Renal lymphoma may be accompanied by involvement of other abdominal organs and lymph nodes (peripheral, abdominal and mediastinal). In cats presenting with renal lymphoma, subsequent progression to central nervous system lymphoma is common, whilst cases with nasopharyngeal lymphoma may subsequently progress to renal lymphoma. The initial response to chemotherapy may be good but the long-term prognosis is guarded.

Hereditary multifocal renal cystadenocarcinoma and nodular dermatofibrosis (RCND) is an inherited disorder in German Shepherd Dogs, and is transmitted in an

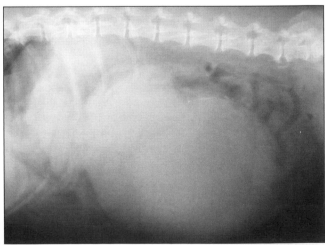

4.18 Right lateral abdominal radiograph of an anaplastic sarcoma causing dramatic unilateral renomegaly, altered shape and altered position in a 7-year-old Bassett Hound bitch.
(Courtesy of Anna Newitt and Laura Blackwood, University of Liverpool)

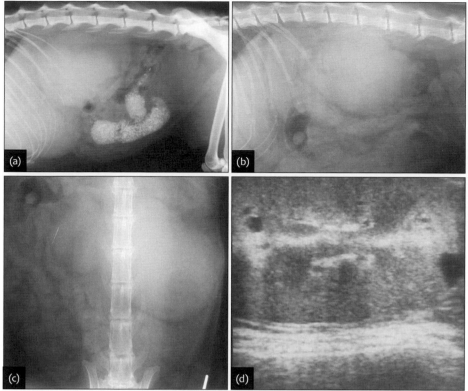

4.19 Renal lymphoma. (a) Right lateral abdominal radiograph of a Domestic Shorthaired Cat with bilateral renomegaly caused by lymphoma. Small intestinal impaction (from ingestion of cat litter) was the result of concurrent pica. (b) Right lateral and (c) ventrodorsal abdominal radiographs of a 14-year-old Domestic Shorthaired Cat with unilateral renomegaly caused by lymphoma. (d) Ultrasonogram of the left kidney of an 11-year-old neutered male Persian cat with bilateral renal lymphoma. There is renomegaly (left kidney = 5.6 cm) and poor corticomedullary definition. Two cysts are also present within the renal cortex, probably secondary to concurrent polycystic kidney disease.

(a, Courtesy of Dr Penney Barber; b–c, Courtesy of Anna Newitt and Rachel Steen, University of Liverpool; d, Courtesy of Anna Newitt and Dan Batchelor, University of Liverpool)

autosomal dominant fashion. As the name suggests, affected dogs can develop renal cystadenocarcinomas accompanied by cutaneous and subcutaneous nodules. Affected entire bitches can also develop uterine leiomyosarcomas. The disease has similarities with RCND in humans, and a disease-associated mutation in exon 7 of the Birt–Hogg–Dube protein has been described (Lingaas *et al.*, 2003). The condition is usually seen in middle-aged to older animals, and clinical signs include polydipsia, weight loss and anorexia.

Prognosis of diseases causing abnormal renal morphology

The overall prognosis for patients with morphological renal abnormalities is variable, and depends upon the specific cause (see Figure 4.2). Some abnormalities are incidental findings (e.g. renal duplication, ectopic kidney) and have no major consequences for the patient. In others the prognosis is favourable, as long as appropriate therapy is provided; examples include unilateral hydronephrosis, perinephric pseudocysts and localized renal neoplasms, which are all amenable to surgical correction. In contrast, many (if not most) diseases have a guarded prognosis, although the rate of progression can be variable. Given such a spectrum of possible outcomes, it is important for the clinician to obtain a definitive diagnosis, so that correct advice can be given to the owner, and correct therapy can be provided.

In summary, abdominal palpation is a key step in the initial examination of any patient with suspected renal disease. Changes in renal morphology can be recognized, which may provide information on the underlying pathological processes of a particular disease condition. Such alterations most commonly imply a pathological process, and the most common abnormalities include renomegaly, decreased size and abnormal shape. In most cases, if a

morphological abnormality is identified, further investigations are warranted in order to determine the exact cause and, ultimately, the prognosis.

References and further reading

Barr FJ, Holt PE and Gibbs C (1990) Ultrasonographic measurement of normal renal parameters. *Journal of Small Animal Practice* **31**, 180–184

Choi H, Won S, Chung W *et al.* (2003) Effect of intravenous mannitol upon the resistive index in complete unilateral renal obstruction in dogs. *Journal of Veterinary Internal Medicine* **17**, 158–162

Cowgill LD and Francey T (2005) Acute uremia. In: *Textbook of Veterinary Internal Medicine, 6th edn*, ed. SJ Ettinger and EC Feldman, pp. 1731–1751. WB Saunders, St. Louis

Ettinger SJ and Feldman EC (2005) *Textbook of Veterinary Internal Medicine, 6th edn*. WB Saunders, St. Louis

Holdsworth A, Bradley K, Birch S, Browne WJ and Barberet V (2014) Elastography of the normal canine liver, spleen and kidneys. *Veterinary Radiology and Ultrasound* **5(66)**, 620–627

Hood JC, Savige J, Hendtlass A *et al.* (1995) Bull Terrier hereditary nephritis: a model for autosomal dominant Alport syndrome. *Kidney International* **47**, 758–765

Lees GE, Helman RG, Kashtan CE *et al.* (1998) A model of autosomal recessive Alport syndrome in English Cocker Spaniel dogs. *Kidney International* **54**, 706–719

Lingaas F, Comstock KE, Kirkness EF *et al.* (2003) A mutation in the canine BHD gene is associated with hereditary multifocal renal cystadenocarcinoma and nodular dermatofibrosis in the German Shepherd Dog. *Human Molecular Genetics* **12**, 3043–3053

Rivers BJ, Walter PA, Polzin DJ and King VL (1997) Duplex Doppler estimation of intrarenal Pourcelot resistive index in dogs and cats with renal disease. *Journal of Veterinary Internal Medicine* **11**, 250–260

Waller KR, O'Brien RT and Zagzebski JA (2007) Quantitative contrast ultrasound analysis of renal perfusion in normal dogs. *Veterinary Radiology and Ultrasound* **48(4)**, 373–377

Watson ADJ, Lefebvre HP, Concordet D *et al.* (2002) Plasma exogenous creatinine clearance test in dogs: comparison with other methods and proposed limited sampling strategy. *Journal of Veterinary Internal Medicine* **16**, 22–33

Young AE, Biller DS, Herrgesell EJ, Roberts HR and Lyons LA (2005) Feline polycystic kidney disease is linked to the PKD1 region. *Mammalian Genome* **16**, 59–65

Zheng K, Thorner PS, Marrano P, Baumal R and McInnes RR (1994) Canine X chromosome-linked hereditary nephritis: a genetic model for human X-linked hereditary nephritis resulting from a single base mutation in the gene encoding the alpha 5 chain of collagen type IV. *Proceedings of the National Academy of Sciences USA* **91**, 3989–3993

Case example 1: Domestic Shorthaired Cat with ethylene glycol toxicosis

SIGNALMENT

A 6-year-old neutered male Domestic Shorthaired Cat.

HISTORY

A 24–36-hour history which started with altered behaviour, ataxia, hysterical vocalization and tremors. Polydipsia, vomiting and collapse developed in the last 24 hours.

PHYSICAL EXAMINATION

Marked bilateral renomegaly, with smooth contours.

HAEMATOLOGY

No abnormality detected.

SERUM BIOCHEMISTRY

- Marked azotaemia (urea 164 mmol/l; reference interval = 3.5–6.0 mmol/l; creatinine 3290 μmol/l; reference <140 μmol/l).
- Hypocalcaemia (2.03 mmol/l; reference interval = 2.10–2.60 mmol/l).
- Hyperphosphataemia (6.70 mmol/l; reference interval = 1.10–2.30 mmol/l).
- Mild hyperkalaemia (5.65 mmol/l; reference interval = 3.80–5.30 mmol/l).

URINALYSIS

Specific gravity 1.015, suggesting inappropriate renal concentrating ability in the face of such marked azotaemia. Sediment analysis revealed calcium oxalate crystals.

ACID–BASE STATUS

High anion-gap metabolic acidosis.

ABDOMINAL RADIOGRAPHY

Bilateral renomegaly (Figure 4.20a).

ABDOMINAL ULTRASONOGRAPHY

Bilateral renomegaly with some loss of corticomedullary definition (Figure 4.20b).

OUTCOME

At this stage the most likely differential diagnosis was ethylene glycol intoxication causing acute nephrosis (e.g. compatible history, presence of hypocalcaemia, presence of high anion-gap metabolic acidosis, calcium oxalate crystalluria and findings on abdominal ultrasonography). Given that clinical signs had been evident for >12 hours, specific therapy for ethylene glycol was not indicated; instead, symptomatic therapy (e.g. intravenous fluids, antimicrobials, gastric protectants) was administered. There was little change 24 hours after admission, and the owner elected to have the cat euthanased, and submitted for post-mortem examination. The owners subsequently located a potential source of ethylene glycol exposure.

POST-MORTEM EXAMINATION

This revealed a mild to moderate periglomerular mixed inflammatory cell infiltrate; there was mild vacuolation of tubular epithelial cells, and multiple pale yellow crystals were evident within the tubular lumen (Figure 4.20c). Such findings confirmed acute nephrosis, secondary to ethylene glycol intoxication.

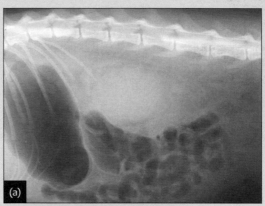

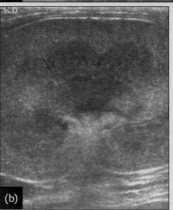

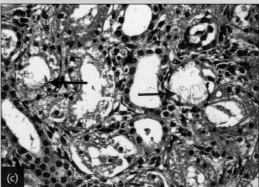

4.20 (a) Right lateral abdominal radiograph demonstrating bilateral renomegaly. (b) Ultrasonogram of the left kidney, demonstrating renomegaly with some loss of corticomedullary definition. (c) Photomicrograph demonstrating mild vacuolation of renal tubular epithelial cells, and elongated pale yellow crystals within the tubular lumen (arrowed). (H&E stain; original magnification X400)
(a–b, Courtesy of Anna Newitt, University of Liverpool; c, Courtesy of Gail Leeming, University of Liverpool)

Case example 2: Weimaraner with pyelonephritis

SIGNALMENT

A 9-year-old neutered female Weimaraner.

HISTORY

Marked polydipsia and polyuria, nocturia and anorexia.

PHYSICAL EXAMINATION

Discomfort on palpation of the craniodorsal abdomen.

HAEMATOLOGY

No abnormality detected.

SERUM BIOCHEMISTRY

- Mild azotaemia (urea 6.8 mmol/l; reference interval = 3.5–6.0 mmol/l; creatinine 124 μmol/l; reference interval = 20–110 μmol/l).

URINALYSIS

Urine was collected by cystocentesis and was turbid on gross examination (see Figure 4.17b). Biochemical assessment demonstrated:

- pH 9.0
- Blood (+++)
- Protein 0.3 g/l
- An active sediment containing massive numbers of leucocytes (neutrophils) and bacterial rods and cocci (see Figure 4.17b). Intracellular bacteria were present in some of the leucocytes.

Bacterial culture demonstrated a heavy, pure growth of haemolytic *Escherichia coli*, resistant to ampicillin and clindamycin, but sensitive to other antimicrobials, including fluoroquinolones.

ABDOMINAL ULTRASONOGRAPHY

Renal pelvis dilatation was evident in both kidneys, and both had poor corticomedullary definition.

OUTCOME

A presumptive diagnosis of pyelonephritis was made. The dog was treated with a 4-week course of enrofloxacin. Clinical signs rapidly resolved, and follow-up urine culture was negative both 7 days after the commencement of treatment, and 7 days after discontinuation.

Chapter 5

Proteinuria

Xavier Roura, Jonathan Elliott and Gregory F. Grauer

Persistent proteinuria with inactive urine sediment has long been a clinicopathological hallmark of chronic kidney disease in dogs and more recently cats. Beyond this diagnostic utility, potential pathophysiological consequences of persistent proteinuria in dogs and cats include decreased plasma oncotic pressure, hypercholesterolaemia, systemic hypertension, hypercoagulability, muscle wasting and weight loss. The importance of proteinuria in canine and feline chronic kidney disease as a prognostic indicator and therapeutic target has been increasingly recognized, and the level of protein in the urine which is considered normal has been revised downwards. Proteinuria is a sensitive early marker for diagnosis of kidney disease in dogs and to a lesser extent in cats. Glomerular lesions are common in renal diseases in dogs and uncommon in cats (Syme *et al.*, 2006), which means that proteinuria is often at a higher level in dogs. Low-level proteinuria is a predictive marker of kidney disease in cats at a population level but, owing to overlap with the normal population, it lacks specificity for the individual cat. Nevertheless, persistent low-level proteinuria in cats (and dogs) warrants monitoring because it can precede (and so indicate) deterioration in renal function in both non-azotaemic (Jepson *et al.*, 2009) and azotaemic cats (Chakrabarti *et al.*, 2012). This chapter will discuss the importance of assessing and classifying proteinuria in the patient with kidney disease, the disorders which may cause proteinuria in the dog and cat and the mechanisms by which it may cause progressive renal injury. The therapeutic approaches that may be used to treat significant proteinuria in dogs and cats will be considered in Chapters 23 and 24.

Physiology of urine formation

The glomerular filter consists of the fenestrated endothelium of the glomerular capillary, the basement membrane and the epithelium (podocytes) lining the visceral aspect of the glomerular capillary wall (Figure 5.1; Patrakka and Tryggvason, 2010). Of these three structures, the endothelium prevents passage of cells into the glomerular filter, the basement membrane provides the structural stability of the filter, anchoring cells in the correct position and contributing to the size and charge permselectivity of the glomerular capillary wall, while the transmembrane proteins of the podocytes (glomerular epithelium), which form the slit diaphragm, act as another charge- and size-selective filtration barrier. Despite being

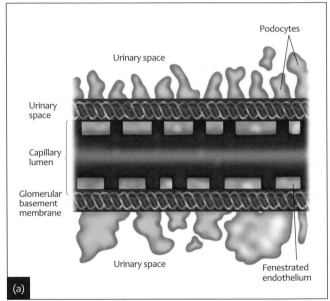

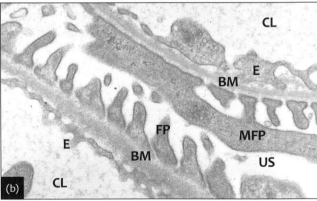

5.1 (a) Structure of the glomerular filter, showing the three components that the fluid elements of the blood have to transverse to move from the capillary to the urinary space. These consist of the capillary wall (fenestrated endothelium), the glomerular basement membrane and the visceral epithelium (podocytes with slit pores). (b) Transverse electron micrograph of a normal glomerulus. BM = basement membrane; CL = capillary lumen; E = endothelial cell; FP = foot process; MFP = major foot process; US = urinary space. (b, © Gregory F. Grauer)

the most abundant plasma protein, albumin appears in the ultrafiltrate at low concentrations because of its size. The molecular weight of albumin (69,000 Daltons) is right at the limit for filtration in terms of size. Nevertheless, data suggest that there is a significant transglomerular

BSAVA Manual of Canine and Feline Nephrology and Urology, third edition. Edited by Jonathan Elliott, Gregory F. Grauer and Jodi L. Westropp. ©BSAVA 2017

flux of albumin such that more of this protein appears in the glomerular filtrate of normal kidneys than was once recognized.

Proteins of molecular weight less than 70,000 Daltons can be filtered at the glomerulus, however, the electrical charge of the protein also has a role in filtration. The glomerular basement membrane has a net negative electrical charge, as does albumin, and therefore albumin tends to be repelled away from the filtration barrier. The albumin that is filtered is largely reabsorbed from the glomerular filtrate as it passes through the proximal convoluted tubule. The reabsorptive process is termed pinocytosis. Tubular cells then break down the albumin into its constitutive amino acids. The apical membrane receptors for protein, megulin and cubilin (Christensen *et al.*, 2013), probably play important roles in the pinocytosis process. Filtered albumin is not completely reabsorbed, therefore albumin is the major urinary protein in healthy dogs and cats as well as in those with renal proteinuria. Loss of protein in the urine in normal healthy dogs and cats usually does not exceed 10–20 mg/kg/day and 30 mg/kg/day, respectively. In addition to small amounts of albumin, urine protein excretion also results from the secretion of enzymes, mucoproteins and immunoglobulins by epithelial cells of the tubules and the lower urinary and genital tracts. These secreted proteins may account for as much as 50% of the proteins that are normally present in urine.

Detection of protein in the urine

Screening tests

Screening tests for proteinuria usually involve some form of dipstick test. These tests are semi-quantitative, depending on the ability of the amino groups of proteins to combine with indicator dyes (e.g. tetrabromophenol blue), which then change colour (Figure 5.2). The degree of binding depends on the number of free amino groups in the protein and, because albumin has more free amino groups than globulins or haemoglobin, the tests are usually 2 to 3 times more sensitive to albumin in the urine. The individual tests vary in their limits of detection but usually produce a positive reaction only if protein is present at a concentration above 30 mg/dl. False-positive results (decreased specificity) may be obtained if the urine is alkaline, the urine sediment is active (pyuria, haematuria and/or bacteriuria), the urine has been contaminated with quaternary ammonium compounds, or the dipstick is left in contact with the urine long enough to leach out the citrate buffer that is incorporated in the filter paper pad. False-positive results with the dipstick test occur much more frequently in cats than in dogs (Lyon *et al.*, 2010) but are commonly reported in both species. In entire male cats it is important to remember that cauxin, the enzyme that produces the pheromone felinine, is a significant contributor to the feline proteome, such that the urine protein to creatinine (UPC) ratio in sexually mature entire male cats is much higher than that in queens and neutered cats (a UPC ratio ≤0.6 can be normal) (Miyazaki *et al.*, 2003). Low levels of cauxin cross-react with tetraphenol blue and are thought to be responsible for the high level of false-positive results seen in queens and neutered cats, and it has been suggested that selective removal of cauxin (by affinity chromatography) from urine prior to assessment of proteinuria by the dipstick test would improve its specificity (Miyazaki *et al.*, 2011).

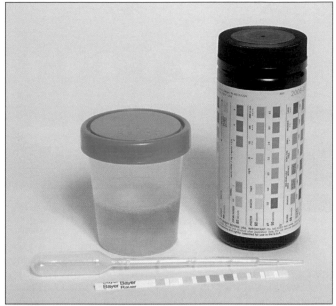

5.2 Conventional semi-quantitative tests are used to screen for protein in the urine.

False-negative results (decreased sensitivity) may occur in the setting of Bence Jones proteinuria, low concentrations of albuminuria and/or dilute or acidic urine. However, a recent publication (Zatelli *et al.*, 2010) demonstrated that, for practitioners, a urine dipstick test together with measurement of urine specific gravity (USG) is reliable, rapid and useful as a screening test for proteinuria in dogs. Irrespective of USG, a negative urine dipstick result (0+) can be safely used by veterinary surgeons (veterinarians) to classify dogs as non-proteinuric, thus eliminating the need for further determination of the UPC ratio. Dogs that have urine dipstick results ≥100 mg/dl (2+), at any urine concentration, are very likely to be proteinuric, and the loss of protein should be quantified with the UPC ratio (Lyon *et al.*, 2010). Finally, the higher the USG for dogs with 30 mg/dl (1+) protein on a urine dipstick test, the more likely it is that the UPC ratio will demonstrate them to be non-proteinuric; however, measurement of the UPC ratio is recommended to determine the degree of proteinuria. Interpretation of the dipstick results could be influenced by the population of dogs sampled and/or the geographical prevalence of infectious disease leading to proteinuric chronic kidney disease (CKD) (e.g. areas of southern Europe where leishmaniosis has a high prevalence).

An alternative screening test is the sulphosalicylic acid (SSA) turbidimetric test. This involves addition of an equal volume of 3–5% SSA to the urine sample and subjective assessment of the turbidity of the sample (0 to 4+) (see Chapter 6). In addition to albumin, the SSA test can detect globulins and Bence Jones proteins. False-positive results may occur if the urine contains radiographic contrast agents, penicillins, cephalosporins, sulfisoxazole or the urine preservative thymol. The protein content may also be overestimated with the SSA test if uncentrifuged, turbid urine is tested. False-negative results are less common in comparison with the conventional dipstick test owing to the increased sensitivity of the SSA test (>5 mg/dl). As the varying degrees of precipitation turbidity are usually not standardized and interpretation of the degree of turbidity is subjective, results may vary among individuals and laboratories. Figure 5.3 shows how this test can be standardized.

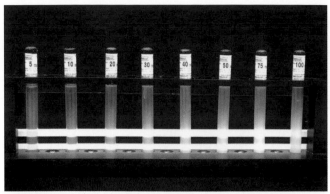

5.3 A set of standards demonstrating the increasing turbidity (from left to right) that develops when 3–5% SSA is mixed with urine containing increasing protein concentrations.

Microalbuminuria is defined as concentrations of albumin in the urine that are greater than normal but below the limit of detection of the dipstick urine protein screening methodology (i.e. <30 mg/dl; see above). Measurement of albumin in canine and feline urine was initially offered commercially through semi-quantitative species-specific dipstick technology. This has been replaced by quantitative species-specific enzyme-linked immunosorbent assays (ELISAs). Owing to the sensitivity of the conventional dipstick test, the upper end of urine albumin concentration that is considered to be microalbuminuria is 30 mg/dl or 30 mg/g (albumin/creatinine). Urine albumin concentrations above this limit are called overt albuminuria and can often be detected using the UPC ratio. The lower end of the microalbuminuria range (1.0 mg/dl) has been less easily defined because of the requirement that this concentration is greater than 'normal' and the necessity that this concentration be reliably detected. Urine albumin concentrations can be adjusted for differences in urine concentration by dividing by urine creatinine concentrations, or the urine sample can be diluted to a uniform specific gravity (e.g. 1.010) prior to measuring the urine albumin concentration. The previous edition of this Manual discussed the interest, at the time of publication, in whether microalbuminuria might be used as a test to identify kidney disease at an early stage in dogs and cats and it was speculated as to the prognostic utility of this test and presented preliminary data from ongoing studies. This research has shown subsequently that there are many systemic disease states that are associated with microalbuminuria, including chronic inflammatory disease (e.g. chronic stomatitis/gingivitis) and neoplastic conditions, and that transient and physiological albuminuria can occur in outwardly healthy dogs and cats. This means that demonstration of significant microalbuminuria requires a thorough search for chronic medical diseases that may be associated with it and demonstration of persistence of the albuminuria. Persistent microalbuminuria is an indication of kidney pathology, which may occur in association with other systemic diseases (e.g. as a result of immune complex disease). Where the quantitative test is available, it could possibly be used in dogs in order to increase the suspicion of kidney disease (International Renal Interest Society (IRIS) CKD Stage 1) in those cases with no evidence of proteinuria on the dipstick test or UPC ratio. However, quantifying microalbuminuria appears to add no further value to the use of the UPC ratio for diagnostic or prognostic purposes in cats, provided the borderline proteinuria category (UPC ratio 0.2–0.4) is viewed as abnormal (Jepson *et al.*, 2009).

Proteinuria detected by the semi-quantitative screening methods (dipstick tests and SSA test) has historically been interpreted in light of the USG and urine sediment. For example, a positive dipstick reading of trace or 1+ proteinuria in hypersthenuric urine has often been attributed to urine concentration rather than abnormal proteinuria. In addition, a positive dipstick reading for protein in the presence of haematuria or pyuria was often attributed to urinary tract haemorrhage or inflammation. In both examples, the interpretation may not be correct. Given the limits on the sensitivity of the conventional semi-quantitative tests, any positive result for protein regardless of urine concentration could be abnormal, and measurement of the UPC ratio is required to quantify proteinuria. Likewise, pyuria has an inconsistent effect on urine albumin concentrations; not all dogs with pyuria have albuminuria but any pyuria obviates the utility of the UPC ratio. By contrast, haematuria has to be severe enough to lead to pink discoloration of urine before effects on the UPC ratio are seen (Vaden *et al.*, 2004). This means that, from a clinical point of view, for any evaluation of true renal proteinuria it is mandatory to rule out the presence of pre- and post-renal proteinuria by measurement of serum total proteins and urine sediment examination (Zatelli *et al.*, 2010), with the proviso that microscopic haematuria does not interfere with interpretation of the UPC ratio or microalbuminuria. A summary of this diagnostic approach is presented in Figure 5.4.

Quantitative tests to confirm the significance of proteinuria

If the results of the screening tests show proteinuria that is consistently present in two or three urine samples collected over a 2-week period, urine protein excretion should be quantified. This helps to evaluate the severity of renal lesions and to assess the response to treatment or the progression of disease. In dogs, renal proteinuria occurs primarily as a result of lesions involving the glomerulus or, in some cases, tubular disease; whereas in cats the primary pathology is usually in the tubulointerstitial compartment with secondary changes in the glomeruli. Even in the presence of altered glomerular permeability or tubular disease, the quantity of proteinuria does not change significantly from day to day. What does change on a daily basis is the 24-hour urine volume and therefore the concentration of the urine.

The gold standard for assessing urinary protein loss would be to collect all the urine passed by the animal for a 24-hour period, measure its volume and protein concentration accurately and calculate the amount of protein lost (in mg protein in urine/kg bodyweight) in the 24-hour period. This technique is only used in the research setting because facilities to allow 24-hour urine collection are not usually available in clinical practices.

Measurement of the UPC ratio is used in veterinary practice as an alternative to measurement of 24-hour urine protein excretion. Inasmuch as the production of creatinine is constant (muscle mass is stable on a day-to-day basis) and it is freely filtered by the glomeruli without significant secretion or reabsorption by the renal tubules, the amount of creatinine excreted day-to-day in urine remains stable and so its concentration varies proportionately with urine volume. By dividing the urine protein concentration (in mg/dl) by the urine creatinine concentration (in mg/dl; to convert creatinine concentration from μmol/l to mg/dl divide by 88.7), the effect of the variation in urine volume

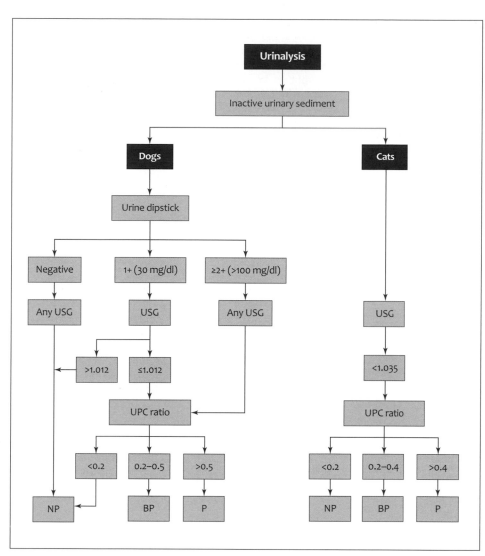

5.4 Flow diagram for the diagnosis of proteinuria in dogs and cats. Urine dipstick screening is not recommended for cats because of the high level of false-positive results. A negative value (which is a rare result for a cat) may be useful in ruling out proteinuria. BP = borderline proteinuria; NP = non-proteinuria; P = proteinuria; UPC = urine protein to creatinine ratio; USG = urine specific gravity.

on the urine protein concentration is negated. A spot urine sample obtained by any means can be used to calculate the UPC ratio as long as the urine sediment is normal/inactive. It may be best performed after a period of confinement (overnight) such that the volume of urine upon which it is based is as large as possible. Laboratories offering this test will measure creatinine and protein by quantitative analyses and express the concentration of both analytes in mg/dl (or g/l) and calculate the ratio of analyte concentrations. Such an approach has been shown to give results in cats and dogs which correlate well with 24-hour urine protein excretion measured under research conditions.

It is not possible to use most standard practice chemistry analysers to measure urine protein and creatinine levels. Most machines are calibrated for plasma, where the concentration of protein is 500 to 1000 times higher than in urine. Cross-contamination of urine with plasma from the previous sample measured is a real issue in quality control of the results. Furthermore, creatinine concentrations are 25 to 100 times higher in urine than in plasma, making it necessary to dilute urine samples considerably before the creatinine concentration is within the working range of the machine. However, Vet-Test® has recently introduced a cartridge to allow the UPC ratio to be measured within the practice. Quality control standards should be run to ensure accuracy in the practice environment. Reference ranges for the UPC

ratio, indicating mild and severe proteinuria are presented in Figure 5.5.

Most studies have shown that normal urine protein excretion in dogs is approximately 10 mg/kg/24h and that a normal UPC ratio is <0.2. Initially recommended normal values for the canine UPC ratio of <1.0 were probably conservative and have recently been lowered. Today, a UPC ratio >0.5 is considered to be abnormal (proteinuric)

UPC ratio in dogs[a]	UPC ratio in cats[a]	Interpretation	Comments
<0.2	<0.2	Normal in humans	Expect values <0.2 in healthy cats[b]
0.2–0.5	0.2–0.4	Borderline proteinuria	Should be monitored longitudinally
>0.5–<1.0	>0.4–<1.0	Proteinuric (mild to moderate)	Could be indicative of glomerular or tubular dysfunction
>1.0	>1.0	Proteinuric (severe)	The higher the UPC, the more likely this involves primary glomerular disease

5.5 Interpretation of the urine protein to creatinine (UPC) ratio measurements in canine and feline urine based on the International Renal Interest Society (IRIS) guidelines (see Chapter 12). [a]The UPC ratio does not have units, provided the protein and creatinine concentrations are expressed in the same units of mass per volume concentration. [b]Entire male cats can have a UPC ratio of up to 0.6.

and a UPC ratio of 0.2–0.5 is considered to be borderline proteinuric (Lees *et al.*, 2005). It is likely, however, that this definition will continue to change with additional research. For example, even the ultra-low level, single-nephron proteinuria that occurs secondary to intraglomerular hypertension in hypertrophied nephrons in CKD is abnormal.

The day-to-day variability of the UPC ratio needs to be taken into account. For example, in the dog, UPC values close to 0.5 need to change by more than 80% before worsening of proteinuria can be concluded (Nabity *et al.*, 2007). Published data on the day-to-day variability in the UPC ratio in the cat are not available but the same principles are likely to apply, and it should be noted that severe proteinuria is unusual in cats so demonstration of the persistence of mild proteinuria is important (see Figure 5.5). This inherent variability needs to be taken into account when:

- Making an assessment of the magnitude of proteinuria in order to stage CKD
- Following the UPC ratio as an indicator of progression of CKD
- Assessing the response to treatment of renal proteinuria.

It is important to standardize the way in which urine samples are handled for serial measurements. Microscopic urine sediment examination must be undertaken for all urine samples to aid in the interpretation of the UPC ratio. As discussed above, pyuria and macroscopic haematuria may influence the UPC ratio and, if present, the UPC ratio should not be measured, because the post-renal addition of protein to the urine complicates its interpretation. The UPC ratio must be measured as soon as samples are collected or, alternatively, the supernatant of the sample should be immediately frozen to increase its stability and minimize the risk of misclassification of proteinuria (Rossi *et al.*, 2012). Moreover, variations in the UPC ratio with or without treatment should be evaluated cautiously, particularly when the absolute UPC ratio at diagnosis of proteinuria is close to 0.5. Here, large percentage changes in the UPC ratio can occur spontaneously as a result of day-to-day variability (Nabity *et al.*, 2007). At this level of proteinuria, it is very important to demonstrate persistence of the UPC ratio >0.5 in three samples collected over a 2-week period to establish a baseline. Alternatively, the UPC ratio of three samples collected over this period mixed together (in equal volumes) to give a single sample could be measured and so provide an average UPC ratio for the three samples. The higher the UPC ratio is in a single sample the more certain the diagnosis of proteinuria. Similar considerations should be taken into account when assessing response to treatment (see Chapters 23 and 24).

Aetiopathogenesis of proteinuria

If a screening test is positive for proteinuria, it is important to determine the source of the proteinuria. Proteinuria can be classified as physiological or pathological, urinary (renal or post-renal) or non-urinary (pre-renal or post-renal) in origin.

Physiological proteinuria

Physiological or benign proteinuria is often transient and abates when the underlying cause is corrected. Strenuous exercise, seizures, fever, exposure to extreme heat or cold, and stress are examples of conditions that may cause physiological proteinuria. The mechanism of physiological proteinuria is not completely understood; however, relative renal vasoconstriction, ischaemia and congestion are thought to be involved. Decreased physical activity may also affect urine protein excretion in dogs; one study showed that urinary protein excretion was higher in dogs confined to cages than in dogs with normal activity levels (McCaw *et al.*, 1985).

Pre-renal proteinuria

Pre-renal proteinuria implies that significantly abnormal concentrations of protein are being presented to the kidney in the plasma. If these proteins are of low molecular weight they will be filtered and may overwhelm the reabsorptive processes. Examples of proteins which are readily filtered include immunoglobulin light chains, and haemoglobin and myoglobin that are not bound to haptoglobin. The detection of these proteins in excess in the plasma and their detection in the urine (see below), in combination with other clinical signs of the diseases that give rise to these proteins, will aid in the diagnosis of the underlying condition. Both free haemoglobin and myoglobin in urine will give a positive reaction on the haem pad on the urine dipstick test (see Chapter 6) and lead to discoloration of the urine and plasma.

Post-renal proteinuria

Post-renal proteinuria implies that protein is added to the urine in the urinary tract after the kidney (in the ureter, bladder or urethra). Inflammation of these parts of the urinary tract, most commonly due to bacterial infection, should be considered as a possible cause of proteinuria. Other causes of inflammation include the presence of uroliths and tumours, both of which may be associated with bacterial infection. In many cases, the cat or dog will show signs of lower urinary tract disease, such as stranguria, dysuria and pollakiuria. Microscopic examination shows that the urine sediment is likely to be active, with evidence of haematuria, inflammatory cells and possibly bacteria (Figure 5.6). Some authors suggest that samples of relatively dilute urine (urine specific gravity <1.020) should be routinely submitted for bacterial culture (even in the

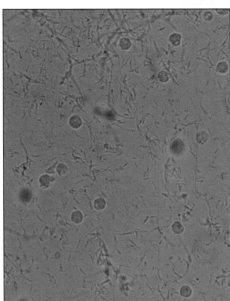

5.6
Unstained urine sediment viewed by light microscopy. The field of view shows >20 leucocytes and numerous chains of rod-shaped bacteria, suggesting urinary tract inflammation secondary to a bacterial urinary tract infection. (Original magnification X400)

absence of lower urinary tract signs and microscopic evidence of inflammation) to rule out subclinical urinary tract infections, although definitive published evidence that this is necessary is lacking.

Renal proteinuria

This implies that defective renal function and/or inflammation of parenchymal kidney tissue is the cause of the appearance of protein in the urine. Active (acute) renal parenchymal inflammation is likely to be associated with acute kidney diseases (pyelonephritis, acute tubular necrosis) and this will be reflected in the history of presentation and the active microscopic urine sediment findings. Localization of the disease to the kidney may be possible on physical examination (painful swollen kidneys on palpation) or on the presence of tubular casts on urine microscopy. However, in some instances (e.g. chronic disease) these signs may be very subtle and localization of the disease to the kidney can be difficult even when advanced imaging techniques are used. In addition to renal inflammation, defective glomerular and tubular function may result in renal proteinuria, e.g. increased glomerular permeability (glomerular proteinuria) and decreased tubular reabsorption (tubular proteinuria).

If pre-renal and post-renal causes of proteinuria have been ruled out, and there are no signs of active inflammation on urine sediment examination in an animal with persistent proteinuria, renal proteinuria is likely to be of either glomerular or tubular origin (see below). This being the case, it is worthwhile quantifying the proteinuria more accurately (see above).

Glomerular proteinuria can occur because of primary glomerular pathology leading to a defective filtration process. Examples of primary glomerular diseases include:

- Glomerulopathies due to developmental abnormalities in the components of the basement membrane and slit diaphragm (well recognized in human patients and a number of breeds of dog (see Chapter 14) but not reported in cats)
- Membranoproliferative glomerulonephritis with immune complex deposition in the glomerulus. This form of primary glomerular disease is much more common in dogs than cats; it is usually idiopathic but it may commonly be associated with infectious diseases in some areas of the world (Dambach *et al.*, 1997; Costa *et al.*, 2003; Zatelli *et al.*, 2003; Figure 5.7)
- Amyloid deposition in the glomerulus.

A feature of primary glomerular diseases that may be helpful in distinguishing them from other causes of renal proteinuria is that the degree of proteinuria, particularly once the disease has become established, tends to be high (UPC ratio >2.0 and often above 5–10). Higher UPC values (>10) may well be associated with the nephrotic syndrome. Dogs, in particular, with severe proteinuria are not always azotaemic when their kidney disease is diagnosed. Many will become azotaemic if they remain proteinuric because persistent proteinuria of this severity leads to progressive renal injury in most cases (see below).

Low-level proteinuria (UPC ratio >0.4 but <1.0 in cats and UPC ratio >0.5 but <1.0 in dogs; see Figure 5.5) could be caused by an inability of the tubules to reabsorb the filtered protein (indicating tubular disease/dysfunction) or by an increased protein flux across the glomerulus. Increased transglomerular flux of proteins (particularly albumin) may occur because of:

Dogs	Geographical areas with higher prevalence
• *Anaplasma* spp. • *Bartonella* spp. • *Borrelia burgdorferi* • *Babesia* spp. • *Brucella canis* • *Ehrlichia* spp. • Heartworm disease • *Hepatazoon americanum* • *Leishmania* spp.* • *Leptospira* spp.	Common in Europe and the USA; uncommon in the UK
• *Mycoplasma* spp. • *Rickettsia rickettsii*	Common in the USA; uncommon in Europe
Cats	
• *Bartonella* spp. • Feline infectious peritonitis (FIP) • Feline immunodeficiency virus (FIV) • Feline leukaemia virus (FeLV)	Common in Europe and the USA
• *Cytauxzoon felis*	Common in the USA; uncommon in Europe

5.7 Infectious diseases associated with glomerulonephritis in dogs and cats. *Not common in the USA.

- Increased glomerular capillary pressure (glomerular capillary hypertension) secondary to loss of functioning nephrons (adaptive response in CKD)
- Structural glomerular disease leading to abnormal development of the glomerulus (e.g. hereditary nephropathies; see Chapter 14)
- Early or late immune complex deposition involving the glomerulus that produces glomerulonephritis.

In addition, proteinuria resulting from increased transglomerular flux of proteins can be exacerbated by tubular cell dysfunction (associated with a number of disease states, including CKD, possibly as a result of oxidative stress), which impairs the ability of proximal tubular cells to deal with filtered proteins.

In the canine or feline azotaemic patient with CKD, assessment of the degree of proteinuria is an important part of classifying the disease and appears to provide information of prognostic value (see below). In addition, early identification and treatment of proteinuria is important in dogs because it may lead to early identification and treatment of an underlying infectious disease. Moderate to severe proteinuria (UPC ratio >1.0) appears to be predictive of progressive renal injury in dogs, although recently the limit of proteinuria to be treated has been lowered to >0.5 in azotaemic dogs (IRIS Stages 2, 3 and 4; see Chapters 23 and 24) and in non-azotaemic dogs testing positive for infectious diseases (IRIS Stage 1) (IRIS GDSG Goldstein *et al.*, 2013). However, the majority of cats with azotaemic CKD appear to have either normal levels of protein in their urine or have borderline or mild proteinuria (UPC ratio >0.2 but <1.0). The significance of borderline or mild proteinuria in non-azotaemic dogs and cats is that it can act as a marker of a number of systemic diseases (see above) that if allowed to persist may chronically damage the kidney. Persistent low-level proteinuria in the cat certainly seems to be a marker of progression of CKD and is associated with tubulointersitial nephritis and glomerular hypertrophy (Jepson *et al.*, 2009; Chakrabarti *et al.*, 2012). Whether the proteins in the filtrate drive tubular pathology to occur or their presence indicates that this pathology is ongoing remains to be determined.

Pathological processes of kidney disease associated with proteinuria

Pathological processes of CKD with primary glomerulonephritis

Several infectious diseases that result in glomerulonephritis in dogs are prevalent around the world (see Figure 5.7). Most of them manifest with a wide range of clinical signs involving multiple organs, especially the kidneys. Several studies have documented a variable prevalence of kidney disease associated with systemic infectious disease, which ranges from 2% to 52% of dogs naturally infected with the organisms listed in Figure 5.7 (Littman, 2011; IRIS GDSG Littman et al., 2013; Pierantozzi et al., 2013). Infectious disease associated nephropathy is mainly characterized by glomerular damage primarily attributed to intraglomerular deposition of circulating immune complexes formed by antigens of the organism and antibodies produced against it. Glomerular lesions associated with several infectious diseases have been classified histologically as membranous glomerulonephritis, membranoproliferative glomerulonephritis, mesangial glomerulonephritis and focal segmental glomerulosclerosis and appear to be the main causes of proteinuria, CKD and death of affected dogs (Roura et al., 2013). These dogs can initially suffer from a moderate to severe proteinuria in the absence of azotaemia. Moreover, the risk of developing these adverse outcomes increases as the magnitude of proteinuria increases. As glomerular disease progresses, tubulointerstitial lesions, azotaemia and CKD (IRIS CKD Stages 2–4) may develop.

Pathological processes of CKD in the absence of primary glomerular disease

The most common histological finding in the ageing feline kidney is chronic interstitial fibrosis with mild inflammatory interstitial infiltrate, which is thought to occur secondary to tubulointerstitial disease (DiBartola et al., 1987). This interstitial fibrous pathology is also common in dogs, accounting for approximately 50% of CKD (MacDougall et al., 1986); however, glomerular lesions leading to glomerulosclerosis are thought to be the primary pathological process. Irreversible damage to any portion of the nephron results in fibrous scar tissue replacement and expansion of the interstitium. Evidence of active primary glomerular disease is usually absent. In the ageing dog and cat with CKD, following loss of a critical amount of renal mass due to primary extrinsic damage (cause often unknown), the remaining functioning nephrons are thought to adapt in response to local changes within the kidney. These adaptive changes lead to hyperfiltration secondary to glomerular capillary hypertension, possibly as a result of activation locally of the renin–angiotensin system (RAS). Angiotensin II drives the hyperfiltration process by selective constriction of the efferent arteriole. In addition, angiotensin II stimulates nephron hypertrophy. Ultimately, these adaptive changes are detrimental and are thought to lead to further interstitial fibrosis and inflammation, with further nephron loss occurring even in the absence of any extrinsic factors which damage the kidney (the so-called intact nephron hypothesis leading to intrinsic progressive nephron loss).

One would predict, from the above discussion, that dogs and cats with CKD where intrinsic progression was occurring would have higher levels of protein in their urine than dogs and cats where the kidney disease was stable and non-progressive. This is because the severity of the proteinuria might be indicative either of the degree of glomerular lesion, hypertension and hyperfiltration (increasing transglomerular protein flux per nephron) or of the degree of tubular dysfunction (leading to reduced tubular uptake of filtered protein).

Maladaptive glomerular capillary hypertension occurs in the canine and feline kidney, as documented in experimental remnant kidney models (Brown et al., 1993; Brown and Brown, 1995). It is associated with an increase in protein excretion as assessed by measurement of the UPC ratio. This form of secondary (maladaptive) glomerular dysfunction is usually associated with low-level proteinuria. For example, in the remnant kidney model referred to above, prior to removal of kidney tissue the cats had a UPC ratio of 0.07 ± 0.01 on average, and after subtotal nephrectomy and time for compensatory hypertrophy, this increased to an average of 0.31 ± 0.06 (Brown and Brown, 1995). This change in protein excretion was associated with approximately a 10% rise in glomerular capillary pressure measured by micropuncture techniques. Chronic maintenance of this model is associated with development of interstitial fibrosis, moderate inflammatory infiltrate of the interstitium and glomerulosclerosis. Evidence from clinical patients supports the intact nephron hypothesis leading to hyperfiltration and exacerbating proteinuria. For example, in cats, the stage of CKD (plasma creatinine) and hypertension are risk factors for proteinuria (Syme et al., 2006; see below).

Definitive evidence that hyperfiltration driving transglomerular flux of proteins is involved in progressive nephron loss requires intervention studies that reduce hyperfiltration and transglomerular protein flux. To date, intervention studies in laboratory animals and human patients (e.g. Maschio et al., 1996) support the intact nephron hypothesis and its role in driving intrinsic progression. Similar level I evidence from intervention studies in veterinary patients is lacking to date.

Association between proteinuria and progressive renal injury – cellular mechanisms

Plasma proteins that have crossed the glomerular capillary wall can accumulate within the glomerular tuft and stimulate mesangial cell proliferation and increased production of mesangial matrix. In addition, excessive amounts of protein in the glomerular filtrate can be toxic to tubular epithelial cells and can lead to interstitial inflammation, fibrosis and cell death. Proximal tubular cells normally reabsorb protein from the glomerular filtrate by pinocytosis. Albumin and other proteins accumulate in lysosomes and are then degraded into amino acids. In proteinuric conditions, excessive lysosomal processing can result in swelling and rupture of lysosomes, causing enzymatic damage to the cytoplasm. Tubular injury may also occur as a consequence of tubular obstruction with proteinaceous casts. Increased glomerular permeability to plasma proteins allows tubular cell contact with transferrin, complement and lipoproteins. Transferrin increases iron uptake by epithelial cells. Once inside the cell the iron ions catalyse the formation of reactive oxygen species that can cause peroxidative injury. Complement proteins can be activated on the brush border of proximal tubular cells, resulting in insertion of a membrane attack complex followed by cytoskeletal damage and cytolysis. Reabsorbed lipoproteins can release lipid moieties that can accumulate into lipid droplets or be oxidized to toxic radicals. All of these processes could irreversibly damage the proximal tubule and interstitium, resulting in activation of resident fibroblasts to become myofibroblasts, recruitment of circulating marrow-derived myofibroblasts or, more rarely, transdifferentiation of epithelial cells into myofibroblasts (Benali *et al.*, 2014; Mack and Yanagita, 2015). Excessive fibrosis resulting from myofibroblast activation drives subsequent nephron loss.

Association between proteinuria and progressive renal injury – molecular mechanisms

In vitro studies have shown that exposure of proximal tubular cells grown in cell culture to albumin and transferrin in concentrations which overwhelm the ability of these cells to digest the proteins within their lysosomes, will lead to activation of nuclear factor κB (NF-κB), which turns on the expression of genes in these cells and causes them to secrete mediators from their basolateral cell surfaces (i.e. towards the interstitium). These mediators include endothelin-1 (ET-1), monocyte chemoatractant protein-1 (MCP-1) and the immunoregulatory cytokine regulated on activation, normal T cell expressed and secreted (RANTES). Expression and secretion of these proteins can be demonstrated *in vivo* in animal models of proteinuric renal disease. Interventions that reduce proteinuria in these models also reduce the expression of these and other cytokines involved in the progressive interstitial fibrosis (Donadelli *et al.*, 2000). These molecular details may explain why proteinuria is an independent risk factor for progression of kidney disease in human medicine and why drugs such as angiotensin converting enzyme (ACE) inhibitors and angiotensin receptor blockers successfully slow progression in proteinuric kidney diseases, independent of their effects on systemic arterial blood pressure, in humans (Cravedi and Remuzzi, 2013). Figure 5.8 presents these concepts in a schematic diagram (see Remuzzi and Bertani, 1998 for review).

Risk factors for proteinuria in feline and canine CKD

Renal proteinuria is not common in cats in clinical practice. Cats with kidney disease that are non-azotaemic and proteinuric are infrequent, with the possible exceptions of cats positive for feline leukaemia virus (FeLV) or feline immunodeficiency virus (FIV) (see Figure 5.7). On the other hand, cats that are mildly or moderately azotaemic (serum creatinine 140–400 µmol/l) may be non-proteinuric (UPC ratio <0.2), borderline proteinuric (UPC ratio 0.2–0.4) or mildly proteinuric (UPC ratio >0.4 to <1.0). Risk factors associated with proteinuria have been identified in large cross-sectional epidemiological studies. They include serum creatinine concentration (the higher the creatinine the more likely the cat is to be proteinuric) and systolic arterial blood pressure (the higher the blood pressure the more likely the cat is to be proteinuric) (Syme *et al.*, 2006; King *et al.*, 2007). These observations (along with remnant kidney model studies) provide circumstantial evidence to support the hypothesis that cats with naturally occurring CKD hyperfiltrate, particularly as they lose more functioning nephrons. If they have systemic hypertension, the protein loss is greater, presumably because of the inability of diseased kidneys to autoregulate.

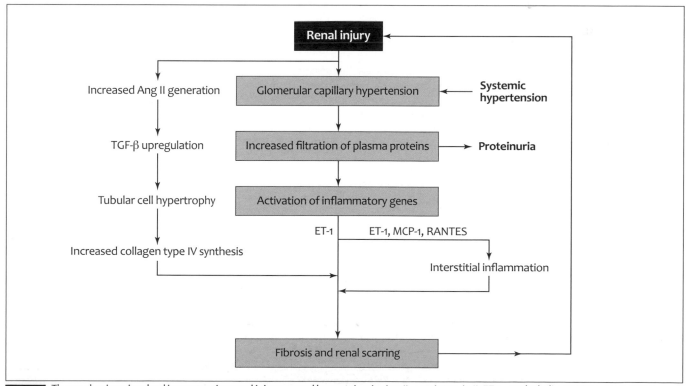

5.8 The mechanisms involved in progressive renal injury caused by proteinuria. Ang II = angiotensin II; ET-1 = endothelin-1; MCP-1 = monocyte chemoatractant protein-1; RANTES = immunoregulatory cytokine regulated on activation, normal T cell expressed and secreted; TGF-β = tissue growth factor-beta.
(Adapted from Remuzzi and Bertani, 1998)

The cats included in the cross-sectional epidemiological study conducted in the UK were also enrolled in a longitudinal survival study (Syme *et al.*, 2006). A Cox proportional hazards model was used to determine the predictive values of age, sex, plasma creatinine concentration, systolic arterial blood pressure and UPC ratio on all-cause mortality. In this study, log UPC ratio as a continuous variable proved to be significantly and independently associated with survival (all-cause mortality), as were age and plasma creatinine concentration. No association was found between gender or systolic blood pressure and survival.

This observation suggests that measurement of the UPC ratio could be used as a prognostic indicator in cats with naturally occurring kidney disease, for all-cause mortality. About 50% of the deaths (including euthanasia) occurring in the population of cats suffering from CKD are the result of progressive kidney disease or acute decompensation of the azotaemic (uraemic) crisis. Further studies involving cats have shown that very low level (borderline) proteinuria (UPC ratio 0.2–0.4) is predictive of the development of azotaemic CKD in geriatric cats undergoing health screens (Jepson *et al.*, 2009) and is predictive of progression (25% increase in plasma creatinine concentration) within the next 12 months in azotaemic cats at the initial diagnosis of CKD (Chakrabarti *et al.*, 2012).

In dogs, proteinuria is more common than in cats, owing to a greater prevalence of glomerular lesions. In dogs with naturally occurring CKD, proteinuria resulting in a UPC ratio ≥1.0 was associated with a three-fold greater risk of the development of uraemic crises and death when compared with dogs with a UPC ratio <1.0 (Jacob *et al.*, 2005). The relative risk of an adverse outcome was approximately 1.5 times higher for every 1-unit increase in the UPC ratio. In addition, dogs with a UPC ratio ≥1.0 had a decrease in renal function that was greater in magnitude than that observed in dogs with a UPC ratio <1.0 (Jacob *et al.*, 2005).

It might be concluded from the available evidence that interventions designed to reduce urinary protein excretion would slow progressive renal injury and, therefore, improve survival in dogs and cats with CKD. This conclusion assumes that protein in the urine of dogs and cats is damaging to the remaining functioning nephrons and so leads to progressive renal injury. Another interpretation of these findings, however, is that the appearance of protein in the urine is merely a marker that progressive renal injury is occurring. In this case, while renoprotective interventions might be expected to reduce protein excretion because they slow progressive renal injury, reducing urine protein excretion by any method will not necessarily prove to be renoprotective. However, all these data indicate to clinicians that the evaluation of proteinuria should improve the management of CKD in dogs and cats because it adds an additional marker to serum creatinine for the evaluation of the progression of the disease. Thus:

- A stable creatinine value with a significant decrease of proteinuria is thought to be a positive response to treatment
- An increase of proteinuria despite a stable serum creatinine concentration could mean worsening of CKD.

It should be noted, however, that severe glomerular disease associated proteinuria (UPC ratio >2) may reduce as the disease progresses purely because of a decrease in the number of functioning nephrons through which protein can be lost.

Summary

Proteinuria is a common disorder in the dog, and to a lesser extent in the cat, that can indicate the presence of renal disease prior to the onset of azotaemia. Proteinuria is a renal disease marker for an early diagnosis in dogs and a marker of progression of CKD in both the dog and the cat. Although a direct pathogenic link between glomerular disease, proteinuria and progressive renal damage has not been established in the dog or cat, attenuation of proteinuria has been associated with decreased renal functional decline in several studies. There is a need to continue to increase our understanding of the effects of proteinuria on the glomerulus, the tubule and the interstitium in dogs and cats. In addition to being a diagnostic marker of renal disease, proteinuria may also contribute to the progressive nature of canine and feline renal disease, making it an important therapeutic target. Proteinuria is commonly associated with primary glomerular diseases, however the loss of renal autoregulation that occurs secondary to nephron loss due to any cause (e.g. vascular, tubular, interstitial, as well as glomerular) can also result in intraglomerular hypertension and proteinuria. Treatments shown to reduce proteinuria are discussed in Chapters 23 and 24.

References and further reading

Benali SL, Lees GE, Castagnaro M *et al.* (2014) Epithelial mesenchymal transition in the progression of renal disease in dogs. *Histology and Histopathology* **29**, 1409–1414

Brown SA and Brown CA (1995) Single-nephron adaptations to partial renal ablation in cats. *American Journal of Physiology* **269**, 1002–1008

Brown SA, Walton CL, Crawford P *et al.* (1993) Long-term effects of antihypertensive regimens on renal hemodynamics and proteinuria. *Kidney International* **43**, 1210–1218

Chakrabarti S, Syme HM and Elliott J (2012) Clinicopathological variables predicting progression of azotemia in cats with chronic kidney disease. *Journal of Veterinary Internal Medicine* **26**, 275–281

Christensen EI, Nielsen R and Birn H (2013) From bowel to kidneys: the role of cubilin in physiology and disease. *Nephrology Dialysis Transplant* **28**, 274–281

Costa FAL, Goto H, Saldanha LCB *et al.* (2003) Histopathologic patterns of nephropathy in naturally acquired canine visceral leishmaniasis. *Veterinary Pathology* **40**, 677–684

Cravedi P and Remuzzi G (2013) Pathophysiology of proteinuria and its value as an outcome measure in chronic kidney disease. *British Journal of Clinical Pharmacology* **76**, 516–523

Dambach DM, Smith CA, Lewis RM *et al.* (1997) Morphologic, immunohistochemical, and ultrastructural characterization of a distinctive renal lesion in dogs putatively associated with *Borrelia burgdorferi* infection: 49 cases (1987–1992). *Veterinary Pathology* **34**, 85–96

DiBartola SP, Rutgers HC, Zack PM and Tarr MJ (1987) Clinicopathologic findings associated with chronic renal disease in cats: 74 cases (1973–1984). *Journal of the American Veterinary Medical Association* **190(9)**, 1196–1202

Donadelli R, Abbate M, Zachi C *et al.* (2000) Protein traffic activates NF-kB signaling and promotes MCP-1-dependent interstitial inflammation. *American Journal of Kidney Diseases* **36**, 1226–1241

Hanzlicek AS, Roof CJ, Sanderson MW *et al.* (2012) Comparison of urine dipstick, sulfosalicylic acid, urine protein-to-creatinine ratio and a feline-specific immunoassay for detection of albuminuria in cats with chronic kidney disease. *Journal of Feline Medicine and Surgery* **14**, 882–888

IRIS Glomerular Disease Study Group: Goldstein RE, Brovida C, Fernández-Del Palacio MJ *et al.* (2013) Consensus recommendations for treatment for dogs with serology positive glomerular disease. *Journal of Veterinary Internal Medicine* **27(Suppl 1)**, 60–66

IRIS Glomerular Disease Study Group: Littman MP, Daminet S, Grauer GF *et al.* (2013) Consensus recommendations for the diagnostic investigation of dogs with suspected glomerular disease. *Journal of Veterinary Internal Medicine* **27(Suppl 1)**, 19–26

Jacob F, Polzin DJ, Osborne CA *et al.* (2005) Evaluation of the association between initial proteinuria and morbidity rate or death in dogs with naturally occurring chronic renal failure. *Journal of the American Veterinary Medical Association* **226**, 393–400

Jepson RE, Brodbelt D, Vallance C *et al.* (2009) Evaluation of predictors of the development of azotemia in cats. *Journal of Veterinary Internal Medicine* **23**, 806–813

King JN, Tasker S, Gunn-Moore DA *et al.* (2007) Prognostic factors in cats with chronic kidney disease. *Journal of Veterinary Internal Medicine* **21**, 906–916

Lees GE, Brown, SA, Elliott J *et al.* (2005) Assessment and management of proteinuria in dogs and cats: 2004 ACVIM Forum Consensus Statement (Small Animal). *Journal of Veterinary Internal Medicine* **19**, 377–385

Littman MP (2011) Protein-losing nephropathy in small animals. *Veterinary Clinics of North America: Small Animal Practice* **41**, 31–62

Lyon SD, Sanderson MW, Vaden SL *et al.* (2010) Comparison of urine dipstick, sulfosalicylic acid, urine protein-to-creatinine ratio, and species-specific ELISA methods for detection of albumin in urine samples of cats and dogs. *Journal of the American Veterinary Medical Association* **236**, 874–879

MacDougall DF, Cook T, Steward AP and Cattell V (1986) Canine chronic renal disease: prevalence and types of glomerulonephritis in the dog. *Kidney International* **29(6)**, 1144–1151

Mack M and Yanagita M (2015) Origin of myofibroblasts and cellular events triggering fibrosis. *Kidney International* **87**, 297–307

Maschio G, Alberti D, Janin G *et al.* (1996) Effect of the angiotensin-converting-enzyme inhibitor benazepril on the progression of chronic renal insufficiency. The Angiotensin-Converting-Enzyme Inhibition in Progressive Renal Insufficiency Study Group. *New England Journal of Medicine* **334**, 939–945

McCaw DL, Knapp DW and Hewett JE (1985) Effect of collection time and exercise restriction on the prevention of urine protein excretion using urine protein/creatinine ratio in dogs. *American Journal of Veterinary Research* **46**, 1665–1669

Miyazaki M, Fujiwara K, Suzuta Y *et al.* (2011) Screening for proteinuria in cats using a conventional dipstick test after removal of cauxin from urine with a Lens culinaris agglutinin lectin tip. *The Veterinary Journal* **189**, 312–317

Miyazaki M, Kamiie K, Soeta S, Taira H and Yamashita T (2003) Molecular cloning and characterization of a novel carboxylesterase-like protein that is physiologically present at high concentrations in the urine of domestic cats (*Felis catus*). *Biochemical Journal* **370**, 101–110

Nabity MB, Boggess MM, Kashtan CE *et al.* (2007) Day-to-day variation of the urine protein:creatinine ratio in female dogs with stable glomerular proteinuria caused by X-linked hereditary nephropathy. *Journal of Veterinary Internal Medicine* **21**, 425–430

Patrakka J and Tryggvason K (2010) Molecular make-up of the glomerular filtration barrier. *Biochemical and Biophysical Research Communications* **396**, 164–169

Pierantozzi M, Roura X, Paltrinieri S *et al.* (2013) Variation of proteinuria in dogs with leishmaniasis treated with meglumine antimoniate and allopurinol: retrospective study. *Journal of the American Animal Hospital Association* **49**, 231–236

Remuzzi G and Bertani T (1998) Pathophysiology of progressive nephropathies. *New England Journal of Medicine* **339**, 1448–1456

Rossi G, Giori L, Campagnola S *et al.* (2012) Evaluation of factors that affect analytic variability of urine protein-to-creatinine ratio determination in dogs. *American Journal of Veterinary Research* **73**, 779–788

Roura X, Fondati A, Lubas G *et al.* (2013) Prognosis and monitoring of leishmaniasis in dogs. *The Veterinary Journal* **198**, 43–47

Syme HM, Markwell PJ, Pfeiffer DU *et al.* (2006) Survival of cats with naturally occurring chronic renal failure is related to severity of proteinuria. *Journal of Veterinary Internal Medicine* **20**, 528–535

Vaden SL, Pressler BM, Lappin MR and Jensen WA (2004) Effects of urinary tract inflammation and sample blood contamination on urine albumin and total protein concentrations in canine urine samples. *Veterinary Clinical Pathology* **33(1)**, 14–19

Zatelli A, Borgarelli M, Santilli R *et al.* (2003) Glomerular lesions in dogs infected with *Leishmania* organisms. *American Journal of Veterinary Research* **64**, 558–561

Zatelli A, Paltrinieri S, Nizi F *et al.* (2010) Evaluation of a urine dipstick test for confirmation or exclusion of proteinuria in dogs. *American Journal of Veterinary Research* **71**, 235–240

Chapter 6

Complete urinalysis

Rick Alleman and Heather Wamsley

A complete urinalysis (Figure 6.1) includes assessment of both the physical and chemical properties of urine. It requires minimal specialized equipment and can be routinely performed by trained individuals in general veterinary practice. With proper sample handling and appropriate testing, urinalysis can provide vital information about the urinary tract and can also be an indicator of disease states in the liver, peripheral blood or endocrine system. Some indications for urinalysis are found in Figure 6.2.

To avoid potential misinterpretation of laboratory results, all components of a complete urinalysis (Figure 6.1) should ideally be performed. For example, knowledge of the urine specific gravity (USG) is necessary for effective interpretation of the serum urea, serum creatinine, urine protein and urine bilirubin concentrations. In addition, microscopic examination of the urine sediment for signs of active inflammation or infection is required to determine the significance of proteinuria by aiding in its localization (e.g. renal *versus* lower urinary tract).

- Gross inspection of the urine
- Specific chemical testing of the urine
- Microscopic examination of the urine sediment

6.1 Components of complete urinalysis.

- Aids in interpretation of elevated serum urea nitrogen and creatinine concentrations
- Screen for occult disease in clinically normal patients:
  - Annual health screening
  - Pre-anaesthetic
  - Geriatric
- Minimum laboratory database for diseased patients:
  - Clinical signs referable to the urinary system
  - Clinical signs referable to other body systems:
    - Endocrine (e.g. detect glucosuria or urinary tract infection)
    - Hepatic (e.g. detect bilirubinuria or ammonium biurate crystals)
    - Haematological (e.g. help localize haemolysis as intravascular by detecting haemoglobinuria)
    - Neurological (e.g. detect bacteriuria associated with discospondylitis)
    - Toxicosis (e.g. ethylene glycol)
    - Polyuric/polydipsic disorders
- Tool for monitoring:
  - Progression of renal disease
  - Response to therapy for urinary tract disease
  - Safety of potentially nephrotoxic drugs

6.2 Indications for and uses of complete urinalysis.

Urine sample collection method, timing and handling prior to analysis

Urinalysis results and the interpretation of those results can be influenced by the urine collection method, the timing of urine collection, administration of therapeutic or diagnostic agents prior to collection and sample handling prior to analysis. There are several methods of urine collection, each with advantages and disadvantages (Figures 6.3 and 6.4). Ideally at least 6 ml of urine should be collected for analysis and, if possible, the sample should be collected prior to the administration of fluids or diuretics. Either naturally voided urine collected midstream into a sterile container or urine obtained by cystocentesis is preferred. It is sometimes necessary to retrieve a voided sample from the top of an examination table or from the floor. If this is necessary, the smallest gauge needle should be attached to a syringe in order to aspirate the urine sample. A urine sample collected by this method will probably be contaminated by disinfectants, cleansers or residues from other cleaning products. Some chemical tests (e.g. glucose, haem, pH, protein) may be affected by these residues. The collection method should always be recorded because results can be significantly affected by the method used to obtain the sample.

Urinalysis results are also affected by the timing of urine collection relative to ingestion of water or a meal, or by how long the urine has been stored within the bladder (Figure 6.5). As with the collection method, the intended purpose of

---

- General:
  - Sterile, sealable, opaque, plastic sample cup
  - 6 ml sterile syringe
- Natural voiding (feline):
  - Non-absorbent plastic granular litter
- Catheterization:
  - Sterile urinary catheter in good condition
  - Sterile gloves
  - Sterile lubricant
- Cystocentesis:
  - Dogs: 22 G sterile needle, 38 mm (1.5 inch) to 76 mm (3 inch), depending on patient size
  - Cats: 23 G sterile needle, 16 mm (0.625 inch) to 25 mm (1 inch), depending on patient size
- If intended for urine culture:
  - Culture tube

6.3 Materials that may be used during urine collection.

Collection method	Advantages	Disadvantages/precautions
Midstream, naturally voided	• Non-invasive, relatively easy technique (in dogs) • Can be performed by clients and is therefore useful to collect the first morning, maximally concentrated, urine samples from outpatients • Unlike cystocentesis or catheterization, is not associated with iatrogenic haematuria • Although not ideal, a freshly voided sample can be used for urine culture, as long as a quantitative urine culture is performed	• Likely to be contaminated by a variable amount of material from the lower genitourinary tract (e.g. bacteria, epithelial cells, blood, sperm, debris), perineum (e.g. *Trichuris* ova) or environment (e.g. pollen), which may be observed during microscopic examination of the urine sediment • Cleanser residues or microorganisms within the collection vessel may affect results. Urine should be collected into a sterile single-use urine collection cup rather than a reusable container provided by the client or veterinary practice • Avoid manual bladder compression to induce micturition, which may cause reflux of urine into other organs (e.g. kidneys, prostate) or iatrogenic haematuria
Transurethral catheterization	• Useful collection method when an indwelling urinary catheter is already present for another reason • Although not ideal, sample can be used for urine culture, as long as a quantitative urine culture is performed	• Risk of traumatic catheterization, which may injure the patient and contaminate the sample with blood • Risk of iatrogenic infection, especially in patients predisposed to urinary tract infection (e.g. lower urinary tract disease, kidney disease, diabetes mellitus, hyperadrenocorticism) • Should be performed aseptically and atraumatically by a trained, experienced individual • Urine sample may be contaminated by variable numbers of epithelial cells, bacteria and debris from the lower genitourinary tract, which may be observed during microscopic examination of the urine sediment • Catheters that are chemically sterilized may contain residue of the antiseptic solution, which can irritate mucosal linings and affect results of urinalysis and urine culture • Catheterization may be technically challenging in female patients. Use of a vaginal endoscope may facilitate collection
Antepubic cystocentesis	• Avoids lower genitourinary tract contamination of urine sample • Ideal sample for urine culture • Less risk of iatrogenic infection than with transurethral catheterization • Easier than collection of a voided sample from cats • Better tolerated than catheterization, especially by cats and bitches	• Contraindicated in patients with a bleeding diathesis (e.g. thrombocytopenia), may be performed with great caution after cystotomy • An adequate volume of urine within the bladder is required • Blind cystocentesis without at least manual localization and immobilization of the bladder is not recommended. Ultrasound-guided needle placement is helpful, though not mandatory • Misdirection of the needle can lead to a non-diagnostic or contaminated sample (e.g. enterocentesis) • A variable degree of iatrogenic microscopic haematuria, which cannot be readily distinguished from pathological, disease-induced haematuria, may be caused by this collection method. This type of contamination can be particularly pronounced when the bladder wall is inflamed or congested. Iatrogenic haematuria may limit the utility of this collection method when monitoring the progression of disease in a patient that has pathological haematuria

6.4 The advantages and disadvantages of different methods of urine collection.

Collection time	Advantages	Disadvantages
First morning urine – urine is formed after a period of several hours of nil by mouth	• Represents the patient's maximally concentrated urine and is therefore ideal for assessing the ability of the renal tubules to concentrate urine • Microscopic sediment will be more concentrated • Postprandial alterations unlikely (e.g. postprandial alkalinuria) • Urine more likely to be acidic, so casts may be better preserved (proteinaceous structures dissolve in alkaline urine)	• Urine present within bladder for a relatively prolonged period • May alter cellular morphology observed during microscopic examination • May decrease viability of fastidious microorganisms, resulting in false-negative culture results
Postprandial	• Useful to assess the effect of diets intended to modulate urinary pH when collected 3–6 hours postprandially • More likely to detect hyperglycaemic glucosuria when collected 3–4 hours postprandially	• pH may be elevated by postprandial alkaline tide when collected within 1 hour postprandially
Randomly timed urine sample – represents urine that has accumulated within the bladder for minutes to hours or urine that has been diluted by recent ingestion of water	• Microscopic cellular morphology and viability of fastidious microorganisms may be better preserved because urine is stored within the bladder for relatively less time	• If the urine is isosthenuric or minimally concentrated, no conclusion can be drawn about renal tubular concentrating ability

6.5 Timing of urine sample collection, indications and potential effects upon urinalysis results.

the sample is a useful factor to consider when selecting the timing of urine collection. For example, culture of a randomly collected urine sample may be more useful than culture of the first morning urine. First morning urine typically is held within the bladder overnight for several hours, which may decrease the viability of fastidious microorganisms and cause a false-negative urine culture. Similarly, cellular morphology may be better preserved in a randomly collected urine sample, rather than in urine which has been held overnight within the bladder, because urine pH and nitrogenous waste materials may cause cells to degenerate.

A key goal of urine sample collection is to obtain and analyse a sample that most closely represents the urine *in vivo*. One step in achieving this goal is to handle urine samples in a way which minimizes the effects of post-collection *in vitro* artefacts (Figure 6.6). Ideally, urine should be collected into a sterile opaque sealable labelled container and analysed within 60 minutes of collection. If it is not possible to analyse the sample within 60 minutes or if it must be shipped to a diagnostic laboratory, the sample should be preserved by refrigeration soon after collection for up to approximately 12 hours (e.g. overnight). Samples intended for routine urinalysis should not be frozen. In addition, although numerous chemical preservatives of urine exist (e.g. boric acid, formalin, Mucolexx®), routine use of these preservatives is not recommended, because each may affect different components of the urinalysis.

Refrigeration is the optimal preservation method because it prevents bacterial overgrowth, preserves cellular and cast morphology and does not affect chemical testing as long as the sample is returned to room temperature prior to analysis. However, refrigeration can cause artefactual changes, particularly crystal formation (i.e. calcium oxalate dihydrate, magnesium ammonium phosphate), which increases as the duration of storage increases (Albasan *et al.*, 2003). To minimize refrigeration artefacts, samples should be allowed to warm to room temperature prior to urinalysis. Furthermore, if crystalluria is observed in a sample that has been refrigerated or that has been stored for more than 6 hours regardless of the storage temperature, the finding should be confirmed with a freshly obtained, non-refrigerated urine sample that will be analysed within 30–60 minutes of collection.

Urinalysis method

During complete urinalysis several physical and chemical characteristics of urine are evaluated (see Figure 6.1). A list of the materials needed and a detailed method of routine urinalysis are provided in Figures 6.7 and 6.8. Urinalysis may yield erroneous results if laboratory materials are used incorrectly, if materials have been stored improperly or if materials are used that have not been validated in veterinary species.

Urine dipsticks

Urine dipstick multiple chemical test strips have various reagents impregnated within each test pad. Guidelines for appropriate use and storage of urine dipsticks are provided in Figure 6.9. Many of the dipstick reagents will be damaged by exposure to light or to disinfectant cleansers, which can cause false-positive or false-negative results, depending upon the test. To prevent inactivation of the reagents, urine dipsticks should be stored with the lid tightly sealed in the container provided by the manufacturer or another airtight container that completely obstructs light. If urine dipsticks are desired at more than one workstation, empty used containers provided by the manufacturer may be refilled and placed at each workstation, as long as the same type of dipstick is used to refill the container (i.e. the urine dipstick must correspond to the interpretation key printed on the outside of the container).

- Ideal urine sample handling:
  - Urine should be collected in a sterile, opaque, airtight, labelled container
  - Either analysis should occur within 1 hour of collection or the sample should be refrigerated until the time for analysis (for up to 12 hours)
  - If the sample has been refrigerated, it should be warmed to room temperature prior to analysis to minimize artefacts caused by cooling of the sample
- Potential artefacts associated with refrigeration:
  - *In vitro* crystal formation (especially calcium oxalate dihydrate) increases with the duration of storage. When clinically significant crystalluria is suspected, it is best to confirm the finding with a freshly collected urine sample that has not been refrigerated and which is analysed within 1 hour of collection
  - A cold urine sample may inhibit enzymatic reactions in the dipstick (e.g. glucose), leading to falsely decreased results
  - The specific gravity of cold urine may be falsely increased, because cold urine is denser than room temperature urine
- Potential artefacts associated with prolonged storage at room temperature:
  - Bacterial overgrowth can cause:
    - Increased urine turbidity
    - Altered pH:
      o Increased pH, if urease-producing bacteria are present
      o Decreased pH, if bacteria use glucose to form acidic metabolites
    - Decreased concentration of chemicals that may be metabolized by bacteria (e.g. glucose, ketones)
    - Increased number of bacteria in urine sediment
    - Altered urine culture results
  - Increased urine pH, which may occur because of loss of carbon dioxide from the sample or bacterial overgrowth, can cause:
    - False-positive dipstick protein reaction
    - Degeneration of cells and casts
    - Alteration of the type and amount of crystals present
- Other potential artefacts:
  - Evaporative loss of volatile substances (e.g. carbon dioxide, ketones, urine water). Avoid this artefact by using an airtight sample container
  - Photodegradation of light-sensitive chemicals (e.g. bilirubin, urobilinogen). Avoid this artefact by using a sample container that does not transmit light (i.e. an opaque sample container)

6.6 Ideal conditions for urine sample handling and potential *in vitro* artefacts associated with urine storage.

- Sterile single-use translucent 15 ml polystyrene conical centrifuge tubes with lids
- Translucent test tubes
- Test tube rack
- Disposable transfer pipettes
- Clean glass microscope slides
- Clean 22 x 22 mm glass coverslips
- Temperature-compensated veterinary refractometer, ideally one with a feline urine specific gravity scale
- Timer that indicates seconds
- Urine dipstick multiple chemical test strip
- Centrifuge
- Microscope with X10 and X40 objectives
- Optional items:
  - Portable pH meter
  - 5% sulphosalicyclic acid
  - Rapid aqueous stain (e.g. new methylene blue, Sedi-Stain™)
  - Diff Quick® or other aqueous-based modified Wright's stain

6.7 Materials needed for complete urinalysis.

1. Ideally collect at least 6 ml of urine by cystocentesis or midstream during natural micturition into a sterile, opaque, sealable container.
2. Record the following in the medical record and on the sample submission form, if a referral laboratory is to be used:
   - Urine collection method
   - Time of urine collection
   - Volume of urine collected
   - Method of preservation, if applicable (e.g. refrigeration, chemical)
   - Medications (e.g. antibiotics, diuretics, glucocorticoids), prescription diet or diagnostic agents administered (e.g. radiographic contrast medium)
   - Whether or not the patient was fasted.
3. Ensure that the container holding the urine, not just the lid, is adequately labelled (e.g. patient identification, date, collection method).
4. If the sample has been refrigerated, allow it to warm to room temperature before performing the urinalysis.
5. Mix the sample well and then transfer 5 ml of urine into a labelled conical centrifuge tube. Save the remaining urine in the refrigerator for additional or confirmatory tests, if indicated.
6. In a well-lit area, against a white background, perform a gross inspection of the urine in the conical tube:
   - Record the urine colour (e.g. light yellow, yellow, dark yellow, red–brown)
   - Record the clarity of the urine (e.g. cloudy, slightly cloudy, clear).
7. Perform biochemical evaluation using a urine dipstick multiple chemical test strip and a timer that indicates seconds:
   - Wet each pad of the test strip either by briefly immersing the strip in the urine sample or by using a pipette to place individual drops of urine on each test pad and then start the timer. Avoid oversaturation or prolonged contact of the test pads with urine. Dab excess urine from the test pads. Do not allow urine from adjacent pads to mix
   - Observe colour changes at the times indicated on the bottle, compare to the coloured squares on the bottle and record the results.
8. Centrifuge the sample to prepare for additional biochemical tests and microscopic examination of the sediment:
   - Centrifuge the 5 ml aliquot of urine in the conical tube (from Step 5) for 5 minutes at 400 x g (1500 rpm)
   - After centrifugation, observe the tube for the presence of a lipid layer floating at the top of the supernatant. If lipid is present, record its approximate volume, remove it from the supernatant and discard it
   - Remove and save in a separate tube 4 ml of the supernatant (or 80% of the original volume, if the initial aliquot volume was less than 5 ml (at Step 5)) for additional biochemical tests. Save the sediment and remaining 1 ml (i.e. 20%) of supernatant for microscopic examination.
9. Perform additional biochemical tests on the 4 ml aliquot of supernatant:
   - Determine the urine specific gravity using a refractometer. Place one or two drops of urine supernatant on the refractometer and determine the specific gravity using the appropriate scale. If the indicated specific gravity is greater than the upper limit of the refractometer scale (usually 1.050 or 1.060), the sample should be diluted and re-read to obtain a more precise measurement if one is desired:
     – Dilute the sample 1-to-1 with distilled water and mix well
     – Place one or two drops of diluted urine on the refractometer and determine the specific gravity using the appropriate scale. This value must be adjusted for the dilution factor before it is reported
     – Adjust the indicated specific gravity for the dilution by multiplying the last two digits by 2 and report the adjusted value (e.g. if the specific gravity of the diluted sample is 1.035, report the specific gravity as 1.070)
   - (Optional) Perform the 5% sulphosalicylic acid precipitation test for protein:
     – Completely mix equal parts (approximately 0.5 ml each) of urine supernatant and 5% sulphosalicylic acid in a translucent test tube
     – In a well-lit area, against a dark background, inspect the tube for the formation of white precipitate (e.g. cloudy white with or without flocculation) and interpret according to a standard scale (see Figure 6.24).
10. Prepare the sediment for microscopic examination:
    - Resuspend the sediment pellet in the remaining 1 ml of supernatant that was left in the conical tube (at Step 8) (or resuspend the pellet in the remaining 20% of the original volume, if the initial aliquot volume was less than 5 ml (at Step 5))
    - Mix the solution by gentle agitation of the conical tube (e.g. by finger-flicking the bottom) or by aspirating the remaining 1 ml of fluid and gently expressing it back into the tube a few times using a transfer pipette. Casts are fragile, so it is imperative to mix the solution well, while avoiding overly aggressive agitation (e.g. vortexing)
    - Prepare a wet mount of the sediment solution. Pipette a single drop of the sediment solution on to one end of a clean glass microscope slide and coverslip. The slide is ready for examination. If the slide will not be examined immediately, the slide should be stored in a humidified Petri dish, as described below
    - (Optional) Stain the sediment solution and prepare a wet mount of the stained solution. Mix 2 drops of the sediment solution and 1 drop of new methylene blue (or other rapid aqueous stain) in a separate test tube and gently mix. Pipette a single drop of this solution on to the other end of the clean glass microscope slide. The slide, which now holds two wet mounts, is now ready for examination
    - If there will be a delay between the time that the sediment wet mount is prepared and the time that it is examined, the wet mount should be stored in a humidified Petri dish to prevent evaporation of the sample:
      – Place a dampened thin piece of absorbent material (e.g. paper towel, gauze, filter paper) in the bottom portion of a Petri dish
      – Place wooden sticks prepared from the broken handle of a cotton-tipped applicator on top of the moist absorbent material
      – Place the microscope slide with the sediment wet mount on top of the wooden sticks
      – Cover the Petri dish with the provided lid. The wet mount will be stable for up to an hour. Multiple sediments can be prepared and examined in a batch if this procedure is followed.
11. Perform systematic microscopic examination of sediment using reduced illumination:
    - Reduce the illumination of the microscope slide either by lowering the microscope's condenser to a couple of centimetres below the stage or by partially closing the aperture of the iris diaphragm within the condenser. (Both lowering the condenser and closing the iris diaphragm will reduce the light excessively and should not be done)
    - Examine 10 microscopic fields of the slide under low power using the X10 objective for the presence of the following things and provide an assessment of their amounts in the unstained wet mount:
      – Crystals: record type(s) present, and qualitative impression of the amount of each type of crystal (none, few, moderate number, many)
      – Casts: may be better visualized at the margins of the coverslip. Record type(s) present (e.g. hyaline, cellular, granular, waxy, lipid, haemoglobin) and record the number of each type of cast per X10 low power field (lpf) as a range (e.g. 0–2/lpf)
      – Epithelial cells: record type(s) present and the number of each type of epithelial cell per X10 lpf as a range (e.g. 0–2/lpf). Observe cellular morphology for the presence of dysplastic or neoplastic changes
      – Mucus threads: record qualitative impression of the number of mucus threads (none, few, moderate number, many)
      – Helminth ova, larva, adult worms or other parasites: record qualitative impression of the number of parasite structures (none, few, moderate number, many)

6.8 Method for routine analysis. (continues) ▶

- Examine 10 microscopic fields of the slide under higher power using the X40 objective. Scrutinize the morphology of structures observed at low power. Confirm the identification of the structures observed at low power. Again, inspect epithelial cells for dysplastic or neoplastic morphological changes. Inspect the slide for the presence of the following things and provide an assessment of their amounts in the unstained wet mount:
  - Erythrocytes: record the number or erythrocytes per X40 high power field (hpf) as a range (e.g. 2–4/hpf)
  - Leucocytes: record the number of leucocytes per X40 hpf as a range (0–3/hpf)
  - Microorganisms (e.g. bacteria, yeast, fungi, algae): record morphology of bacteria (e.g. cocci, bacilli, filamentous, spore-forming) and qualitative impression of the number of each type of microorganism (none, few, moderate number, many)
  - Lipid droplets: lipid droplets need to be distinguished from erythrocytes. They are variably sized, refractile and often float above the focal plane. Record qualitative impression of the number of lipid droplets (none, few, moderate number, many)
  - Sperm: record qualitative impression of the number of sperm (none, few, moderate number, many)
  - Other structures or unidentified structures: identify the structures or describe their morphology and record qualitative impression of the number of these structures (none, few, moderate number, many)

6.8 (continued) Method for routine analysis.

Oversaturation of test pads with urine can dilute the reagents and cause false results (e.g. false-positive dipstick protein). Also, urine should not be allowed to flow from one test pad to another. This can cause reagents in one test pad to intermingle with those in the adjacent pad, invalidating the results. For example, on the Multistix® dipstick, the pH test pad is immediately adjacent to the protein test pad, which contains an acidic buffer. If the acidic buffer from the protein test pad contaminates the pH test pad, the measured pH will be falsely decreased. Suggested ways to avoid oversaturation and cross-contamination of test pads are provided in Figures 6.9 and 6.10.

- Store urine dipsticks sealed in the container provided by the manufacturer
- If the urine sample has been refrigerated, allow the aliquot of the sample that will be tested to warm to room temperature before urinalysis
- Mix the sample well so that materials (e.g. erythrocytes) which may have sedimented due to gravity are in solution
- Avoid oversaturating the dipstick test pads with urine and do not allow urine to mix between dipstick test pads (see Figure 6.11):
  - Wet each pad of the test strip either by briefly immersing the strip in the urine sample or by using a pipette to place individual drops of urine on each test pad and then start the timer. If a pipette is used, make sure that the surface tension of the urine drops is disrupted so that the urine soaks completely into the test pad
  - Dab excess urine from the test pads by laying the dipstick horizontally on a paper towel and gently elevating one edge of the dipstick along its axis so that excess urine is pulled by gravity and capillary action into the paper towel
- Observe test pad colour changes at the interpretation times designated by the manufacturer on the label, not before or after
- The following dipstick reactions are not valid or useful in dogs and cats and should be ignored if they are present on the dipstick:
  - Leucocytes: specific but insensitive in dogs; invalid in cats
  - Nitrite
  - Specific gravity
  - Urobilinogen

6.9 Guidelines for appropriate use and storage of urine dipstick multiple chemical test strips.

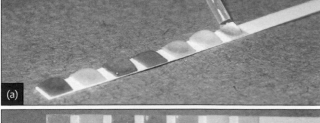
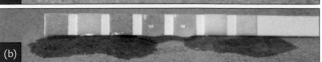

6.10 Application of urine to the urine dipstick pad. (a) Placement of individual drops of urine on to each test pad, breaking the surface tension of each drop after placement. (b) Careful removal of excess urine to avoid oversaturation of the test pads and intermingling of reagents between test pads.

Interpretation of urine dipsticks is based upon the colour change that occurs within a specific time after urine is applied to the test pad (Figure 6.11). Colour will continue to develop beyond the indicated interpretation time, therefore results observed after the designated interpretation times are invalid. Cold urine will slow enzymatic reactions that occur in some of the test pads on the dipstick (e.g. glucose) and cause falsely decreased results. To avoid this artefact of refrigeration, allow the sample to warm to room temperature before urinalysis. Abnormally coloured urine will also affect interpretation of some tests (e.g. bilirubin, ketones). Well maintained (regularly calibrated and serviced) automated urine strip readers will provide standardized assessment of these simple tests and produce an electronic record to go into the patient files.

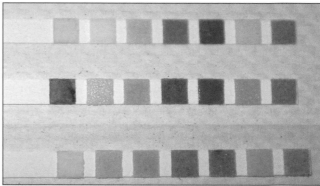

6.11 Interpretation of urine dipstick test reactions is based upon the colour change that develops within the specific amount of time designated by the manufacturer. Distilled water was placed on the top dipstick for comparison with the lower two dipsticks, to which urine from two different patients was applied. The middle dipstick exhibits a strongly positive reaction for glucose and haem and moderate reaction for protein. The bottom dipstick reveals a weakly positive reaction for haem and protein.

Refractometer

Guidelines for appropriate use and storage of refractometers are provided in Figure 6.12. Refractometers are used to estimate the USG, which is an indication of how much solute is dissolved in the urine (i.e. the concentration of the urine). Refractometric estimation of USG is performed to determine the ability of the renal tubules to conserve water and produce well concentrated urine. Refractometers take advantage of the fact that a beam of light is bent when it passes from air into water. The degree to which the beam of light is bent is directly proportional to the number of molecules that are dissolved in solution. However, the light beam is also bent by other materials (e.g. cells, crystals, mucus, bacteria) that are present within the urine. The presence of these other materials causes overestimation of the USG determined by refractometry and, therefore, overestimation of the renal tubular

- Store refractometers away from heating and cooling vents
- If the urine sample has been refrigerated, allow the aliquot of the sample that will be tested to warm to room temperature before urinalysis
- Measure the urine specific gravity of the supernatant formed after centrifugation
- Use a veterinary refractometer with canine and feline scales. Alternatively, for feline urine samples, use the formula to convert human urine specific gravity values to the corresponding feline value:

Feline specific gravity = (0.846 x human specific gravity) + 0.154

6.12 Guidelines for use and storage of refractometers.

ability to conserve water and produce concentrated urine. This potential inaccuracy can be avoided by measuring the SG of the supernatant after centrifugation of the urine, which causes cells, crystals, etc. to collect in the sediment pellet (see Figure 6.8).

Most newer refractometers are temperature-compensated and are designed to be used at ambient temperatures. Refractometers should be stored away from heating and cooling vents, as this may cause spurious results. Also, cold fluids are denser than warm fluids. Therefore, the USG determined by refractometry is falsely increased in urine that is cold. To avoid this artefact of refrigeration, allow the sample to warm to room temperature before urinalysis.

Feline urine is naturally more refractive than canine and human urine. Consequently, feline USG will be slightly overestimated to a variable degree when a refractometer designed for humans is used (i.e. by approximately 0.002–0.005 units). There are two possible ways to prevent this inaccuracy. Feline USG can be measured using a veterinary refractometer that has separate scales for canine and feline samples. Alternatively, feline USG can be calculated using a formula to convert the USG indicated by a human refractometer to the equivalent feline value (George, 2001). The conversion formula for feline USG is as follows:

Feline USG = (0.846 x human USG) + 0.154

Urine sediment evaluation

Guidelines for urine sediment preparation and evaluation are provided in Figure 6.13. Because increased concentrations of cells, casts, microorganisms or crystals may indicate underlying urinary tract disease, one goal of urine sediment evaluation is to determine semiquantitatively the concentration of these materials within the urine. In addition to the patient's urinary tract health, the concentrations of these materials are directly affected by how the sediment is prepared.

Given that cells, crystals, etc. will spontaneously sediment due to gravity, it is necessary to mix the urine sample well before removing an aliquot for centrifugation to ensure that the urine sediment wet mount is fully representative of the whole urine sample. Also, the concentration of the sediment is affected by the starting urine aliquot volume that is centrifuged to form the sediment pellet and the volume of supernatant urine that is used to resuspend the sediment pellet prior to wet mounting. For example, if two aliquots of urine, one containing 10 ml and one containing 5 ml, were centrifuged, there would be twice as much material in the sediment formed from the 10 ml urine aliquot as in the sediment formed from the 5 ml urine aliquot. If the sediment pellets of both urine aliquots were resuspended in an equal volume of supernatant (e.g. 1 ml), then the sediment prepared from the 10 ml urine aliquot would give the false impression of

1. Since cells, crystals, casts etc. will spontaneously sediment due to gravity, mix the whole urine sample well before removing an aliquot for centrifugation to ensure that the urine sediment wet mount is representative of the whole urine sample.
2. Use a standard volume aliquot of urine for centrifugation (e.g. 5 ml).
3. Use a standard volume of urine supernatant to resuspend the sediment pellet (i.e. 20% of the original aliquot volume):
   - If centrifuged 5 ml of urine, remove 4 ml of supernatant and resuspend the pellet in the remaining 1 ml
   - If centrifuged 4 ml of urine, remove 3.2 ml of supernatant and resuspend the pellet in the remaining 0.8 ml
   - If centrifuged 3 ml of urine, remove 2.4 ml of supernatant and resuspend the pellet in the remaining 0.6 ml
   - If centrifuged 2 ml of urine, remove 1.6 ml of supernatant and resuspend the pellet in the remaining 0.4 ml
4. Examine a standard number of microscopic fields (i.e. 10 fields) using both the X10 and X40 objectives.
5. Determine the concentration of materials within the sediment in the unstained wet mount (e.g. cells per high power field as a range, i.e. 0–2), since the addition of stain dilutes the sediment.
6. Stain (e.g. new methylene blue) is helpful for identification of nucleated structures, but may form crystals or may be contaminated with microorganisms. If crystals or microorganisms are observed in a stained sediment wet mount, confirm their presence in an unstained wet mount of the sediment.

6.13 Guidelines for urine sediment preparation and evaluation.

increased concentrations of cells, microorganisms, etc. and may lead one to conclude wrongly that urinary tract disease exists. To avoid this type of error, a standard urine volume should be used as an aliquot for centrifugation and the resultant pellet should be resuspended in a standard volume of supernatant.

Reference values for interpretation of urine sediment concentrations of cells and casts are based upon sediment pellets that were resuspended in 20% of the original urine aliquot volume; 5 ml is generally recommended as a reasonable urine aliquot volume for centrifugation, and it is generally recommended that a pellet formed by centrifugation of 5 ml of urine be resuspended in 1 ml of supernatant, which represents 20% of the original volume. If 5 ml of urine is not available for analysis, the volume of supernatant used to resuspend the pellet will need to be adjusted down to account for the smaller volume of urine available for centrifugation. The volume of supernatant used should be adjusted down to 20% of whatever the original urine aliquot volume is (e.g. resuspend the pellet formed from a 4 ml urine aliquot in 0.8 ml of supernatant, rather than 1 ml) (Figure 6.13). There are commercial urinalysis centrifugation systems (e.g. StatSpin® Urine Sediment Analysis System) that use smaller urine volumes to prepare urine sediments for microscopic examination. Follow the manufacturer's usage and maintenance guidelines to ensure uniform, standardized results.

Since the concentrations of materials observed in urine are reported as a range per microscopic field (e.g. 0–2 leucocytes per high power field), a standard number of microscopic fields (i.e. ten fields) should be evaluated using both the X10 and X40 objectives for each urine sample. A stained wet mount (e.g. new methylene blue) may be helpful to identify nucleated cells; however, addition of stain will dilute the concentration of the sediment. If necessary, nucleated cells can be identified in a stained wet mount, but they should be counted in the unstained wet mount (Figure 6.14). Also, if there will be a delay between when the urine sediment is prepared and when it will be examined, the slide can be stored in a humidified Petri dish (Figure 6.15).

Stain may form crystals or may be contaminated by microorganisms (Figures 6.16). To avoid false urinalysis

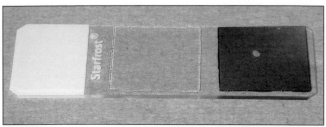

6.14 Unstained and new methylene blue stained urine sediment wet mounts. If desired, both the unstained and stained wet mounts can be prepared on a single microscope slide.

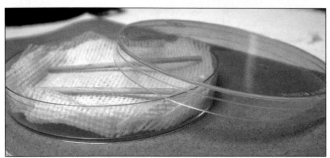

6.15 Humidified Petri dish to preserve wet mounts. If there is to be a significant delay between the time that the sediment wet mount is prepared and the time that it is examined, it can be preserved in a humidified Petri dish created by moistening absorbent material at the bottom of the dish. Details on its construction are provided in Figure 6.8 (Step 10).

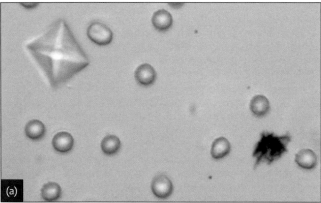

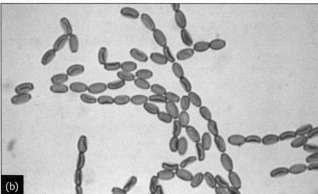

6.16 New methylene blue stained urine sediment wet mounts. (a) Two crystals are present: a calcium oxalate dihydrate crystal (left) and a contaminating crystal from the new methylene blue (right). When crystals are observed in a stained wet mount, they should be verified in the unstained preparation. Note the numerous pale orange erythrocytes in the background, which are swollen by water uptake within the relatively hypotonic, dilute urine. (New methylene blue stain; original magnification X500) (b) Numerous budding yeasts are observed as contaminants in a new methylene blue-stained wet mount. When microorganisms are observed in a stained wet mount, they should be verified in the unstained preparation. (New methylene blue stain; original magnification X400)

results, any crystals or microorganisms that are identified in a stained wet mount should be confirmed in the unstained wet mount, which will not contain contaminants that may be present in the stain. Cytological examination of the urine sediment pellet that has been aspirated from the conical centrifuge tube, smeared on to a microscope slide and stained, similarly to the process for a fine-needle aspirate, is also useful for verification, detection and identification of microorganisms (Swenson *et al.*, 2004). The method for preparing direct smears of the urine sediment pellet is described later in the chapter.

Urinalysis interpretation

Gross inspection of the urine

Normal urine may be various shades of yellow due to the presence of natural urine pigments, referred to as urochromes. Well concentrated urine may be a darker shade of yellow, but this is not always true. If present, bilirubinuria may impart a dark yellow–orange colour and give the false impression of concentrated urine. Also, urine may become darker yellow with exposure to light, which causes urochrome degradation. Therefore, urine colour should not be used to assess renal tubular concentrating ability. Urine colour may also be altered by the presence of substances that are not normally found in urine, such as haemoglobin or myoglobin (Figure 6.17).

Finding	Cause
Colour	
Pale yellow	• Normal
Yellow	• Highly concentrated urine
Dark yellow	• Highly concentrated urine • Bilirubinuria • Photodegradation of urine pigments
Orange–yellow	• Highly concentrated urine • Bilirubinuria
Red–orange	• Haematuria
Red	• Haemoglobinuria
Dark red–brown	• Myoglobinuria
Pink	• Haematuria • Haemoglobinuria • Porphyrinuria (rare)
Brown to black	• Methaemoglobin from haemoglobin or myoglobin breakdown • Bile pigments
Green	• Biliverdin (green) – can form due to *in vitro* degradation of bilirubin • Urobilin (green) – can form due to oxidation of urobilinogen in acidic urine
Blue	• Various drugs and drug metabolites
Clarity	
Clear Slightly cloudy	• Normal
Cloudy	• Cells • Crystals • Casts • Microorganisms • Lipid • Mucus • Semen

6.17 Potential findings during gross inspection of urine, and their common causes.

Normal urine is clear (i.e. transparent) or slightly cloudy owing to the presence of epithelial cells or crystals. In fresh, well mixed urine of dogs and cats, increased cloudiness is an abnormal but non-specific finding that can occur because of the presence of cells, crystals, casts, micro-organisms, lipid, mucus or semen. Even if urine is not cloudy, abnormalities may still be detected during micro-scopic evaluation of the sediment. Therefore, urine clarity should not be used as the sole method to detect cells, crystals, and so on.

Specific chemical testing of the urine

Urine specific gravity

The USG primarily reflects renal tubular ability to respond to antidiuretic hormone stimulation and conserve water by producing well concentrated urine (see Chapter 2). USG values may be classified into four categories based upon the value relative to the SG of glomerular filtrate, which ranges from 1.008–1.012 and represents urinary filtrate that has not yet been modified by the renal tubules (Figure 6.18). To determine the clinical significance of a given USG measurement, the value must be interpreted in light of the patient's age, hydration status, concurrent diseases, serum urea nitrogen and creatinine concentrations, urine glucose and protein concentrations, and recent admin-istration of therapeutic agents (e.g. parenteral fluids, glucose, diuretics, anticonvulsants). For example, a USG of 1.020 in a euhydrated dog would probably represent a normal physiological variation in response to recent water ingestion; however, the same value in a dehydrated, azo-taemic dog would indicate renal tubular concentrating dysfunction that could indicate renal dysfunction. Severe proteinuria or glucosuria both increase the measured USG; therefore, the value will not be entirely represen-tative of renal tubular concentrating function (Figure 6.18).

The USG is relatively insensitive for the detection of early kidney disease (see Chapter 10). In an azotaemic patient, USG should be used to help localize the cause of azotaemia as pre-renal, renal or post-renal (Figure 6.19; see Chapter 21). With pre-renal azotaemia, adequately functioning kidneys respond to decreased perfusion by conserving water and producing concentrated urine that has a high SG. However, there are some instances of pre-renal azotaemia where the underlying disease compro-mises tubular concentrating ability (see Chapter 2). Renal azotaemia is typically associated with inadequate renal tubular water conservation and production of dilute urine that is minimally concentrated or even isosthenuric. How-ever, some cats with renal azotaemia, which indicates that kidney function is at or below 25% of optimum, maintain

Localization of azotaemia	Urine specific gravity		Causes of azotaemia
	Dogs	Cats	
Pre-renal	≥1.030	≥1.035 and usually >1.045	• Decreased delivery of nitrogenous waste to the kidneys due to renal hypoperfusion • Increased generation of nitrogenous waste
Renal	1.008–1.029	1.008–1.034 occasionally >1.045	• Decreased removal of nitrogenous waste from circulation due to primary renal dysfunction
Post-renal	Variable	Variable	• Decreased elimination of nitrogenous waste due to urethral obstruction or bladder rupture

6.19 Use of urine specific gravity to aid in anatomical localization and identifying causes of azotaemia.

Classification	Urine specific gravity		Significance
	Dogs	Cats	
Well concentrated	≥1.030	≥1.035	• Renal tubules can produce well concentrated urine • Urine may be less concentrated in clinically normal juvenile animals
Range of minimal concentration	1.013–1.029	1.013–1.034	• Could represent an appropriate variation due to recent ingestion of water or administration of fluids • Inappropriate value in dehydrated or azotaemic patients • Can be observed in patients with kidney disease
Isosthenuria	1.008–1.012	1.008–1.012	• Could represent an appropriate variation due to recent ingestion of water or administration of fluids • Inappropriate value in dehydrated or azotaemic patients • Can be observed in patients with kidney disease

Hyposthenuria	<1.008	<1.008	• Indicates that renal tubules can produce dilute urine, reducing the likelihood of kidney disease
			• Inappropriate value in dehydrated or azotaemic patients
			• Can be observed with various conditions[a]:
			  • Polyuria due to various aetiologies, causing loss of renal medullary solute concentration gradient
			  • Hyperadrenocorticism/hypercortisolaemia
			  • Hypercalcaemia
			  • Hepatic disease
			  • Pyometra due to endotoxin exposure
			  • Psychogenic polydipsia
			  • Diabetes insipidus (central or primary renal)
			  • Therapeutic agent administration:
			    – Anticonvulsants
			    – Diuretics
			    – Fluid therapy
			    – Glucocorticoids
			    – Excessive thyroxine supplementation

6.18 Classification of urine specific gravity measurements and clinical significance. Note that for each 55.5 mmol/l (1000 mg/dl) of glucose, the specific gravity is increased by 0.0004–0.0005, and for each 10 g/l (1000 mg/dl) of protein, the specific gravity is increased by 0.0003–0.0005.
[a] In these conditions the action of ADH on the renal tubule is inhibited (see Chapter 2) or the amount of water ingested/administered means production of dilute urine is appropriate. With the exception of diabetes insipidus and psychogenic polydipsia, many of these conditions will result in urine of variable USG, which will occasionally be in the hyposthenuric range.

their ability to conserve water and can have concentrated urine with a SG ≥1.035. The USG associated with post-renal azotaemia is variable. Other clinical findings, such as oliguria or anuria with a firm, possibly distended bladder, can be used to diagnose this cause of azotaemia.

Bilirubin

Normal metabolism of haemoglobin from senescent erythrocytes results in hepatic formation of conjugated bilirubin, which is removed from the body primarily in bile via the gastrointestinal tract and, to a lesser extent, in urine via the kidneys. Chemical testing of urine for the presence of bilirubin is performed as a screen to detect haemolytic or hepatobiliary diseases (i.e. intrahepatic or posthepatic cholestasis) (Figure 6.20). However, this screening test has reduced utility in dogs. Clinically normal dogs, especially entire male dogs, form conjugated bilirubin in renal tubular epithelial cells and excrete a small amount into concentrated urine (USG >1.030) in the absence of diseases associated with hyperbilirubinaemia. To determine the clinical significance of bilirubinuria in dogs, the bilirubin concentration must be interpreted in the context of the USG. More concentrated urine with a higher USG may have a greater amount of bilirubin, whereas less concentrated urine should have a lower amount of bilirubin. For example, a 2+ urine bilirubin in a dog that has a USG of 1.040 is unlikely to be clinically

Urine biochemical finding	Causes of urine biochemical finding	Causes of false-negative results or decreases	Causes of false-positive results or increases
Bilirubinuria	• Normal in concentrated urine of dogs (urine specific gravity (USG) >1.030) • Haemolytic disease • Cholestatic diseases (hepatic or posthepatic) • Mild increase with prolonged anorexia or fever • Test is sensitive to conjugated bilirubin, but not unconjugated bilirubin (i.e. bilirubin bound to albumin); therefore, albuminuria caused by glomerular disease is not a cause of detectable bilirubinuria	• Photodegradation of bilirubin due to exposure of the urine sample to light for more than 30 minutes • Oxidation of bilirubin to bilverdin, which is green. Oxidation occurs spontaneously and is accelerated by exposure of the urine sample to air • Discoloured urine may mask test pad colour change • Centrifugation of the urine sample prior to bilirubin test may cause bilirubin to precipitate • Drugs: ascorbic acid	• Drugs: etodolac metabolites; phenothiazines (large doses, reported in humans); phenazopyridine (makes urine red)
Glucosuria	*Persistent or transient hyperglycaemia:* • Diabetes mellitus • Extreme stress in cats (glucosuria may temporarily persist after resolution of hyperglycaemia) • Hyperadrenocorticism (<10% of cases) • Acute pancreatitis • Rare causes: acromegaly; dioestrus; hyperglucagonaemia; hyperthyroidism; phaeochromocytoma • Drugs or toxins: dextrose-containing fluids; adrenocorticotrophic hormone; adrenaline; glucocorticoids; ethylene glycol; megestrol acetate; morphine; phenothiazines; progesterone; thiazide diuretics; potentially other drugs that cause hyperglycaemia (e.g. dexmedetomidine, ketamine, propranolol, xylazine) *Acquired or congenital proximal renal tubular disease:* • Fanconi syndrome • Primary renal glucosuria • Aminoglycoside toxicity • Acute kidney injury with severe tubular pathology (e.g. infection, ischaemia, toxicosis)	• Cold urine sample applied to test pad • Outdated dipsticks • Dipsticks exposed to sunlight • Discoloured urine may mask test pad colour change • *In vitro* bacterial overgrowth may decrease glucose; numerous bacteria will be present in the sediment • In samples with low glucose concentration, moderate ketonuria (2+ (0.4 g/l)) will cause a false-negative result • Very high specific gravity • Drugs: in samples with low glucose concentration, ascorbic acid will cause a false-negative result; tetracyclines due to ascorbic acid formation (above); formaldehyde formed from methenamine (hexamine)	• Contamination of dipsticks or urine sample with oxidizing chemicals (e.g. bleach, hydrogen peroxide) • Prolonged exposure of dipsticks to air (days) • Urinary haemorrhage in a patient with mild hyperglycaemia (i.e. <10.0 mmol/l (180 mg/dl) in dogs; <15.5 mmol/l (280 mg/dl) in cats) • One report observed 'pseudoglucose' in cats with urethral obstruction • Drugs: cefalexin (Chemstrips 10 SG)
Haem reaction	• Pathological or iatrogenic haematuria (erythrocytes may not be observed in urine sediment owing to lysis in dilute urine (USG <1.008), very alkaline urine (pH >9) or moderately alkaline (pH >7.5) or very concentrated urine (USG >1.035)) • Haemoglobinuria due to destruction of erythrocytes that occurs either outside or within the urinary tract • Myoglobinuria due to myocyte injury	• Failure to mix the urine sample well prior to testing in order to resuspend sedimented erythrocytes • Outdated dipsticks • Very high specific gravity • Possible but unlikely: large amount of nitrate from bacteria in urinary tract infection • Drugs: ascorbic acid, captopril; formaldehyde formed from methanamine (hexamine)	• In a voided sample, genital tract haemorrhage and oestrus are sources of intact erythrocytes • Contamination of dipsticks or urine sample with oxidizing chemicals (e.g. bleach, hydrogen peroxide) • Contamination of urine sample with digested haemoglobin in flea excrement ('flea dirt') • High urine bilirubin • Possible but unlikely: peroxidases from bacteria, leucocytes, epithelial cells or sperm; large amount of bromide or iodide (e.g. KBr administration)

6.20 Interpretation of urine biochemistry results determined by urine dipstick. Causes of false-positive or false-negative results vary with different test methods; consult product documentation for specific details. (continues) ▶

Urine biochemical finding	Causes of urine biochemical finding	Causes of false-negative results or decreases	Causes of false-positive results or increases
Urobilinogen reaction	• This test has minimal clinical significance in veterinary medicine • A small amount (0.2 mg/l) is normal, though normal animals may have none owing to diurnal variation *Increased amount:* • Usually spurious • May be seen with haemolytic or hepatobiliary disease *Decreased amount:* • Spurious • Diurnal variation • Bile duct obstruction	• Photodegradation of urobilinogen due to exposure of the urine sample to light • Oxidized by acidic urine to urobilin (green) • Drugs: formaldehyde formed from methanamine (hexamine)	• Outdated dipsticks • Improper storage of dipstick near a heat source • Drugs: aminosalicylic acid; aminobenzoic acid; phenazopyridine; sulphonamides
Ketonuria	*Hyperglycaemic ketonuria:* • Uncontrolled diabetes mellitus (a common and important cause) *Normo- or hypoglycaemic ketonuria (most are uncommon causes):* • Prolonged anorexia/starvation (the more likely cause in young animals) • Severe carbohydrate restriction • Strenuous exercise • Extreme cold • Fever • Hyperglucagonaemia due to liver disease causing reduced hepatic clearance of glucagon • Glycogen storage disease • Lactation • Methylmalonic acidaemia (reported in a family of Maltese dogs) • Postpancreatectomy • Pregnancy • Renal glucosuria • Hyperthyroidism (ketonuria documented in humans) *Uncommon endocrinopathies associated with variable blood glucose:* • Acromegaly • Adrenal tumours • Glucagonoma • Insulinoma • Pituitary adenomas • Drugs: aspirin intoxication; growth hormone administration; streptozotocin	• Predominant ketone is beta-hydroxybutyrate, which is poorly detected by dipstick • Improper storage of dipsticks (exposure of reagent to light, heat, moisture) • Improper storage of urine sample which can allow evaporation of ketones • Ketones in the sample can be decreased by bacteria that are present owing to urinary tract infection or *in vitro* contamination	• Discoloured urine • Low pH may cause trace reaction • High specific gravity may cause trace reaction • Presence of the amino acid cysteine in urine due to proximal renal tubular disease • Presence of pyruvate in urine due to mitochondrial myopathy • Drugs or diagnostic agents: N-acetylcysteine; bromosulphophthalein; captopril; dimercaprol; methionine; levodopa metabolites; mesna; D-penicillamine; phenazopyridine; tiopronin (2-MPG); valproic acid; others
pH	*High pH >7.5:* • Postprandial alkaline tide (1 hour postprandially) • Urinary tract infection caused by urease-producing bacteria (e.g. *Staphylococcus*, *Proteus*) that generate ammonia • High vegetable content diet • Alkalosis, usually metabolic (e.g. due to vomiting) • Renal tubular acidosis (rare). Early proximal renal tubular acidosis due to bicarbonate loss into urine; later develop aciduria once bicarbonate depleted. Distal renal tubular acidosis: pH is inappropriately high (>6) given the presence of concurrent metabolic acidosis caused by failure to excrete hydrogen ions • Alkalinizing therapy (see Figure 6.22) *Low pH <7:* • Normal in carnivores (usually between 5.5 and 7.5) • Urinary tract infection caused by acid-producing bacteria	• Overflow of urine between test pads, causing contamination of pH test pad by acid buffer from protein test pad • *In vitro* overgrowth of bacteria that use glucose to form acidic metabolites, numerous bacteria will be present in the sediment • Discoloured urine may interfere with interpretation of colour change • Dipstick pH measurements *estimate* pH within ± 1 pH unit of that determined by pH meter. Feline urine pH determined by dipstick is consistently lower than pH determined by meter	• Contamination of dipsticks or urine sample with cleanser residues (e.g. quaternary ammonium compounds) • Improper storage of urine sample which can allow loss of carbon dioxide, raising pH • *In vitro* overgrowth of urease-producing bacteria that generate ammonium, numerous bacteria will be present in the sediment • Discoloured urine may interfere with interpretation of colour change • Dipstick pH measurements estimate pH within ± 1 pH unit of that determined by pH meter

6.20 (continued) Interpretation of urine biochemistry results determined by urine dipstick. Causes of false-positive or false-negative results vary with different test methods; consult product documentation for specific details. (continues) ▶

Urine biochemical finding	Causes of urine biochemical finding	Causes of false-negative results or decreases	Causes of false-positive results or increases
pH (continued)	**Low pH <7: (continued)** • High meat content diet • Increased protein catabolism (e.g. fever, anorexia) • Acidosis, usually metabolic (e.g. diabetic ketoacidosis, lactic acidosis, uraemic) • Hypokalaemia • Severe diarrhoea • Metabolic alkalosis with paradoxic aciduria associated with severe vomition, upper gastrointestinal obstruction, etc. • Proximal renal tubular acidosis (rare) once bicarbonate depleted • Acidifying therapy (see Figure 6.22)		
Proteinuria	**Preglomerular:** • Physiological proteinuria (transient): fever; seizures; stress; temperature extremes; venous congestion • Dysproteinaemia causing tubular overload: severe hyperglobulinaemia (i.e. mono- or polyclonal gammopathy); Bence Jones proteinuria; myoglobinuria; excessive plasma administration **Glomerular:** • Primary glomerular proteinuria: immune-mediated destruction; glomerular haematuria; inflammatory; neoplastic • Secondary glomerular proteinuria: amyloidosis (dogs); glomerular hyperfiltration; hyperadrenocorticism; immune complex deposition **Postglomerular:** • Urogenital tract disease: haemorrhagic; inflammatory; ischaemic; neoplastic; traumatic • Normal genital secretions • Acquired or congenital proximal renal tubular disease (e.g. Fanconi syndrome, nephrotoxic drug administration (e.g. aminoglycoside))	• Low-level albuminuria (microalbuminuria) or proteinuria associated with proteins other than albumin (e.g. haemoglobin, Bence Jones proteins)	• False-positive results, particularly in cats, resulting from high levels of cauxin found in some feline urine samples (see Chapter 5) • In order to attribute proteinuria to haemorrhage alone, the dipstick haem reaction must be ≥3+, and haematuria should be visible grossly • Elements in the sediment (cells, casts, microorganisms) may be the cause of a positive reaction • Moderately alkaline, well concentrated urine or extremely alkaline (pH >9) urine • Oversaturation of the urine test pad which dilutes a necessary buffer from the test pad • Contamination of the urine sample or dipsticks with cleanser residues (e.g. quaternary ammonium compounds, chlorhexidine) • Improper storage of dipsticks (exposure to moisture) • Drugs: phenazopyridine
Miscellaneous	• Nitrate • Leucocytes • Specific gravity These dipstick reactions are not valid or useful in dogs and cats and should be ignored if they are present on the dipstick	• The dipstick leucocyte test is specific (93%), but insensitive (46%) in dogs	• The dipstick leucocyte test is positive in many feline urine samples even if they do not contain leucocytes (34% specificity) and is therefore invalid in cats

6.20 (continued) Interpretation of urine biochemistry results determined by urine dipstick. Causes of false-positive or false-negative results vary with different test methods; consult product documentation for specific details.

significant. The same urine bilirubin concentration in a dog that has a USG of 1.020 should raise concern for diseases associated with hyperbilirubinaemia.

In cats, the renal threshold for bilirubin excretion is nine times greater than it is in dogs. Therefore, any amount of bilirubinuria is clinically significant in cats and should raise concern for diseases associated with hyperbilirubinaemia. In both species, it is generally accepted that with diseases that cause jaundice, excess bilirubin first accumulates within urine; it subsequently increases in plasma and ultimately is visible at mucous membranes. However, owing to a relatively high rate of false-negative bilirubin reactions, the absence of bilirubinuria should not be used to exclude the possibility of diseases associated with hyperbilirubinaemia (i.e. haemolytic or hepatobiliary diseases), and other tests, such as serum biochemistry, should also be performed.

Glucose

Glucose is a small molecule that freely passes through the glomerulus into the filtrate; however, virtually all of the glucose that is present within the initial glomerular filtrate is efficiently removed from the urine and conserved by properly functioning renal tubules. Screening urine for the presence of glucose is done to detect diseases that cause an excess amount of glucose to be present in the glomerular filtrate (i.e. hyperglycaemia) or to detect diseases that cause proximal renal tubular dysfunction with failure to remove glucose from the glomerular filtrate.

There are several potential causes of glucosuria (see Figure 6.20), however diabetes mellitus and stress-induced transient hyperglycaemia in cats are the most common. Serum biochemistry, potentially with evaluation of serum fructosamine, is indicated in the diagnosis and management of patients with diabetes mellitus. Fructosamine is a glyco-sylated protein whose serum concentration is directly proportional to the serum glucose concentration over the preceding 2–3 weeks. Fructosamine evaluation is useful in cats to distinguish diabetic hyperglycaemia from transient stress hyperglycaemia (Plier *et al.*, 1998) and can be used as an indicator of glycaemic control during the medical management of diabetic dogs and cats.

Persistent glucosuria, as is seen with diabetes mellitus, predisposes patients to urinary tract infections that may not be apparent during urine sediment evaluation, and urine culture is necessary in patients with persistent gluco-suria to exclude underlying urinary tract infection. Diabetic patients can be immunocompromised and may develop urinary tract infections, which are associated with dimin-ished inflammatory response by leucocytes (see Figure 6.41). Consequently, the infections are referred to as silent, because pyuria may not be observed. Also, glucose is an osmotic diuretic, causing formation of large volumes of dilute urine. The dilution of cells and bacteria in the sedi-ment may decrease their concentration to a level that is below the detection limit by light microscopy. Therefore, even if bacteriuria is not observed, urine culture is neces-sary to exclude urinary tract infection in patients with per-sistent glucosuria.

In two studies, it was determined that 20% to 30% of dogs with clinical leptospirosis infections, of various serogroups, had glucosuria without hyperglycaemia. This was presumably due to damage to the proximal tubules resulting in a decreased ability to reabsorb glucose in the glomerular filtrate (Goldstein *et al.*, 2006; Tangeman *et al.*, 2013).

Haem reaction

The haem reaction is performed to screen urine for the presence of intact erythrocytes, free haemoglobin from lysed erythrocytes or free myoglobin from damaged myo-cytes (see Figure 6.20). A low number of erythrocytes (<5 per high power field) is a normal microscopic finding in urine and does not cause a positive haem reaction. An increased number of urine erythrocytes may be observed due to:

- Iatrogenic haematuria caused by collection
- Pathological haematuria due to urinary tract haemorrhage
- Genital sources of erythrocytes (e.g. oestrus) if the sample is voided.

Chapter 1 provides additional information about haematuria. Free haemoglobin and free myoglobin are not seen in normal urine. Free haemoglobin may be observed in urine during systemic haemolytic diseases and is an indicator of intravascular haemolysis. It may also be found when previously intact erythrocytes are lysed within urine that is either dilute (USG <1.008) or very alkaline. Persistent haemoglobinuria in the absence of systemic haemolytic disease should prompt further evaluation of the patient for occult urinary tract haemorrhage (e.g. diagnostic imaging). Myoglobinuria due to myocyte injury (e.g. ischae-mic, toxic, traumatic) occurs uncommonly in dogs and cats.

Positive haem reactions are most commonly due to haematuria. However, a positive haem reaction is a non-specific finding and additional information obtained from urinalysis and the peripheral blood is necessary to discriminate the cause of a positive reaction. With some urine dipsticks, intact erythrocytes will cause a stippled green colour change (Figure 6.21). Centrifugation and observation of urine colour facilitate identification of the

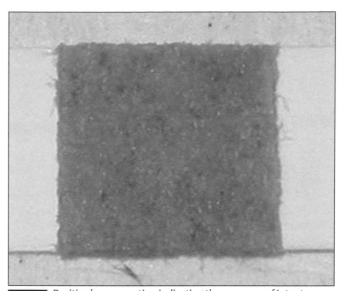

6.21 Positive haem reaction indicating the presence of intact erythrocytes. The positive haem reaction in this case indicates the presence of intact erythrocytes by its speckled green appearance. Compare this colour change to the diffusely green 3+ positive haem reaction of the middle dipstick in Figure 6.11, which could either be due to intact erythrocytes, free haemoglobin or free myoglobin.

source of a positive haem reaction. Urine that contains erythrocytes, haemoglobin or myoglobin may be various shades of red–brown. Centrifugation will cause red blood cells to sediment and the supernatant to become more yellow; if haemoglobin or myoglobin is present, the colour of the supernatant will be unchanged. Sediment evalu-ation can be used to detect intact erythrocytes, as long as the urine is not dilute or extremely alkaline (both can cause erythrocyte lysis). If erythrocytes are not observed in the sediment, the positive haem reaction is likely to be due to haemoglobinuria or myoglobinuria.

A complete blood cell count (CBC) and serum bio-chemistry may be used to distinguish haemoglobinuria and myoglobinuria. Pink or red plasma can be observed with haemoglobinuria, but not with myoglobinuria. Methae-moglobinaemia, associated with Heinz body haemolytic anaemia, which is an uncommon cause of haemo-globinuria, will cause blood to be chocolate brown. CBC abnormalities that are suggestive of haemolytic disease include regenerative anaemia and abnormal erythrocyte morphology (e.g. spherocytes, schistocytes, erythrocyte ghosts). Concurrent with myoglobinuria, the serum cre-atine kinase concentration should be markedly elevated. Creatine kinase is muscle specific and will not be elevated with *in vivo* haemolysis. If necessary, additional special-ized tests are available at referral laboratories to differenti-ate haemoglobinuria from myoglobinuria (e.g. ammonium sulphate precipitation, electrophoresis).

Ketones

Ketones are small organic acids that are normally produced in very small quantities when fatty acids are catabolized to produce energy. Ketones are not detected in the urine of healthy animals that are receiving adequate, balanced nutrition. In diseases or conditions associated with aber-rant carbohydrate metabolism (e.g. diabetes mellitus, renal glucosuria, pregnancy), alternative sources of energy are required. A compensatory increase in the rate of fat cata-bolism (i.e. lipolysis), which generates additional ketone byproducts, occurs in an attempt to meet energy demands. Increased ketone production is usually first detected as ketonuria (see Figure 6.20), which typically precedes the development of ketonaemia, because ketones are readily removed from the circulation via the kidneys.

Ketonuria is uncommonly observed in dogs and cats (1.9% of dogs, 2.6% of cats) (Osborne and Stevens, 1999) and is most often detected in poorly regulated diabetic patients that are glucosuric and either ketotic or keto-acidotic. The latter is characterized by the concurrent presence of ketosis with ketonuria, increased anion gap metabolic acidosis, consistent clinical signs (e.g. dehydration, lethargy) and often disease of another organ (e.g. infection, pancreatitis, kidney disease) in a patient with diabetes mellitus.

Urine screening for ketones is typically performed to aid in the diagnosis of diabetes mellitus and to regulate insulin therapy, even though commonly used dipstick reagents do not detect the ketone that is usually most abundant in dogs and cats, beta-hydroxybutyrate. Other ketones (i.e. acetone and acetoacetic acid) are detected by the urine dipstick and are usually present in urine along with beta-hydroxybutyrate.

Similar to glucosuria, ketonuria has a diuretic effect, causing formation of large volumes of dilute urine, which may dilute urine sediment constituents (e.g. cells, casts; see 'Glucose'). Also, excretion of ketones into urine causes concurrent loss of sodium and potassium into the urine and predisposes the patient to hyponatraemia and hypokalaemia. Careful monitoring of serum electrolytes (e.g. magnesium, phosphorus, potassium, sodium) in patients with diabetic ketoacidosis is helpful to monitor for complications associated with the disease and treatment.

pH

Urine pH measurement (see Figures 6.20 and 6.22) provides a rough assessment of systemic acid–base status and facilitates diagnosis of urinary tract infections and uncommon renal tubular diseases (i.e. renal tubular acidoses). Urine pH values are stable for up to 24 hours in urine that has been refrigerated (Raskin et al., 2002; Albasan et al., 2003). Urine dipsticks estimate pH to within 1 pH unit above or below that measured by a pH meter. In cats, urine pH is consistently underestimated by urine dipsticks; in dogs, there is no consistent direction of this error (Heuter et al., 1998). Therefore, when more precise measurement of urine pH is required (e.g. during management of urolithiasis), measurement of pH using a properly calibrated and maintained pH meter is necessary. Hand-held, portable pH meters can be purchased for this purpose. However, electrodes may need to be replaced every 6 months (Raskin et al., 2002), which would probably

render their use impractical in general veterinary practice. If necessary, shipment of refrigerated urine within 24 hours of collection to a referral diagnostic laboratory that has a pH meter may be a more feasible option.

Effective interpretation of urine pH requires knowledge of the patient's acid–base status, therapeutic agent administration, timing of urine collection relative to ingestion of a meal, and urine sediment findings. Inappropriate pH values may fall within the reference range (5–7.5); therefore, measurement of serum total carbon dioxide concentration or blood pH are helpful to determine whether a given urine pH value is physiologically inappropriate. It is uncommon for pH measurements to exceed the limits of the reference range. Extreme pH values of undetermined cause should prompt investigation for an underlying abnormality (most commonly urinary tract infection) or artefact (e.g. contamination of the dipstick or sample container with cleanser residues).

Consideration of the urine pH is helpful when interpreting other components of the urinalysis (e.g. dipstick protein, sediment). Urine that is either markedly (pH >9) or moderately alkaline (pH >7.5) and highly concentrated (USG >1.035) will probably cause a false-positive dipstick protein reaction. Highly alkaline urine also causes cells and tubular casts to degenerate more rapidly, so they may be absent from the sediment. Acidic urine is inhospitable to leptospires, and may cause false-negative leptospire culture. Urine pH has a direct effect upon the type of crystals that may be observed in the sediment, and it can also be used to predict urolith mineral content while awaiting the results of proper urolith analysis.

Protein

Urine dipstick protein testing is performed to screen for diseases that cause excess protein loss by the kidneys (i.e. renal proteinuria) or, less likely, that cause excess systemic production of protein with overflow into urine (e.g. multiple myeloma). However, because other non-pathological or pathological causes of proteinuria occur more commonly, a positive protein reaction should be interpreted judiciously. Figure 6.20 and Chapter 5 provide additional information about proteinuria.

The dipstick protein reaction is most sensitive to albumin. Other proteins (e.g. haemoglobin, immunoglobulin light chains (Bence Jones proteins)) must be present at very high concentrations to react with dipstick reagents and cause a positive reaction. The sulphosalicylic acid protein precipitation test is a simple method that screens for all types of protein and permits verification of dipstick results (see Figures 6.8 (Step 9), 6.23 and 6.24). The test is very easy to perform and the single reagent used in the test has a long shelf life. All types of protein may be detected by this method, therefore Bence Jones proteinuria, which would most likely go undiagnosed by urine dipstick, can be identified.

Additional data from the urinalysis (i.e. USG, pH, sediment examination) are needed to determine the significance of proteinuria detected by the dipstick reaction. A positive protein reaction should be interpreted in the context of the USG, because a small amount of protein (trace to 1+, <0.30 g/l) can be a normal finding in a single well concentrated urine sample (USG >1.035); however, persistent trace or 1+ proteinuria should prompt further investigation (Lees et al., 2005). A similar protein concentration in dilute urine, or in an animal receiving potentially nephrotoxic drugs, regardless of urine concentration would be abnormal.

Agents that increase pH
• Carbonic anhydrase inhibitors (e.g. acetazolamide)
• Alkalinizing prescription diets
• Citrate salts (e.g. potassium citrate)
• Sodium salts (e.g. acetate, bicarbonate, lactate)
• Thiazide diuretics (e.g. chlorothiazide)

Agents that decrease pH
• Ammonium chloride
• Ascorbic acid
• Acidifying prescription diets
• Loop diuretics (e.g. furosemide)
• Methanamine (hexamine)
• Methionine
• Phosphate salts (ammonium, potassium, sodium)

6.22 Therapeutic agents that may affect urine pH.

Interpretation	Amount of precipitate formed
Negative	No cloudiness
Trace	Cloudiness just perceptible against a dark background
1+	Cloudiness is distinct, but not granular
2+	Cloudiness is distinct and granular
3+	Cloudiness is heavy with distinct clumps
4+	Cloudiness is dense with large clumps
False-negative reactions	• Highly alkaline urine
False-positive or increased reactions	• Testing uncentrifuged urine (the test should only be performed on the supernatant urine after centrifugation) • Co-precipitation of crystals due to acid pH • Administration of radiocontrast medium or massive doses of some antibacterial drugs

6.23 Standard scale for interpretation of sulphosalicylic acid protein precipitation and causes of spurious results.

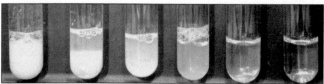

6.24 Sulphosalicylic acid precipitation of a serially diluted protein solution. Sulphosalicylic acid protein precipitation has been performed on solutions containing a known amount of protein, demonstrating the semiquantitative results obtained by sulphosalicylic acid protein precipitation. A white precipitate is formed in protein-containing solutions. The amount of precipitate formed is directly proportional to the protein concentration. Here, the amount of protein present in each tube is decreasing from 4+ in the leftmost tube to negative in the rightmost tube.

Furthermore, recent advances in our understanding of proteinuria have prompted re-evaluation of what protein concentration should be considered normal and have called into question the utility of the dipstick protein test, particularly in cats (see below and Chapter 5), possibly due to the high levels of the enzyme cauxin found in feline urine.

Consideration of the urine pH is necessary, because urine that is either markedly (pH >9) or moderately alkaline (pH 7.5) and well concentrated (USG >1.035) will be likely to cause a false-positive protein reaction on the dipstick. In one study, false-positive reactions were more common in cats than in dogs (Lyon *et al.*, 2010). The specificity of the dipstick protein reaction was 31% in cats and 69% in dogs when compared with a species-specific albumin enzyme-linked immunosorbent assay (ELISA). False-positive reactions may have occurred owing to the presence of non-albumin proteins or other interfering substances. Contamination of the urine sample with cleanser residues or improper dipstick usage or storage can also cause false-positive reactions (see Figure 6.20).

Knowledge of the urine sediment is requisite for accurate interpretation of urine dipstick protein. The most common pathological causes of increased urine protein concentration are urinary tract inflammation, infection, haemorrhage, or some combination of the three that most often arises from the lower urinary or genital tracts. In these instances, microscopic examination of the urine sediment will probably reveal pyuria, bacteriuria or haematuria. In order to attribute dipstick proteinuria entirely to haemorrhage, the haem reaction must be at least 3+ (large) and macroscopic haematuria should be present. If the haem reaction is less than 3+, no other causes of a persistently positive protein reaction (e.g. pyuria, bacteriuria, spurious) are detected and pre-renal causes of proteinuria (e.g. multiple myeloma) are ruled out, then the presence of a protein-losing nephropathy (e.g. nephrotic syndrome, proximal renal tubular defect) should be investigated (see Chapter 5).

Urine protein to creatinine ratio: When significant dipstick proteinuria has been verified as persistent on the basis of a second urinalysis and when other sources of a positive protein reaction (e.g. pyuria with or without bacteriuria; pre-renal causes) have been excluded, measurement of the urine protein to creatinine ratio (UPC) is necessary to determine more precisely the severity of proteinuria. The American College of Veterinary Internal Medicine (ACVIM) consensus statement (Lees *et al.*, 2005) defines proteinuria as a UPC >0.5 in the dog and >0.4 in the cat. Persistent renal proteinuria is a hallmark of active kidney disease and the patient should be investigated to try to identify an underlying cause and monitored carefully.

A UPC >1.0 in a sample obtained by cystocentesis should arouse concern for glomerular disease (e.g. glomerulonephritis, glomerulosclerosis or canine amyloidosis), Bence Jones proteinuria or, much less commonly, tubular proteinuria. Serum biochemistry and serum or urine protein electrophoresis are useful initial tests that will help localize the cause of proteinuria to preglomerular *versus* renal causes, and these results may direct the course of future diagnostic testing (e.g. bone marrow biopsy *versus* renal biopsy). Chapters 5 and 13 provide additional detailed information on this topic.

Serial measurement of the UPC can be used to stage the progression of renal disease and to evaluate the response to therapy. Determination of the UPC may also be performed to help establish the prognosis for newly diagnosed cases of canine (Jacob *et al.*, 2005) and feline chronic kidney disease (CKD) (Syme *et al.*, 2006; Chakrabarti *et al.*, 2012). In dogs a UPC >1.0 at the time of initial CKD diagnosis is a negative prognostic indicator. Compared with patients with a UPC <1.0, canine CKD patients with a UPC >1.0 experience more rapid progression of renal disease, greater likelihood of uraemic crisis and greater risk of death due to either renal or non-renal causes. The rate of disease progression and risk of complications were directly proportional to the magnitude of UPC elevation. Similarly, proteinuria predicts the development of azotaemic CKD in healthy, non-azotaemic cats (Jepson *et al.*, 2009) and reduced survival time in cats with chronic kidney disease (Syme *et al.*, 2006). UPC, analysed as a continuous variable, in healthy non-azotaemic cats or in cats with CKD was a positive independently significant predictor of the development of azotaemia and reduced survival time, respectively, in these two studies.

Microalbuminuria: An assay to detect microalbuminuria is available where albumin is quantified using a species-specific ELISA (Heska and Antech) following dilution of urine to a USG of 1.010. Microalbuminuria refers to increased urine albumin that remains beneath the detection limit of the urine dipstick protein reaction (i.e. urine albumin >1 mg/dl but <30 mg/dl). The prevalence of microalbuminuria has been reported as 15–19% in clinically normal dogs (Jensen *et al.*, 2001; Gary *et al.*, 2004) and 14% in clinically normal cats. Increased prevalence has been reported with older age or the presence of non-renal disease (Heska Corporation, unpublished data). Persistent microalbuminuria is an early sign of kidney dysfunction, either resulting from altered glomerular perm-selectivity or reduced ability of the proximal tubules to reabsorb albumin that has crossed the glomerular barrier. These two situations cannot be distinguished in the microalbuminuric patient. Detection of microalbuminuria is an indication to search for medical conditions that may be associated with this problem (e.g. chronic inflammatory disease, neoplasia) and to treat these conditions if possible. Serial monitoring of the urine albumin concentration and renal function is recommended to determine whether proteinuria is worsening with time and if this is associated with progressive decline in renal function. If this situation is recognized, antiproteinuric therapy may be indicated (see Chapters 23 and 24).

Microscopic examination of the urine sediment

Microscopic evaluation of the urine sediment is performed to detect increased concentrations of cells, casts, microorganisms or crystals, which may indicate underlying urinary tract disease. The concentration of the sediment and the preservation of cellular morphology are directly affected by the technique used to prepare and examine the sediment (see Figure 6.13), potential contaminants from staining (see Figure 6.16) and by urine biochemistry (Figure 6.25). Therefore, it is important to consider the results of the urine dipstick tests when evaluating the sediment. For example, within dilute urine (USG <1.008) erythrocytes will probably be lysed. Highly alkaline urine may reduce the numbers of cells and casts observed in the sediment, and urine pH also strongly influences crystal formation (Figure 6.26).

Crystalluria

Crystalluria occurs when urine is saturated with dissolved minerals or other crystallogenic substances that precipitate out of solution to form crystals. Crystals may form *in vivo* for either pathological or non-pathological reasons, or crystals may precipitate in urine *ex vivo* as a result of cold temperature or prolonged storage, post-collection alterations of urine pH or evaporation of water from the sample (Figure 6.27). To increase the likelihood that

Crystal	Acidic urine	Neutral urine	Alkaline urine
Ammonium biurate	✓	✓	
Bilirubin	✓		
Calcium carbonate (not reported in dogs and cats)			✓
Calcium oxalate dihydrate	✓	✓	✓ (in stored samples)
Calcium oxalate monohydrate	✓	✓	
Cystine	✓	✓	
Magnesium ammonium phosphate (struvite)		✓	✓
Amorphous phosphates			✓
Sulphonamide metabolites	✓		
Amorphous urates	✓		
Uric acid	✓		

6.26 Influence of pH on the formation of commonly observed urine crystals.

Crystal	Causes
Magnesium ammonium phosphate (struvite)	• Refrigerated storage for more than 1 hour • Commonly seen in clinically normal animals • Urinary tract bacterial infection involving urease-producing bacteria • Alkaline urine for reasons other than infection (e.g. diet, recent meal, renal tubular ammoniagenesis in cats, post-collection artefact) • Sterile or infection-associated uroliths of potentially mixed mineral composition
Calcium oxalate dihydrate	• Storage for more than 1 hour with or without refrigeration • Acidic urine (e.g. diet, post-collection artefact) • May be seen in clinically normal animals • Calcium oxalate urolithiasis • Hypercalciuria (e.g. due to hypercalcaemia or hypercortisolaemia) • Hyperoxaluria (e.g. ingestion of oxalate-containing vegetation, ethylene glycol or chocolate)
Calcium oxalate monohydrate	• Hyperoxaluria (e.g. ingestion of ethylene glycol or chocolate)
Calcium carbonate	• Not reported in dogs and cats • Sulphonamide crystals with similar morphology may be mistaken for calcium carbonate
Bilirubin	• A low number commonly found in concentrated canine urine, especially in males • Altered bilirubin metabolism (e.g. haemolytic or hepatobiliary diseases)
Amorphous phosphates	• Insignificant finding in clinically normal animals
Amorphous urates	• Portovascular malformation • Severe hepatic disease
Uric acid	• Ammonium biurate urolithiasis
Ammonium biurate	• Breed associated: Dalmatians, English Bulldogs; a low number of crystals is an insignificant finding
Cystine	• Defect in proximal renal tubular transport of amino acids
Iatrogenic	• Sulphonamide crystals (sulpha-containing antibiotic administration) • Xanthine crystals (allopurinol administration) • Radiocontrast medium crystals • Fluoroquinolone and other drug crystals (reported in humans)

6.27 Potential causes of commonly observed urine crystals.

Urine specific gravity (USG)
- Very concentrated (>1.035):
  - Shrinkage and crenation of erythrocytes
  - Shrinkage of leucocytes
- Hyposthenuric (<1.008):
  - Erythrocyte and leucocyte swelling or lysis
  - Usually associated with larger urine volumes so sediment constituents may be diluted

Bilirubinuria
- Casts may be orange–yellow due to bilirubin
- The number of bilirubin crystals will be increased

Glucosuria
- Has a diuretic effect so larger urine volumes are produced which dilutes sediment constituents
- Secondary urinary tract infection is common, therefore pyuria and bacteriuria may be observed

Ketonuria
- Has a diuretic effect so larger urine volumes are produced which dilutes sediment constituents

Alkalinuria
- Cell lysis
- Cast degeneration
- Promotes formation of crystals that form in alkaline urine

Aciduria
- Casts may be better preserved
- Promotes formation of crystals that form in acidic urine

6.25 Effects of abnormal urine biochemistry on sediment evaluation.

crystals present in the urine sample represent those formed *in vivo*, fresh non-refrigerated urine samples should be analysed within 1 hour of collection.

In most instances, crystalluria does not necessarily indicate the presence of uroliths or even a predisposition to form uroliths. For example, a small number of magnesium ammonium phosphate or amorphous phosphate crystals are frequently observed in clinically normal dogs and cats. Detection of crystalluria may be diagnostically useful in the following situations:

- When pathological crystal types are identified (e.g. ammonium biurate, calcium oxalate monohydrate, cystine)
- When large aggregates of magnesium ammonium phosphate or calcium oxalate dihydrate crystals are found
- When crystalluria is observed in a patient that has confirmed urolithiasis.

Evaluation of the type of crystals present may be useful to estimate the mineral component of the urolith(s), while awaiting results of complete urolith analysis. Uroliths are often heterogeneous; therefore, crystalluria is not a definitive indicator of urolith mineral content. Sequential evaluation of crystalluria may aid in monitoring a patient's response to therapy for urolith dissolution. Specific types of common urine crystals are discussed here. Further details, including uncommon types of crystalluria, can be found in texts devoted entirely to urinalysis (e.g. Osborne and Stevens, 1999).

Magnesium ammonium phosphate crystals: These are referred to as struvite crystals, triple phosphate crystals (a misnomer) or infection crystals (an older term) (Figure 6.28a). They are colourless and frequently form variably sized casket cover-shaped crystals. They also form three- to eight-sided prisms, needles or flat crystals with oblique ends. Magnesium ammonium phosphate crystals most commonly form in alkaline urine, which often occurs in association with bacterial infection. They may develop after collection in refrigerated urine samples (Albasan *et al.*, 2003), or in those that become alkaline during storage, for example as a result of bacterial overgrowth

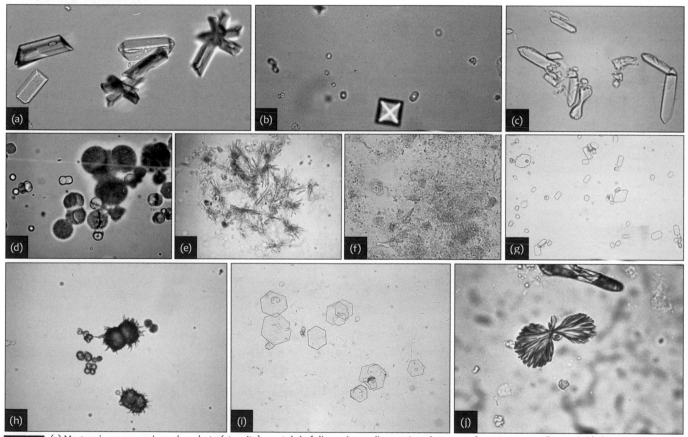

6.28 (a) Magnesium ammonium phosphate (struvite) crystals in feline urine sediment. A casket cover form is present (lower left). (Unstained; original magnification X500.) (b) Calcium oxalate dihydrate crystals in canine urine sediment. (c) Calcium oxalate monohydrate in feline urine sediment. Two morphologies are present: most crystals resemble picket fence boards and a single dumbbell-shaped crystal is found near the centre of the field. The picket fence board morphology is highly suggestive of recent ethylene glycol ingestion. This form appears similar to magnesium ammonium phosphate crystals, but calcium oxalate monohydrate crystals are always flat, while magnesium ammonium phosphate crystals form three-dimensional prisms (a). (Unstained, original magnification X400) (d) Calcium carbonate crystals forming spheres with radial striations in equine urine sediment. These crystals have not been reported in dogs or cats. Sulphonamide crystals may form globules with radial striations and could be mistaken for calcium carbonate crystals. (e) Bilirubin crystals in canine urine sediment. Copious sheaves of needle-like, dark orange bilirubin crystals are found clumped within urine sediment from a dog with hepatobiliary disease. (f) Amorphous phosphate crystals in urine sediment from alkaline urine from a clinically normal dog. Compare with the amorphous urate crystals in Figure 6.40a. (g) Uric acid crystals in canine urine sediment. Several flat, six-sided, diamond-to-rectangular shaped uric acid crystals are present in acidic urine from a clinically normal Dalmatian. (h) Ammonium biurate crystals. Dark golden-brown spheroids and sarcoptic mange-like ammonium biurate crystals are identified in urine sediment from a patient with hepatoencephalopathy caused by portovascular malformation. (i) Cystine crystals in canine urine sediment. Cystine crystals, which are never a normal sediment finding, form flat hexagons with unequal sides in acidic urine. They most commonly occur in male dogs of certain breeds with proximal renal tubular disease and are a risk factor for cystine urolithiasis. Note the large number of sperm in the background. (j) Sulphonamide crystals in canine urine sediment after administration of sulpha-containing antibiotic. A sheaf of pale yellow needle-like sulphonamide crystals is seen surrounded by a few yellow globular forms. (b, d–j unstained; original magnification X100)

or contamination of the sample with cleanser residues. When magnesium ammonium phosphate crystals are detected in a stored urine sample, the finding should be verified by prompt examination of a freshly obtained urine sample that has not been refrigerated.

Magnesium ammonium phosphate crystals are very commonly seen in dogs and occasionally in cats. When found in significant number, they are most frequently associated with bacterial infection caused by urease-producing bacteria, such as *Staphylococcus* spp. or *Proteus* spp. However, in cats, they can occur in the absence of infection, probably due to ammonia excretion by the renal tubules. Magnesium ammonium phosphate crystals may also be seen in clinically normal animals that have alkaline urine for reasons other than infection (e.g. diet, recent meal), animals that have sterile or infection-associated uroliths of potentially mixed mineral composition, or with urinary tract disease in the absence of urolithiasis.

Calcium oxalate crystals: These occur in two forms, dihydrate and monohydrate (see Figures 6.16a and 6.28bc). Calcium oxalate dihydrate crystals occur much more commonly. They are colourless, variably sized octahedrons that resemble a small envelope or a Maltese cross and most commonly form in acidic urine. They may develop after collection in stored urine samples with or without refrigeration (Albasan *et al.*, 2003) or in those that become acidic during storage due to bacterial overgrowth, for example. When calcium oxalate dihydrate crystals are detected in a stored urine sample, the finding should be verified by prompt examination of freshly obtained urine that has not been refrigerated. Calcium oxalate dihydrate crystals may be seen in clinically normal animals. They also occur with calcium oxalate urolithiasis, hypercalciuria (e.g. due to hypercalcaemia or hypercortisolaemia) or hyperoxaluria (e.g. ingestion of vegetation high in oxalates (e.g. Brassica family), ethylene glycol or chocolate). They have been reported with increased frequency in cats as a complication of urine acidification used to manage magnesium ammonium phosphate formation.

Calcium oxalate monohydrate crystals are colourless and variably sized. They may be flat with pointed ends and resemble picket fence boards. They may also form spindle- or dumbbell-shaped crystals. Although either calcium oxalate monohydrate or dihydrate crystals can be seen with acute ethylene glycol intoxication, the monohydrate form with picket fence board morphology is more diagnostic of intoxication, because this form is usually only seen during acute ethylene glycol toxicity. Formation of these crystals is time dependent and occurs only during the early phase of intoxication. Crystalluria may be observed within 3 hours of ingestion in cats and within 6 hours in dogs and may last up to 18 hours after ingestion. Calcium oxalate monohydrate crystals with spindle or dumbbell morphology are uncommonly observed with other causes of hyperoxaluria (e.g. chocolate ingestion).

Calcium carbonate crystals: These are variably sized yellow–brown or colourless variably shaped crystals (tic-tac-shaped, dumbbell-shaped or spheres with radial striations) that are found individually or in clusters usually within alkaline urine (Figure 6.28d). They are seen in clinically normal horses, elephants, goats, rabbits and guinea pigs. Anecdotally, they may very rarely be seen in dogs. Sulphonamide crystals, which can be seen in dogs and cats after administration of sulpha-containing antibiotics, may form globules with radial striations and could be mistaken for calcium carbonate crystals.

Bilirubin crystals: These may precipitate as orange to reddish-brown granules or needle-like crystals (Figure 6.28e). A low number of crystals are routinely observed in canine urine, especially in highly concentrated samples from male dogs. When bilirubin crystals are found in other species or in persistently large quantities in a canine patient, a disease associated with icterus (i.e. haemolytic or hepatobiliary disease) may be present.

Amorphous phosphate and amorphous urate crystals: These are similar in shape and may form amorphous debris or small spheroids (Figure 6.28f). Amorphous phosphates are distinguished from amorphous urates in two ways: phosphates are colourless or light yellow and form in alkaline urine, while urates are yellow–brown to black and form in acidic urine. Amorphous phosphates are commonly observed in alkaline urine of clinically normal animals, and they are not clinically significant. Conversely, amorphous urates are an uncommon abnormal finding in most breeds. They may be seen in animals with portovascular malformation, severe hepatic disease or ammonium biurate urolithiasis. Amorphous urates are routinely found in Dalmatians and English Bulldogs and may represent a predisposition for urate urolithiasis in these breeds.

Compared with other breeds, Dalmatians excrete a larger amount of uric acid in their urine and are therefore prone to form uric acid crystals or ammonium biurate crystals (Figure 6.28g). Uric acid crystals are colourless, flat, variably but often diamond-shaped six-sided crystals. Most other breeds convert uric acid to a water-soluble compound (allantoin) for excretion. Dalmatians have diminished hepatocellular uptake of uric acid, preventing this conversion, so that uric acid is excreted in its native form into the urine. In addition, Dalmatians have decreased tubular reabsorption of uric acid compared with other breeds. Uric acid crystals or ammonium biurate crystals can also occasionally be seen in English Bulldogs. They are rarely seen in other dog breeds or cats and, when observed, have the same significance as amorphous urate or ammonium biurate crystals.

Ammonium biurate crystals: These are golden-brown and spherical with irregular protrusions, giving a thorn-apple or sarcoptic mange-like appearance (Figure 6.28h). In cats, they may form smooth aggregates of spheroids. Ammonium biurate crystals are seen in animals with portovascular malformation, severe hepatic disease, ammonium biurate urolithiasis and, uncommonly, in clinically normal Dalmatians and English Bulldogs.

Cystine crystals: These are colourless flat hexagons that may have unequal sides (Figure 6.28i). Cystine crystalluria is an abnormal finding seen in animals that are cystinuric owing to an inherited defect in proximal renal tubular transport of several amino acids (i.e. arginine, cysteine, lysine, ornithine). Crystals are prone to develop in cystinuric patients that have concentrated, acidic urine. Cystinuria predisposes to the development of cystine urolithiasis, though not all cystinuric individuals develop uroliths. Among dogs, male Dachshunds, Basset Hounds, English Bulldogs, Yorkshire Terriers, Irish Terriers, Chihuahuas, Mastiffs, Rottweilers and Newfoundlands are affected with increased frequency. Uroliths often lodge at the base of the os penis and may be missed on survey radiographs because they are relatively radiolucent. Bitches and other breeds may also be affected. In cats, this disease has been recognized in male and female Siamese and American Domestic Shorthairs.

Iatrogenic crystalluria: This can be seen with administration of some antibacterial drugs, allopurinol and radiocontrast medium. Sulphonamide crystals (Figure 6.28j) are pale yellow crystals and may form haystack-like bundles or globules with radial striations. The latter morphology may be mistaken for calcium carbonate crystals.

Renal tubular casts and pseudocasts

Renal tubular casts are formed by proteinaceous plugs of dense, mesh-like mucoprotein (Tamm–Horsfall mucoprotein) that accumulate within the distal portion of the nephron (i.e. the loop of Henle, distal tubule, collecting duct). A low number (<2 per high power field) of these proteinaceous hyaline casts can occasionally be observed in the urine of normal animals (Figure 6.29). Diuresis of dehydrated animals or proteinuria of preglomerular or renal aetiology can cause an increased number of hyaline casts to be present in the urine. Renal tubular epithelial cells that die and slough into the tubular lumen can be entrapped within the dense mucoprotein matrix (Figure 6.30). If present, inflammatory cells associated with renal tubulo-interstitial inflammation may also be entrapped.

During microscopic evaluation of sediment, cellular casts are further classified as either epithelial, leucocyte or erythrocyte casts, if the constituent cells can be discerned. Once locked within the proteinaceous matrix, cells continue to degenerate, progressing from intact cells, to granular cellular remnants, and finally to a waxy cholesterol-rich end-product. A cast may dislodge from a given renal tubular lumen at any time during this degenerative process and may be observed in the urine sediment. However, in clinically normal animals only hyaline casts are rarely found (<2 per high power field). Other material can lodge within the proteinaceous matrix, such as lipid from degenerated renal tubular epithelial cells, haemoglobin during haemolytic disease and bilirubin (Figure 6.31).

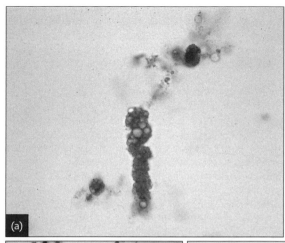
(a)

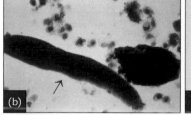
(b)

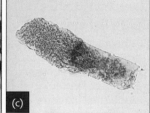
(c)

6.31 (a) Fatty renal tubular cast in feline urine sediment, consisting of granular cellular remnants admixed with non-staining spherical lipid droplets. Feline renal tubular epithelial cells are relatively lipid rich; therefore, these casts are more commonly seen in cats. (New methylene blue stain; original magnification X100) (b) Haemoglobin renal tubular cast (arrowed) in canine urine sediment. The haemoglobin content of the cast imparts a dark reddish-brown colour. When observed in patients with haemolytic disease, this finding specifically indicates intravascular haemolysis, rather than extravascular haemolysis. (c) Bright orange bilirubin-containing mixed granular and waxy renal tubular cast in canine urine sediment. The cellular material is more degenerated in the right portion of the cast. (b–c unstained; original magnification X400)

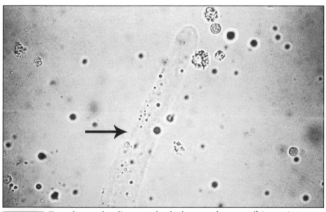

6.29 Translucent hyaline renal tubular cast (arrowed) in canine urine sediment. Note the evenly separated, parallel sides and rounded end of the cast, which allows this cast to be distinguished from a mucus thread (see Figure 6.32c). A transitional epithelial cell is touching the cast. A few smaller leucocytes are also seen in the background. (Unstained; original magnification X400)

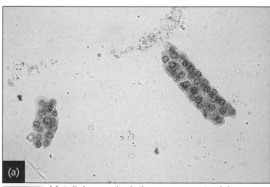
(a)

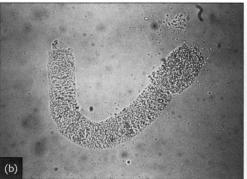
(b)

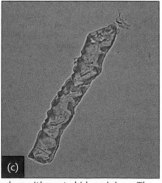
(c)

6.30 (a) Cellular renal tubular cast comprised desquamated renal tubular epithelial cells in the urine sediment of a dog with acute kidney injury. The cells within the cast are well preserved, suggesting that the cast had recently formed and was dislodged from the renal tubule before appreciable cellular degeneration occurred. (New methylene blue stain; original magnification X400) (b) Granular renal tubular cast in feline urine sediment. Although the cast is curvilinear, note the evenly separated parallel sides. Falling between intact cellular casts and aged waxy casts, granular casts represent an intermediate stage of cellular degeneration. A low number of granular casts are occasionally seen in urine from clinically normal animals. (c) Cholesterol-rich waxy renal tubular cast in feline urine sediment, indicating that a chronic renal tubular lesion is present. These casts have characteristic sharply broken, blunt ends and are less translucent than hyaline casts. (b–c unstained; original magnification X400)

The number of casts observed in the sediment does not correlate with the severity of kidney disease or its reversibility, and the absence of casts from urine sediment cannot be used to exclude the possibility of kidney disease, especially because casts are fragile and prone to degeneration, particularly in alkaline urine. When hyaline or granular casts are present in increased numbers or when other cast types are observed, one can only conclude that the renal tubules are involved in an active pathological process of unknown severity or reversibility. When present, the type of cast observed may provide additional information. Leucocyte casts indicate active renal tubulointerstitial inflammation. Waxy casts reflect a chronic tubular lesion. To recognize the onset of nephrotoxicity in patients receiving aminoglycoside antibiotic therapy, it is useful to monitor urine sediment for the appearance of tubular epithelial cell casts, which should prompt withdrawal of the antibiotic. Other abnormalities seen with aminoglycoside-induced nephrotoxicity include isosthenuria, proteinuria, glucosuria and aminoaciduria, all of which may precede the onset of azotaemia (see Chapter 21).

Structures such as mucus threads or fibres may resemble casts and should not be mistaken for them during microscopic examination (Figure 6.32). Mucus threads are distinguished by their variable width and tapered ends. Fibres are typically much larger than the surrounding cells and may contain a repetitive internal structure, suggesting a synthetic origin.

Epithelial cells

Epithelial surfaces along the length of the genitourinary tract undergo constant turnover, therefore it is routine to see a low number of epithelial cells (fewer than five per low power field) in normal urine samples. Using wet-mount preparations, it can be challenging to distinguish the different types of epithelial cell, because transitional cells are highly pleomorphic and all epithelial cells will become rounded within a fluid milieu and degenerate when exposed to urine. Cell morphology is best appreciated in freshly formed and collected urine that is promptly analysed. When evaluation of cell morphology is critical, the sediment pellet can be evaluated by routine cytology, similar to that performed with a fine needle aspirate (Figure 6.33). A larger number of epithelial cells are seen in urine samples collected by catheterization or in patients with inflamed, hyperplastic or neoplastic mucosa. Methods to diagnose structural lesions within the urinary tract (e.g. ultrasonography, catheter biopsy) that are more reliable and conclusive than urinalysis are available.

1. Centrifuge the urine as for wet mounting (see Figure 6.8, Step 8).
2. Use a transfer pipette to aspirate the pellet from the bottom of the conical centrifuge tube.
3. Place a small drop of the aspirated material on to a clean glass microscope slide.
4. Allow the slide to air dry. Heat fixation is not necessary and will alter cell morphology.
5. Stain as for routine cytology using Diff Quik® or other similar stain. Alternatively, the slide can be stored in a covered container at room temperature and sent to a referral diagnostic laboratory for evaluation.

6.33 Method used to prepare urine sediment for dry mounting and routine cytological examination.

Squamous epithelial cells: These line the distal third of the urethra, the vagina and the prepuce. They are large flat or rolled cells that have angular sides and usually a single small condensed nucleus, or they may be anucleate (Figure 6.34). A variable number of squamous epithelial cells is most commonly observed with lower urinary tract contamination of voided or catheterized samples. Squamous epithelial cells should not be present in samples collected by cystocentesis. A significant number of squamous epithelial cells is very rarely seen in cystocentesis samples in patients with squamous cell carcinoma of the bladder or squamous metaplasia of the bladder, which can occur with transitional cell carcinoma or chronic bladder irritation. Squamous epithelial cells may also be found if the uterine body of an intact female is unintentionally penetrated during urine sample collection.

Transitional epithelial cells: These line the renal pelves, ureters, bladder and proximal two thirds of the urethra. They are highly pleomorphic, variably sized cells that are smaller than squamous epithelial cells and 2–4 times larger than leucocytes (see Figures 6.34b and 6.35a). They may be round, oval, pear-shaped, polygonal or caudate, and often have granular cytoplasm with a single nucleus that is larger than that of squamous epithelial cells. There should be fewer than five transitional epithelial cells per low power field in normal urine sediment. A larger number of transitional epithelial cells are seen in urine samples collected by catheterization or in patients with inflamed, hyperplastic or neoplastic mucosa. Transitional epithelial cells with caudate morphology specifically line the renal pelves (Figure 6.35b). These cells are rarely observed in urine sediments and are an abnormal finding that can sometimes be seen in patients with pyelonephritis, renal pelvic calculi or other pathology involving the renal pelves.

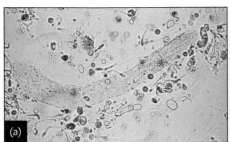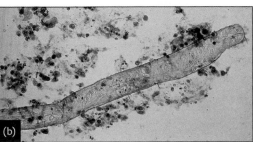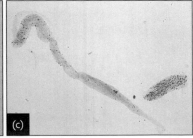

6.32 (a) Curved hyaline renal tubular cast within an active canine urine sediment. The cast is surrounded by several pale orange erythrocytes and some leucocytes and transitional epithelial cells. There are also several bacteria and sperm in the background. Note the size of the cast relative to the surrounding cells and the difference in magnification of this image compared with (b). (Unstained; original magnification X400) (b) Large, synthetic fibre within an active canine urine sediment. The fibre, which could be mistaken for a cast, is surrounded by numerous cells that are much smaller than the fibre. Note the uneven irregular separation of the parallel sides, the repetitive internal structure and the dull blunt end of the fibre. (Unstained; original magnification X100) (c) Mucus thread in feline urine sediment. Mucus threads could be mistaken for hyaline casts, but are distinguished by their irregularly spaced twisting parallel sides and pointed wispy ends. (New methylene blue stain; original magnification X100)

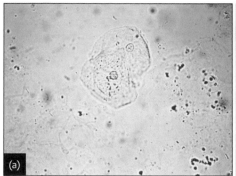

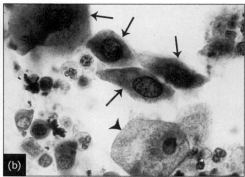

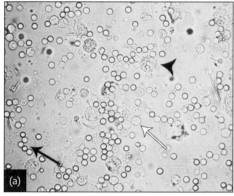

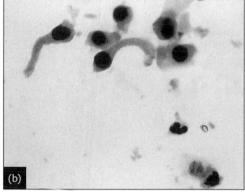

6.34 (a) Squamous epithelial cells in canine urine sediment. Note their angular borders, abundant translucent cytoplasm and single condensed nucleus. (Unstained; original magnification X400) (b) Mixed population of epithelial cells and leucocytes in canine urine sediment. Four transitional epithelial cells are visible (arrowed). Note their pleomorphism and relatively large nuclei. An angular squamous epithelial cell is present (arrowhead). Some leucocytes with segmented nuclei and fewer small round cells are scattered throughout the field. (SediStain™; original magnification X400)

6.35 (a) Size comparison of cells in an active canine urine sediment. Erythrocytes are the smallest cells (black arrow), leucocytes are larger than erythrocytes (white arrow) and transitional epithelial cells are larger than leucocytes (arrowhead). Squamous epithelial cells are the largest cells (not pictured). (Unstained; original magnification X400) (b) Caudate transitional epithelial cells (top) exfoliated from the renal pelvis of a cat with pyelonephritis. Beneath the epithelial cells, two smaller neutrophils are found. (New methylene blue stain; original magnification X400)

Renal tubular epithelial cells: Cuboidal to low columnar renal tubular epithelial cells often become small round cells once they have exfoliated into urine (Figure 6.36a) and are not always easily distinguished from leucocytes or small transitional epithelial cells. Unless they are found within a tubular cast, the presence of renal tubular epithelial cells is not considered a dependable indicator of renal disease, because a low number of tubular cells are sloughed normally and because other similarly sized cells (e.g. small transitional epithelial cells, leucocytes) may be mistakenly identified as renal tubular epithelial cells in wet-mount preparations. Observation of a large number of these cells with their cuboidal to low columnar morphology intact is a rare abnormal finding, however, that would indicate active renal tubular disease (Figure 6.36b).

Neoplastic epithelial cells: These are occasionally identified in urine sediment (Figure 6.37). In a patient that has a bladder or urethral mass, the urine sediment finding of atypical transitional epithelial cells in the absence of inflammation is suggestive of transitional cell carcinoma. Neoplastic transitional epithelial cells may exfoliate in cohesive sheets or individually. They are identified by their malignant features, such as high nuclear:cytoplasmic ratio, variable cell and nuclear size, clumped chromatin with prominent nucleoli, and mitotic activity. However, when inflammation is present, it is not possible to distinguish hyperplastic epithelial cells, which develop similar cytological features, from neoplastic epithelial cells. It is quite common for bladder tumours to become inflamed secondarily, and therefore definitive diagnosis using urine cytology alone is often not possible. In these instances, additional diagnostic information (e.g. imprint cytology or histology of catheter biopsy material) may be helpful in making a definitive diagnosis. Other less commonly observed tumours include rhabdomyosarcoma, urothelial papilloma and squamous cell carcinoma.

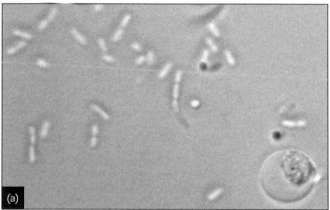

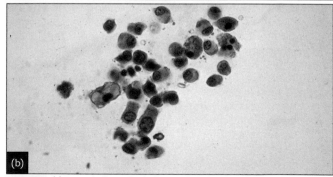

6.36 (a) Rounded renal tubular epithelial cell and bacteria in canine urine sediment. A small round cell is present (lower right) that can be presumptively identified as a renal tubular epithelial cell on the basis of the eccentric placement of its round nucleus. There are several bacilli in the background. (Unstained; original magnification X500) (b) A large number of cuboid to low columnar renal tubular epithelial cells in feline urine sediment. Most cells are cuboidal or low columnar with eccentric nuclei. Fewer cells are rounded. Though not identified within a cast, this large number of renal tubular epithelial cells is abnormal and suggests an active tubular lesion. (New methylene blue stain; original magnification X400)

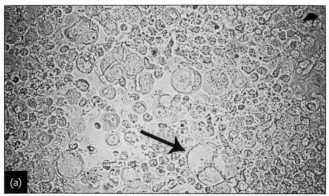

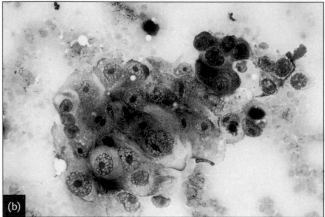

6.37 (a) A large number of neoplastic epithelial cells in canine urine sediment. It is apparent that the nuclear:cytoplasmic ratio is markedly increased, although a stained preparation would improve visualization of nuclear details. The arrow is pointing to a cohesive cell cluster. (Unstained; original magnification X400) (b) Neoplastic epithelial cells in a dry-mounted canine urine sediment prepared for routine cytology as described in Figure 6.33. There is a cohesive sheet of neoplastic transitional epithelial cells. Note the absence of inflammation and the presence of morphological changes consistent with malignancy (i.e. variation in cell and nuclear sizes, very high nuclear:cytoplasmic ratio, open chromatin pattern and prominent, large nucleoli). Compare the morphology of these cells with the non-neoplastic transitional epithelial cell in Figure 6.41b. Several erythrocytes are also present in the background. (Diff Quik®stain; original magnification X500)

The veterinary bladder tumour antigen (v-BTA) test is a rapid latex agglutination assay that is designed to be used as a screening test for early diagnosis of transitional cell carcinoma by detecting an antigen that is produced by the tumour and released into the urine. This test is associated with a high rate of false-positive results, which may occur due to haematuria, pyuria, 4+ glucosuria or 4+ proteinuria. Therefore, this test would not be useful in patients that have an advanced transitional cell carcinoma associated with haematuria and pyuria, which often occur secondary to bladder neoplasia. To decrease the possibility of false-positive reactions, the test should be performed upon the supernatant of centrifuged urine. However, some investigators feel that the test has an unacceptable number of false-positive reactions, even in dogs with normal urine sediment. Using the supernatant of centrifuged urine, the specificity of the test has been reported as 46% in unhealthy patients with urinary tract disease other than transitional cell carcinoma. The specificity increased to approximately 86% in clinically normal animals or in animals with non-urinary tract disease (Henry *et al*., 2003).

In its current form, this assay is unlikely to be useful as a screening test for use in the general canine population. Because of the low incidence of bladder tumours in dogs (<2% of canine cancers) and the high frequency of false-positive test reactions, an unacceptable number of animals may be subjected to invasive and costly diagnostic procedures in order to prove a false reaction. However, this test may have some utility in selected at-risk canine populations, such as obese, geriatric dogs from urban areas with lower urinary tract signs and breed predisposition for transitional cell carcinoma (e.g. Scottish Terriers, Shetland Sheepdogs, Beagles, Wire-Haired Fox Terriers, West Highland White Terriers) (Mutsaers *et al*., 2003), when a negative result can be used to help exclude the possibility of transitional cell carcinoma in a high-risk individual.

Blood cells, infectious agents and other sediment findings

Highly alkaline or dilute urine or improper sample storage may significantly reduce the number of cells in the urine sediment (see Figures 6.6 and 6.25). During microscopic examination care should be taken to distinguish erythrocytes from lipid droplets. Lipid droplets are quite variably sized, refractile, greenish discs that are usually smaller than erythrocytes, often float above the plane of focus and never exhibit the biconcave appearance of erythrocytes (Figure 6.38). They are frequently observed in feline urine. Beyond their potential to be misidentified as erythrocytes, they are of little significance.

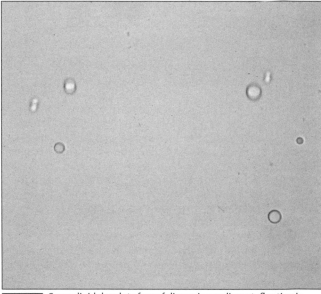

6.38 Seven lipid droplets from feline urine sediment, floating in different focal planes. Note their variable size, refractile, jewel-like appearance and greenish hue, all of which are features that distinguish them from erythrocytes (not pictured). (Unstained; original magnification X400)

Erythrocytes: Erythrocytes are quite translucent and may be pale orange owing to their haemoglobin content. Erythrocyte shape varies with the tonicity of the urine. They may:

- Maintain their biconcave disc morphology
- Shrivel, becoming crenated, in concentrated urine
- Swell, becoming rounded, in dilute urine (Figure 6.39).

There should be fewer than five erythrocytes per high power field. However, the number observed can be influenced by the collection method (see Figure 6.4). Haematuria can be a component of pathology seen with haemorrhagic diathesis (e.g. thrombocytopenia), infection, inflammation, necrosis, neoplasia, toxicity (e.g. cyclophosphamide) or trauma (see Chapter 1).

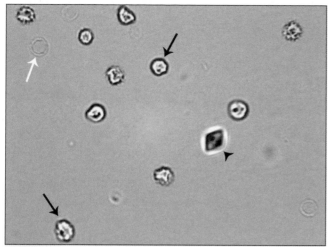

6.39 Variable erythrocyte morphology in canine urine sediment. Ten pale orange crenated erythrocytes (black arrows) are present along with three colourless erythrocyte ghosts (white arrow). Compare with Figures 6.16a and 6.35a. A single diamond-shaped calcium oxalate dihydrate crystal (arrowhead) is in the middle of the field. (Unstained; original magnification X500)

Leucocytes: In a sample collected by cystocentesis, there should be fewer than three leucocytes per high power field. In a sample collected by catheterization or midstream voiding, there should be fewer than eight leucocytes per high power field. Being larger than erythrocytes and smaller than epithelial cells, leucocytes are intermediate in size compared with other cells that may be present in the sediment (see Figure 6.35a). They are usually round with a stippled appearance and greyish internal structure that transmits less light than erythrocytes; segmented nuclei are frequently visualized (see Figures 6.34b and 6.40). Some leucocytes contain granules that are occasionally visible as refractile structures within the leucocyte. These cells may be referred to as glitter cells.

Observation of pyuria with concurrent bacteriuria indicates active urinary tract inflammation with either primary or secondary bacterial infection (Figure 6.40). Urine culture is useful to identify microorganisms definitively and to determine their antimicrobial sensitivities. Pyuria is also seen with other causes of genitourinary tract inflammation, such as urolithiasis, neoplasia, prostatitis, pyometra and less common infections involving viruses, mycoplasmas or ureaplasmas. Cystocentesis may avoid contamination of the urine sample by leucocytes from the genital tract and aid in localizing the source of pyuria.

Bacteria: The absence of pyuria does not exclude the possibility of a urinary tract infection, therefore urine sediment evaluation alone cannot be used to exclude definitively the possibility of infectious urinary tract disease. Silent urinary tract infections (i.e. those lacking a detectable inflammatory response) can be seen with hyperadrenocorticism/hypercortisolaemia, diabetes mellitus and other immunosuppressed states (Figure 6.41). Also, leucocytes and bacteria may be diluted below the detection limit of light microscopy in polyuric conditions when large volumes of dilute urine are produced (e.g. pyelonephritis). At least 10,000 bacilli/ml or 100,000 cocci/ml are required for detection by light microscopy.

Bacteria may be observed in urine sediment for reasons other than urinary tract infection (e.g. overgrowth after collection) (Figure 6.42). When microorganisms are observed in stained wet mounts, it is necessary to distinguish them from contaminants (see Figure 6.16b) by confirming their presence in unstained wet mounts or by cytological examination of the dry-mounted sediment pellet (Figure 6.41b). The latter is a more sensitive and specific method to detect bacteria than wet mounting and permits more accurate identification of bacterial morphology (Swenson et al., 2004). Urine cultures can occasionally be negative even though bacteria were detected during urinalysis (Figure 6.43). Also,

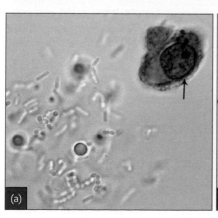

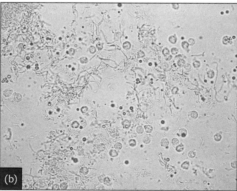

6.40 (a) Pyuria, bacteriuria and amorphous urate crystalluria in urine sediment from a Dalmatian. A leucocyte that has a segmented nucleus is present (black arrow). Note that it is stippled grey and transmits less light than an erythrocyte (not pictured). There are several bacilli in the background (arrowhead) and two aggregates of brownish-black amorphous urate crystals (white arrows). Compare these with the amorphous phosphate crystals in Figure 6.28f. (Unstained; original magnification X500) (b) Pyuria and bacteriuria in canine urine sediment. Several leucocytes and bacilli are surrounding a bacterial microcolony (upper left corner) in urine sediment from a dog with bacterial cystitis. (Unstained; original magnification X400)

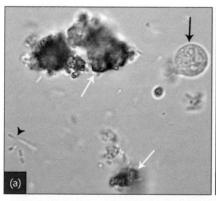

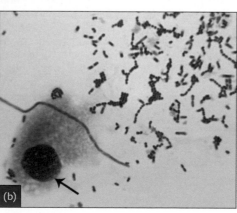

6.41 Bacteriuria in urine sediment from a Miniature Schnauzer with glucosuria. The dog was isosthenuric (specific gravity 1.008) and mildly glucosuric (5.6 mmol/l). (a) A mixed population of bacteria (bacilli and cocci) is present near a transitional epithelial cell (arrowed). Note the absence of pyuria. (New methylene blue stain; original magnification X500) (b) Bacteriuria in dry-mounted urine sediment from the same dog. This slide was prepared using the method described in Figure 6.33. Several cocci, small bacilli and large bacilli are present with a single transitional epithelial cell (arrowed). This method of slide preparation improves visualization of bacterial morphology and increases the sensitivity and specificity for the detection of bacteriuria. (Wright–Giemsa stain; original magnification X500)

- Urinary tract infection
- Sample contamination during micturition or catheterization
- Sample contamination during processing (e.g. by staining)
- *In vitro* bacterial overgrowth

6.42 Causes of bacteriuria.

- The observed bacteria represent contaminants of the urine sample incurred during collection or processing
- The observed bacteria may actually be non-bacterial structures in the sediment that were mistakenly identified as bacteria during urinalysis
- The observed bacteria may not be viable because of:
  - Prior antimicrobial administration
  - Prolonged urine storage
  - Fastidious nutritional and culture requirements (e.g. *Mycoplasma* or *Ureaplasma* spp.)
- The observed bacteria may not grow because of improper culture technique

6.43 Potential causes of a negative urine culture despite identification of bacteria in the urine sediment.

uncommon infections by viruses or highly fastidious micro-organisms (e.g. *Mycoplasma* or *Ureaplasma* spp.) may result in a negative urine culture although a urinary tract infection is present.

Urine culture: Cystocentesis is the ideal collection method for urine culture. The likelihood of representative culture results may be enhanced by collection of a randomly timed urine sample (which will probably consist of freshly formed urine that has not stagnated within the bladder) along with inoculation of a culture tube immediately after collection. Afterwards, the culture tube should be refrigerated to prevent overgrowth of robust bacteria.

With routine urine culture, results are reported that simply identify the bacteria present and their respective antimicrobial sensitivities. Quantitative urine culture is an alternative that may be helpful to determine whether the bacteria cultured from a urine sample are likely to represent a true infection or are likely to be contaminants of the sample. In addition to bacterial identification and elucidation of their antimicrobial sensitivities, quantitative culture enumerates the bacteria as colony-forming units (cfu)/ml; this is done by serial dilution and plating. Quantitative urine culture can be most beneficial when the urine sample has been collected by transurethral catheterization or by collection of midstream voided urine (Figure 6.44).

Other sediment findings

Depending on geography, other infectious agents are occasionally identified in urine sediment (Figure 6.45), such as fungi (e.g. *Candida* spp., *Aspergillus* spp., *Blastomyces dermatitidis*, *Cryptococcus* spp.), algae (e.g. *Prototheca* spp.) and nematode ova, larvae or adults (e.g. *Capillaria* spp., *Dirofilaria immitis* and *Dioctophyma renale*). *Trichuris* spp. (whipworm) parasite eggs appear very similar to the eggs of *Capillaria* spp. These two types of egg can

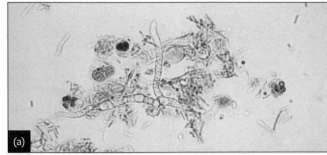

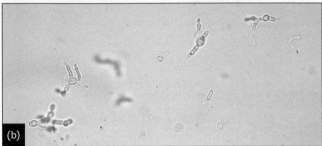

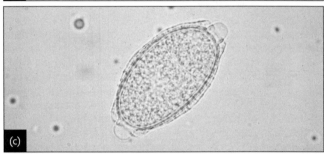

6.45 (a) Fungal hyphae, bacteriuria and pyuria in canine urine sediment. Septate branching fungal hyphae are present, surrounded by leucocytes and numerous bacteria. (SediStain™; original magnification X400) (b) Budding pseudohyphae of *Candida* in canine urine sediment. (c) *Capillaria* ovum in canine urine sediment. A single amber ovum is present surrounded by a few lipid droplets. Note the placement of the bipolar caps, which are slightly askew, and the granular texture of the outer shell, distinguishing this ovum from that of *Trichuris*. (b–c unstained; original magnification X400)

be distinguished by the positioning of their bipolar caps and the texture of their outer shells. The bipolar caps of *Capillaria* spp. ova are slightly askew, rather than being perfectly bipolar as they are in *Trichuris* ova. Also, the shells of *Capillaria* ova have a granular appearance, rather than being perfectly smooth as they are in *Trichuris* ova. *Capillaria* are usually an incidental finding in the urine of asymptomatic cats. However, *Capillaria* eggs are very occasionally identified in cats that present with haematuria, which resolves after fenbendazole administration.

Common contaminants of urine samples include sperm, talc, glass chips, plant pollen, hair and fibres (Figure 6.46; see also Figures 6.28i and 6.32). Aside from sperm, these contaminants can be mistaken for urine crystals (e.g. talc, glass chips), transitional epithelial cells (e.g. plant pollen) or casts (e.g. hair, fibres).

Collection method	Significant (cfu/ml)		Questionable (cfu/ml)		Contamination (cfu/ml)	
	Dog	Cat	Dog	Cat	Dog	Cat
Cystocentesis	>1000	>1000	100–1000	100–1000	<100	<100
Catheterization	>10,000	>1000	1000–10,000	100–1000	<1000	<100
Voided	>100,000	>10,000	>10,000	1000–10,000	<10,000	<1000

6.44 Guidelines for the interpretation of quantitative urine cultures (see Chapter 30).

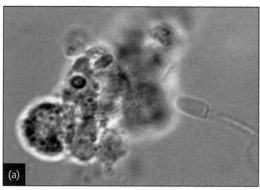 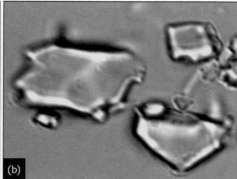

6.46 (a) Pyuria and sperm in the urine of a Persian cat with bilateral renomegaly. An aggregate of leucocytes (left) and a single sperm (right) are present. Sperm are a potential contaminant of voided samples. (Unstained; original magnification X1000) (b) Glass chip contaminants in canine urine sediment. Glass chips are common contaminants of urine sediments that may be mistaken for crystalluria. (Unstained; original magnification X500)

References and further reading

Albasan H, Lulich JP, Osborne CA *et al.* (2003) Effects of storage time and temperature on pH, specific gravity, and crystal formation in urine samples from dogs and cats. *Journal of the American Veterinary Medical Association* **222**, 176–179

Chakrabarti S, Syme HM and Elliott J (2012) Clinicopathological variables predicting progression of azotemia in cats with chronic kidney disease. *Journal of Veterinary Internal Medicine* **26(2)**, 275–281

Gary AT, Cohn LA, Kerl ME and Jensen WA (2004) The effects of exercise on urinary albumin excretion in dogs. *Journal of Veterinary Internal Medicine* **18**, 52–55

George JW (2001) The usefulness and limitations of hand-held refractometers in veterinary laboratory medicine: a historical and technical review. *Veterinary Clinical Pathology* **30**, 201–210

Goldstein RE, Lin RC, Langston CE, *et al.* (2006) Influence of infecting serogroup on clinical features of leptospirosis in dogs. *Journal of Veterinary Internal Medicine* **20**, 489–494

Henry CJ, Tyler JW, McEntee MC *et al.* (2003) Evaluation of a bladder tumor antigen test as a screening test for transitional cell carcinoma of the lower urinary tract in dogs. *American Journal of Veterinary Research* **64**, 1017–1020

Heuter KJ, Buffington CA and Chew DJ (1998) Agreement between two methods for measuring urine pH in cats and dogs. *Journal of the American Veterinary Medical Association* **213**, 996–998

Jacob F, Polzin DJ, Osborne CA *et al.* (2005) Evaluation of the association between initial proteinuria and morbidity rate or death in dogs with naturally occurring chronic renal failure. *Journal of the American Veterinary Medical Association* **226**, 393–400

Jensen WA, Grauer GF and Andrews J (2001) Prevalence of microalbuminuria in dogs. *Journal of Veterinary Internal Medicine* **15**, 300 [abstract 113]

Jepson RE, Brodbelt D, Vallance C, Syme HM and Elliott J (2009) Evaluation of predictors of the development of azotemia in cats. *Journal of Veterinary Internal Medicine* **23(4)**, 806–813

Lees GE, Brown SA, Elliot J, Grauer GF and Vaden SL (2005) Assessment and management of proteinuria in dogs and cats: 2004 ACVIM forum consensus statement (small animal). *Journal of Veterinary Internal Medicine* **19**, 377–385

Lyon SD, Sanderson MW, Vaden SL *et al.* (2010) Comparison of urine dipstick, sulfosalicylic acid, urine protein-to-creatinine ratio, and species-specific ELISA methods for detection of albumin in urine samples of cats and dogs. *Journal of the American Veterinary Medical Association* **236(8)**, 874–879

Mutsaers AJ, Widmer WR and Knapp DW (2003) Canine transitional cell carcinoma. *Journal of Veterinary Internal Medicine* **17**, 136–144

Osborne CA and Stevens JB (1999) *Urinalysis: A Clinical Guide to Compassionate Patient Care, 1st edn*, pp. 1–214. Veterinary Learning Systems, Bayer Corporation, Shawnee Mission, Kansas

Plier ML, Grindem CB, MacWilliams PS and Stevens JB (1998) Serum fructosamine concentration in nondiabetic and diabetic cats. *Veterinary Clinical Pathology* **27**, 34–39

Raskin RE, Murray KA and Levy JK (2002) Comparison of home monitoring methods for feline urine pH measurement. *Veterinary Clinical Pathology* **31**, 51–55

Stockham SL and Scott MA (2002) Urinary system. In: *Fundamentals of Veterinary Clinical Pathology*. Iowa State Press, Ames

Swenson CL, Boisvert AM, Kruger JM and Gibbons-Burgener SN (2004) Evaluation of modified Wright-staining of urine sediment as a method for accurate detection of bacteriuria in dogs. *Journal of the American Veterinary Medical Association* **224**, 1282–1289

Syme HM, Markwell PJ, Pfeiffer D and Elliott J (2006) Survival of cats with naturally occurring chronic renal failure is related to severity of proteinuria. *Journal of Veterinary Internal Medicine* **20(3)**, 528–535

Tangeman LE and Littman MP (2013) Clinicopathologic and atypical features of naturally occurring leptospirosis in dogs: 51 cases (2000–2010). *Journal of the American Veterinary Medical Association* **243**, 1316–1322

Chapter 7

Diagnostic imaging of the urinary tract

Rachel E. Pollard and Kathryn L. Phillips

Kidneys and ureters

Radiography

Survey radiography can provide information regarding the size, number, location, margination and opacity of the kidneys in dogs and cats with adequate retroperitoneal fat. The kidneys may be poorly visualized in emaciated animals and those with fluid in the retroperitoneal or peritoneal cavities, owing to reduced contrast. A three-view radiographic study is recommended. The right lateral radiographic view maximizes renal visualization as it encourages the right kidney to slide cranially thereby minimizing renal superimposition. The left lateral radiographic view reduces renal positional changes induced by body position that might alter interpretation of size and margination. The ventrodorsal (VD) view allows individual assessment of the kidneys but there is greater superimposition of other abdominal viscera so that the right and occasionally the left kidney may be difficult to visualize in their entirety.

Normal kidneys are bean-shaped, smoothly marginated structures located dorsally in the retroperitoneal space. Renal size is typically assessed in comparison with an internal reference, the most common of which is the length of the second lumbar vertebrae (L2) on the VD view. In the dog, normal renal length is 2.75–3.25 times L2 (Feeney *et al.*, 1979; Shiroma *et al.*, 1999). In the cat, normal renal length is 1.9–2.6 times L2 if neutered and 2.1–3.2 if entire (Feeney *et al.*, 1979; Shiroma *et al.*, 1999). The kidneys should be paired, with the right kidney positioned more cranially than the left. In the dog, the cranial margin of the right kidney is nestled within the renal fossa of the caudate lobe of the liver, making visualization challenging. The right kidney is usually level with the T12–L1 vertebrae. The left kidney is more caudally and ventrally located, with the descending colon residing ventral to its ventral margin at the level of L2–4. Feline kidneys tend to be more mobile and rounder in comparison with those of the dog.

The ureters reside within the retroperitoneal space and when normal are only rarely visualized radiographically.

Excretory urography

Excretory urography (EU) can provide information about renal morphology and internal architecture. However, the same information can be gleaned less invasively using ultrasonography, so EU is rarely performed for that purpose. EU is typically used as a method to visualize the ureters and to provide a rough assessment of renal function (Feeney *et al.*, 1981).

All animals should be adequately hydrated prior to EU. Food should be withheld for 12–24 hours before the procedure. A cleansing enema should be performed approximately 2 hours prior to EU (Feeney *et al.*, 1981, 1982). Right lateral and VD survey radiographs are performed prior to administration of intravenous contrast material. To minimize the risk of adverse reactions, the use of non-ionic iodinated contrast media such as iopamidol or iohexol at a dose of 880 mg iodine per kilogram bodyweight is advised (Pollard *et al.*, 2008; Pollard and Puchalski, 2011). Contrast media should be delivered rapidly through a cephalic or other indwelling catheter because extravasation can be irritating to regional tissues. Right lateral and VD radiographs are obtained immediately and then at 5, 10, 20 and 40 minutes after contrast administration. Oblique views of the ureteral terminus and/or negative contrast cystography may be added to the radiographic study obtained at 5 minutes after contrast administration if ureteral ectopia is suspected. Abdominal compression in the form of a tight elastic wrap applied to the caudal abdomen has been historically reported to increase opacification of the renal pelves. Care should be taken to observe the animal closely for evidence of an adverse reaction for at least 1 hour after administration of intravenous contrast media of any kind. Adverse reactions are rare in animals but can range in severity from mild (nausea, urticaria), to moderate (vomiting, hypotension, collapse) or severe (cardiac or respiratory failure) (Pollard *et al.*, 2008; Pollard and Puchalski, 2011).

Excretory urography may be performed in azotaemic and non-azotaemic animals provided that hydration is adequate. A higher dose of contrast media (up to a 10% increase in dose) may be necessary as renal compromise progresses in order to reach adequate renal and ureteral opacification (Wallack, 2003). A temporary reduction in renal function may follow EU. A less common outcome of EU is contrast-induced renal failure, which has only been sporadically reported in the veterinary literature. Readers are referred elsewhere for a discussion of treatment for contrast-induced renal failure (Ihle, 1991).

Excretory urography can be divided into the nephrogram (opacification of the functional renal parenchyma) and the pyelogram (opacification of the renal pelvis, pelvic recesses and ureters) phases. Initially, the renal cortex is more opacified than the medulla. However, approximately 10–30 seconds into the nephrogram phase, the kidney is typically homogeneously and intensely contrast

BSAVA Manual of Canine and Feline Nephrology and Urology, third edition. Edited by Jonathan Elliott, Gregory F. Grauer and Jodi L. Westropp ©BSAVA 2017 enhancing. A steady reduction in the degree of contrast enhancement should be seen over time. Renal size, shape and margination are unchanged relative to the survey radiographs. Persistent or progressive opacification of the nephrogram indicates severe hypotension or contrast-induced nephropathy (Figure 7.1).

During the pyelogram phase (2–3 minutes after contrast administration), the renal pelvis, pelvic recesses and ureters should exceed the opacification of the renal parenchyma. The renal pelvis and pelvic recesses should not exceed 1–2 mm in diameter in the dog (values have not been reported for cats). In general, the proximal ureter should not exceed 2–3 mm in diameter although it is important to recognize that ureteral diameter will vary with peristalsis.

Nephropyelography

Antegrade pyelography is a technique that has been described in both dogs and cats for identifying ureteral obstruction (Rivers *et al.*, 1997; Adin *et al.*, 2003). It is particularly useful in animals whose renal function is impaired to the point that EU does not result in adequate pelvic and ureteral opacification. Moreover, the risk of contrast medium nephrotoxicity is avoided, because systemic contrast is not administered. When a diagnostic study can be obtained, antegrade pyelography has 100% sensitivity and specificity for identifying ureteral obstruction in cats, far surpassing ultrasonography or radiography alone (Adin *et al.*, 2003).

To perform the procedure, the animal is anaesthetized and the ventral abdomen is shaved and aseptically cleansed. A 25 G, 2.5 inch (6.25 cm) spinal needle is directed into the dilated renal pelvis from a ventrolateral approach under ultrasound guidance, taking care to avoid the arcuate arteries located at the corticomedullary junction. A moderate degree of pelvic dilation should be present to minimize the likelihood of lacerating the collecting system. Typically, 1–2 ml of urine is removed for aerobic bacterial urine culture and then iodinated contrast medium

is injected into the pelvis. The volume of contrast medium administered is arbitrarily determined, based on the degree of resistance to injection, but should be roughly equal to the quantity of urine removed. Serial radiography or fluoroscopy is subsequently used to determine whether ureteral obstruction is present.

The most common complication is leakage of contrast material through the needle tract, rendering the study non-diagnostic. Renal pelvic laceration, and intrapelvic and retroperitoneal haemorrhage are also possible complications (Adin *et al.*, 2003).

Ultrasonography

Ultrasound assessment of the kidneys and ureters is very rarely performed in isolation. It is important to recognize that evaluation of the entire abdomen is essential because findings in one organ system will often influence the interpretation of findings in another.

Before the ultrasound evaluation begins the clinician must ensure that the animal is comfortable. It is recommended that the ultrasound examination should be performed in a dimly lit room with as little traffic as possible. Restraint of the patient is typically achieved by having assistants hold the animal's legs and head. A foam pad cut into a wedge (V-trough) works well as a positioning device to hold an animal on its back during the procedure. If an animal is highly stressed or aggressive, or the ultrasound examination is lengthy, chemical restraint is indicated.

For adequate ultrasound scanning, the hair needs to be clipped from the ventral abdomen to reduce artefacts and provide better visualization of the abdominal organs. The hair should be clipped from the xiphoid caudally to the inguinal region with the lateral margins of the clip following the costal arch and extending roughly halfway up the flank. Subsequently, alcohol or a water solution is applied to moisten the skin, displace hair associated with the hair follicles and remove the surface layer of grease which can be present on the skin surface. The final preparation includes

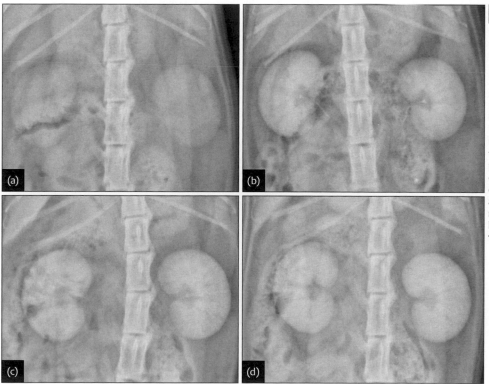

7.1 Ventrodorsal images of a normal cat being screened for kidney donation. (a) A survey radiograph shows smoothly marginated, symmetrical kidneys. (b) An image obtained immediately after the administration of intravenous iodinated contrast medium shows the parenchymal blush of the nephrogram phase and early filling of the collecting system indicative of the beginning of the pyelogram phase. (c) An image obtained 10 minutes later shows that the pyelogram phase has not progressed and renal parenchymal opacification has persisted. (d) An image obtained 20 minutes after contrast administration shows a persistent nephrogram, indicative of severe hypotension or contrast-induced renal failure.

applying liberal amounts of coupling gel to the abdomen. The ultrasonographic gel should be manually worked into the shaved skin surface for optimal acoustic coupling.

A high frequency (7.5–10 MHz) transducer should be selected for all but the largest dogs. The image orientation dot or symbol on the screen should be positioned on the left side of the image display. This dot correlates to a mark, line, dot or light on the transducer. This indicator should be directed towards the head of the animal for the longitudinal scan plane and directed toward the animal's right side (towards the machine and sonographer) for the transverse scan plane. When performing the ultrasound scan, the transducer should not be lifted from the skin when moving to another region; instead, slide the transducer along the abdomen until the next area of interest is encountered.

While the kidneys are not the first organ to be scanned, a complete discussion of abdominal ultrasonography is beyond the scope of this chapter (see *BSAVA Manual of Canine and Feline Abdominal Imaging*). To locate the left kidney, the transducer is placed in the longitudinal imaging plane along the lateral surface of the mid-left abdomen caudal to the costal arch. The kidney is located caudal to the head of the spleen and lateral to the abdominal aorta. Once the left kidney is located, imaging the organ in the longitudinal plane initially is usually easiest and most informative. This plane allows the sonographer to evaluate the size and shape of the kidney along with visualization of the corticomedullary definition. The transducer is then rotated counterclockwise to produce a transverse image of the kidney. The transverse plane of the kidney is the most sensitive image for detecting renal pelvic dilatation.

In the dog the best way to visualize the right kidney is to place the transducer directly medial to the 13th rib and direct the sound beam cranially and perhaps a little laterally. In the cat the right kidney is usually easily seen and can be imaged directly from the right side without the interference of the ribs and the associated costal arch. Complete evaluation of the right kidney consists of both the longitudinal and transverse views. Transducer pressure should be moderate for evaluation of the kidney, because the overlying small intestine needs to be displaced to limit imaging artefacts secondary to intestinal gas.

In both dogs and cats, ultrasonography allows evaluation of the peri-renal tissues, cortex, medulla, hilus and blood vessels. Kidneys can be evaluated for size, shape, location, number, echogenicity and architecture. In the cat, kidney length ranges from 3 to 5 cm when measured in the longitudinal imaging plane (DeBruyn *et al.*, 2012).

Considerably more variability exists in the dog. There is a loose linear relationship between renal length and bodyweight (see Chapter 4) but a large standard deviation exists and there is marked variation in kidney length among normal dogs of similar size (Barr *et al.*, 1991). The renal cortex in dogs is close in echogenicity to that of the liver and slightly less than that of the spleen. Renal cortical echogenicity is variable in the cat and can be similar to that of liver or spleen, with entire male cats frequently having subjectively hyperechoic renal cortices as a normal finding. The renal medulla is less echogenic than the cortex in both cats and dogs. In some animals, a thin hyperechoic line is seen at the interface of the cortex and the medulla. This line, known as the 'medullary rim sign' represents mineral material in the proximal tubules and, in the absence of other renal changes, is typically incidental (Mantis and Lamb, 2000) (Figure 7.2).

The renal hilus contains fat and fibrous connective tissue so that it appears ultrasonographically bright. The thick-walled interlobar and arcuate arteries are easily visualized and may result in mild acoustic shadowing, which should not be confused with parenchymal mineralization. The renal pelvis and ureters are typically not seen unless they are distended. It is important to note that anything that causes increased urine production can cause mild renal pelvic dilatation (up to 2 mm) so that a hypoechoic sliver of urine is visible displacing the renal hilus from the papilla. If a tubular structure is visible exiting the kidney, travelling through the retroperitoneal space and/or dorsal to the urinary bladder, colour Doppler may be useful to determine whether it is vascular or ureteral in origin.

Doppler techniques can be useful for evaluating blood flow to the kidneys. Colour or power Doppler can be used to confirm the presence of blood flow when renal infarction or vascular avulsion is suspected, or to evaluate solid lesions to distinguish vascular from avascular masses. Pulsed-wave Doppler is occasionally used to measure resistive index (RI) as a specific (but not very sensitive) indicator of renal disease. Resistive index is measured from the interlobar or arcuate arteries and calculated by the ultrasound machine as follows:

$$RI = \frac{\text{Peak systolic velocity} - \text{End diastolic velocity}}{\text{Peak systolic velocity}}$$

This unitless measure is considered elevated when >0.70, which is most commonly seen in acute interstitial disease, ureteral obstruction and rejection of a transplanted kidney (Figure 7.3).

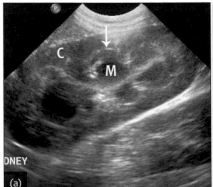
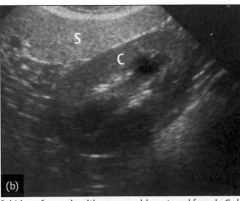
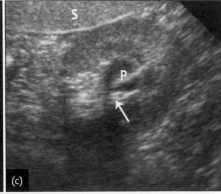

7.2 (a) Sagittal ultrasound image of the left kidney from a healthy 7-year-old neutered female Golden Retriever. The outer cortex (C) is more echogenic than the inner medulla (M). There is a thin hyperechoic line (arrowed) near the corticomedullary junction, representing an incidental medullary rim sign. (b) Sagittal ultrasound image of the left kidney of a healthy 5-year-old West Highland White Terrier allows comparison of the renal cortex (C) with the adjacent spleen (S), confirming that the spleen is more echogenic. (c) The transverse image of the left kidney from the same dog as in (b) shows that the renal papilla (P) is in contact with the hyperechoic fat and fibrous connective tissue in the hilus (arrowed). The spleen (S) is in the near field.

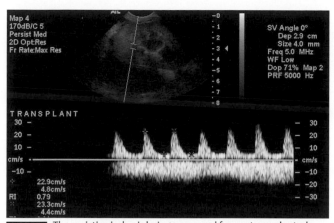

7.3 The resistive index is being measured from a transplanted kidney in a 4-year-old neutered male German Shorthaired Pointer. The callipers are placed over the arcuate arteries of the kidney and the resistive index is calculated from the Doppler waveform.

In recent years, ultrasound contrast agents have been developed and used for the evaluation of parenchymal organs. Ultrasound contrast agents are microbubbles encapsulated in a synthetic shell that are injected intravenously (Chomas *et al.*, 2001). They result in a marked increase in sound reflection and therefore make vascular structures appear bright. Although there is very little information on the use of ultrasound contrast agents for the evaluation of veterinary patients, the enhancement pattern of the normal canine kidney has been reported (Waller *et al.*, 2007). Preliminary data exist to support that quantitative ultrasound contrast techniques can identify changes in renal blood flow in dogs with hypercortisolism and after renal biopsy (Haers *et al.*, 2010; 2011). The role of ultrasound contrast agents in veterinary urology remains to be established.

Computed tomography

While ultrasonography plays a significant role in the evaluation of the upper urinary tract, there are a number of limitations that can be overcome with other cross-sectional imaging techniques. Most notably, visualization of the terminus of the ureters can be nearly impossible, particularly if they reside within the pelvic canal or they are of normal diameter. Moreover, ultrasonography is incapable of assessing renal function. For these reasons, contrast-enhanced computed tomography (CT) has a place in evaluation of the kidneys and ureters. CT image generation follows the same principles as conventional radiography in that X-rays and iodinated contrast media are used to acquire images. One can evaluate renal size, shape, density, location and number. Once contrast medium has been administered, ureteral diameter, thickness, location, peristalsis and termination can be visualized. With the superior anatomical detail and contrast resolution that CT can offer, sensitivity and specificity of lesion detection is improved over conventional radiography.

In general, animals are anaesthetized for the CT examination. The animal is placed in dorsal recumbency on a moving table within the CT unit. The X-ray source and detectors rotate around the animal in either a helical or single slice configuration. As with conventional radiography, ionizing radiation is the basis for image acquisition, so radiation safety precautions are required for the protection of the personnel involved in the procedure. Collimator settings determine the slice thickness such that thinner slices provide superior image resolution but deliver

a higher total radiation dose. Within limits, the table movement can be increased while maintaining a given collimation thickness to increase the volume of anatomy imaged. The relationship of table travel to X-ray tube rotation is termed the 'pitch'. As pitch increases, a greater length of the patient's anatomy can be imaged with a given number of images of fixed collimation thickness.

Both pre- and post-contrast images are obtained for comparison. This is of particular importance when urinary tract calculi are suspected because contrast media will appear of similar density to radiodense uroliths and may mask their visualization if pre-contrast images are not available for comparison. As with EU, non-ionic iodinated contrast medium is recommended at a dose of 880 mg iodine per kilogram of bodyweight to minimize the risk of untoward effects. Contrast medium should be administered into a peripheral indwelling catheter as rapidly as possible and ideally with a pressure injector. Post-contrast images are obtained immediately following the administration of contrast medium and then every few minutes until ureteral opacification and visualization are satisfactory.

Should information regarding renal function be desired, sequential images of the kidneys can be obtained during contrast media injection. As with EU, CT image acquisition can be timed to evaluate the initial vascular enhancement, nephrogram and pyelogram phases. Qualitative assessment of renal function can be made by evaluating the rapidity and degree to which the kidneys contrast enhance and by evaluating transit to and through the collecting system. Quantitative estimates of glomerular filtration rate (GFR) can also be obtained, although CT has been shown to underestimate GFR when compared with nuclear scintigraphy and plasma clearance tests, and is therefore not the test of choice for evaluating GFR (O'Dell-Anderson *et al.*, 2006). Furthermore, if renal function is severely impaired (e.g. with a complete ureteral obstruction), adequate pelvic and ureteral opacification will not be obtained and GFR cannot be estimated.

Image post-processing allows the user to manipulate the three-dimensional CT dataset in all directions. Image reformatting in the dorsal and sagittal planes can allow multiplanar assessment of organs. Three-dimensional surface or volume rendering and maximum intensity projection reconstruction facilitate surgical planning and allow for improved understanding of complex anatomical details.

Magnetic resonance imaging

There is very little information in the literature regarding the use of magnetic resonance imaging (MRI) for evaluation of the upper urinary system. This is probably the result of the greater expense, limited availability and long acquisition times associated with MRI. Given the utility of radiography, ultrasonography and contrast CT for imaging the urinary system, the limitations of MRI mostly outweigh its advantages.

That said, MRI is a high-contrast cross-sectional imaging technique that can be used to obtain both anatomical and functional information about the urinary system. The animal must be anaesthetized and is placed within the core of the unit. A strong magnetic field aligns the hydrogen atoms within the patient, and then temporary disruptions of the proton alignment are induced using radiofrequency waves. The radiofrequency waves are pulsed in predefined sequences intended to emphasize different types of tissue. The most common predefined sequences result in T1- and T2-weighted images. As the protons in the animal realign, they generate their own radiofrequency signal that is recorded and mapped so as to yield a three-dimensional image of the area of interest. The intensity of each pixel is related to proton density and the chemical properties of the tissue. Intravenous contrast agents can be administered to evaluate the vascularity of tissue. The most common MRI contrast agents are small molecular gadolinium agents that increase the signal intensity on T1-weighted images. While ionizing radiation is not used, there are still risks associated with the powerful magnetic field so that safety precautions are imperative.

As with CT, magnetic resonance images can provide multiplanar and three-dimensional reconstruction to facilitate surgical planning and accurately represent complex anatomical regions. Dynamic magnetic resonance sequences can be performed during intravenous contrast agent administration to evaluate renal function in the dog (Fonseca-Matheus et al., 2011).

Nuclear scintigraphy

Nuclear scintigraphy refers to the use of radioactive elements or radionuclides for diagnostic purposes. The radionuclide is bound to another compound to create a radiopharmaceutical that will travel throughout the body and concentrate in the area of interest. The detection of radiopharmaceutical uptake is performed by a gamma camera that counts radioactive emissions. If a dynamic study is performed, the change in uptake over time can be measured.

Nuclear scintigraphy has limited application in veterinary patients because very few facilities have access to a gamma camera. Moreover, the handling and storage of radiopharmaceuticals and monitoring of radioactive animals are heavily regulated and can only be performed by licensed operators.

In veterinary nephrology, nuclear scintigraphy is typically used to assess renal function because anatomical resolution is poor. The GFR can be estimated using plasma clearance of radionuclides (e.g. technetium 99m-diethylene-triaminepentaacetic acid; Tc 99m-DTPA). This technique can estimate global as well as individual kidney GFR; however, global GFR evaluations are not considered reliable and this technique is most often performed prior to unilateral nephrectomy to assess the function of the apparently healthy kidney.

Congenital absence of a kidney

Unilateral absence of a kidney is an occasional finding, with the right kidney being more frequently absent than the left.

Radiography

- Absence of one kidney with compensatory hypertrophy of another (should be confirmed by EU, contrast CT or nuclear scintigraphy).
- The remaining kidney is enlarged with normal architecture.

Ultrasonography

- Changes as for radiography.
- Absence may be further confirmed by showing that the renal artery and vein are not present.

Renal dysplasia and juvenile nephropathies

Familial nephropathies are present in certain breeds such as the Alaskan Malamute and Miniature Schnauzer, and typically affect both kidneys (Figure 7.4).

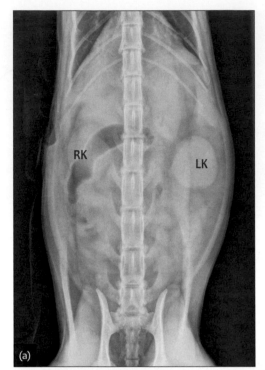

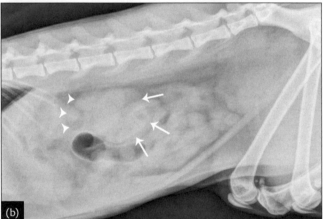

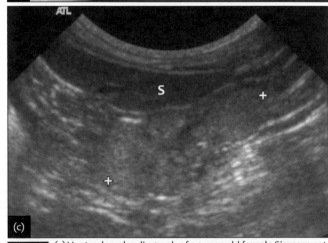

7.4 (a) Ventrodorsal radiograph of a 1-year-old female Siamese cat with renal azotaemia. The kidneys are bilaterally small, measuring less than two lengths of L2. (b) Right lateral radiograph of the same cat as in (a). The caudal margin of the left kidney (arrowed) and the cranial margin of the right kidney (arrowheads) are irregular. (c) Sagittal ultrasound image of the left kidney of a 4-year-old neutered female Yorkshire Terrier with renal dysplasia. The kidney (between callipers) is small and irregular with reduced corticomedullary distinction and increased cortical echogenicity in comparison with the adjacent spleen (S). These findings are suggestive, but not pathognomonic, for renal dysplasia.

Radiography

- The kidneys are small and have either a smooth or irregular contour.
- Excretory urography can confirm kidney size and shape and there will be delayed or poor opacification.
- Renal secondary hyperparathyroidism may manifest as demineralization of the skull and dystrophic calcification of soft tissues such as gastric rugae and major blood vessels (see Chapter 11).

Ultrasonography

- Findings do not allow differentiation from other chronic or endstage renal diseases, although young age and breed may be suggestive.
- The kidneys are small and may be smooth or irregular, have reduced corticomedullary differentiation, parenchymal hyperechogenicity (fibrosis and mineralization) and/or small parenchymal cyst formation.

Acute kidney injury

The kidneys may be affected unilaterally or bilaterally depending upon the underlying disease.

Radiography

- Usually normal or slightly enlarged. Retroperitoneal detail may be reduced owing to regional inflammation.
- Excretory urography may show poor or absent opacification, depending on functional ability.

Ultrasonography

- May appear normal.
- May see an increase in size with cortical hyperechogenicity, mild pelvic dilatation and perinephric effusion or hazy retroperitoneal fat (suggestive for inflammation)
- Specific aetiologies may have distinct changes, as follows:
  - Ureteric obstruction will yield hydronephrosis and hydroureter along with peri-renal fluid accumulation and a hazy appearance to regional fat due to inflammation
  - Leptospirosis typically causes renomegaly with mildly increased cortical echogenicity, renal pelvic dilatation and perinephric effusion (Figure 7.5). A broad distinct well marginated hyperechoic band in the medulla is strongly suggestive of this disease
  - *Aspergillus* nephritis often results in moderate renal pelvic dilatation with thickening of the collecting system and echogenic debris in the renal pelvis (Figure 7.6). Granulomas may be seen affecting the renal parenchyma.

Chronic kidney disease

Most commonly a bilateral disease process although the degree of change may be asymmetrical (Figure 7.7).

Radiography

- May be normal.
- May see small, irregular or misshapen kidneys with mineralization or calculi.
- Excretory urography confirms kidney size and shape, along with poor opacification.

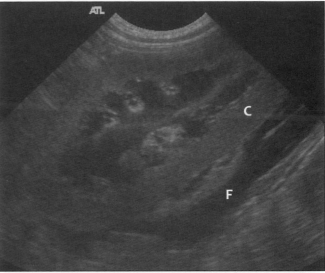

7.5 Sagittal ultrasound image of the left kidney of a 1-year-old neutered male Labrador Retriever with leptospirosis. There is perinephric fluid (F) and the renal cortex (C) is subjectively hyperechoic, which was confirmed by comparison with the spleen (not shown).

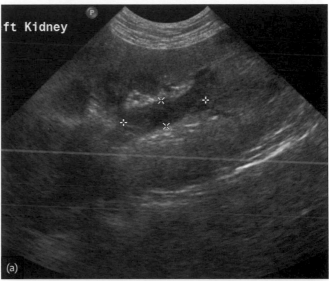

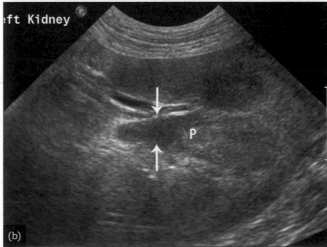

7.6 Ultrasound images of the left kidney of a 3-year-old neutered male German Shepherd Dog with systemic aspergillosis. (a) The sagittal image shows reduced corticomedullary distinction and dilatation of the renal pelvis (between callipers). (b) The transverse image confirms dilatation of the renal pelvis (arrowed) with echogenic fluid and a blunted appearance to the renal papilla (P).

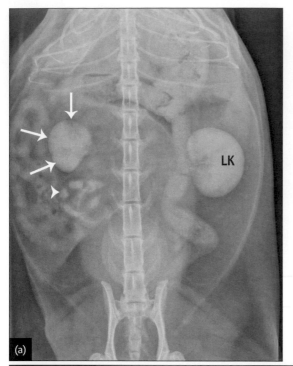

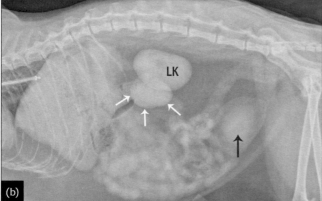

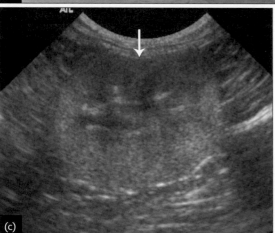

Ultrasonography

- May appear normal.
- Parenchymal mineralization or collecting system calculi may appear as hyperechoic foci with acoustic shadowing.
- May see reduced corticomedullary differentiation.
- Reduced or increased cortical thickness relative to the medulla.
- Diffuse uniform or patchy increased cortical echogenicity often combined with wedge-shaped hyperechoic regions of chronic infarction.
- May see reduced renal size with smooth or irregular margination.
- Mild renal pelvic dilatation may result from polyuria.
- Endstage kidneys may be difficult to identify as renal tissue. Location aids in organ identification.

Pyelonephritis

One or both kidneys may be affected (Figure 7.8). This disease may be seen concurrently with ureteral ectopia or other causes of hydroureter.

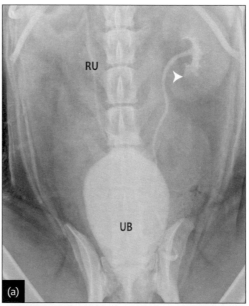

7.7 (a) Ventrodorsal 10-minute excretory urogram of an 11-year-old neutered female Domestic Shorthaired (DSH) Cat with chronic right-sided nephritis. The right kidney (arrowed) is small with an irregular outer margin. Contrast medium is seen in the small intestine (arrowhead), which is the alternative method of excretion when renal function is compromised. (b) The right lateral radiograph of the same cat as in (a) again shows the irregular and small right kidney (white arrows). Some contrast medium is seen in the urinary bladder and there is a central filling defect (black arrow) consistent with a radiolucent stone or blood clot. (c) Sagittal ultrasound image of the left kidney of an 8-year-old neutered female DSH with chronic kidney disease. There is reduced corticomedullary distinction and the outer margin of the kidney is slightly irregular (arrowed). The kidney is small, measuring 2.2 cm in length.

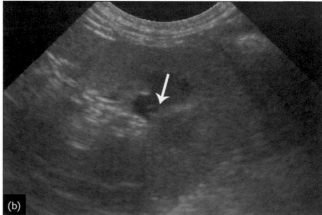

7.8 (a) Ventrodorsal 20-minute excretory urogram of a 5-year-old neutered male Pyrenean Mountain Dog with pyelonephritis. The left renal pelvis is mildly dilated and the pelvic diverticuli are blunted (arrowhead). The left ureter is slightly greater in diameter than the right (RU), suggesting ureteritis. UB = urinary bladder. (b) Transverse ultrasound image of the left kidney of a 12-year-old neutered female Beagle with pyelonephritis. The renal pelvis is mildly dilated and the renal papilla is invaginated (arrowed), indicative of necrosis.

Radiography

- The kidneys may appear normal, enlarged or small and irregular depending upon severity and chronicity.
- Renal calculi may also be present.
- Excretory urography will show mild dilatation of the renal pelvis and proximal ureter with filling defects that represent clumped debris.

Ultrasonography

- May appear normal.
- Acute pyelonephritis may cause mild renomegaly and pelvic dilatation.
- Reduced corticomedullary differentiation with uniform or patchy cortical hyperechogenicity in the more chronic stage.
- Focal hyperechoic regions may be seen in the renal crest and medulla.
- Mild renal pelvic dilatation may accompany flattening or invagination of the renal crest and visible echogenic debris in the pelvis.

Renal calculi

Most renal calculi in companion animals (Figure 7.9) are composed of struvite or calcium oxalate and are radiodense. Urate and cystine calculi, while less common, are radiolucent (see Chapter 26), depending upon their size and precise composition. All mineral material (and therefore all calculi) creates a hyperechoic interface with varying levels of acoustic shadowing when assessed ultrasonographically. Nephroliths are frequently seen in animals with other renal diseases such as pyelonephritis or chronic kidney disease.

Radiography

- Mineralized opacities seen in the renal pelvis on orthogonal views.
- Large calculi may extend into the diverticuli and down the proximal ureter (stag-horn calculi are often composed of struvite).
- Calculi may be present elsewhere in the urinary tract.
- Excretory urography may obscure radiodense calculi but radiolucent calculi will appear as filling defects.

Ultrasonography

- Nephroliths have a hyperechoic interface with distinct, clean (hard) acoustic shadowing.
- Calculi may be difficult to differentiate from parenchymal mineralization. Calculi often accompany pelvic dilatation and can be definitively differentiated from parenchymal mineralization when they are surrounded by pelvic fluid.

Feline infectious peritonitis

One or both kidneys may be affected by feline infectious peritonitis (FIP) (Figure 7.10). It is important to look for changes in other organs and lymph nodes, and for free fluid in the abdomen.

Radiography

- The kidneys may be enlarged and irregular.
- An uneven nephrogram may be seen on EU.

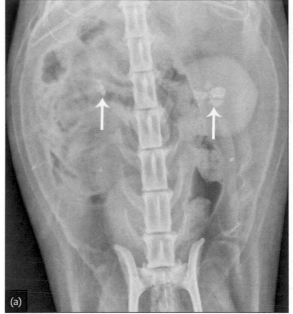

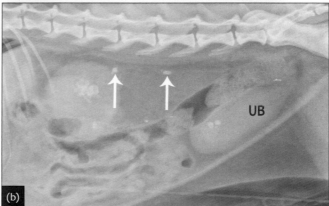

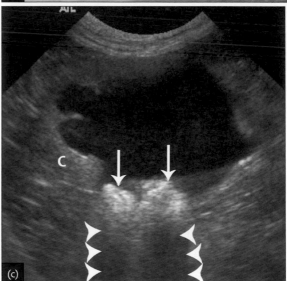

7.9 An 8-year-old neutered female Domestic Shorthaired Cat with renal calculi. (a) The ventrodorsal radiograph confirms that calculi are in the region of the pelves (arrowed) and are not likely to be parenchymal. The left kidney appears rounded, suggestive of hydronephrosis. (b) The right lateral radiograph shows that calculi are superimposed over the kidney shadows in the region of the pelves. Calculi are seen elsewhere in the urinary tract including the ureters (arrowed) and urinary bladder (UB). (c) The sagittal ultrasound image of the left kidney shows severe hydronephrosis with minimal remaining cortex (C). Hyperechoic structures (arrowed) with acoustic shadowing (arrowheads) are seen in the dependent aspect of the pelvis, consistent with calculi.

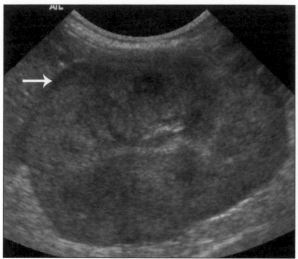

7.10 Sagittal ultrasound image of the left kidney of a 6-month-old neutered male Domestic Longhaired Cat with feline infectious peritonitis. The corticomedullary distinction is reduced. The kidney is enlarged, measuring 5 cm in length. There is scant subcapsular fluid/infiltrate (arrowed).

Ultrasonography

- The kidneys may be enlarged and irregular.
- Focal hyperechoic nodules (granulomas) or diffuse mottling of the parenchyma may occur.
- Hypoechoic perinephric fluid/infiltrate may be seen.
- Diffuse ultrasonography findings appear similar to those of renal lymphoma and the two diseases cannot be differentiated without cytological assessment.

Renal trauma

Excretory urography (radiographic or with computed tomography) may be superior to ultrasonography for confirming renal and ureteral rupture (Figure 7.11).

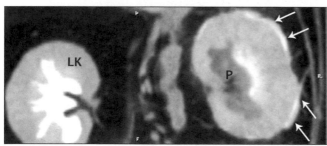

7.11 Dorsally reconstructed post-contrast computed tomography image of the kidneys of a 2-year-old neutered female Domestic Shorthaired Cat with right renal rupture. Note that contrast has accumulated around the right kidney (arrowed) and very little contrast is located within the right renal pelvis (P) when compared with that of the left kidney (LK). Right renal parenchymal enhancement confirms that the vascular supply has not been compromised.

Radiography

- The kidney may change shape if ruptured, or appear enlarged if perinephric haemorrhage/urine accumulates.
- Retroperitoneal or peritoneal detail may be reduced owing to haemorrhage or urine leakage.
- Excretory urography may show an absent nephrogram if the renal artery is compromised. The nephrogram may show uneven enhancement with parenchymal trauma or contrast extravasation with rupture.

Ultrasonography

- Renal rupture will appear as distortion or loss of normal architecture.
- Haematomas may appear as anechoic, hypoechoic or complex masses within the renal parenchyma or outside the kidney.
- Echogenic or anechoic fluid may reside within the retroperitoneal or peritoneal space if haemorrhage or urine leakage has occurred.
- Subcapsular fluid may be anechoic or echogenic with perinephric haemorrhage.

Renal lymphoma

Most commonly, both kidneys are affected by renal lymphoma (Figure 7.12). The kidneys may be the only organs affected or widespread lymphoma may occur so that evaluation of other organs and lymph nodes is essential.

Radiography

- The kidneys may be enlarged and irregular or appear normal.
- An uneven nephrogram may be seen on excretory urography.

Ultrasonography

- The kidneys may be enlarged and irregular.
- Focal, hyperechoic nodules (granulomas) or diffuse mottling of the parenchyma may occur.
- Hypoechoic perinephric fluid/infiltrate may be seen.
- Diffuse ultrasonography findings appear similar to FIP and the two diseases cannot be differentiated without cytological assessment.

Renal neoplasia (other than lymphoma)

Malignant tumours are more common than benign but cannot be differentiated with imaging (Figure 7.13). Cytology is required to determine cell type. Both primary and metastatic renal lesions are possible. Thoracic radiographs are indicated to assess for metastatic disease.

Radiography

- Unilateral or bilateral renal enlargement and/or contour irregularity.
- The colon can be displaced ventrally.
- Sometimes only one renal pole is affected.
- Dystrophic mineralization can occur.
- Excretory urography will confirm that the mass is renal in origin:
  - The nephrogram may be patchy with areas of poor enhancement
  - The renal pelvis and proximal ureter may be distorted or dilated with filling defects that represent neoplastic tissue or haemorrhage.

Ultrasonography

- Heterogeneous tissue causes expansile enlargement of the kidney(s) with contour irregularity and loss of normal shape.
- The entire kidney may be replaced with abnormal tissue.

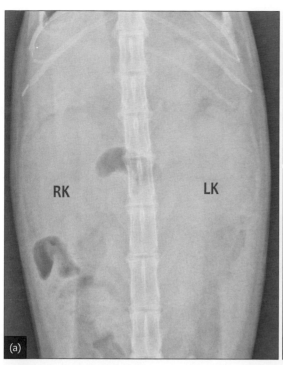

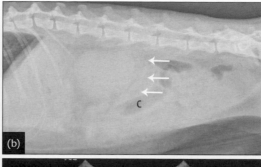

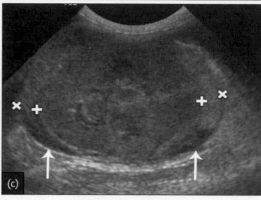

7.12 A 14-year-old neutered male Domestic Shorthaired Cat with renal lymphoma. (a) The ventrodorsal radiograph shows that both kidneys (RK and LK) are enlarged, measuring approximately three lengths of L2. Mid-abdominal serosal detail is reduced suggesting ascites, inflammation or lymphadenomegaly. (b) The right lateral radiograph confirms renomegaly, with the left kidney (arrowed) displacing the colon (C) ventrally. (c) The sagittal ultrasound image of the left kidney shows that corticomedullary distinction is reduced. The kidney is enlarged, measuring 5.4 cm in length. There is scant subcapsular fluid/infiltrate (arrowed), which is more echogenic near the poles (between callipers).

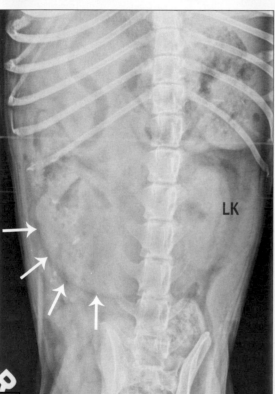

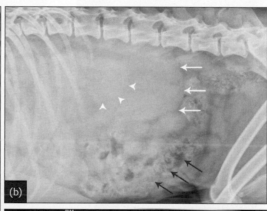

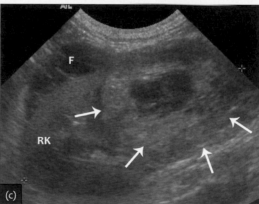

7.13 (a) Ventrodorsal radiograph of an 8-year-old neutered male Beagle with a right renal carcinoma. The caudal margin of the right kidney (arrowed) extends all the way into the caudal abdomen. The left kidney (LK) is displaced laterally and caudally. (b) The right lateral radiograph of the same dog as in (a) confirms right renomegaly (white arrows) with ventral deviation of the faeces-filled colon (black arrows). The left kidney (arrowheads) can be seen summating with the mass. (c) Sagittal ultrasound image of the right kidney of a 15-year-old neutered female Domestic Longhaired Cat with a right renal carcinoma. The cranial pole of the right kidney (RK) appears fairly normal. However, the caudal pole has been replaced by a cavitated mass (arrowed), resulting in distortion of the shape of the kidney. Perinephric fluid (F) is seen and may represent haemorrhage or urine.

- Primary tumours are often solitary complex solid masses that cause focal disruption of the normal architecture.
- Renal cystadenomas/cystadenocarcinomas are usually bilateral in German Shepherd Dogs, with variable anechoic/hypoechoic cysts and nodules.

Contrast CT

- Contrast CT may be useful for surgical planning and assessing for invasion of renal tumours into surrounding musculature and organs.

- Quantitative assessment of the contralateral kidney using nuclear scintigraphy may give a rough estimate of GFR if surgical removal of the affected kidney is planned.

Renal cysts

Solitary renal cysts are often incidental in dogs and cats but polycystic kidney disease is a progressive bilateral process in Persian cats and related breeds (Figure 7.14) (see Chapter 14). Incidental renal cysts are often seen with contrast CT performed for other reasons.

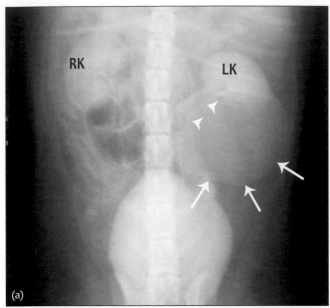

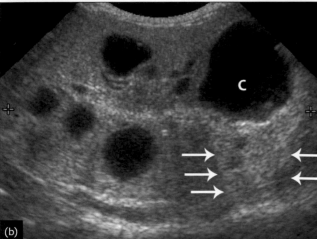

7.14 (a) Ventrodorsal image obtained 20 minutes post-excretory urogram in a 9-year-old neutered female Akita with a solitary left renal cyst. The nephrogram phase of the right kidney (RK) and the cranial pole of the left kidney (LK) appear normal. The caudal pole of the left kidney is enlarged and the parenchyma has been replaced by a non-contrast-enhancing lesion (arrowed) consistent with a cyst. The cyst is displacing the left ureter (arrowheads) medially and the renal pelvis is moderately distorted. (b) Sagittal ultrasound image of the right kidney (between callipers) of a 12-year-old neutered male Persian cat with polycystic kidney disease. There are multiple variably sized cysts throughout the parenchyma, the largest of which (C) shows acoustic enhancement (arrowed), thereby confirming that it contains fluid. The remaining parenchyma is subjectively hyperechoic, and corticomedullary distinction is reduced. The kidney is enlarged, measuring 4.9 cm in length.

Radiography

- May appear normal with small or single cysts.
- Numerous or large cysts can cause renomegaly and contour irregularity.
- Excretory urography shows spherical filling defects in the renal parenchyma, which may distort the renal pelvis.

Ultrasonography

- Most cysts appear as round thin-walled well defined structures with anechoic contents and acoustic enhancement.
- Occasionally cysts will contain echoic debris or mineralization (hyperechoic regions with shadowing) but should always appear thin walled and well defined.

- Polycystic kidney disease often begins as one or more 1–2 mm cysts in a kitten a few weeks after birth. Cysts enlarge and become more numerous with age and eventually efface the normal parenchyma. Lesions may be cortical, corticomedullary or medullary. At advanced stages, the kidneys are enlarged with irregular outer margins.
- Pelvic dilatation may occur if cysts of any kind encroach upon the renal pelvis.

Renal abscess/granulomas/haematomas

Lesions may be solitary or multifocal, unilateral or bilateral (Figure 7.15).

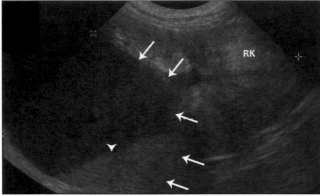

7.15 Sagittal ultrasound image of the right kidney of a 1-year-old female Boxer with a renal abscess. The caudal pole of the right kidney (RK) is normally shaped but displays reduced corticomedullary distinction suggestive of chronic inflammation. There is a fluid-filled mass distorting the cranial pole of the kidney (arrowed). Echogenic debris is seen suspended within the fluid, some of which has settled to the dependent portion of the abscess cavity (arrowhead).

Radiography

- Small lesions may be undetectable.
- Numerous or large lesions can result in renomegaly and contour irregularity.
- Excretory urography will show enhancement defects when haematomas and/or abscesses are present but patchy parenchymal enhancement is often present with granulomas.

Ultrasonography

- Abscesses appear as focal or multifocal thick-walled, fluid-filled lesions with echogenic contents. Peri-renal fluid may be seen, and regional fat is often hazy if inflammation is present. Evidence of pyelonephritis may also be present (see above).
- Haematomas may appear similar to abscesses and be difficult to differentiate without cytological assessment.
- Granulomas appear as solid focal or multifocal heterogeneous or hyperechoic nodules.
- Systemic aspergillosis in German Shepherd Dogs often causes hyperechoic multifocal renal nodules with fungal pyelonephritis (see above).

Contrast CT

Differentiation of renal abscesses, granulomas and haematomas from renal tumours may be challenging. Contrast CT can provide superior images of the lesions without superimposition of overlying structures, and thereby facilitates differentiation of these lesions. Cytology is often still necessary.

Perinephric pseudocysts

Accumulation of modified transudate in the subcapsular space often occurs in association with chronic kidney disease (CKD) and is often bilateral (although not always symmetrical) (Figure 7.16). Older male cats are predisposed.

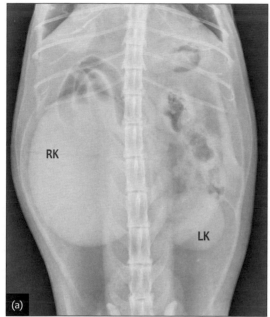

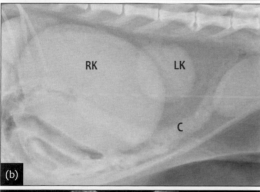

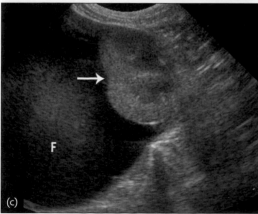

7.16 A 13-year-old neutered Domestic Shorthaired Cat with bilateral perinephric pseudocysts. (a) The ventrodorsal radiograph shows severe enlargement of the right renal silhouette (RK), which has resulted in displacement of the bowel cranially and medially. The left kidney (LK) is small but appears round and is displaced caudally. Note that the margins of both kidneys remain smooth and well defined. (b) The right lateral radiograph confirms severe right renal enlargement with ventral displacement of the colon (C). (c) The sagittal ultrasound image of the right kidney shows a large accumulation of fluid (F) focally located around the kidney. The kidney has reduced corticomedullary distinction and an irregular outer margin (arrowed) suggestive of chronic kidney disease.

Radiography

- Smooth and often severe enlargement of the renal shadow(s) is seen.
- The enlarged renal shadow exerts a mass effect on regional organs.
- Excretory urography demonstrates that the kidney itself is only a small part of the renal shadow.

Ultrasonography

- Circumscribed anechoic fluid is seen surrounding the kidney(s) in varying quantity. A thin hyperechoic capsule is seen surrounding the fluid. Occasionally septations are present attached to the renal surface.
- The kidney(s) often show imaging signs of CKD (see above).

Hydronephrosis

Hydronephrosis (Figure 7.17) can be unilateral or bilateral and results from pyelonephritis or partial or complete obstruction of the ureters (ureteroliths, trigonal neoplasia). It is often seen with ureteral ectopia.

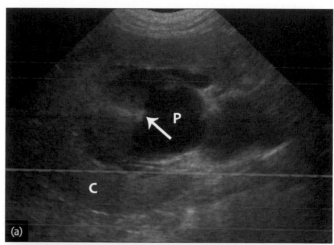

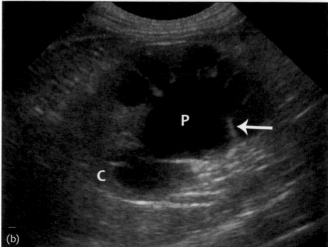

7.17 (a) Transverse ultrasound image of the right kidney of a 6-year-old neutered male Swiss Mountain Dog with hydronephrosis. The renal pelvis (P) is moderately dilated with anechoic fluid. The renal papilla is blunted (arrowed). The remaining cortex (C) appears normal. (b) Sagittal ultrasound image of the left kidney of an 11-year-old neutered female Domestic Shorthaired Cat with hydronephrosis. There is a large quantity of anechoic fluid in the renal pelvis (P) and very little normal cortex (C) remains. Hyperechoic linear structures extend into the centre of the fluid-filled pelvis (arrowed) and represent the support for the arcuate arteries.

Radiography

- Kidney size may be normal, enlarged or small (in cases of chronic partial obstruction).
- The renal outline may be rounded with loss of the hilar notch (bean shape).
- Excretory urography of mild and moderate hydronephrosis shows distension and rounding of the pelvis and diverticuli. Renal opacification may not occur or may appear as a thin rim of peripheral enhancement with severe hydronephrosis. Dilatation of the ureter is often present depending on the cause of the hydronephrosis. Contrast may not be taken up by the kidney if complete obstruction is present.

Ultrasonography

- Anechoic fluid resides within the renal pelvis, resulting in displacement of the renal crest away from the hyperechoic fat in the hilus (seen best in the transverse plane).
- Diverticuli are widened and cortical thinning occurs in varying degrees depending upon the severity and duration of disease.
- Ureteral dilatation often accompanies hydronephrosis and the dilated fluid-filled ureter can be seen exiting the renal hilus. Ultrasonography can be used to trace the ureter distally toward the bladder in search of obstruction.

Ethylene glycol intoxication
Radiography

- The kidneys may appear normal.
- Renomegaly and/or diffuse increased opacity results from mineral deposition in the kidney.

Ultrasonography

- Increased cortical echogenicity (at 4 hours) is followed by increased medullary echogenicity. Echogenicity may equal or exceed that of spleen (Figure 7.18). A relatively less increased echogenicity at the corticomedullary junction may result in a hypoechoic band (halo sign) at the corticomedullary junction, which is reported to be a poor prognostic indicator.

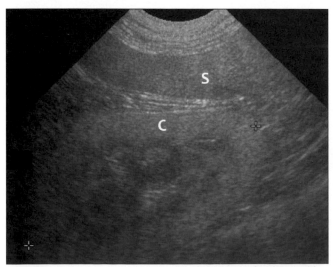

7.18 Sagittal ultrasound image of the left kidney of an 8-year-old neutered female mixed-breed dog with a known history of ethylene glycol ingestion. The renal cortex (C) is seen to be substantially more echogenic than the adjacent spleen (S). The kidney is enlarged, measuring 8.5 cm in length.

Nephrocalcinosis

Nephrocalcinosis has various causes including CKD, hyperadrenocorticism, hypercalcaemia and hypervitaminosis D. Ultrasonography is more sensitive than radiography for detecting subtle mineralization.

Radiography

- Patches and lines of mineralization are superimposed over the renal silhouettes on both views.
- If associated with CKD, the kidneys may be small and irregular (see above).
- May be difficult to differentiate from small calculi.

Ultrasonography

- Hyperechoic foci are present within the renal parenchyma with varying degrees of acoustic shadowing depending on size (small lesions may not have significant shadowing).
- Often seen in association with CKD (see above).

Renal infarcts

Renal infarcts (Figure 7.19) may be single or multiple and are often seen with CKD. Care should be taken to search for a source for the infarcts. Incidental renal infarcts are often seen with contrast CT performed for other reasons.

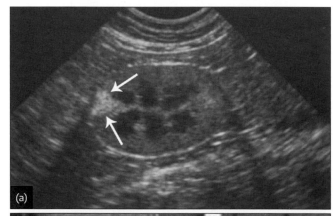

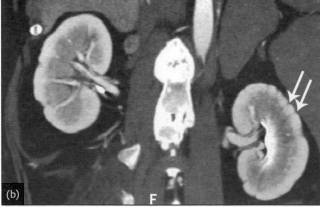

7.19 (a) Sagittal ultrasound image of the left kidney of a 12-year-old Domestic Shorthaired Cat with a renal infarct secondary to hypertrophic cardiomyopathy. There is a hyperechoic wedge-shaped lesion (arrowed) in the cranial pole of the kidney consistent with fibrosing change of a chronic infarct. (b) Dorsally reformatted post-contrast computed tomography image of the kidney of a 10-year-old neutered female Labrador Retriever with renal infarcts. The outer margin of the kidneys is irregular bilaterally and there are wedge-shaped regions of reduced parenchymal contrast enhancement seen affecting the left kidney (arrowed).

Radiography

- The kidneys usually look normal. Occasionally contour defects will be seen with large infarcted regions.
- Excretory urography shows wedge-shaped areas lacking opacification during the nephrogram phase.

Ultrasonography

- Wedge-shaped lesions with the apex towards the medulla.
- Acute infarcts are hypoechoic and visible within 24 hours of occurrence.
- Subacute and chronic infarcts are hyperechoic and often associated with a depression in the surface of the kidney.
- Chronic infarcts are a common finding in older animals and may be incidental.

Idiopathic renal haemorrhage

This is a rare condition with no findings on radiography or ultrasonography. Imaging is used to rule out other causes of haematuria.

Amyloidosis
Radiography

- The kidneys may be small, normal or enlarged.

Ultrasonography

- The kidneys may be small, normal or enlarged.
- Cats often have increased medullary echogenicity.
- Dogs often have increased cortical echogenicity and irregular cortical margins (Figure 7.20).

Ureteral ectopia

Ectopic ureters (Figure 7.21) are usually congenital and can be unilateral or bilateral (see Chapters 9 and 30). Ectopic ureters usually terminate in the urethra or bladder and may tunnel through the bladder and urethral wall. Secondary changes such as hydronephrosis, hydroureter and evidence of pyelonephritis may be seen and are circumstantial evidence for ectopia even if the ureteral opening is not clearly identified.

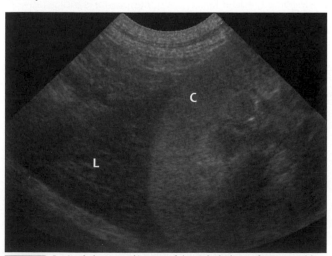

7.20 Sagittal ultrasound image of the right kidney of a 3-year-old neutered male Shar Pei with amyloidosis. The renal cortex (C) is thick and hyperechoic in comparison with the adjacent liver (L).

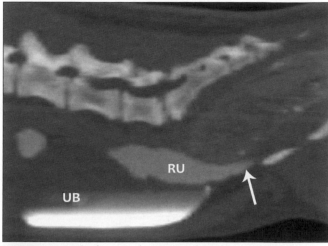

7.21 Sagittal reformatted contrast-enhanced computed tomography image of the caudal abdomen of a 6-month-old neutered female Welsh Corgi with right-sided ectopic ureter. The right ureter (RU) is severely enlarged and the terminal aspect of the ureter (arrowed) bypasses the urinary bladder (UB).

Radiography

- Usually normal, although severe ureteral enlargement can sometimes be seen as a linear soft tissue dense tube in the retroperitoneal space.
- Excretory urography with pneumocystography highlights the ureters and allows the best visualization of the ureteral terminus:
  - Peristalsis may necessitate multiple radiographs in order to view the terminus. In dogs, the ureters may appear to have the normal terminal 'hook' but then continue caudally, tunnelling through the wall of the bladder and urethra
  - Ectopic ureters are frequently dilated as a result of strictures at the opening or chronic infection
  - Absence of contrast accumulation in the bladder indicates bilateral ectopia. However, the presence of contrast medium in the bladder does not rule out bilateral ectopia because urine can leak forwards into the bladder.
- Reterograde (vagino)urethrography can be used to define ureteral openings.

Ultrasonography

- Ectopic ureters can be visualized if hydroureter exists.
- Terminal ureters are most easily visualized as thin-walled tubes residing dorsal to the urinary bladder in the retroperitoneal space. Peristalsis can often be seen.
- If the ureter can be seen to terminate in an abnormal location then a definitive diagnosis can be made. In some cases, the exact terminus is too far caudal in the pelvic canal or is difficult to visualize owing to regional gas. Additional imaging is then warranted.
- Visualization of ureteric jets arising from two discrete normally positioned ureterovesicular junctions makes ureteral ectopia unlikely.

Contrast CT

- Contrast CT (as well as cystoscopy, see Chapter 8) may be the best way definitively to identify ureteral termination prior to correction of the ectopic ureter. Multiple post-contrast sequences with three-dimensional reformatting are often necessary to identify the exact location of the terminal ureter.

Ureterocele

Ureteroceles (Figure 7.22) are defined as regions of congenital localized ureteric dilatation, usually located in the bladder wall. They may be seen with ureteral ectopia.

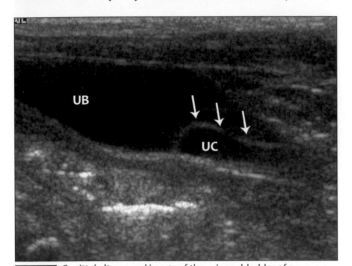

7.22 Sagittal ultrasound image of the urinary bladder of a 3-month-old female Beagle with a right-sided ureterocele. There is anechoic urine in the urinary bladder (UB) and a mural ureterocele (UC). The wall of the ureterocele is visible (arrowed), separating the two compartments.

Radiography

- Often unremarkable.
- Excretory urography shows focal ureteral dilatation, occasionally with secondary hydroureter and hydronephrosis.
- Cystography may show a filling defect arising from the bladder wall in the trigone region.

Ultrasonography

- Focal, cystic dilatation of the ureter is present, which may be within the bladder wall or adjacent to the bladder neck.
- Hydronephrosis and hydroureter may also be present.

Hydroureter

This is ureteric dilatation (Figure 7.23) due to partial or complete obstruction (ureteral calculi, trigonal tumour) or ascending infection.

Radiography

- If dilatation is severe, a tubular soft tissue opacity is seen in the retroperitoneal space.
- Excretory urography shows the ureter to be enlarged, tortuous and lacking in peristaltic breaks.
- Hydronephrosis often accompanies hydroureter.
- Depending on the cause, other radiographic features (e.g. ureteral calculi) may be seen.

Ultrasonography

- A fluid-filled thin-walled tube is visible and can be traced between the kidney and the bladder. Peristalsis is often present.
- Colour Doppler can be useful to ensure the structure is not actually a blood vessel.

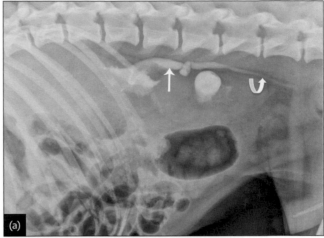

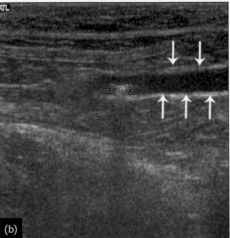

7.23 (a) Right lateral radiograph following a bilateral nephropyelogram in a 1-year-old neutered male Boxer with bilateral hydronephrosis and right-sided hydroureter of unknown cause. The proximal right ureter (arrowed) is moderately enlarged while the distal ureter (curved arrow) is of a more normal diameter. (b) Sagittal ultrasound image of the right ureter of a 10-year-old neutered male Domestic Shorthaired Cat with hydronephrosis secondary to obstructive calculi. Echogenic debris (between callipers) is seen within the lumen of the dilated ureter (arrowed). Obstruction must be present further distally because ureteral dilatation is present caudal to the echogenic debris.

- Hydronephrosis often accompanies hydroureter.
- Assessment for luminal contents (e.g. calculi) and trigonal bladder lesions (e.g. neoplasia) is indicated when hydroureter is seen.

Ureteric calculi

Calculi (Figure 7.24) may also be present elsewhere in the urinary tract (kidneys, bladder).

Radiography

- Radiolucent calculi may not be visible.
- Small, mineralized opacities are seen in the region of the ureters. Orthogonal views are necessary to localize and lateralize the calculi.
- Excretory urography confirms the ureteral location of the density and can identify hydronephrosis and hydroureter proximally.
- Radiolucent calculi can only be seen following intravenous contrast administration.
- Calculi may accompany or result in stricture of the ureters (see below).

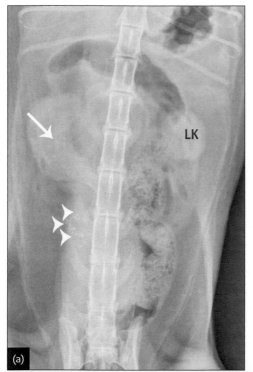

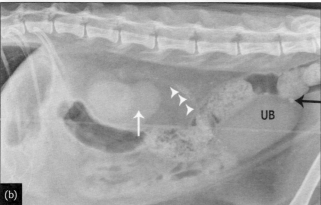

7.24 An 11-year-old neutered female Domestic Shorthaired Cat with ureteral calculi. (a) The ventrodorsal view shows a large number of calculi in the right ureter (arrowheads) and calculi in the renal pelvis (arrowed). The left kidney (LK) is small and irregular, indicating chronic kidney disease. (b) The right lateral view confirms the presence of calculi in the ureter (arrowheads) and the right renal pelvic region (white arrow). Calculi can also be seen at the ureterovesicular junction (black arrow) and in the urinary bladder (UB).

Ultrasonography

- Calculi of all mineral compositions are seen as hyperechoic structures with acoustic shadowing distally.
- Hydronephrosis and hydroureter can be identified and ultrasonography used to trace the dilated ureter in search of obstructive luminal contents.
- Perinephric urine accumulation (urinoma) may occur with chronic or complete ureteral obstruction.
- Care should be taken to continue tracing the ureter if dilatation continues past the first calculus because multiple calculi may be present within the same ureter.

Contrast CT

- Contrast CT can be useful to differentiate complete from partial ureteral obstruction because very small amounts of contrast in the ureter distal to the calculus may be visible with CT but not with radiography.

Ureteric rupture

Rupture of a ureter (Figure 7.25) can occur with trauma or iatrogenically at laparotomy.

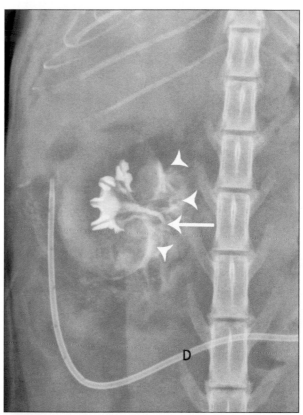

7.25 Ventrodorsal view following a right-sided nephropyelogram in an 8-month-old neutered male Domestic Shorthaired Cat with a traumatic ureteral rupture. Contrast medium can be seen in the renal pelvis and proximal ureter (arrowed). Contrast medium can also be seen outside the collecting system (arrowheads) and around the kidney. A peritoneal drain is in place (D).

Radiography

- Increased opacity and reduced retroperitoneal detail may be present from urine or blood accumulation.
- Excretory urography shows leakage of contrast into the retroperitoneal space:
  - The distal ureter may fail to opacify
  - The ureter proximal to the site of rupture may be dilated as a result of ureterospasm.

Ultrasonography

- Fluid may be seen in the retroperitoneal space.
- Urinomas may be present, appearing as septated cystic masses containing anechoic fluid in the retroperitoneal space.
- Hydronephrosis and hydroureter proximal to the site of rupture, due to ureterospasm, may be visible.
- The exact site of rupture is rarely seen.

Contrast CT

- Contrast CT can detect leakage of small amounts of contrast from the ureter and may be the best way to detect ureteral rupture. The exact location of the rupture can be determined using contrast CT.

Ureteral stricture (following trauma, calculus or tumour)

Radiography

- Severe or chronic stricture may result in renomegaly due to hydronephrosis; a small kidney may be present when the disease is endstage.
- The kidney may appear normal.
- A soft tissue dense tubular structure may be seen in the retroperitoneal space, representing a dilated ureter proximal to the stricture, if severe.
- Excretory urography will confirm a stricture (Figure 7.26) but multiple images may be necessary to differentiate stricture from peristalsis:
  - The ureteral lumen may be smooth or irregular at the site of narrowing, with the latter suggesting mucosal proliferation or infiltration.
- Depending on the cause, other findings such as ureteral calculi may be seen.

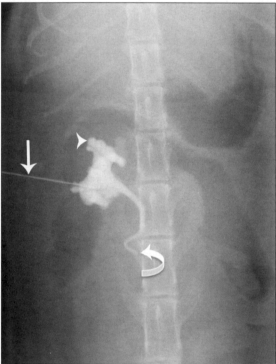

7.26 Ventrodorsal view following right-sided nephropyelogram in a 7-year-old neutered male Siamese cat with a ureteral stricture. A needle (arrowed) is seen passing through the abdominal wall and into the renal pelvis. The renal pelvis is dilated and filled with contrast medium. There is blunting of the pelvic diverticuli (arrowhead) consistent with hydronephrosis. The ureter can be seen to terminate abruptly (curved arrow) at the level of L4.

Ultrasonography

- Hydronephrosis and hydroureter proximal to the stricture may be seen.
- Depending on the cause, other findings such as ureteral calculi may be seen.

Contrast CT

- Contrast CT can determine the exact location of a stricture and will occasionally identify small stones that are difficult to see radiographically.

Bladder and urethra

Radiography

Indications

Radiographs provide an efficient overall evaluation that includes the presence or absence of the urinary bladder, the surrounding peritoneal detail and osseous structures of the spine and pelvis. Radiographs provide information regarding the size, shape, position and opacity of the urinary bladder. The big picture overview that radiographs provide is valuable for assessing multisystemic disease processes such as poly-trauma and osseous metastases from urogenital carcinomas (Figure 7.27). Plain radiographs are often thought to be limited in evaluating the urinary bladder, because they do not allow evaluation of the bladder wall. This is because soft tissue and fluid are the same radiographic opacity, making the bladder wall indistinguishable from fluid within the lumen. However, the serosal (outside) margin of the urinary bladder can normally be identified if the urinary bladder is surrounded by fat. The urinary bladder may not be radiographically detectable if it is empty, surrounded by peritoneal fluid causing border effacement or if there is a lack of intra-abdominal fat.

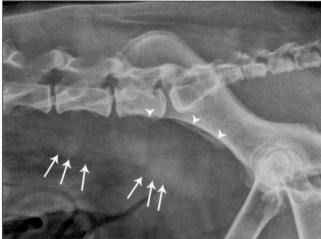

7.27 Lateral radiograph of a 10-year-old neutered male Labrador Retriever with transitional cell carcinoma of the urethra and prostate. There is an irregular margin along the ventral margin of the ilium and L7, representing polyostotic aggressive bone lesions (arrowheads). The undulating soft tissue structure in the caudodorsal retroperitoneal region (arrowed) is consistent with sublumbar lymphadenopathy. These findings are consistent with metastatic transitional cell carcinoma.
(Courtesy of North Carolina State University College of Veterinary Medicine)

Techniques

The urinary bladder is best seen on lateral radiographs, where there is the least superimposition. However, orthogonal radiographs will alter superimposition and help to triangulate structures, which can be valuable because cutaneous debris such as dirt or cat litter can be inconveniently superimposed over the urinary tract. Two or more radiographs should always be obtained unless there is a reason, such as possible spinal instability, which dictates that the patient should not be manipulated.

Small intestinal loops in the caudal abdomen can be superimposed on the urinary bladder and obscure small cystic calculi. Gentle external compression with the use of a wooden spoon or air-filled paddle can be used to displace the intestinal loops and help to separate these structures (Figure 7.28).

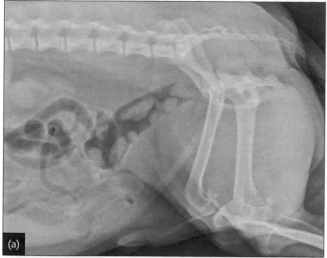

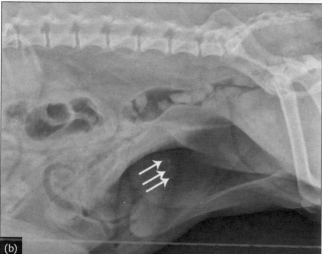

7.28 (a) Lateral radiograph of a 5-year-old neutered male Miniature Schnauzer. (b) External compression applied using a wooden spoon when taking a lateral radiograph helps to displace structures of the caudal abdomen, so that the cystoliths (arrowed) are not obscured by overlying bowel loops.
(Courtesy of North Carolina State University College of Veterinary Medicine)

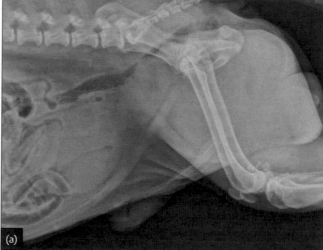

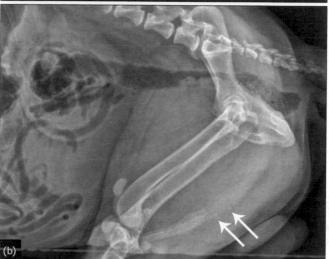

7.29 In male dogs, an additional radiographic view with the pelvic limbs pulled forward allows complete evaluation of the penile urethra. (a) Radiograph centred over the caudal abdomen of an 11-year-old male American Staffordshire Terrier. (b) When the pelvic limbs are pulled forward, a stack of uroliths at the base of the os penis (arrowed) are revealed. These were obscured by the femurs in (a).
(Courtesy of North Carolina State University College of Veterinary Medicine)

When using radiographs to evaluate for urinary calculi it is important to image the entire urinary tract, including the penile urethra, with as little superimposition as possible. In male dogs this requires an additional lateral view that is centred caudally with the pelvic limbs moved cranially so that the femurs are not superimposed on the penile urethra (Figure 7.29).

Normal bladder and urethra

The size of the urinary bladder varies greatly within normal physiological limits. Thus, the size of the urinary bladder should be assessed in conjunction with the clinical signs. Severe bladder distension can indicate an inability to urinate due to mechanical (e.g. urethroliths) or functional (e.g. reflex dssynergy) obstruction or increased production of urine as with diuresis.

The normal urinary bladder is ovoid in shape with smooth serosal margins. The apex of the urinary bladder refers to the cranial margin, while the neck or trigone of the urinary bladder indicates the caudal portion where the ureterovesicular junctions and urethra are located. In dogs, the neck of the urinary bladder gradually tapers into the urethra. In the male dog there is a small triangle of fat

along the ventral aspect that outlines the neck of the urinary bladder and cranial margin of the prostate. The transition from the neck of the urinary bladder to the urethra is more abrupt in cats and they have a longer portion of the urethra that extends into the caudal abdomen. The intra-abdominal segment of the urethra can be visualized if surrounded by fat.

The urinary bladder lies between the ventral body wall and colon, and in entire female patients it is ventral to the uterus. The caudal portion of the urinary bladder can lie within the pelvic canal, especially when it is underdistended, and will extend further into the caudal abdomen with distension. Displacement of the urinary bladder occurs with traumatic body wall hernias, degenerative perineal hernias and masses.

The urinary bladder and urethra should be of homogeneous soft tissue opacity. A small linear mineralized structure in the perineal region of some male cats represents a normal os penis and should not be mistaken for mineralized urethral grit (Piola *et al.*, 2011).

The prostate gland encircles the internal urethral sphincter in male dogs. In cats the prostate is small, lies just dorsolateral to the urethra, further caudally than in dogs, and is not identified radiographically. In dogs the size of the prostate is variable, depending on the age and reproductive status of the patient. In patients that were neutered at a young age a normal prostate gland will not be detected on survey radiography, while the prostate will be larger in entire dogs and increase in size with age. A normal prostate gland should not exceed 70% of the pubic to sacral promontory height (Feeney *et al.*, 1987).

Cystography
Positive-contrast cystography

Indications: Retrograde positive-contrast cystography is an inexpensive and readily available test to determine the location and integrity of the urinary bladder. Positive-contrast cystography is the imaging test of choice to evaluate for urinary bladder leakage or rupture and is frequently performed in patients with trauma to the caudal abdomen. Contrast cystography also provides information regarding the thickness of the bladder wall and outlines intra-luminal space-occupying structures such as radiolucent cystoliths and mass lesions. Indications for positive-contrast cystography include:

- Excellent test to evaluate for bladder leakage or rupture
- Identification of the urinary bladder when not visualized, displaced, or to differentiate it from a caudal abdominal mass or paraprostatic cyst
- Provides back-pressure for retrograde urethrography
- Outlines the shape and mucosal margin of the urinary bladder
- Evaluation for intraluminal space-occupying structures.

Technique: To optimize visualization of the lower urinary tract the descending colon must be evacuated. This can be facilitated by withholding food the night before, ensuring the patient has been walked and administering enemas until the colon is empty. A lateral radiograph of the caudal abdomen can be used to ensure complete emptying of the descending colon before anaesthetizing the patient. This can be done in conjunction with survey radiographs. Survey radiographs are acquired and inspected prior to any contrast study. If a cause for the clinical signs is identified then the contrast study does not need to be performed.

Retrograde contrast studies require catheterization and manipulation of the patient to obtain multiple radiographic views. General anaesthesia or an appropriate level of sedation with adequate analgesia is required to decrease discomfort of the patient, prevent repeat catheterizations and trauma to the urethra, ease manipulation of the patient and decrease radiation exposure to personnel.

Technique for positive-contrast cystography:

1. The external urethral opening is cleaned and a urinary catheter is placed using aseptic technique. A Foley catheter works well because the balloon can be inflated once in the urinary bladder and then moved caudally to tuck into the neck of the bladder, preventing leakage of contrast media around the catheter.

2. The urinary bladder is emptied, the volume noted and samples collected for urinalysis and culture if this has not been previously submitted for analysis. It is important to obtain these samples before introducing contrast media, which will change the specific gravity and may alter urine bacterial culture results (Blake and Halasz, 1995).

3. Water-soluble iodine-based contrast medium is then slowly infused into the bladder. Undiluted contrast medium is more opaque than cystoliths and will obscure luminal filling defects. It is not necessary to have a precise concentration, but approximately 50–100 mg iodine per millilitre is sufficient. This can be achieved by making a 4 parts saline to 1 part iodine contrast solution. Barium should never be used in the urinary tract.

4. The total volume that is injected into the bladder may vary depending on the underlying disease process. In healthy animals, the bladder capacity is approximately 5 ml/kg and therefore this is the volume that should be made readily available before the procedure begins. As the contrast medium is injected, the clinician should carefully palpate the bladder. Instillation of the contrast should be discontinued if the bladder becomes turgid or if there is rebound in the syringe, to prevent rupture of the urinary bladder. The volume of urine that was removed at the beginning of the study can serve as a reference for a safe volume to instil. Several radiographs can be acquired throughout this process to ensure that adequate bladder distension is achieved, because inadequate bladder distension may lead to an inaccurate diagnosis.

5. A lateral, VD and two 45-degree oblique radiographic views should be obtained. The oblique views will allow more thorough evaluation along the wall of the urinary bladder (Figure 7.30).

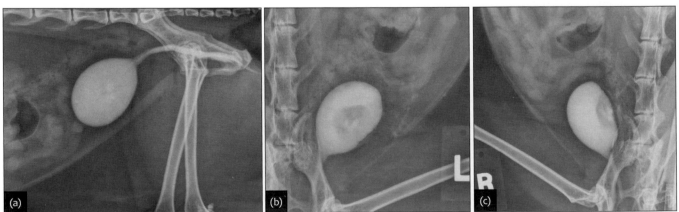

7.30 (a) A positive-contrast cystourethrogram has been performed in a 12-year-old neutered male Domestic Shorthaired Cat. (b–c) Oblique ventrodorsal views allow the urinary bladder to be moved away from the spine and provide more thorough detail of the mucosal surface. This patient has a broad-based filling defect and irregular surface along the left side of the urinary bladder that was cytologically diagnosed as transitional cell carcinoma by traumatic catheterization.
(Courtesy of North Carolina State University College of Veterinary Medicine)

Negative-contrast cystography

Indications: Negative-contrast cystography uses gas rather than positive contrast media. It is an inexpensive way to localize the urinary bladder but does not provide as much information as other imaging techniques and is rarely used alone. Using pneumocystography in conjunction with an excretory urogram to outline the trigone of the urinary bladder greatly improves visualization of the terminal ends of the ureters and gives increased confidence in diagnosing ectopic ureters compared with EU alone (Mason *et al.*, 1990) (Figure 7.31). If CT or cystoscopy (see Chapter 8) is available then a pneumocystogram is usually not needed to trace the shape of the caudal ureters.

Insufflating the bladder with gas is not as sensitive for detecting bladder leakage as positive-contrast cystography, because interpretation of peritoneal gas can be confounded by overlying intestine. Rare instances of fatal air embolization have been reported in veterinary medicine following a pneumocystogram or double-contrast cystogram (Zontine and Andrew, 1978). It is hypothesized that air can move from the bladder lumen into the low-pressure venous capillary system; this is reported more frequently in patients with active haemorrhage. For this reason, negative-contrast studies are contraindicated for patients with haematuria.

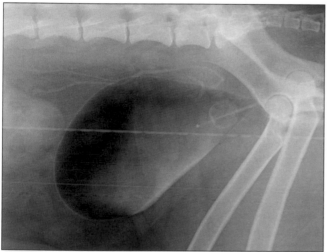

7.31 A pneumocystogram and excretory urogram have been performed to identify the terminal ureters in a 1-year-old neutered female Labrador Retriever with urinary incontinence. The ureters contain contrast medium and have the normal 'J' hook shape before entering the urinary bladder. The bladder contains gas from the pneumocystogram and contrast medium from the ureters.
(Courtesy of North Carolina State University College of Veterinary Medicine)

Indications for negative-contrast cystography:

- In conjunction with an excretory urogram to determine the location of the terminal ureters
- Localization of the bladder.

Technique: Negative-contrast cystography is performed in the same way as positive-contrast cystography but the iodinated contrast media is replaced with gas.

- This procedure should not be performed in patients with haematuria owing to the increased risk of a fatal air embolism (Figure 7.32).
- Room air is most commonly used for this procedure, however there are gases that are more soluble in blood and thus safer to use, such as carbon dioxide (CO_2) or nitrous oxide (N_2O).

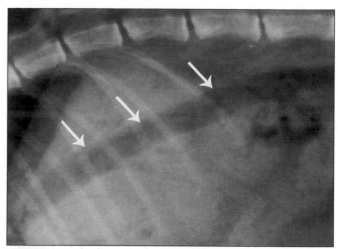

7.32 Lateral radiograph of a Domestic Shorthaired Cat following a double-contrast cystogram. The abdominal caudal vena cava is filled with gas and streaks of gas (arrowed) radiating through the liver represent gas within the intrahepatic veins.

- During this procedure the patient should be positioned in left lateral recumbency; this will lower the pulmonary artery, so that if an air embolism does occur it is less likely to become entrapped within the right ventricular outflow tract. If an air embolism is suspected the patient should remain in left lateral recumbency and the head be lowered to encourage the gas to rise away from the brain and respiratory system.
- The gas should be injected slowly while the clinician carefully palpates the urinary bladder to ensure safe and appropriate distension. If CO_2 or N_2O is used, a pressurized system must not be attached directly to the urinary catheter.

Double-contrast cystography

Indications: Double-contrast cystography provides information regarding the lumen and wall of the urinary bladder. Although this procedure provides more information about the bladder wall than the other contrast studies it has been largely replaced by abdominal ultrasonography, which has even better resolution and is non-invasive.

Indications for double-contrast cystography:

- Outlines luminal and mural lesions
- Assessment of wall thickness and mucosal irregularities.

Technique: Following aseptic placement of a urinary catheter, the urine should be removed from within the bladder, and a small volume (approximately 1–6 ml) of undiluted iodinated contrast medium injected into the bladder. The patient is then rotated to help distribute the contrast medium evenly within the urinary bladder. Finally, the urinary bladder is inflated with gas while palpating the bladder from the ventral abdomen to ensure appropriate safe filling. The precautions for an air embolism are the same as for a pneumocystogram (see above). Lateral, VD and at least two oblique radiographs should be obtained.

Normal findings in cystography

Contrast cystography will delineate the mucosal margin of the urinary bladder, allowing evaluation of the overall thickness of the bladder wall. The wall of the urinary bladder should be uniformly thin (1–2 mm) and the mucosal margin should be smooth and rounded along all margins. The wall of the urinary bladder can appear artefactually thickened if the bladder is underdistended. An underdistended bladder will appear flaccid, because the margins will not be rounded and filled out.

Gas bubbles introduced during catheterization or in double-contrast cystography can appear similar to filling defects and complicate interpretation. Multiple small gas bubbles will tend to accumulate around the margins, similar to froth along the edges of a coffee cup. Large gas bubbles are more likely to reside centrally, have rounded margins and remain in the most independent portion of the urinary bladder as the patient is repositioned.

Contrast media refluxing retrograde into the distal ureters can imply ureterovesicular sphincter incompetency, however this can also occur in normal patients when using a pressurized system. This makes interpretation of uretero-vesicular reflux more difficult, but the size of the distal ureters and degree of distension of the urinary bladder can aid in interpretation because normal ureters are very thin and reflux should only occur when the bladder is under maximal distension.

Urethrography

Indications

Urethrography uses positive-contrast media to examine the integrity, location, mucosal margin and lumen of the urethra. It is frequently used to evaluate for a rupture or tear of the urethra following pelvic trauma or a difficult urethral catheterization. As urethrography highlights the diameter of the urethra, it can also be used to identify regions of compression by adjacent masses, or focal stricture. Likewise, luminal filling defects or regions of obstruction will be further anatomically localized.

Indications for urethrography include:

- Identify tears or rupture of the urethra
- Localize luminal filling defects such as urethroliths, urethral plugs and mass lesions
- Evaluate luminal diameter
- Outline the urethral mucosal margin.

Technique

Patient preparation is similar to that for cystography. Any overlying faeces within the descending colon and rectum will hinder interpretation and should be evacuated by defecation or cleansing enemas. Survey radiographs including the entire urethra should be acquired and examined prior to any contrast studies. A plan should be made to minimize personnel radiation exposure while maintaining an aseptic urinary catheter. Extension sets allow increased distance from the radiation, and shielding can be applied using sheets of lead. This, combined with careful collimation, is recommended in order to decrease radiation exposure to personnel. Patients should be sedated or anaesthetized. Catheterization of female patients is more challenging and general anaesthesia is usually required.

1. Aseptic technique should be used when handling urinary catheters. Foley catheters or red rubber catheters can be used in dogs and red rubber or tomcat catheters can be used in cats.
2. Only water-soluble iodinated contrast media should be used for urethrography. Negative-contrast (air) should be avoided owing to the possibility of urethrocavernous reflux (Figure 7.33).

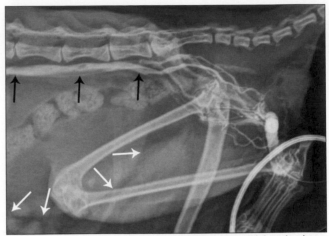

7.33 A retrograde urethrogram was attempted and there has been urethrocavernous reflux of contrast medium into the penile venous drainage and caudal vena cava (black arrows). The patient sustained previous pelvic limb trauma and the limbs cannot be extended, thus they are superimposed on the caudal abdomen. The urinary bladder is severely distended (white arrows).

3. A more concentrated contrast medium is used for urethrography than for cystography, because the urethra is a much smaller structure. The concentration of the contrast medium should be approximately 150 mg iodine per ml. The concentration does not need to be exact because it is a retrograde study and the most convenient way to prepare it is to mix a 50:50 solution of 240 or 350 mg I/ml commercially available iodinated contrast medium with sterile saline.
4. The urinary catheter should be primed prior to injecting the contrast material to minimize gas bubbles. This can be done by combining the procedure with a cystogram or by filling the catheter with contrast medium or saline before passing it into the urethra.
5. A distended bladder will provide mild back pressure to help distend the urethra. A cystogram is often performed first and therefore the bladder is distended before the urethrogram is performed.
6. In both male and female patients, small aliquots of contrast medium can be injected as the catheter is incrementally retracted through the urethra, with multiple radiographs acquired throughout the procedure. The volume of contrast medium will vary, based on the length of urethra that needs to be opacified, but should range from 2 to 10 ml. Radiographic images should be acquired as the injection is ending. This is challenging in female patients because of their shorter urethras and requires tiny movements of the catheter.
   - Alternatively, in male patients, a retrograde contrast urethrogram can be obtained by placing the tip of the catheter in the distal urethra, and a Foley balloon can be gently inflated for a short period of time to prevent backflow as contrast medium is injected into the urethra. Normograde urethrography has been described in female patients but is infrequently performed because it is challenging to time the acquisition of radiographs while the urethra is distended. It also increases personnel radiation exposure as the bladder is manually expressed by abdominal compression while the images are acquired.
   - In female patients, the urethra can also be evaluated using a retrograde vaginocystourethrogram, which is described below.

7. The majority of this examination and the images obtained will be in lateral recumbency (right or left) because this is the view with the least superimposition. Orthogonal views can be obtained, especially with male patients. For male dogs, slightly oblique ventrodorsal views are valuable to prevent the urethra from being superimposed on itself.

Vaginocystourethrography

Indications: Vaginocystourethrography is another way to evaluate the female urethra because it outlines part of the vestibule, the vagina, urethra and urinary bladder.

Technique: To perform a vaginocystourethrogram the patient must be anaesthetized and the rectum devoid of faeces. Multiple absorbent pads should be stacked under the perineal region of the patient so they can be removed as they become contaminated by refluxed contrast media and not obscure the image. The tip of a Foley balloon-tip catheter should be cut off just beyond the inflatable cuff. The catheter is then passed just beyond the vulvar lips and the balloon is inflated within the vestibule. The vulvar lips are closed around the balloon to prevent backflow of contrast medium using atraumatic forceps such as Doyens or Allis tissue forceps. A tighter seal can be obtained by positioning the catheter in the ventral commissure of the vulva and retracting the catheter so that the balloon fits snugly against the vulvar lips. Despite all of this, some contrast medium will leak during this examination and will need to be cleaned intermittently from the perineal region of the patient and the workspace. As contrast medium is injected, the vagina will fill first and, as pressure increases, the urethra and bladder will act as a 'pop-off valve' and contrast will then pass into the urethra. As the pressure builds within the vagina, the contrast medium must be able to move into and fill the urethra. This is why the tip of the catheter is cut short to prevent it from extending too far into the vagina and occluding the external urethral orifice. Serial radiographs can be obtained throughout the procedure to ensure proper catheter placement and appropriate distribution of contrast medium.

Normal appearance on urethrography

The male urethra is divided into three radiographic anatomical regions: the prostatic urethra from the bladder through the prostate; the membranous urethra through the pelvic canal; and the penile urethra caudal to the ischium. In cats, the penile urethra is very narrow compared with the membranous and prostatic urethra. A thin longitudinal filling defect along the dorsal border of the prostatic urethra is normal and represents the colliculus seminalis in dogs and the urethral crest in cats. Occasionally, small amounts of contrast medium will reflux into normal prostatic ducts and will appear as a thin arborizing pattern of contrast medium branching off from the prostatic urethra.

A vaginocystourethrogram will outline the vestibule, the urethral papilla between the vagina and urethra, the vagina, cervix and urethra. A small narrowing at the junction of the vestibule and vagina is normal and focal stricture or perforate hymen is present in some bitches at this site.

Gas bubbles introduced during catheterization can confound interpretation but will easily move with subsequent injections. If a filling defect is identified, repeating the process with an additional aliquot of contrast medium will help eliminate any false-positive findings caused by gas bubbles (Figure 7.34).

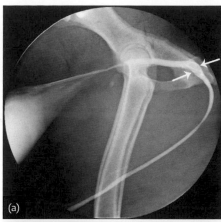
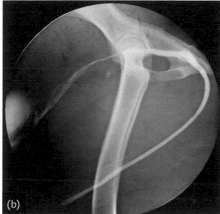

7.34

Two lateral radiographs obtained during positive-contrast urethrography in a 7-year-old neutered male Akita with stranguria. (a) This image shows a radiolucent filling defect in the urethral contrast at the level of the ischium (arrowed). (b) A second contrast injection demonstrates that the radiolucent filling defect was transient indicating that it was actually a gas bubble.

Ultrasonography

Ultrasonography is non-invasive, readily available and provides superb resolution of the urinary bladder. Ultrasonography allows the bladder to be imaged in conjunction with the remainder of the urinary system, including the kidneys, sublumbar lymph nodes, the proximal portion of the urethra and the prostate.

The highest frequency probe available that allows visualization of the structures of interest should be selected. The urinary bladder is easily imaged from either the ventral or lateral abdomen. When trying to discern whether a structure is associated with the bladder wall or simply adjacent to the wall, changing the patient's position to take advantage of gravity can be beneficial. This technique is also useful in overcoming near-field artefacts, when the resolution of the bladder wall in the far field is better than that of the bladder wall in the near field. The urethra is a challenge to image as it courses through the pelvic canal. As much as possible of the proximal portion of the urethra should be imaged by angling the probe caudally from a transabdominal window. The distal portion of the urethra can be evaluated from a perineal window and by tracing the penile urethra as the urethra lies within a groove along the ventral aspect of the os penis (Figure 7.35). Despite this additional window, a short segment of the urethra remains incompletely evaluated. A caudodorsal approach from between the sacrum and ischium can be used to gather crude information regarding the pelvic canal but gas within the more dorsally located rectum typically obscures the urethra.

Ultrasonography allows excellent evaluation of the wall of the urinary bladder and with a high-frequency probe this includes discernible wall layering. The mucosal and serosal layers should appear as thin hyperechoic lines sandwiching a hypoechoic muscular layer. The normal

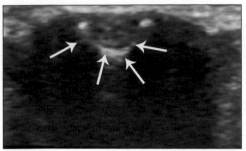

7.35 Transverse ultrasound image from the ventral aspect of a normal os penis in a 14-year-old male terrier cross. The penile urethra runs through the shallow trough along the ventral aspect of the os penis (arrowed).
(Courtesy of North Carolina State University College of Veterinary Medicine)

bladder wall is thin (1–3 mm) but the thickness of the bladder wall changes with distension and can appear artificially thickened owing to underdistention. If the bladder is underdistended at the time of evaluation, examine the remainder of the abdomen and return to the urinary bladder at the end of the procedure. Alternatively, evaluate the patient later in the day, but this can be difficult in patients that are pollakiuric.

Another artefact that can be incorrectly interpreted is caused by refraction of the ultrasound beam along the cranial curvature of the bladder wall, resulting in what appears to be discontinuity of the bladder wall. This typically occurs in patients with peritoneal effusion and can be incorrectly interpreted as bladder rupture. This artefact can be minimized by using compound imaging, where structures are imaged from multiple angles of insonation and data compounded to form the image.

The ureteral papillae can be identified as two focal mounds of tissue at the trigone of the urinary bladder. Ureteral jets of urine can often be seen periodically on greyscale images; this is due to a difference in the specific gravity of the ureteral jet compared with the luminal contents of the bladder. Colour Doppler can be used to enhance detection of these ureteral jets.

The prostate is located at the pelvic inlet, and the majority of prostate can be imaged in most dogs from a transabdominal window by angling the ultrasound probe caudally. There is great variability in the size of the prostate gland but it should be symmetrical in shape. In patients neutered at a young age the prostate will appear as a small bulge along the proximal urethra. In entire dogs, the prostate will appear as two symmetrical lobes that are hyperechoic compared with the spleen and renal cortices and will be noted on either side of a hypoechoic urethra. Small intraparenchymal cysts can be seen in older patients as benign prostatic hyperplasia results in epithelial cell hyperplasia and hypertrophy of the ductal space. These prostatic cysts can become quite large and the normal columnar epithelium can undergo squamous metaplasia, predisposing the patient to abscesses (see Chapter 25).

Computed tomography

Ultrasonography is typically utilized for imaging the urinary bladder prior to more invasive techniques such as computed tomography (CT). However, the pelvic canal limits ultrasonography of the urethra. Contrast-enhanced CT is an excellent modality to evaluate the structures within the pelvic canal, including the trigone of the urinary bladder and urethra. The axial imaging of CT allows visualization of these structures without superimposition. The excellent contrast resolution of CT provides visualization of small structures such as the terminal ureters. Intravenous contrast administration improves visualization of these structures and can be used as an excretory urogram to evaluate for ectopic ureters with minimal patient preparation and without performing a simultaneous pneumocystogram (Rozeard and Tidwell, 2003). CT has decreased the number of retrograde contrast studies that need to be performed, but all of the previously described contrast studies can still be performed with CT rather than radiography if further characterization is needed. The lack of superimposition makes these studies easier to interpret and more sensitive for the detection of small lesions. For retrograde CT contrast studies of the urinary tract, the iodinated contrast medium must be very dilute. Therefore, approximately a 5% (1 in 20) dilution of commercially available 240–350 mg I/ml iodinated contrast medium is used. The increased contrast resolution of CT will allow visualization of this very dilute contrast solution and will minimize artefacts caused by strongly attenuating substances.

Patient preparation and positioning will vary, based on the case. CT allows rapid and complete evaluation for poly-trauma cases, and in these instances the patient may be strapped to a board in lateral recumbency. The isovolumetric acquisition allows post-processing and multiplanar reconstructions that can overcome crooked positioning and aid in surgical planning. For non-emergent cases, patient preparation is standard for an anaesthetic procedure and similar to radiographic studies in that the descending colon should be evacuated. The pelvic limbs should be extended to minimize beam-hardening and edge artefact. To help separate out structures, the patient can be imaged in sternal recumbency with the pubis elevated by a pad so that the caudal abdomen has room to drape ventrally without compression.

Cystoliths
Radiography

- Struvite, calcium oxalate and calcium phosphate calculi are radiopaque and visible on plain radiographs (see Chapters 26 and 27).
- Cystine and urate calculi are often radiolucent (variability in radiodensity exists, depending on the size of the urolith as well as other minerals that may be present within the calculus).
- Compound or mixed composition uroliths will have variable radiodensity and visibility on plain radiographs will depend upon the predominant mineral present.
- Urate urolithiasis is a frequent finding in patients with portosystemic shunts (Figure 7.36) and may be seen in dogs with genetic hyperuricosuria.

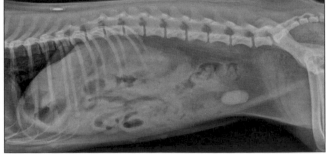

7.36 Radiographs allow overview of the whole patient. In this single lateral radiograph of a 2-year-old neutered female Yorkshire Terrier there is a large cystolith within the urinary bladder, bilateral renomegaly and severe microhepatia with cranial displacement of the gastric axis. This patient has a congenital portosystemic shunt and has developed an ammonium urate cystolith.
(Courtesy of North Carolina State University College of Veterinary Medicine)

- If cystoliths are detected or suspected, radiographs that include the entire urinary tract (including the distal urethra) should be obtained.
- Radiographs are recommended to ensure complete removal of all calculi that may be within the urinary tract after the chosen procedure for calculus removal (using either surgery or other minimally invasive techniques).
- External compression using a wooden spoon can be helpful to visualize cystic calculi by displacing overlying small intestinal loops.
- Non-diluted contrast medium is so opaque that it can obscure cystoliths. Contrast media should be diluted with sterile water or saline to approximately 20% (1 in 5) solution.

Ultrasonography

Mineral appears as a hyperechoic interface at its margin and creates a distal acoustic shadow.

- Ultrasonography is sensitive for evaluation of small cystoliths and mineralized debris.
- All types of calculi are detectable ultrasonographically, including radiolucent calculi.
- Typically cystoliths are gravity-dependent and will move as the patient changes position; however, small calculi can be adhered to the bladder wall.
- Evidence of cystitis can occur as a sequela to cystoliths, or bacterial cystitis can be a concurrent or predisposing factor for calculi.
- Twinkle artefact creates a mosaic of colour when colour Doppler is applied over areas of mineralization.

Urethroliths
Radiography

- Well defined calculi or mineralized debris is seen along the urethra.
- Superimposition of osseous structures such as the pelvis and femurs can inhibit detection. Orthogonal radiographs and an additional view with the femurs moved off the penile urethra in dogs should be acquired.
- Calculi tend to accumulate at the ischial arch and the base of the os penis
- Urethrography can outline intraluminal filling defects and any strictures that may have developed secondary to urethroliths.

Ultrasonography

- Urethroliths are hyperechoic and create a distal acoustic shadow (Figure 7.37).
- They can be detected along the intra-abdominal and penile urethra.
- The urethra may be distended secondary to obstruction (Figure 7.38).
- Urethritis may occur secondary to abrasive trauma caused by a urethral calculus.

Haematomas

Blood clots can create large filling defects within the urinary bladder. This finding is typically seen in conjunction with gross haematuria. The haemorrhage may originate from either the urinary bladder, as with cyclophosphamide-associated sterile hemorrhagic cystitis, the kidneys or systemic coagulopathy.

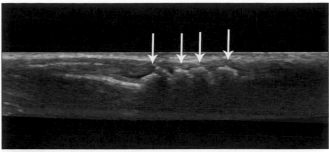

7.37 Longitudinal ultrasonographic view of the penile urethra in a 9-year-old neutered male Miniature Poodle. A stack of four urethroliths is present at the base of the os penis (arrowed).
(Courtesy of North Carolina State University College of Veterinary Medicine)

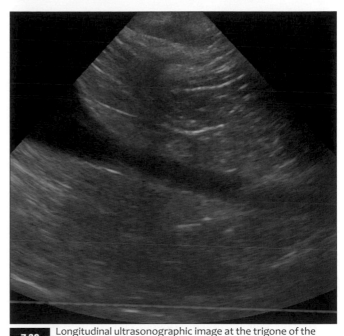

7.38 Longitudinal ultrasonographic image at the trigone of the urinary bladder. The patient is an 8-year-old neutered female Pyrenean Mountain Dog that was presented for stranguria. A distended urinary bladder is present and is confluent with a distended proximal urethra. This is consistent with a distal urethral obstruction.
(Courtesy of North Carolina State University College of Veterinary Medicine)

Radiography

- Haematomas are not detected on plain radiographs.
- Cystography will reveal a filling defect with poorly delineated margins.
- The blood clot may be broken up during the examination and change shape throughout the study.

Ultrasonography

- An echogenic structure is seen within the lumen of the urinary bladder (Figure 7.39).
- Needs to be distinguished from a mural mass:
  - Change the patient's position to determine whether the structure moves with gravity or whether a stalk attaching it to the mucosal wall can be identified
  - No blood flow is detected with Doppler interrogation.

Computed tomography

- The blood clot will not contrast enhance.
- Will create a luminal filling defect after intravenous contrast medium collects within the urinary bladder.

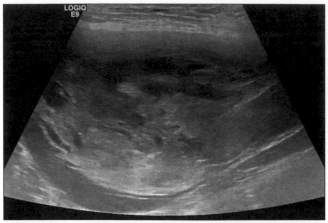

7.39 Longitudinal ultrasonographic image of the urinary bladder in a 12-year-old neutered female American Eskimo Dog with renal haematuria. There is a large blood clot within the lumen of the urinary bladder.
(Courtesy of North Carolina State University College of Veterinary Medicine)

Cystitis
Radiography

- Can be normal.
- Thickening of the urinary bladder wall cannot be identified on plain radiographs because the wall of the bladder silhouettes with fluid in the lumen of the bladder.
- Contrast cystography can demonstrate thickening of the bladder wall and irregularities along the mucosal surface.
- Intramural accumulation of contrast medium may be caused by mucosal lifting and subsequent dissection of contrast medium into the bladder wall, which is more common in cats with cystitis. More common in cats with idiopathic cystitis. Typically no long-term ill effects.

Ultrasonography

- Can be normal.
- Echogenic debris may be present within the lumen that includes punctate echoes that swirl with agitation. The debris may eventually settle with gravity along the dependent portion of the bladder wall. Blood clots can be present, especially with cyclophosphamide-induced haemorrhagic cystitis.
- The most common finding is thickening of the bladder wall.
- Cystitis can be diffuse or focal. Focal cystitis is usually seen at the apex of the urinary bladder, in contrast to bladder wall tumours, which are typically located at the trigone of the urinary bladder.
- The thickness of the bladder wall changes in response to distension of the urinary bladder, and under-distension will artefactually thicken the wall of the urinary bladder.
- Ultrasonography facilitates sampling of urine via ultrasound-guided cystocentesis.

Emphysematous cystitis

Emphysematous cystitis is gas within the wall of the urinary bladder. It is often associated with diabetes mellitus as glycosuria provides a medium for bacterial growth (Figure 7.40).

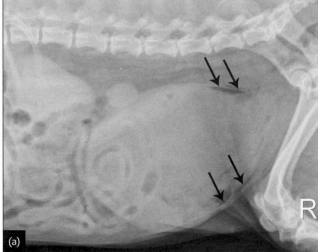

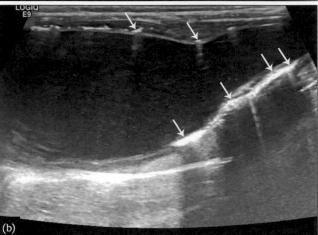

7.40 Emphysematous cystitis. Streaks of gas are evident along the margin of the urinary bladder both (a) radiographically and (b) ultrasonographically (arrowed). Ultrasonographically, gas within the wall of the bladder creates a hyperechoic interface with reverberation artefact deep to the surface along both the near and the far wall of the urinary bladder.
(Courtesy of North Carolina State University College of Veterinary Medicine)

Radiography

- Streaks of gas may run along the margin or completely outline the urinary bladder.
- If present on survey radiographs, there is no indication for subsequent contrast studies.

Ultrasonography

- Gas in the wall of the urinary bladder will create a hyperechoic margin and reverberation artefact that obscures deeper structures.
- Reverberation artefact appears as multiple repeating hyperechoic lines deep to the gas interface.

Polypoid cystitis

Polypoid cystitis is a form of severe chronic cystitis with mucosal proliferation.

Radiography

- The condition is not detectable on plain radiographs.
- Contrast cystography will outline the irregular mucosal margin and filling defects, usually at the apex of the urinary bladder.

Ultrasonography

- Thinly stalked fronds extend from the mucosa into the lumen of the urinary bladder (Figure 7.41).
- These are seen typically at the apex or body of the urinary bladder, in contrast to bladder wall neoplasms which occur more frequently at the trigone of the bladder.
- Can be very prolific and fill a large portion of the lumen.
- Requires biopsy to differentiate from bladder wall neoplasia.

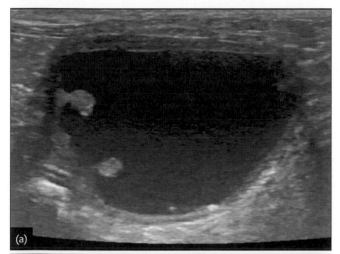
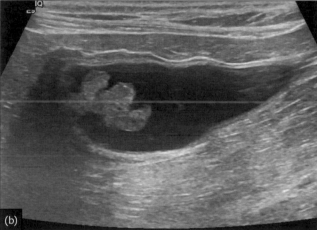

7.41 (a–b) Longitudinal ultrasound images of a 9-year-old neutered male English Cocker Spaniel. Polypoid cystitis appears as stalks of proliferative mucosa extending into the lumen of the urinary bladder. Polypoid cystitis typically occurs at the apex of the urinary bladder. The cranial aspect of the urinary bladder (the apex) is on the left of the image with the caudal aspect on the right.
(Courtesy of North Carolina State University College of Veterinary Medicine)

Urethritis

Radiography

- Survey radiographs will be normal.
- Urethrography may demonstrate an irregular mucosal margin.

Ultrasonography

- Can be normal.
- The most common finding is urethral wall thickening. The differential diagnosis is urethral neoplasia or proliferative urethritis.
- The surrounding fat may be hyperechoic, representing regional steatitis.

Prostatitis

Radiography

- Acute prostatitis may cause mild prostatomegaly, while chronic prostatitis may result in fibrosis and a small prostate with an irregular shape (see Chapter 25).
- In severe cases there can be decreased serosal detail of the caudal abdomen caused by regional peritonitis.

Ultrasonography

- May be normal.
- The prostate may be mildly enlarged, heterogeneous in echogenicity, and the capsule may be unclear.
- If regional inflammation is present, steatitis will appear as hyperechoic surrounding fat and there may be small amounts of fluid in adjacent facial planes.
- Punctate mineralization of the prostate may represent dystrophic mineralization from chronic prostatitis if seen in entire male dogs or dogs recently neutered.

Prostatic abscess

Radiography

- May cause prostatic enlargement and asymmetry.
- If the abscess has ruptured there will be regional peritonitis.

Ultrasonography

- Cystic structures of varying echogenicity are noted in the prostate; they may contain echoic sediment to very hypoechoic fluid.
- The cystic structures within the prostate may be thin walled or have thick capsules. They can be surrounded by parenchyma or bulge beyond the margin of the prostate.
- Diffuse or focal heterogeneous parenchyma, with asymmetrical enlargement, may be seen.
- Regional inflammation is frequently but not necessarily present.
- Ultrasound-guided drainage of the abscess is diagnostic as well as therapeutic.

Benign prostatic hyperplasia

As the animal ages there is a natural alteration in androgen ratios; a relative increase in oestrogen sensitizes the prostatic cells to testosterone. This increased sensitivity to testosterone results in benign prostatic hyperplasia (BPH).

Radiography

- Variable degrees of prostatomegaly may be seen.
- When severely enlarged the prostate may cause cranial displacement of the urinary bladder and dorsal displacement of the colon.
- The margins of the prostate remain smooth and it maintains a bilobed shape.

Ultrasonography

- The prostate maintains a normal bilobed shape with the urethra centrally located.
- The capsule remains intact and the margins clearly defined.
- Small parenchymal cysts are often present within the prostate.
- The prostatic parenchyma may be hyperechoic and slightly mottled.

Squamous metaplasia

Squamous metaplasia occurs secondary to excess androgens and oestrogen, which leads to metaplasia of normal columnar epithelium into squamous epithelium. This metaplasia predisposes the patient to cysts and abscess formation.

Radiography

- Prostatomegaly is most notable when the patient is a neutered male.
- Gynaecomastia – enlargement of the mammary chain – may be seen.
- There may be an abdominal mass representing a Sertoli cell tumour in a retained testicle or an adrenal mass.

Ultrasonography

- Ultrasonography can be used to search for the source of excess androgens; for example, an adrenal mass or retained testicular mass.

Paraprostatic cysts

Cysts form within the prostate as part of the spectrum of benign prostatic hyperplasia as the ducts increase in size. Once these cysts become so large that they are no longer surrounded by prostatic tissue they are called paraprostatic cysts. These cysts are usually sterile but are prone to infection and an abscess may be present.

Radiography

- Paraprostatic cysts may become quite large, extending into the abdomen, and can be difficult to differentiate from the urinary bladder because they can look like a rounded mass in the caudal abdomen (Figure 7.42).
- Paraprostatic cysts may have a thin-walled shell of mineralization (Figure 7.43).
- Contrast cystography may be used to differentiate the cyst from the urinary bladder:
  - The cysts become large when they do not communicate with the prostatic ducts and urethra, therefore contrast medium from retrograde studies does not typically fill paraprostatic cysts.

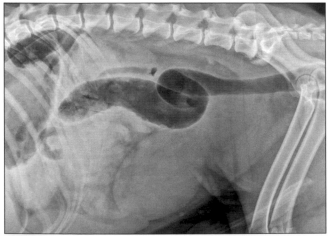

7.42 Lateral radiograph of a 9-year-old male mixed-breed dog. There are two rounded soft tissue structures in the caudal abdomen. One is the urinary bladder and the other represents a paraprostatic cyst. These structures cannot be differentiated without additional imaging, such as ultrasonography or a cystourethrogram.
(Courtesy of North Carolina State University College of Veterinary Medicine)

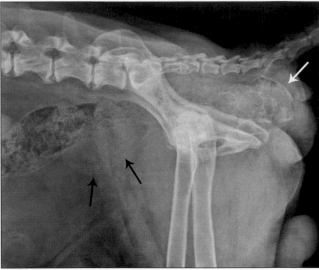

7.43 A 10-year-old male Golden Retriever with several thin-walled mineralized paraprostatic cysts. One of the paraprostatic cysts extends into the caudal abdomen, dorsal to the urinary bladder (black arrows), while several additional mineralized cysts extend caudally into a perineal hernia (white arrow). Entire male patients are more prone to perineal hernias than neutered dogs.
(Courtesy of North Carolina State University College of Veterinary Medicine)

Ultrasonography

- Differentiated large cysts can be difficult to visualize, because the cysts may only have thin stalks connecting them to the prostate.
- When in conjunction with a perineal hernia these cysts can be caudally located between the pelvic canal and the perineum.
- The contents of the cysts may vary as there can be some echogenic sediment.
- The prostate is typically simultaneously enlarged with benign prostatic hyperplasia.

Uterus masculinus

Uterus masculinus is a true form of a paraprostatic cyst that occurs occasionally as a persistent vestigial remnant of the Müllerian ducts. It is a bi-horned or unilateral tubular structure, resembling a uterus, that passes through the cranial margin of the prostate and opens into the urethra through the colliculus seminalis (Lim *et al.*, 2014). The uterus masculinus may be cystic, providing a reservoir for urinary tract infections.

Radiography

- Cystic uterus masculinus can fill with contrast medium during retrograde cystourethrography:
  - It will appear as two blunt-ended thin projections of contrast medium extending cranially from the prostatic urethra.

Ultrasonography

- Uterus masculinus appears as a thin-walled tubular structure extending cranially from the prostate gland.
- It may be cystic and fluid-filled or appear as thin cylindrical structures with no discernible lumen.
- The wall is isoechoic to the urinary bladder wall.
- Can be bi-horned with similar shape to a uterus.
- Variable length.

Diverticula

Several congenital urachal anomalies may occur along the median umbilical ligament. These include: a complete failure to close, resulting in a patent urachus, a small persistent opening at the apex of the urinary bladder; resulting in a vesicourachal diverticulum or urachal remnant (Figure 7.44); and a urachal cyst along the vestigial ligament.

Pathologies causing increased pressure in the bladder can lead to the opening of a microscopic or previously closed vesicourachal diverticulum (Figure 7.45). Traumatic acquired diverticula can also occur as a result of tearing of the serosal and muscular layers with herniation of the bladder mucosa (Figure 7.46). Diverticula are of clinical importance because they create areas of urostasis that may not empty completely when voiding.

Radiography

- Frequently not detected on plain radiographs; however, they may be apparent if the urinary bladder is distended and surrounded by fat.
- Urachal diverticula will appear as cone-shaped extensions along the cranioventral margin of the urinary bladder.
- Traumatic diverticula are seen as a change in the shape of the urinary bladder.
- Contrast cystography will outline diverticula. Multiple views may be needed so that the diverticulum is oriented along the margin of the urinary bladder.

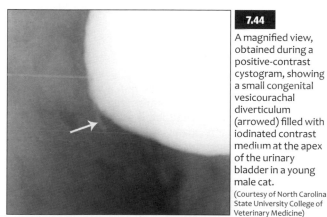

7.44 A magnified view, obtained during a positive-contrast cystogram, showing a small congenital vesicourachal diverticulum (arrowed) filled with iodinated contrast medium at the apex of the urinary bladder in a young male cat.
(Courtesy of North Carolina State University College of Veterinary Medicine)

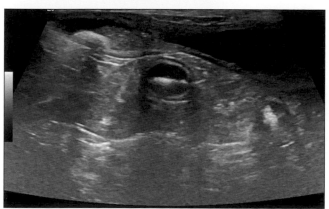

7.45 Longitudinal ultrasound image at the apex of the urinary bladder in a 13-year-old neutered female Shih Tzu. There is a urachal diverticulum that extends from the apex of the urinary bladder towards the ventral body wall. In this example the urachal diverticulum contains both a cystolith and accumulated echogenic debris. The urachal diverticulum opened over time as a large mass developed at the trigone of the urinary bladder and caused partial urethral obstruction.
(Courtesy of North Carolina State University College of Veterinary Medicine)

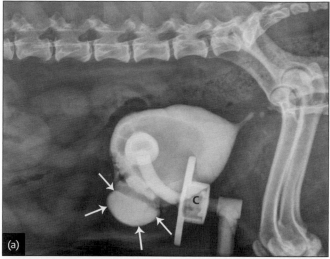

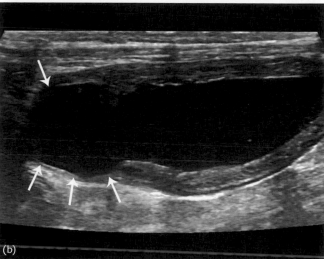

7.46 Traumatic diverticulum in a 9-year-old neutered female Pekingese. (a) Positive-contrast cystography was performed by injecting iodinated contrast medium through a pre-existing cystotomy tube (C). The contrast medium outlines a traumatic diverticulum (arrowed) as a rounded outpouching of the bladder mucosa through a tear in the muscular layer of the bladder. (b) Ultrasound image of the same traumatic diverticulum (arrowed) at the apex of the urinary bladder.
(Courtesy of North Carolina State University College of Veterinary Medicine)

Ultrasonography

- Vesiculourachal diverticula will appear as an extension of the lumen from the apex of the urinary bladder towards the subcutaneous tissues of the umbilicus.
- Traumatic diverticula will vary in appearance depending on size, but typically appear as an outpouching that balloons beyond a focal concentrically smaller opening.

Bladder rupture

Bladder rupture is a frequent sequel to caudal abdominal or pelvic trauma and should always be ruled out in cases of pelvic fracture. The remainder of the lower urinary tract is also subject to traumatic rupture, including the urethra and distal ureters, although this occurs less frequently because these structures are not under pressure at the time of trauma. Lacerations of these structures can result in uroabdomen if the laceration is at the insertion of the urinary bladder (Figure 7.47). Bladder rupture can also occur secondary to urethral obstruction or a diseased bladder wall.

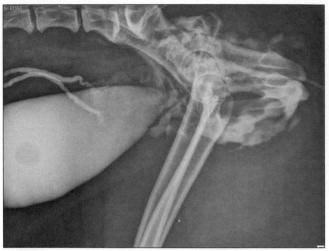

7.47 An excretory urogram and cystourethrogram were simultaneously performed in this 2-year-old Bichon Frise following a traumatic event. There is extravasation of contrast medium from a laceration at the junction of the trigone and the proximal urethra. The ureters are normal.
(Courtesy of North Carolina State University College of Veterinary Medicine)

Radiography

- Small defects of the urinary bladder wall may be overlooked on plain radiographs, if the rupture has not led to a detectable volume of peritoneal fluid.
  - Peritoneal fluid will obscure the normal serosal margins of the urinary bladder. Plain radiographs cannot be used to determine the type of peritoneal fluid, and thus cannot help to differentiate uroabdomen and haemoabdomen.
  - Urine peritonitis disrupts normal gastrointestinal peristalsis and can result in either spastic bowel with a corrugated appearance or functional ileus with distended intestinal loops (Figure 7.48).
- Positive-contrast cystography is an excellent way to evaluate for bladder rupture.

Ultrasonography

- Peritoneal fluid may be seen in the caudal abdomen adjacent to the body wall, small intestines and serosal margin of the urinary bladder.

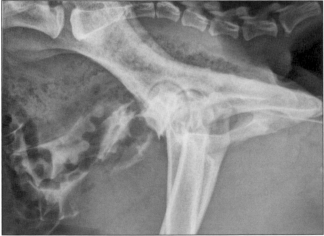

7.48 Retrograde positive-contrast cystography confirms a ruptured bladder in this 1-year-old neutered female German Shepherd Dog. The small intestinal loops are spastic and appear corrugated secondary to the uroabdomen.
(Courtesy of North Carolina State University College of Veterinary Medicine)

- The echogenicity of the peritoneal fluid can be confounding and cytological sampling is recommended:
  - Ultrasound guidance can facilitate diagnostic abdominocentesis.
- The urinary bladder is typically small and may be collapsed and difficult to identify.
- A specific defect in the bladder wall may not be identified.
- Agitated sterile saline can be injected into a urinary catheter, which can be used to confirm bladder rupture if bubbles appear in peritoneal fluid outside the urinary bladder.

Urethral rupture

Radiography

- Urethrography is an ideal way to identify small urethral tears or ruptures as extravasation of contrast medium can be seen in the surrounding tissues.
- Urethral tears may occur all along the urethra, including at the trigone of the urinary bladder.

Ultrasonography

- Tears or ruptures are often not identified ultrasonographically.
- Regional pockets of fluid dissecting through tissue planes may be identified.
- Ultrasonography can facilitate collection of fluid for cytology and culture.

Transitional cell carcinoma

Transitional cell carcinoma (TCC) is a type of urothelial cell carcinoma and is the most common bladder wall neoplasm. Urothelial cell carcinomas typically occur at the trigone of the urinary bladder, and approximately half the cases have urethral involvement. Owing to the location at the trigone, disease can extend into or cause obstruction of the ureterovesicular junctions or the urethra. If a mass is found in the urinary bladder, complete staging is recommended because 37% of patients with TCC have metastatic disease at the time of diagnosis (Norris *et al.*, 1992).

Radiography

- The appearance may be normal, or the tumour may distort the margins of the trigone or cause thickening of the urethra (Figure 7.49).
- The mass may be partially mineralized.
- Sublumbar lymphadenopathy may be present and cause soft tissue masses in the caudal retroperitoneal space.
- Aggressive bone lesions from metastatic disease may be present, which are usually haematogenously distributed and consequently often polyostotic. The caudal lumbar spine may be involved where there is slow vertebral venous blood flow and there can be reactive periostitis adjacent to affected sublumbar lymph nodes.
- Cystography will demonstrate focal thickening of the bladder wall.
- TCC usually occurs at the trigone of the urinary bladder, in comparison with cystitis, which is typically at the apex (Figure 7.50).

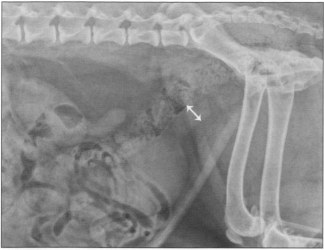

7.49 Lateral radiograph of the caudal abdomen of a 10-year-old neutered female Labrador Retriever that presented for stranguria. The intra-abdominal portion of the urethra is severely thickened (arrowed), creating an abnormal shape at the junction of the bladder and urethra. The patient was cytologically diagnosed with transitional cell carcinoma.
(Courtesy of North Carolina State University College of Veterinary Medicine)

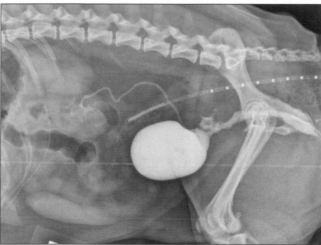

7.50 A lateral radiograph of a positive-contrast cystourethrogram in an 8-year-old neutered female Scottish Terrier. There is an undulating mass at the trigone and proximal urethra. The mass has distorted the ureteral papilla and there is ureterovesicular reflux with contrast medium extending into the left ureter and renal pelvis. A measuring device is present within the colon.
(Courtesy of North Carolina State University College of Veterinary Medicine)

Ultrasonography

- Broad-based mural thickening is observed, with an undulating margin that extends into the lumen of the urinary bladder.
- Subtle thickening of the bladder or urethral wall can be present.
- TCC may arise from the urethra and not be seen along the bladder wall (Figure 7.51).
- TCC may be pedunculated on a thin stalk or have multiple fronds protruding into the lumen but will have blood flow, seen on Doppler interrogation (Figure 7.52).
- Typically, TCC are heterogeneously hypoechoic; they often have a thin hyperechoic mucosal margin.
- Cystic TCC is usually confluent with or involving the muscular (central hypoechoic) layer of the urinary bladder wall (Hanazono *et al.*, 2014).
- Possible hydroureter and/or hydronephrosis may be present if the mass is obstructive at the trigone area.

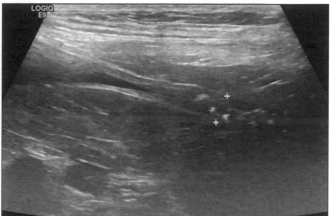

7.51 Longitudinal ultrasound image of the proximal urethra in a 7-year-old neutered female Rat Terrier. There is a transitional cell carcinoma of the urethra, causing thickening of the urethra with multiple hyperechoic foci representing regions of mineralization (between callipers).
(Courtesy of North Carolina State University College of Veterinary Medicine)

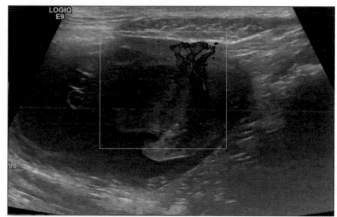

7.52 Transverse ultrasound image of the bladder. Colour Doppler can be used to differentiate mural masses that extend into the lumen and debris or blood clots adherent to the wall of the urinary bladder.
(Courtesy of North Carolina State University College of Veterinary Medicine)

Botryoid rhabdomyosarcoma

Botryoid rhabdomyosarcoma is a rare juvenile tumour that carries a poor prognosis and arises from the urinary bladder wall.

Radiography

- As it is a soft tissue mass, the margins will be effaced by fluid within the lumen of the urinary bladder.
- Contrast cystography may outline a mass with multiple round undulating margins.

Ultrasonography

- Botryoid means 'grape-like'. The tumour appears as a multinodular mass with clusters of cystic structures extending into the lumen of the urinary bladder (Figure 7.53).

Prostatic carcinoma

Prostatic carcinoma can appear very similar to TCC and histopathology is often needed to differentiate them if the lesion is confined to the prostate. Often the disease has progressed by the time of diagnosis, and pulmonary, sublumbar lymph node and/or osseous metastases can be present at diagnosis.

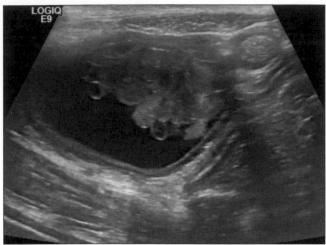

7.53 Ultrasound image of a 10-month-old neutered male Scottish Terrier. Botryoid rhabdomyosarcoma is a bladder tumour of young dogs that has the appearance of a cluster of grapes.
(Courtesy of North Carolina State University College of Veterinary Medicine)

Radiography

- Large prostate detected in a neutered male patient or prostate >90% of the pubic to sacral promontory ratio.
- Prostatic mineralization in neutered male dogs has an extremely high positive predictive value for neoplasia (Bradbury *et al.*, 2009).
- Pulmonary metastatic disease, enlarged sublumbar lymph nodes causing displacement of the descending colon and/or polyostotic aggressive bone lesions may be present.

Ultrasonography

- The prostate may be enlarged, asymmetrical and is often irregularly marginated.
- The parenchyma can be diffusely heterogeneous with course echotexture or there may be a focal nodule.
- There may be areas of extensive mineralization.
- The sublumbar lymph nodes should be evaluated for malignancy.

Malpositioning of the urinary bladder

The urinary bladder may be displaced by adjacent masses or secondary to body wall hernias (Figure 7.54).

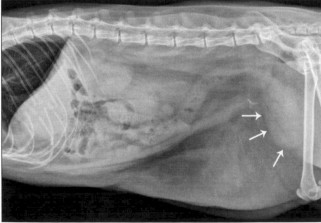

7.54 Lateral radiograph of a 4-year-old neutered male Persian cat. There is a traumatic body wall hernia with ventral herniation of the urinary bladder (arrowed).
(Courtesy of North Carolina State University College of Veterinary Medicine)

Radiography

- When the urinary bladder is markedly displaced, contrast cystography or ultrasonography may be needed to identify its location.
- Rounded masses in the caudal abdomen may be difficult to distinguish from the urinary bladder. Large paraprostatic cysts can displace the urinary bladder in any direction.
- Twenty percent of patients with perineal hernias have caudal displacement and retroflexion of the urinary bladder (Thrall, 2013).

Ultrasonography

- Ultrasonography is useful to help locate the urinary bladder, however it can be difficult to determine the origin of large masses within the pelvic canal.
- A perineal window can be utilized to evaluate a caudally displaced bladder.

Urethral strictures

Strictures can occur at sites of previous mucosal trauma or result from compression of the urethra by external structures.

Radiography

- Urethrography is the ideal way to identify urethral strictures because the contrast column will narrow (Figure 7.55).
- Strictures will be consistent on multiple views and must be differentiated from peristalsis or urethral spasm that will cause transient narrowing.
- Compression from adjacent masses will cause deviation of the urethra or more broad-based narrowing of the urethra with tapering on either end, when compared with primary urethral strictures due to previous mucosal damage.

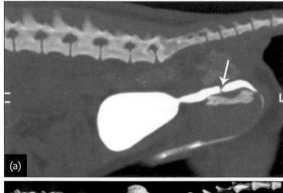

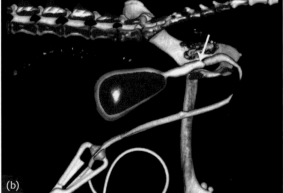

7.55 (a–b) Sagittal computed tomography images of a retrograde contrast cystourethrogram of a 2-year-old neutered male Miniature Poodle. A very focal circumferential narrowing of the membranous urethra persists on multiple scans of the same region, representing a urethral stricture (arrowed).
(Courtesy of North Carolina State University College of Veterinary Medicine)

References and further reading

Adin CA, Herrgesell EJ, Nyland TG *et al.* (2003) Antegrade pyelography for suspected ureteral obstruction in cats: 11 cases (1995–2001). *Journal of the American Veterinary Medicine Association* **12**, 97

Barr FJ, Holt P and Gibbs C (1991) Ultrasonographic measurement of normal renal parameters. *Journal of Small Animal Practice* **31**, 180–184

Blake MP and Halasz SJ (1995) The effects of X-ray contrast media on bacterial growth. *Australian Radiology* **39(1)**, 10–13

Bradbury CA, Westropp JL and Pollard RE (2009) Relationship between prostatomegaly, prostatic mineralization, and cytologic diagnosis. *Veterinary Radiology and Ultrasound* **50(2)**, 167–171

Chomas JE, Dayton P, Allen J, Morgan K and Ferrara KW (2001) Mechanisms of contrast agent destruction. *IEEE Transactions on Ultrasonics, Ferroelectrics and Frequency Control* **48**, 232–248

DeBruyn K, Haers H, Combes A *et al.* (2012) Ultrasonography of the feline kidney: Technique, anatomy and changes associated with disease. *Journal of Feline Medicine and Surgery* **14**, 794–803

Feeney DA, Barber DL and Johnston GR (1982) The excretory urogram: techniques, normal radiographic appearance and misinterpretation. *Compendium on Continuing Education for the Practicing Veterinarian* **4**, 233

Feeney DA, Barber DL and Osborne CA (1981) *Advances in canine excretory urography*. Proceedings of the 30th Gaines Veterinary Symposium, New York

Feeney DA, Johnstone GR, Klausner JS *et al.* (1987) Canine prostatic disease – comparison of radiographic appearance with morphologic and microbiologic findings: 30 cases (1981–1985). *Journal of the American Veterinary Association* **190(8)**, 1018–1026

Feeney DA, Thrall DE, Barber DL, Culver DH and Lewis RE (1979) Normal canine excretory urogram: effects of dose, time and individual dog variation. *American Journal of Veterinary Research* **40**, 1596–1604

Fonseca-Matheus JM, Perez-Garcia CC, Ginja MM *et al.* (2011) Contrast-enhanced dynamic magnetic resonance nephrography in healthy dogs. *Veterinary Journal* **189**, 341–345

Haers H, Smets P, Pey P, Piron K, Daminet S and Saunders JH (2011) Contrast harmonic ultrasound appearance of consecutive percutaneous renal biopsies in dogs. *Veterinary Radiology and Ultrasound* **52**, 640–647

Haers H, Vignoli M, Paes G *et al.* (2010) Contrast harmonic ultrasonographic appearance of focal space-occupying renal lesions. *Veterinary Radiology and Ultrasound* **51**, 516–522

Hanazono K, Fukumoto S, Endo Y *et al.* (2014) Ultrasonographic findings related to prognosis in canine transitional cell carcinoma. *Veterinary Radiology and Ultrasound* **55(1)**, 79–85

Ihle SL and Kostolich M (1991) Acute renal failure associated with contrast medium administration in a dog. *Journal of the American Veterinary Medical Association* **199(7)**, 899–901

Lim CK, Heng HG, Hui TY *et al.* (2014) Ultrasonographic features of uterus masculinus in six dogs. *Veterinary Radiology and Ultrasound* **56(1)**, 1–7

Mantis P and Lamb CR (2000) Most dogs with medullary rim sign on ultrasonography have no demonstrable renal dysfunction. *Veterinary Radiology and Ultrasound* **41**, 164–166

Mason LK, Stone EA, Biery DN *et al.* (1990) Surgery of ectopic ureters: pre and postoperative radiographic morphology. *Journal of the American Animal Hospital Association* **26**, 73–79

Norris AM, Laing EJ, Valli VE *et al.* (1992) Canine bladder and urethral tumors: a retrospective study of 115 cases (1980–1985). *Journal of Veterinary Internal Medicine* **6**, 145–153

Nyland T, Wallack S and Wisner E (2002) Needle-tract implantation following US-guided fine-needle aspiration biopsy of transitional cell carcinoma of the bladder, urethra and prostate. *Veterinary Radiology and Ultrasound* **43**, 50–53

O'Brien R and Barr F (2009) *BSAVA Manual of Abdominal Imaging*. BSAVA Publications, Gloucester

O'Dell-Anderson KJ, Twardock R, Grimm JB, Grimm KA and Constable PD (2006) Determination of glomerular filtration rate in dogs using contrast-enhanced computed tomography. *Veterinary Radiology and Ultrasound* **47**, 127–135

Piola V, Posch B, Aghte P *et al.* (2011) Radiographic characterization of the os penis in the cat. *Veterinary Radiology and Ultrasound* **52(3)**, 270–272

Pollard RE and Puchalski SM (2011) Reaction to intraarterial ionic iodinated contrast medium administration in anesthetized horses. *Veterinary Radiology and Ultrasound* **52**, 441–443

Pollard RE, Puchalski SM and Pascoe PJ (2008) Hemodynamic and serum biochemical alterations associated with intravenous administration of three types of contrast media in anesthetized dogs. *American Journal of Veterinary Research* **69**, 1268–1273

Rivers BJ, Walter PA and Polzin DJ (1997) Ultrasonographic-guided, percutaneous antegrade pyelography: technique and clinical application in the dog and cat. *Journal of the American Animal Hospital Association* **33**, 61–68

Rozeard L and Tidwell A (2003) Evaluation of the ureter and ureterovesicular junction using helical computed tomographic excretory urography in healthy dogs. *Veterinary Radiology and Ultrasound* **44(2)**, 155–164

Scheepens ETF and L'Eplattenier H (2005) Acquired urinary bladder diverticulum in a dog. *Journal of Small Animal Practice* **46**, 578–581

Shiroma JT, Gabriel JK, Carter RL, Scruggs SL and Stubbs PW (1999) Effect of reproductive state on feline renal size. *Veterinary Radiology and Ultrasound* **40**, 242–245

Thrall DE (2013) *Textbook of Veterinary Diagnostic Radiology, 6th edition*. Elsevier Saunders, St Louis

Wallack ST (2003) Excretory urogram/intravenous pyelogram (IVP). In: *The Handbook of Veterinary Contrast Radiography*, ed. TS Wallack, pp. 112–121. San Diego Veterinary Imaging Inc., San Diego

Waller KR, O'Brien RT and Zagzebski JA (2007) Quantitative contrast ultrasound analysis of renal perfusion in normal dogs. *Veterinary Radiology and Ultrasound* **48**, 373–377

Zontine W and Andrew LK (1978) Fatal air embolization as complication of pneumocystography in two cats. *Veterinary Radiology and Ultrasound* **19(1)**, 8–11

Chapter 8

Cystoscopy

Larry Adams

The principal form of endoscopy for the urinary tract in veterinary medicine is transurethral cystoscopy. Although it has been underutilized, transurethral cystoscopy is an integral part of the diagnostic evaluation of dogs and cats with recurrent or persistent lower urinary tract disease (Cannizzo *et al.*, 2001; McCarthy, 2005; Messer *et al.*, 2005). Cystoscopy allows visualization and biopsy of any lesions in the bladder and urethra. The most common indications for cystoscopy are listed in Figure 8.1.

Endourology refers to an area of human medicine involving closed urological surgical procedures (diagnostic and therapeutic) performed using instruments such as cystoscopes, nephroscopes and ureteroscopes. Veterinary surgeons (veterinarians) have also progressed from the use of cystoscopes primarily for diagnostic evaluation of the lower urinary tract to more advanced diagnostic and therapeutic endourological techniques (Berent, 2015).

Equipment

Several rigid and flexible endoscopes designed for use in humans may be used for transurethral cystoscopy in dogs and cats. Figure 8.2 shows the tips of flexible and rigid cystoscopes used in small animals. The size of the patient's urethra dictates the size of cystoscope to be used. Because the urethras of male dogs are long, with small diameters, 2.7 mm diameter (8 Fr), 65–70 cm long flexible ureteroscopes may be utilized for transurethral cystoscopy (Figure 8.2). Rigid cystoscopes used for diagnostic cystoscopy typically

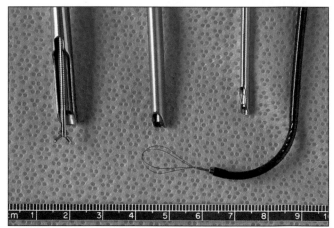

8.2 The tips of rigid and flexible cystoscopes used for cystoscopy. From left to right: 4 mm rigid cystoscope within 19 Fr cystoscopy sheath (5 Fr cup biopsy instrument in working channel); 2.7 mm diameter rigid cystoscope with 14.5 Fr sheath; 1.9 mm diameter cystoscope with 9 Fr sheath; and 2.8 mm diameter flexible ureteroscope with stone basket in the working channel.

Problem	Use of cystoscopy	Comments
Urinary incontinence	• Examine for ectopic ureters or other developmental abnormalities • Injection of peri-urethral bulk-enhancing agents	• More sensitive than contrast radiography • Equally sensitive to contrast computed tomography (CT) • Treatment of refractory urinary incontinence due to urethral sphincter mechanism incompetence
Haematuria	• Determine source of haematuria	• Treatment also possible for idiopathic renal haematuria (sclerotherapy)
Recurrent urinary tract infection (UTI)	• Examine for anatomical abnormalities or uroliths that might contribute to UTI • Obtain mucosal biopsy sample for culture	• Abnormalities of the lower urinary tract are readily detected; more difficult to detect kidney involvement of UTI • Cultures of mucosal samples are more sensitive than urine culture alone
Urinary tract trauma	• Examine integrity of the lower urinary tract • Assist in placement of indwelling catheter past urethral tears	• Cystoscopy is able to detect small perforations or tears of the urinary tract • Placement of guide wire through the cystoscope past urethral tears facilitates catheter placement without enlarging tears
Urolithiasis	• Removal of uroliths via basket retrieval or voiding urohydropropulsion • Obtain uroliths for quantitative analysis or culture via basket retrieval • Fragment larger uroliths via laser lithotripsy	• Cystoscopy is sensitive for detection of small uroliths before and after voiding urohydropropulsion • Basket retrieval allows removal of irregular stones that may be difficult to remove by urohydropropulsion • See Chapter 27 regarding laser lithotripsy
Neoplasia	• Determine extent and location of neoplasia • Obtain biopsy samples for cytology and histopathology	• Cystoscopy is sensitive for detecting bladder and urethral involvement • Stone baskets may be used to biopsy polyp-like projections of masses

8.1 Indications for cystoscopy.

have a 30-degree upward angle view. For bitches weighing 5–20 kg, 2.7 mm diameter (8 Fr), 18 cm long rigid paediatric cystoscopes allow transurethral cystoscopy. For bitches of <5 kg bodyweight and queens, a 1.9 mm diameter (6 Fr), 18 cm long paediatric cystoscope is small enough to pass through the urethra in most animals. For larger bitches, 4 mm diameter (12 Fr), 30 cm long cystoscopes allow access to the cranial aspect of the urinary bladder.

The 8 Fr ureteroscope and 9 Fr paediatric rigid cystoscope sheath each have a 1.2 mm working channel which accepts 3 Fr working instruments. The larger working channels in the 14.5 and 19 Fr cystoscope sheaths accept 5 Fr working instruments. Laser fibres may be passed through the working channel for laser lithotripsy (see Chapter 27). Guide wires may also be passed through the working channels of rigid and flexible cystoscopes for passage proximally in the urinary tract.

Working instruments that are most commonly used during cystoscopy include biopsy forceps, graspers and stone baskets. These instruments are generally available in 3–5 Fr sizes, depending on the size of the working channel within the cystoscope sheath. Use of the largest biopsy forceps that the working channel will accommodate provides larger biopsy specimens.

Flexible-tipped urological guide wires are available in a variety of sizes and designs for endourological procedures. Guide wires may be used as working wires, such that scopes or catheters are passed over the guide wire, or as safety wires to maintain a pathway into the portion of the urinary tract being manipulated. Guide wires may be placed past urethral tears or obstructions under visual guidance via cystoscopy, and then an indwelling catheter can be passed over the guide wire to bypass the tear or obstruction. Without visual placement of the guide wire, retrograde placement of a catheter using a blind technique risks enlarging the urethral tear. Flexible-tipped guide wires can also be passed through the cystoscope into the ureteral orifice to obtain retrograde ureteral access.

Diagnostic techniques

Routine cystoscopic examination of the lower urinary tract

Prior to cystoscopy, the hair around the vulva in bitches and around the prepuce in male dogs is clipped and the skin surrounding the area is cleaned using standard pre-surgical techniques. Bitches and queens may be positioned in dorsal, ventral or lateral recumbency with the vulva positioned at the end of the table. Dorsal and lateral recumbency are the most useful positions for access to the vulva for passage of the cystoscope. Male dogs and cats are placed in lateral recumbency and the penis is exteriorized to access the urethral orifice.

The cystoscope and all related equipment should be sterile. For cystoscopic procedures, aseptic principles are observed, including the wearing of sterile surgical gowns and sterile gloves. The sterile isotonic irrigation solution (e.g. normal saline) should be warmed.

To avoid overlooking any less obvious changes, routine cystoscopy should follow a standard protocol to inspect all aspects of the lower urinary tract before focusing on any obvious abnormalities. In females, the cystoscope may be passed blindly with the blunt obturator using a technique identical to urethral catheterization, or it may be passed under visual guidance with fluid distension of the urethra.

The disadvantages of blind passage include the potential of causing apparent lesions in the urethra or overlooking significant urethral lesions until the cystoscope is withdrawn at the end of the procedure. Therefore, the author prefers to inspect the urethra during initial passage of the cystoscope under visual guidance. The cystoscope should be passed retrograde into the vestibule and into the urethra without entering the body of the vagina to avoid contamination of the scope tip with normal vaginal flora. Once the cystoscope is in the urinary bladder, the urine is drained and the bladder is lavaged with sterile warm isotonic solution and then refilled. This process is repeated as often as necessary to provide clear visualization of the bladder lumen. Overdistension of the urinary bladder should be avoided and the irrigation solution allowed to flow by gravity, with the fluids positioned no higher than 80 cm above the patient. Overdistension may result in bleeding from iatrogenic trauma to the mucosa with resultant impaired visualization of the urinary tract.

Normal bladder mucosa allows easy visualization of submucosal blood vessels (Figure 8.3). Oedema or inflammation of the bladder wall makes the vessels more difficult to visualize and may completely obscure the smaller vessels. Normal ureteral orifices are C-shaped with the opening of the 'C' pointing medially (Figure 8.4). In normal dogs, the ureteral openings are positioned symmetrically

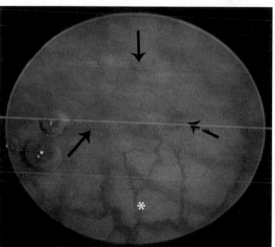

8.3 Appearance of the bladder mucosa in a bitch with calcium oxalate uroliths (uroliths not visible). Note the visibility of the large and small blood vessels in the submucosa of the bladder wall in the normal portion of the urinary bladder (*). In contrast, the vessels are less visible in the cranioventral portion of the urinary bladder owing to oedema and mucosal thickening (arrowed) in response to the uroliths. Three air bubbles are also visible on the left side of the image.

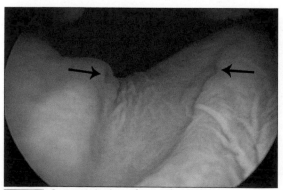

8.4 Cystoscopic view of normal ureteral openings (arrowed) in a bitch placed in dorsal recumbency with minimal bladder distention.

in the trigone approximately 1–3 cm from the vesico-urethral junction, with smoother appearing mucosa between the ureters. The ureteral openings appear to be closer together if the bladder is less distended. In cats, the ureteral orifices are more caudally positioned than in dogs and the ureteral orifices appear to be in the proximal urethra. The positions of both ureteral orifices are identified within the trigone region and urine should be seen entering the bladder from each orifice.

The bladder mucosa should be visually inspected throughout the entire urinary bladder. If a 30-degree view cystoscope is utilized with the animal positioned in dorsal recumbency, the scope should be rotated 180 degrees along the long axis to view the dependent portion of the bladder, in order to inspect for uroliths, masses or other lesions. Figures 8.5 and 8.6 show images from dogs with uroliths and transitional cell carcinoma, respectively.

Masses or polyps

Masses or polyps in the urinary bladder or urethra may be visualized and biopsied during cystoscopy. Transitional cell carcinoma (TCC), the most common neoplasm of the lower urinary tract in dogs and cats, has a highly variable cystoscopic appearance (see Figure 8.6). TCC may involve the bladder, urethra or both. Polypoid cystitis in dogs is a benign lesion that often occurs

secondary to urolithiasis and/or chronic urinary tract infection (Figure 8.7a). Definitive differentiation of TCC from polypoid cystitis requires histopathological evaluation of biopsy samples obtained during cystoscopy. Placement of the biopsy forceps or a stone basket across (or around) the base of pedunculated or papillary lesions (Figure 8.7b) often allows removal of larger biopsy samples from the lesions (Childress *et al.*, 2011).

Urethral masses may also be evaluated using cystoscopy to determine the location and extent of the mass while obtaining specimens for histopathology (see Figures 8.6cd and 8.8). Proliferative urethritis is a benign proliferative lesion that occurs secondary to urinary tract infection (UTI) or uroliths and may result in urethral obstruction (Hostutler *et al.*, 2004). Proliferative urethritis is commonly characterized by side-to-side bands of tissue rather than papillary projections (Figure 8.8). Proliferative urethritis must be differentiated from TCC by histopathology of multiple biopsy samples.

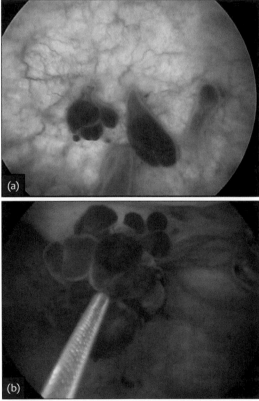

8.5 Calcium oxalate uroliths in the urinary bladder with multiple smaller uroliths. A 550 μm diameter flexible quartz laser fibre is positioned near the surface of the urolith (see Chapter 27).

8.7 Polypoid cystitis in a dog. (a) Polypoid cystitis in the apex of the urinary bladder of a dog. (b) Basket biopsy of polyps from a dog with polypoid cystitis.

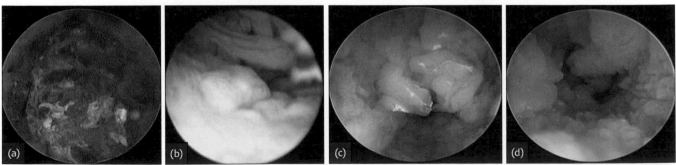

8.6 Variable appearance of transitional cell carcinoma (TCC) in dogs. (a) Large haemorrhagic and partially necrotic mass in the urinary bladder. (b) Papillary structure of TCC. Note the blood vessel extending to the tip of the papillary structure, which is highly suggestive of TCC. (c) Multiple discrete masses in the urethra of a bitch with urethral TCC. Also note that the entire surface of the urethral mucosa is irregular. (d) Urethral TCC resulting in complete urethral obstruction in a bitch.

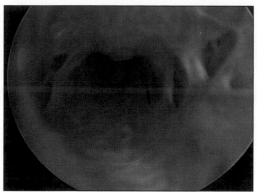

8.8 Proliferative urethritis in a bitch with recurrent urinary tract infection and urinary obstruction. Note the side-to-side bands of tissue, which are more commonly observed with proliferative urethritis than with neoplasia.

Diagnostic evaluation of recurrent urinary tract infection

Cystoscopy is useful for diagnostic evaluation of dogs with recurrent UTI to evaluate for anatomical defects and other comorbidities predisposing to UTI, and to obtain biopsy samples for cytology, histopathology and microbiological culture. Figure 8.2 shows biopsy forceps used to obtain mucosal specimens that have been passed through the working channel of a rigid cystoscope. In two studies comparing urolith cultures and cultures of mucosal samples obtained during cystotomy to routine urine cultures, cultures of mucosal specimens or uroliths were able to detect infections in 18–24% of dogs that were not detected by concurrent urine culture (Hamaide *et al.*, 1998; Gatoria, 2006). In another study, there was no additional benefit from cultures of mucosa obtained by cystoscopy over routine urine culture (Sycamore *et al.*, 2014). While these studies provide contradictory conclusions, the author has observed that cultures of mucosal samples obtained via cystoscopy may detect aerobic bacteria, including *Mycoplasma* spp., not isolated on simultaneous urine cultures. Any lesions present in the lower urinary tract of dogs with recurrent UTI should be also biopsied for culture and histopathology.

Multiple small follicles are often present throughout the lower urinary tract of dogs with chronic UTI; this has been termed follicular cystitis. Biopsy and culture of one or more follicles confirms the chronic nature of the UTI and may facilitate identification of the infecting organism(s). Follow-up cystoscopy can be used to document regression of follicular cystitis after effective management of the UTI, although this is not essential. Uroliths may also be retrieved from the bladder or urethra aseptically for culture using stone baskets.

Ectopic ureters

Recent studies confirm that cystoscopy is more sensitive than excretory urography for identification of ectopic ureters and associated anatomical defects (Cannizzo *et al.*, 2003). Contrast-enhanced computed tomography (CT) is comparable to cystoscopy for diagnosis of ectopic ureters provided the ureter is associated with a functional kidney. The normal ureteral openings should be visualized within the trigone of the urinary bladder (see Figure 8.4), and ectopic ureteral openings are usually detected in the urethra (Figure 8.9a) or in the vaginal vestibule (uncommon). To assist in determining whether ectopic ureters are intramural or extramural, flexible-tipped urological guide wires may be passed retrograde into the ureteral opening

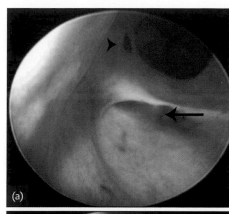

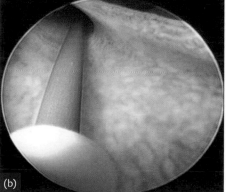

8.9 Bilateral ectopic ureters in a bitch. (a) The right ureteral opening (arrowhead) is located in the proximal urethra just distal to the junction with the urinary bladder. The left ureteral opening is visible in the dorsal aspect of the mid-urethra (black arrow). (b) A urological guide wire is passed through an open-ended ureteral catheter proximally into the left ectopic ureter.

under visual guidance (Figure 8.9b) and retrograde ureterography may be performed using fluoroscopy. Intramural ectopic ureters may be corrected by cystoscopic-guided laser ablation (see Chapter 27) (Berent *et al.*, 2012).

Concurrent urethral malformation is common in dogs with ectopic ureters (Cannizzo *et al.*, 2003). Urethral conformation is evaluated during initial visual passage of the cystoscope, assessing its shape and noting the presence of any ectopic ureteral openings within the urethra. The normal urethra in bitches and queens has a single prominent dorsal ridge extending most of the length of the urethra. In bitches with ectopic ureters, ureteral troughs are often seen as ridges that extend down the urethra from the edge of the ectopic ureteral openings. Abnormalities of the vaginal vestibule such as paramesonephric septal remnants (also called vaginal septae) are also common concurrent developmental abnormalities seen in bitches with ectopic ureters (Cannizzo *et al.*, 2003). These vaginal septae may also be corrected by laser ablation using cystoscopic guidance (Burdick *et al.*, 2014).

Localization of haematuria

During cystoscopy, the source of gross haematuria can usually be definitively localized to the genital tract, urethra, bladder, or the left or right kidney and ureter. This approach is more accurate than predicting the location of haematuria on the basis of when blood is noted during voiding. Haemorrhagic lesions in the lower urinary tract can be confirmed and sometimes treated, depending on the nature of the lesion (e.g. uroliths, neoplasia). Diagnosis of upper tract (kidneys, ureters) haematuria can be determined by direct visualization of gross haematuria from the ureteral orifice (Figure 8.10). Recently, cystoscopic-guided sclerotherapy has been reported as an option for treatment of idiopathic renal haematuria in dogs, as opposed to performing nephrectomy (Berent *et al.*, 2013). Nephrectomy is not

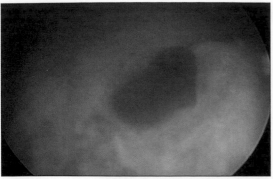

8.10 Gross haemorrhagic urine from the left ureteral orifice in a bitch with unilateral idiopathic renal haematuria.

recommended because 20–30% of dogs with idiopathic renal haematuria may bleed from both kidneys at the time of initial diagnosis or later in life. Ureteral stent placement is recommended following sclerotherapy. If sclerotherapy does not resolve the haematuria, then retrograde ureteroscopy and electocautery may be attempted for direct cauterization of the bleeding vessel inside the renal pelvis. Ureteroscopy is facilitated by the passive ureteral dilation caused by the indwelling ureteral stent.

Therapeutic techniques

Stone baskets

Stone baskets may be used to remove uroliths from the lower urinary tract provided the uroliths are smaller than the dilated urethra. Stone baskets are usually passed through the working channel of the cystoscope (see Figure 8.2), the basket is opened and, once the urolith is engaged in the basket, the basket is closed around the urolith and positioned at the end of the cystoscope (Figure 8.11). The cystoscope and basket containing the urolith are then slowly withdrawn through the urethra (the urethra is distended by infusing sterile saline) under direct visualization to ensure there is no bulging of the urothelium around the urolith edges, which may indicate that the urolith is becoming wedged in the urethra. This technique may be safely used to remove some uroliths that will not readily pass during voiding urohydropropulsion; however, caution is required to avoid getting the urolith wedged in the urethra. If

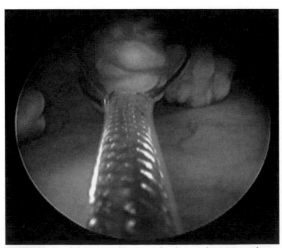

8.11 Urolith trapped in stone basket and positioned near the end of the cystoscope prior to removal. Note additional uroliths adjacent to stone basket.

the urolith is too large for basket extraction, it may be released and broken into smaller fragments by laser lithotripsy using a holmium:YAG (yttrium aluminium garnet) laser (see Chapter 27); alternatively, other minimally invasive techniques have been recommended (Adams *et al.*, 2008).

Peri-urethral injection of bulk-enhancing agents for treatment of urinary incontinence

An alternative therapy for dogs with refractory urinary incontinence due to confirmed urethral sphincter mechanism incompetence includes cystoscopic-guided peri-urethral injection of bulk-enhancing agents (e.g. glutaraldehyde cross-linked collagen) (Arnold *et al.*, 1996; Barth *et al.*, 2005; Byron *et al.*, 2011). Peri-urethral injection of collagen narrows the urethral lumen and allows more effective closure of the urethra by the existing urethral pressure. In one study, 68% of dogs remained continent for an average of 17 months after peri-urethral collagen injection (Barth *et al.* 2005), although repeat cystoscopic injection of collagen is required in some dogs to maintain continence (Byron *et al.* 2011). For further discussion of urethral bulking agents, see Chapter 30.

Removal of polyps or tumours

Cystoscopy is useful for documenting the extent and location of lower urinary tract neoplasia and for obtaining biopsy samples for cytology and histopathology from lesions within the bladder or urethra. Biopsy using stone baskets placed around the base of the mass (see Figure 8.7b) results in larger samples, which are more often diagnostic than pinch biopsy specimens obtained using cup biopsy forceps (Childress *et al.*, 2011). Some polyps or tumours with narrow stalks can be removed using biopsy instruments, electrocautery snares or with a holmium:YAG or diode laser (McCarthy, 2003; Cerf and Lindquist, 2012). It is important to avoid full-thickness injury, resulting in urethral or bladder perforation and resultant uroabdomen. TCC lesions with a narrow-based stalk may be removed using a holmium:YAG or diode laser followed by fulguration of the base. Benign polyps (e.g. polypoid cystitis) may also be removed from the bladder using a holmium:YAG or diode laser.

Urethral stricture dilation

Urethral strictures appear as an abrupt narrowing of the urethral lumen during cystoscopy (Figure 8.12a). If the stricture is too small to allow passage of the cystoscope, a flexible-tipped guide wire may be passed through the strictured area via the working channel of the scope under fluoroscopic guidance (Figure 8.12b). Next, an open-ended catheter may be passed over the guide wire and retrograde contrast studies should be performed to delineate the extent of the urethral stricture and to obtain measurements for interventions to correct the stricture. Alternatively, contrast may be injected through the working channel of a flexible cystoscope to perform retrograde contrast studies. Urethral strictures may be dilated over the guide wire using an appropriately sized balloon dilation catheter (Figures 8.12b–d) (Hill *et al.*, 2014). Urethral strictures will re-stricture to some degree after balloon dilation and may require re-dilation. If the urethral stricture recurrence is severe enough to cause urine retention, then placement of a nitinol self-expanding urethral stent may be required to resolve the urinary retention (Hill *et al.*, 2014).

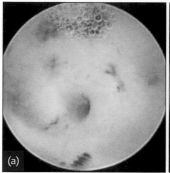 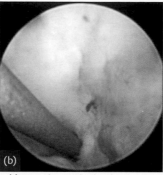 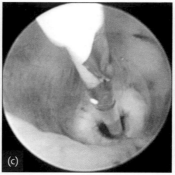 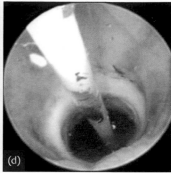

8.12 Urethral stricture in a queen. (a) Note the marked reduction in urethral diameter and firm white appearance of the urethral stricture. (b) Guide wire (0.025 inch diameter) passed through the stricture. (c) Initial stage of balloon dilation of the urethral stricture using a clear balloon catheter passed parallel to the cystoscope over the 0.64 mm guide wire. (d) Complete balloon dilation of the urethral stricture.

Risks and complications

Complications from routine cystoscopy are uncommon; however, potential complications include iatrogenic UTI and trauma to the urinary tract such as perforation or rupture of the urethra or urinary bladder. Passage of rigid cystoscopes should be done as atraumatically as possible and only under visual guidance, to avoid urethral trauma. Insertion of too large a cystoscope for the patient's size is an avoidable error that could lead to urethral trauma.

Iatrogenic UTI can be avoided by use of appropriate aseptic technique and avoiding mucosal trauma. Additionally, irrigation with large volumes of sterile isotonic solutions, normally done to provide clear visualization of the urinary tract, further serves to remove any bacteria introduced by passage of the cystoscope from the non-sterile distal urethra and vaginal vestibule into the urinary bladder. Routine administration of prophylactic antibiotics (e.g. amoxicillin 20 mg/kg orally q12h for 3 days) is not required unless the cystoscope is passed up the urethra multiple times during the procedure or there are additional predisposing factors to the establishment of UTI such as mucosal injury, neoplasia or urethral stricture.

References and further reading

Adams LG, Berent AC, Moore GE et al. (2008) Use of laser lithotripsy for fragmentation of uroliths in dogs: 73 cases (2005–2006). Journal of the American Veterinary Medical Association 232, 1680–1687

Arnold S, Bubler M, Lott-Stolz G et al. (1996) Treatment of urinary incontinence in bitches by endoscopic injection of glutaraldehyde cross-linked collagen. Journal of Small Animal Practice 37, 163–168

Barth A, Reichler IM, Hubler M et al. (2005) Evaluation of long-term effects of endoscopic injection of collagen into the urethral submucosa for treatment of urethral sphincter incompetence in female dogs: 40 cases (1993–2000). Journal of the American Veterinary Medical Association 226, 73–76

Berent AC (2015) Interventional urology: endourology in small animal veterinary medicine. Veterinary Clinics of North America: Small Animal Practice 45, 825–855

Berent AC, Weisse CW, Brantler E et al. (2013) Endoscopic-guided sclerotherapy for renal-sparing treatment of idiopathic renal hematuria in dogs: 6 cases (2010–2012). Journal of the American Veterinary Medical Association 242, 1556–1563

Berent AC, Weisse CW, Mayhew PD et al. (2012) Evaluation of cystoscopic-guided laser ablation of intramural ectopic ureters in female dogs. Journal of the American Veterinary Medical Association 240, 716–725

Burdick S, Berent AC, Weisse CW et al. (2014) Endoscopic-guided laser ablation of vestibulovaginal septal remnants in dogs: 36 cases (2007–2011). Journal of the American Veterinary Medical Association 244, 944–949

Byron JK, Chew DJ and McLoughlin ML (2011) Retrospective evaluation of urethral bovine cross-linked collagen implantation for treatment of urinary incontinence in female dogs. Journal of Veterinary Internal Medicine 25, 980–984

Cannizzo KL, McLoughlin ML, Chew DJ et al. (2001) Uroendoscopy. Evaluation of the lower urinary tract. Veterinary Clinics of North America: Small Animal Practice 31, 789–807

Cannizzo KL, McLoughlin ML, Mattoon JS et al. (2003) Evaluation of transurethral cystoscopy and excretory urography for diagnosis of ectopic ureters in female dogs: 25 cases (1992–2000). Journal of the American Veterinary Medical Association 223, 475–481

Cerf DJ and Lindquist EC (2012) Palliative ultrasound-guided endoscopic diode laser ablation of transitional cell carcinomas of the lower urinary tract in dogs. Journal of the American Veterinary Medical Association 240, 51–60

Childress MO, Adams LG, Ramos-Vara JA et al. (2011) Comparison of cystoscopy versus surgery in obtaining diagnostic biopsy specimens from dogs with transitional cell carcinoma of the urinary bladder and urethra. Journal of the American Veterinary Medical Association 239, 350–356

Gatoria IS (2006) Comparison of three techniques for the diagnosis of urinary tract infections in dogs with urolithiasis. Journal of Small Animal Practice 47, 727–732

Hamaide AJ, Martinez SA, Hauptman J et al. (1998) Prospective comparison of four sampling methods (cystocentesis, bladder mucosal swab, bladder mucosal biopsy, and urolith culture) to identify urinary tract infections in dogs with urolithiasis. Journal of the American Animal Hospital Association 34, 423–430

Hill TL, Berent AC and Weisse CW (2014) Evaluation of urethral stent placement for benign urethral obstructions in dogs. Journal of Veterinary Internal Medicine 28, 1384–1390

Hostutler RA, Chew DJ, Eaton KA et al. (2004) Cystoscopic appearance of proliferative urethritis in 2 dogs before and after treatment. Journal of Veterinary Internal Medicine 18, 113–116

McCarthy TC (2003) Transitional cell carcinoma. Veterinary Medicine 98, 96–96

McCarthy TC (2005) Cystoscopy. In: Veterinary Endoscopy, ed. TC McCarthy, pp.49–135. Elsevier Saunders, St. Louis

Messer JS, Chew DJ and McLoughlin ML (2005) Cystoscopy: techniques and clinical applications. Clinical Techniques in Small Animal Practice 20, 52–64

Sycamore KF, Poorbaugh VR, Pullin SS et al. (2014) Comparison of urine and bladder or urethral mucosal biopsy culture obtained by transurethral cystoscopy in dogs with chronic lower urinary tract disease: 41 cases (2002 to 2011). Journal of Small Animal Practice 55, 364–368

Chapter 9

Diagnostic approach to the incontinent patient

Julie Byron

Urinary incontinence (UI), the involuntary loss of urine through the urethra, is a common problem in small animal veterinary practice. Female neutered dogs are most commonly affected, with up to 20% of neutered female dogs and 30% of those weighing more than 20 kg reported to be incontinent. Urinary incontinence is less common in the male dog and in cats, but has been reported. Urinary incontinence in male dogs, intact bitches and cats is often related to congenital defects such as ureteral ectopia or urogenital sinus malformations. There is a wide range of causes of UI and diagnosis of the underlying disorder is important in determining treatment and prognosis. Careful attention to the history and physical examination, and a systematic approach to diagnostic planning, will ensure that unusual or uncommon disorders will not be missed. In this chapter, a basic diagnostic algorithm is presented for assessment of male dogs and bitches with UI (Figures 9.1 and 9.2) as well as more detailed information on diagnostic imaging and the use of advanced diagnostic techniques in small animal patients.

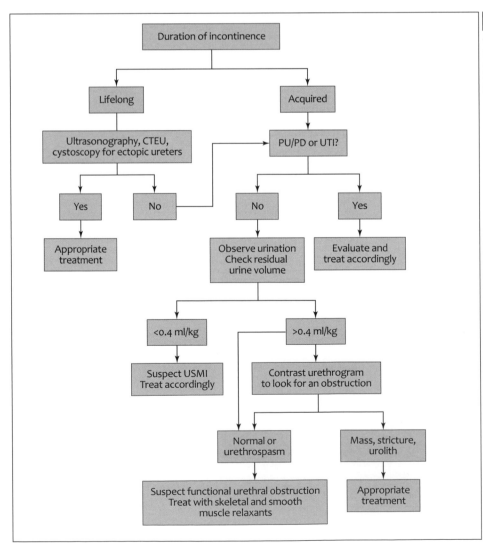

9.1 Diagnostic algorithm for male dogs with urinary incontinence. CTEU = computed tomographic excretory urogram; PU/PD = polyuria/polydipsia; USMI = urethral sphincter mechanism incompetence; UTI = urinary tract infection. (© Julie Byron)

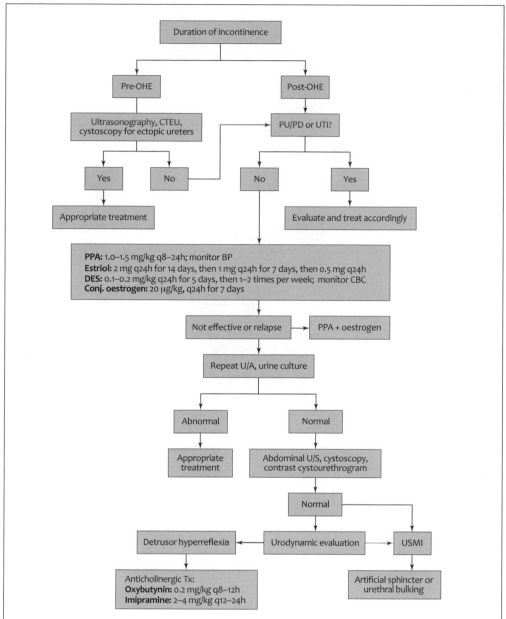

9.2 Diagnostic algorithm for bitches with urinary incontinence. BP = blood pressure; CBC = complete blood count; Conj. = conjugated; CTEU = computed tomographic excretory urogram; DES = diethystilboestrol; OHE = ovariohysterectomy; PPA = phenylpropanolamine; PU/PD = polyuria/polydipsia; Tx = therapy; U/A = urinalysis; U/S = ultrasonography; USMI = urethral sphincter mechanism incompetence; UTI = urinary tract infection.
(© Julie Byron)

Initial evaluation

Diagnostic evaluation of the patient with UI at first presentation has several important parts. These include verifying the presence of urinary incontinence *versus* other urogenital diseases, assessing the duration of the clinical signs, and determining whether the cause is a disorder of storage (e.g. urethral sphincter mechanism incompetence, USMI) or a disorder of emptying (e.g. functional obstruction). Routine urinalysis and urine culture may also be performed. Additional testing for concurrent disease or to monitor for complications is dependent on the patient and may be related to initial therapeutic decisions.

Signalment and history

A careful history must be taken when discussing UI with pet owners. It must be distinguished from behavioural problems, polyuria or pollakiuria, and it is important to establish that the animal is unconsciously voiding urine.

Many owners will use the term 'incontinence' when inappropriate conscious urination occurs (e.g. pollakiuria). Some owners may report finding urine spots in the home, but may not have observed how it occurred. In this situation, it is important to keep in mind the potential for polyuria, pollakiuria or behavioural problems, particularly if the animal does not respond to empirical therapy.

The timing and situational occurrence of UI can also be useful to the veterinary surgeon (veterinarian) in determining the cause. Urinary incontinence varies in frequency among patients. Some animals have only a few episodes a month, while others are persistently leaking urine. Most neutered females with USMI leak urine when relaxed, lying down or sleeping. Occasionally, UI will occur during vigorous physical activity. Some animals are reported to be incontinent after active urination. Since normal urination nearly empties the bladder, this may be a sign of urine retention, either from physical or functional obstruction, particularly in male dogs. In addition, it is thought that some bitches can have 'urine pooling' in either the vagina or the vestibule, although this can be challenging to document.

The age of onset of UI is important to establish in young dogs, to determine the potential for ureteral ectopia or other conformational abnormalities. Breeds such as the Soft-coated Wheaten Terrier, Labrador Retriever, Siberian Husky, Golden Retriever, Newfoundland and English Bulldog have an increased prevalence of ureteral ectopia. Animals with ectopic ureters often have clinical signs of UI, which start prior to neutering, although this may be misinterpreted as poor housetraining by the owners. A small number of dogs with ectopic ureters (particularly males) may not have significant UI until after neutering, so later onset does not rule out the possibility of a congenital malformation. Dogs with early onset of clinical signs should be evaluated for ectopic ureters, particularly if they show little or no response to empirical medical therapy. In addition to ureteral ectopia, several other conformational abnormalities can lead to UI from a young age. Hypoplastic or short urethra, pelvic bladder displacement, and juvenile or 'hooded' vulvar conformation in females have all been associated with either congenital or acquired UI. Dobermanns and Weimaraners have a higher prevalence of pelvic bladder, and older obese neutered bitches may have hooded vulvas.

General historical information such as water and food intake, activity level and evidence of discomfort when urinating can provide clues to the cause of the UI. Patients where UI has developed along with an increase in water intake should be further evaluated for disorders causing polyuria and polydipsia. If an underlying cause, such as hyperadrenocorticism (see Chapter 2), can be identified and treated, it is likely to improve the chances of a response to UI therapy by reducing the overall volume of urine produced and decreasing the bladder pressure exerted on a weak urethral sphincter mechanism. Dogs and cats with neurological disease or orthopaedic pain may have difficulty posturing to urinate and may have urine retention. A history of pain or straining when urinating, or a reluctance to urinate, may indicate such a problem. Finally, it is also important to note the frequency with which the animal is allowed to urinate consciously, and any changes in 'asking to go out' or use of a litterbox or container. This will help to establish bladder capacity expectations or may indicate urinary inflammation or retention.

Physical examination and observation of urination

While a thorough physical examination should be performed on every patient, there are some areas that are particularly important to evaluate in the incontinent animal. Palpation of the bladder, assessing for size, position and pain, and watching for urine loss during palpation may indicate conformational problems, cystitis or severely decreased urethral pressure. Many animals with disorders of emptying and urine retention have palpably overdistended bladders. Rectal examination will allow the clinician to assess the prostate in males and palpate the urethra through the rectal wall. The normal pelvic urethra, even in patients with USMI, is smooth and does not change much in thickness, while irregularity may indicate an obstructive process such as an urethrolith or a mass lesion. Anal tone should also be assessed during rectal examination.

The external genitalia of the animal should be carefully examined. Bitches may have a hooded vulva, leading to perivulvar dermatitis or urine pooling in the vestibule (Figure 9.3). Male animals may have preputial or penile conformational abnormalities, which can impede urine

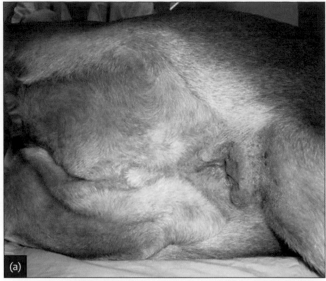

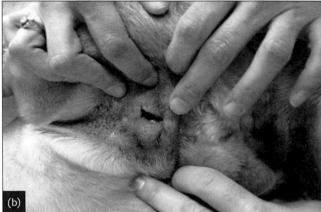

9.3 Juvenile or 'hooded' vulva. (a) This 8-year-old neutered female mixed-breed dog had a 3-year history of urinary incontinence due to urethral sphincter mechanism incompetence (USMI) and recurrent urinary tract infections. (b)There is evidence of perivulvar dermatitis when the perineal folds are retracted. The relationship between a 'hooded' vulva and USMI in neutered bitches is unclear.

flow. Staining of the hair around the prepuce or vulva may be further indication of UI or of excessive grooming of the perineum to remove leaked urine. Some animals with severe long-term UI may have significant urine-induced ulcerative dermatitis around the vulva or prepuce.

An orthopaedic and neurological examination should be performed, including observation of the gait. Particular attention should be paid to the hips and stifles, as well as the thoracolumbar and lumbosacral spine. Pain on posturing can prevent an animal from fully emptying the bladder and lead to overflow incontinence. Bladder and urethral function is impaired with lesions cranial to the first sacral spinal segment (cranial to the 5th lumbar vertebra in the dog and approximately the 3rd lumbar vertebra in the cat) leading to automatic or 'upper motor neuron' bladder. These patients have difficulty emptying their bladders, due to increased urethral sphincter pressure, and may develop chronic overdistension of the urinary bladder. This leads to overflow UI and is considered a disorder of emptying. Alternatively, lesions at the 1st and 2nd sacral spinal segment (5th lumbar vertebra in the dog and 3rd to 5th lumbar vertebrae in the cat) can lead to autonomous or 'lower motor neuron' bladder. This lesion affects the pudendal nerve and decreases urethral, anal and perineal tone. These animals may also have tail paresis or paralysis.

A key point that is often overlooked is the direct observation by the clinician of the animal's urination. This can clarify the owner's description of the clinical signs, and often reveals subtle changes they may not have observed. It is especially important to note the width of the urine stream, particularly in males, and any difficulty maintaining an adequate flow of urine. Most dogs with USMI and other disorders of storage (both male and female) have no difficulty urinating and appear otherwise healthy. However, dogs and cats with disorders of emptying will often display signs of dysuria such as straining, multiple attempts to void and a narrow or 'intermittent' urine stream. Male dogs with detrusor–urethral dyssynergia and functional obstruction may be able to start a urine stream which then will narrow and diminish into a few drops of urine while the patient continues to posture and strain. The urine stream can be difficult to assess in bitches that squat very close to the ground, but watching the urine volume produced on a hard surface may provide the clinician with an estimate of the flow rate. The animal's gait, anxiety level and voiding posture can also be assessed at this time.

In conjunction with observation of voiding, quantification of residual urine volume may be performed after the animal has had an adequate opportunity to urinate. In male dogs with UI this is particularly important. The true prevalence of detrusor reflex dyssynergia (see Chapter 30) and resulting overflow incontinence in males is probably underestimated, and the reported poor response of males to medical therapy for USMI may be due to misdiagnosis of these cases. Residual urine volume should be <0.4 ml/kg (range 0.2–3 ml/kg). This can be objectively measured by catheterization, a relatively easy procedure in the male dog, or subjectively evaluated by ultrasonography or radiography in the male and female cat and the bitch. Palpation of the bladder may also be useful, but only if a significant residual volume is present. The author suggests measuring residual urine volume in all male dogs with UI as part of the initial evaluation. This may be a secondary diagnostic test in bitches and in male and female cats, particularly if therapy for USMI is unsuccessful, provided there are no other indications of urine retention.

Laboratory evaluation

All patients with UI should have a urinalysis with sediment examination and an aerobic bacterial urine culture submitted to a laboratory for evaluation. While the leakage of urine may be exacerbated by a urinary tract infection, the incontinence itself may predispose the patient to bacterial cystitis. A complete blood count and serum chemistry evaluation are indicated if the patient has decreased urine concentration, particularly in the face of dehydration. As noted above, the development of polyuria from any cause can lead to UI in a previously continent patient with a weak urethral sphincter mechanism. If possible, improvement of urine concentration and a decrease in volume produced may improve the frequency and volume of urine leakage. A complete blood count or indirect systolic blood pressure measurement may be performed to establish a baseline value, depending on the clinician's initial treatment choice (see Figures 9.1 and 9.2).

Empirical therapy

Provided that no additional abnormalities are noted on physical examination, urination or laboratory evaluation up to this point, most experts would agree that in an otherwise healthy neutered bitch a tentative diagnosis of USMI can be made and empirical medical treatment is acceptable. Responses to appropriate therapy in male dogs and bitches may confirm the diagnosis of USMI, although other lower urinary tract disease may also exist.

Advanced diagnostic evaluation: imaging

Diagnostic imaging of the lower urinary tract is indicated for animals with lifelong UI, abnormal urogenital conformation or poor response to empirical therapy for USMI. Imaging to evaluate for ectopic ureters is warranted for intact animals, those with UI prior to neutering, and those animals where a thorough history cannot be obtained (e.g. dogs obtained from shelters and rescue facilities). Although ectopic ureters are more often diagnosed in bitches, they can occur in males, and may actually be underdiagnosed owing to a lack of clinical signs of UI. Ectopic ureters have also been reported in the cat.

Radiography

Imaging of the lower urinary tract often begins with radiography. The ureters, bladder, urethra and prostate or vagina are most important to assess in the patient with UI. Plain radiography is useful to identify the size and position of the bladder, as well as the presence or absence of any radiopaque uroliths. The prostate should also be assessed in males. The urethra is not usually visible with plain radiography unless there are uroliths in the lumen. Contrast cystourethrography may need to be performed to better identify the details of the lower urinary tract. The reader is referred to Chapter 7 for detailed information regarding imaging studies for the lower urinary tract.

Excretory urography

Contrast imaging of various parts of the lower urinary tract can be accomplished using several types of studies (Figure 9.4) (Habing and Byron, 2015). Excretory urography has often been used to identify ectopic ureters, with a sensitivity of approximately 80% (Cannizzo et al., 2003; Samii et al., 2004). This is lower than the sensitivity of other modalities such as cystoscopy or computed tomographic excretory urogram (CTEU), but is the most widely available technique, and can be performed in most practice settings. To gain the most information from the images, close attention should be paid to preparing the patient with an enema, adequate sedation, and taking orthogonal views at appropriate time points. Risks associated with this procedure include acute vomiting, urticaria, and facial and pharyngeal/laryngeal oedema, all of which are related to intravenous administration of iodinated contrast media and are usually transient. Contrast-induced nephropathy is a more serious complication leading to acute kidney injury, but is rare in veterinary patients. Reduction of risk is accomplished by ensuring adequate hydration, renal perfusion and blood pressure prior to the use of iodinated contrast. In addition, non-ionic contrast media (240 mg I/ml) should be used for intravascular studies.

Cystourethrography

Contrast cystourethrography provides an image of the distended bladder and urethra. It is most often performed in the male, as a counterpoint to the vaginourethrogram in the female. It is useful to evaluate the patient for urethral

Procedure	Patient preparation	Contrast	Dose/ volume	Technique	Additional considerations
EU (fluoroscopy/ radiography)	• 12–24-hour fast • ± enema • Sedation/ general anaesthesia • Intravenous catheter	Aqueous iodinated (non-ionic preferred, 240 mg/ml)	• 600–880 mg/kg • Increase dose by 20% if renal azotaemia is present	1. Survey RT and VD. 2. Rapid intravenous bolus injection. 3. RL and VD; time 0, 5, 20, 40 minutes. 4. Repeat RT and LT OBL as needed, starting at 5 minutes for UVJ.	• Concurrent negative-contrast cystogram may be performed for ectopic ureter evaluation
CTEU			• 400–880 mg/kg • Increase dose by 20% if renal azotaemia is present	1. Position in sternal recumbency with pelvis elevated. 2. Survey CT (cranial to kidneys to caudal urethra). 3. Rapid intravenous bolus injection. 4. Repeat scan at time 0, 3 minutes 5. Repeat scans from mid bladder to caudal urethra as needed for UVJ.	
Cystourethrogram	• Sedation/ general anaesthesia • Aseptic distal urethral catheterization • ± 2% lidocaine (2–5 ml) injected into urethra to reduce spasm	15% aqueous iodinated (diluted with sterile saline or sterile water)	• 10–15 ml (dog) • 5–10 ml (cat)	1. Survey RL and RL with legs pulled forward (male dogs). 2. Inject 50% of contrast medium. 3. RL with legs forward (image obtained at end of injection). 4. Inject remaining contrast. 5. RL, RL and LT OBL.	• Urinary bladder should be fully distended to facilitate urethral distension • Terminate injection if back pressure is felt on the syringe plunger • Foley catheter is preferred in male dogs • Red rubber or tomcat catheter is used in cats and female dogs
Vaginourethrogram	• General anaesthesia • Aseptic vestibule Foley catheterization	Aqueous iodinated	• 10–15 ml (dog) • 5–10 ml (cat)	1. Survey RL and VD. 2. Inject 50% of contrast medium. 3. RL (image obtained at end of injection). 4. Inject remaining contrast. 5. RL and VD.	• Plastic haemostats are used to clamp vulvar lips around the catheter to prevent contrast leakage • The tip of the catheter should be cut to prevent it from extending into the vagina • Terminate injection if back pressure is felt on the syringe plunger

9.4 Commonly used imaging procedures for diagnostic evaluation of urinary incontinence. CT = computed tomography; CTEU = computed tomographic excretory urogram; EU = excretory urethrography; LL = left lateral; LT = left; OBL = oblique; RL = right lateral; RT = right; UVJ = ureterovesicular junction; VD = ventrodorsal.
(Adapted from Weisse and Berent, 2015)

strictures, masses and other obstructive lesions. It also allows for precise localization of the bladder and subjective assessment of bladder capacity and compliance (Figure 9.5). Occasionally, vesicoureteral reflux can occur during the procedure, particularly if ureteral ectopia is present, thus identifying their distal openings.

9.5 Normal contrast cystourethrogram in a male dog. This 8-year-old male neutered Golden Retriever was evaluated for difficulty urinating and was diagnosed with functional urethral obstruction.

The normal male urethra is smooth and well defined with mild distention at the level of the prostate when it is maximally distended. The diameter of the remainder of the urethra is uniform except for a small amount of tapering that may be seen at the ischial arch. Occasionally, a small filling defect may be seen at the colliculus seminalis. It is important not to misinterpret this as an ectopic ureter.

Vaginourethrography

The vaginourethrogram provides information about the vestibule, vagina and urethra in a bitch or queen. This allows estimation of urethral length, assessment for obstructive processes and, if the bladder is adequately filled, an opportunity to determine capacity and compliance subjectively. There is some evidence that this procedure is better for viewing the distal portion of ectopic ureters than a radiographic excretory urogram. Vesicoureteral reflux due to the abnormal ureteral openings can send contrast material up the ureter towards the renal pelvis, and this leads to more contrast in the ureters than with a traditional excretory urogram.

The contrast should fill the vestibule and vagina, with a small narrowing at the vaginal entrance (Figure 9.6). This is the cingulum and should not be interpreted as a stricture, although narrowed vaginal orifices have been noted

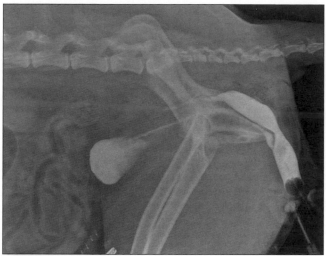

9.6 Normal contrast vaginourethrogram in a 13-year-old neutered female Samoyed with urethral sphincter mechanism incompetence. Radiopaque suture material is secondary to previous overiohysterectomy.

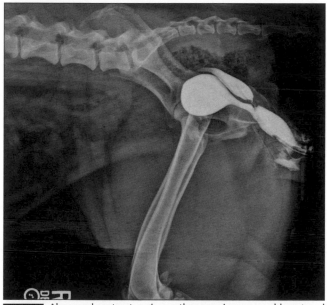

9.7 Abnormal contrast vaginourethrogram in a 1-year-old neutered female Dobermann with urinary incontinence since weaning. Note the hypoplastic urethra, pelvic bladder position and narrow vagina. The bladder capacity in this dog is also subjectively reduced.
(© Julie Byron)

in some animals, due either to persistent mesonephric/ hymenal remnants or to vestibulovaginal stenosis (Figure 9.7). Several studies have indirectly implicated these abnormalities as contributing to UI in bitches, either through urine pooling, or in the frequent comorbid urogenital abnormalities such as ureteral ectopia. Such defects in the vaginal entrance have been noted, however, in clinically normal animals; their relationship to clinical signs of UI remains unclear.

The urethra will also fill and distend with contrast and should be smooth and well demarcated. There should be a clear distinction where the urethra transitions into the bladder neck and trigone. Some studies have correlated measurements such as the vesicourethral angle and vaginal length with the risk of UI; however, others have found this correlation to be unreliable. The use of such measurements is not considered routine and data on their predictive value in continent dogs at risk of developing USMI after neutering is currently lacking.

Ultrasonography

Ultrasonography is considered a reliable way to evaluate the urogenital tract with the exception of the vagina and the middle and distal urethra. In some dogs, where the bladder is located very caudally in the abdomen, it can be hard to evaluate the bladder neck and trigone. In addition, ultrasonographic quality and evaluation are very dependent on the equipment and operator. Therefore, these limitations must be kept in mind when choosing this diagnostic modality to assess an animal with UI. The renal pelves should be identified and the ureters followed as far caudally as possible to their entrance into the bladder. If the bladder is not overly distended, it may be possible to observe normally positioned ureteral papillae and potentially observe small jets of urine from them with colour Doppler signals, or movement of urine sediment.

Ureteral dilatation is seen in approximately 50% of dogs with ectopic ureters, making the ureters easier to identify using ultrasonography than ureters in normal dogs. Ectopic ureters can be followed caudally and are usually seen to enter the serosal surface of the bladder at the level of trigone, and then tunnel intramurally alongside the urethra. The caudal termination of an ectopic ureter is often difficult to identify using ultrasonography owing to the intrapelvic position. The less common extramural ectopic ureters travel alongside the urethra as well, and it can be difficult to distinguish them from intramural ureters with ultrasonography alone.

Other lower urinary tract abnormalities can be identified with ultrasonography. In patients with UI, the presence of urogenital malformation, even if it does not directly affect the continence mechanism, potentially indicates the presence of additional abnormalities not seen. A hypoplastic or short urethra may not be visualized by ultrasonography alone; however, it has been associated with uterine malformations and UI.

Specialized diagnostic testing

Patients with equivocal clinical or imaging results, or that do not respond to appropriate therapy as expected, may need to be referred for more advanced diagnostic testing. This includes advanced imaging using computed tomography, direct visualization and inspection of the urogenital tract with cystoscopy, and functional evaluation of the bladder and urethra.

Computed tomography excretory urography

A CTEU is performed in a manner similar to the radiographic excretory urogram, but computed tomography allows the clinician to see the abdominal structures in more distinct detail and on several planes. The advantages of a CTEU over a traditional excretory urogram include the reduction of summation artefacts and three-dimensional reconstructive capability for examination of the lower urinary tract (Figure 9.8). A lower dose of intravenous contrast material is used, which may be advantageous in patients with underlying renal disease. A CTEU has a higher sensitivity for detecting ectopic ureters (91%) and improved assessment of whether they are intra- or extramural compared with traditional radiographic urography (Samii et al., 2004). Intramural ectopic ureters are much more common than extramural ectopic ureters; it is important to know this detail and identify their path because the

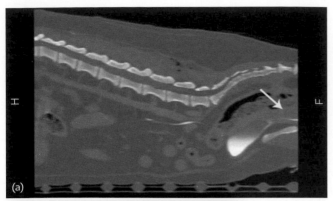

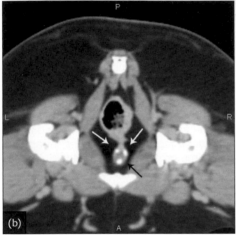

9.8 Computed tomographic excretory urogram of ureteral ectopia in a 3-year-old neutered female Miniature Pinscher with urinary incontinence since weaning. (a) Sagittal plane of the abdomen. Note the contrast enhancement of the ureters caudal to the neck of the bladder (arrowed). The bladder is filling with contrast as it flows retrograde from the ectopic openings. (b) Transverse plane of the abdomen at the level of the proximal urethra. Both ectopic ureters (white arrows) are clearly visible as well as the urethra (black arrow), with a small amount of contrast in the lumen.
(© Julie Byron)

choice of corrective procedure is different for intramural *versus* extramural ectopic ureters (see Chapter 30). Patients with UI are often referred for a CTEU if there is a strong suspicion of ectopic ureters, and the study is frequently performed prior to surgical or cystoscopic correction. Although an uroendoscopic evaluation is possibly more sensitive for detecting ectopic ureters, the CTEU has the advantage of revealing the anatomy of the entire urinary tract, with both luminal and serosal details.

Uroendoscopy

Uroendoscopy is the evaluation under anaesthesia of the urogenital tract using a flexible endoscope in males and a flexible or rigid endoscope in females. This allows the operator to visualize anatomical defects directly that may not be evident on palpation, or are intraluminal and therefore not revealed by other imaging methods. The field of uroendoscopy also includes the use of techniques such as laser tissue ablation and injection of urethral bulking agents, which imparts therapeutic potential to an otherwise diagnostic procedure. For detailed information on uroendoscopy, see Chapter 8.

Patients are generally referred for this procedure if there is a strong suspicion of ectopic ureters or other urogenital malformation such as a hypoplastic urethra (Figure 9.9). As noted above, there are several other ways to diagnose ureteral ectopia; however, laser ablation of an ectopic

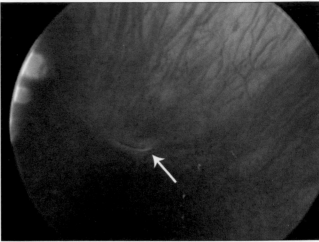

9.9 Cystoscopic view of an ectopic ureter in a 1-year-old neutered female Labrador Retriever with a history of urinary incontinence prior to neutering. The left ureter (arrowed) terminated in the middle third of the urethra and the right ureter terminated at the bladder neck. Laser tissue ablation was used to open the ureters at the level of the trigone.
(© Julie Byron)

ureteral trough can be performed at the time of the diagnostic procedure and reduce the need for additional anaesthesia or more invasive procedures. Patients with acquired urinary incontinence that does not respond to medical treatment are also frequently referred for uroendoscopy to assess for any anatomical causes contributing to the UI. Although currently of very limited availability, the use of injectable bulking agents to improve urethral closure pressure may be an option for these patients. The injections are performed under cystoscopic guidance and, similar to laser ablation, can be performed during the initial diagnostic procedure (see Chapter 30 for further details on these procedures).

It is important to perform the baseline diagnostics discussed previously prior to referring patients with UI for uroendoscopy. Ideally, patients should not have an active urinary tract infection because of the risk of ureteral reflux and resulting pyelonephritis, although this is not always feasible. Most dogs and cats should have imaging of the bladder prior to uroendoscopy. Complications associated with uroendoscopy include mild postoperative discomfort, haematuria, urinary tract infection and trauma to the lower urinary tract. These are uncommon, however, and are less likely if animals undergo previous imaging of the bladder, which may indicate bladder wall friability and an increased risk of iatrogenic damage.

Urodynamic evaluation

Urodynamic studies are a group of tests that quantitatively evaluate the functionality of the continence mechanism. The principle behind them is that the urethral pressure must be higher than the bladder pressure during the storage phase of the micturition cycle in order to maintain urinary continence. There are a number of urodynamic studies that are performed in humans with micturition disorders; however, those performed most often and best characterized in veterinary patients are the urethral pressure profile (UPP) and the cystometrogram (CMG).

The use of urodynamic studies to diagnose the cause of UI is somewhat controversial. The animals must be anaesthetized for the procedure and the data obtained are greatly affected by most of the anaesthetic agents used in veterinary medicine. The most common anaesthetic protocol used in veterinary medicine at the author's institution is a slow rate of propofol infusion. In addition, there is also variability in technique between institutions that perform it, which complicates the determination of 'normal' reference values. In general, urodynamic studies are most often used in a research setting, but indications for their use in clinical patients do sometimes arise.

Urethral pressure profile

The urethral pressure profile (UPP) evaluates the resting pressure of the urethra along its entire length and compares it with the bladder pressure at the same time. A UPP in a dog or cat with UI is usually performed when it is unclear whether the animal has a weak urethral sphincter contributing to the incontinence. This is generally done after the patient has had proper imaging studies to rule out ectopic ureters, and appropriate medical therapy for USMI has been tried with little or no response. In male dogs with no response to USMI treatment, it is important before performing a urethral pressure profile that either a residual urine volume assessment is obtained or a therapeutic trial with an adrenoceptor antagonist (e.g. prazosin) be considered if clinically indicated.

Cystometrography

The cystometrogram (CMG) evaluates the integrity of detrusor function and bladder compliance. The bladder is catheterized and slowly filled while measuring the intravesical pressure. At a threshold pressure there will normally be a detrusor reflex and urination will occur. The change in pressure as the volume of fluid in the bladder increases indicates the compliance of the bladder. The timing and strength of the detrusor reflex assesses its function. A CMG is generally indicated when there is a strong suspicion of low bladder compliance or 'overactive' bladder (OAB). Low bladder compliance can lead to UI by reducing the volume of urine it can hold without discomfort, and this leads to high pressures in the bladder which can overcome the urethral closure pressure and lead to leakage. OAB is the most common cause of UI in women, but is poorly characterized in veterinary patients. A CMG can record spontaneous contractions of the detrusor muscle at low filling volumes and inappropriately low filling pressures. These indicate detrusor hyperreflexia, which can also decrease the overall compliance of the bladder. Identification of dogs and cats that will benefit from CMG evaluation is challenging. Referral for the procedure often occurs when there may be partial response to USMI treatment, with a degree of urgency or leakage when the animal is anxious or active, but not when at rest.

Summary

UI is a difficult problem for owners, and lack of response to empirical therapy can lead to frustration and inappropriate expectations. Although USMI is by far the most common cause of UI, it is important to pursue a methodical diagnostic course, particularly if the patient does not respond to empirical therapy. This will reduce the risk of misdiagnosis and treatment that may exacerbate the incontinence. A thorough history and physical examination, along with observing the patient urinate, are cornerstones to the initial evaluation. Imaging also plays an important role, particularly in patients with suspected congenital abnormalities. Referral for advanced diagnostics in these patients may also afford an opportunity for correction or more targeted therapy.

References and further reading

Cannizzo KL, McLoughlin MA, Mattoon JS et al. (2003) Evaluation of transurethral cystoscopy and excretory urography for diagnosis of ectopic ureters in female dogs: 25 cases (1992–2000). *Journal of the American Veterinary Medical Association* **223**, 475–481

Habing AM and Byron JK (2015) Imaging of the urinary tract. In: *Veterinary Image-Guided Interventions*, ed. C Weisse and A Berent. Wiley-Blackwell, Iowa

Samii VF, McLoughlin MA, Mattoon JS et al. (2004) Digital fluoroscopic excretory urography, digital fluoroscopic urethrography, helical computed tomography, and cystoscopy in 24 dogs with suspected ureteral ectopia. *Journal of Veterinary Internal Medicine* **18**, 271–281

Weisse C and Berent A (ed) (2015) *Veterinary Image-Guided Interventions*. Wiley-Blackwell, Oxford

Chapter 10

Early detection of chronic kidney disease

Natalie Finch and Reidun Heiene

Chronic kidney disease (CKD) in human patients is defined as a sustained reduction in renal function (glomerular filtration rate (GFR) <60 ml/min/1.73 m^2 for >3 months) and/or evidence of renal damage (urine albumin to creatinine ratio >30 mg/g for >3 months). There is no clearly established definition in cats and dogs, however, though similar principles apply. There should be evidence of disease chronicity, functional and/or structural change and/or renal damage.

Structural changes associated with CKD are irreversible and disease progression, although often slow, can lead to end-stage CKD. The total number of functioning nephrons in the kidney is reduced in patients with CKD. This increases the functional demand of the remaining nephrons, recognized as an increase in single nephron GFR (hyperfiltration). Increased single nephron GFR may be associated with glomerular hypertension, hypertrophy and sclerosis. This is termed the 'hyperfiltration theory'. The initial adaptive response in renal haemodynamics and function may be beneficial; however, over time, the changes become maladaptive and contribute to the self-perpetuating (intrinsic) progression of kidney disease. Other factors contributing to the self-perpetuating progression of disease have been suggested in more recent years, among which proteinuria has gained most attention. Early identification of patients with CKD is desirable because, at this stage, the primary disease process may be identified and addressed by treatment. In addition, interventional therapy could be implemented which may attenuate disease progression and prevent secondary metabolic complications. Early identification of CKD may also be important in improved patient monitoring to assess disease stability. What remains unclear in both human and veterinary patients is whether very early stage CKD represents a normal ageing process or is a definite disease process.

The prevalence of early stage CKD is unknown in cats and dogs, but older cats are the population most commonly affected. Indeed, the incidence of development of azotaemic CKD in geriatric cats within 12 months was reported to be 30% in one study (Jepson *et al.*, 2009), suggesting that there are a substantial number of senior cats with undetected early stage CKD. Selection of patients for screening for CKD should include those with risk factors for CKD such as increasing age, breed predisposition, patients receiving nephrotoxic drugs or patients with previous acute kidney injury (AKI) in addition to those with clinical findings suggestive of CKD such as polyuria and polydipsia, weight loss or abnormal renal palpation.

Historical findings

Obtaining a thorough and accurate history is essential for a patient when CKD is suspected and can provide important information to aid the diagnosis. Many clinical signs are nonspecific such as weight loss, inappetence, lethargy and vomiting. Polyuria and polydipsia (PU/PD; see Chapter 2) can develop, with polydipsia being recognized more often than polyuria by owners. Polydipsia is defined as water intake >100 ml/kg/24h and polyuria is defined as urine production >50 ml/kg/24h. However, PU/PD can be present below the threshold defined above, provided the owner recognizes a definite increase in intake relative to the norm for that animal (see Chapter 2). Therefore, if an owner notes any increase for that animal, it may be significant.

Clinical examination

Early in the course of CKD the clinical findings can be normal. A thorough clinical examination is important to identify concurrent disease or predisposing factors for CKD. Reduced body condition may be noted. Renal palpation should be performed, when possible. The kidneys can be palpated in the mid-dorsal abdomen caudal to the ribs, with the left kidney normally identified more caudal than the right. In cats, the kidneys can be very mobile, particularly in older cats. In large or overweight dogs, the kidneys can be difficult to palpate owing to the large abdominal size. Findings on renal palpation which can suggest kidney disease include changes in size and shape, and renal pain (see Chapter 4).

Routine laboratory diagnosis of CKD

Creatinine

Creatinine is freely filtered at the glomerulus with no tubular reabsorption and negligible tubular secretion, hence its clinical utility as a marker of GFR. There is an exponential relationship between creatinine and GFR so that in early CKD there can be large changes in GFR with relatively small changes in creatinine concentration (Figure 10.1).

BSAVA Manual of Canine and Feline Nephrology and Urology, third edition. Edited by Jonathan Elliott, Gregory F. Grauer and Jodi L. Westropp ©BSAVA 2017

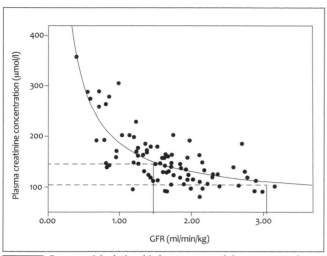

10.1 Exponential relationship between creatinine concentration and glomerular filtration rate (GFR) in cats, indicating that a large decrease in GFR results in only a small corresponding increase in creatinine concentration.
(Adapted from Finch, 2014)

However, in addition to GFR there are other factors that will influence plasma creatinine concentration. Creatinine is a metabolic product of creatine and phosphocreatine, both of which are found almost exclusively in muscle. Thus, the rate of creatinine production is proportional to muscle mass and varies little from day to day. However, endogenous production can change over longer periods of time if there is a change in muscle mass. The conversion of creatine and phosphocreatine is non-enzymatic, irreversible and occurs at an almost constant rate with approximately 2% of the body pool converted to creatinine every day. The amount of creatine derived from ingested meat can be quite high and variability in meat intake can, therefore, also contribute to variability in serum creatinine concentrations. In addition, there may be non-renal excretion of creatinine via the gastrointestinal tract and degradation by colonic bacteria that may be of greater significance in patients with decreased renal excretion of creatinine.

Age, breed and sex may lead to variability in plasma creatinine concentration in dogs and cats, although this is poorly characterized. Often older animals have decreased muscle mass, and any potential effect of age upon GFR to increase creatinine may be partially offset by reduced generation of creatinine due to lower muscle mass, leading to no change in plasma concentrations. There is breed variability in creatinine concentration in dogs and cats. For example, Birman cats have been reported to have higher plasma creatinine concentration than other breeds (Paltrinieri *et al.*, 2014). However, it is unclear whether this reflects a higher prevalence of underlying CKD in the breed or a higher concentration of creatinine in healthy animals. Larger dogs have higher creatinine concentrations, probably due to both larger muscle mass and lower GFR (Bexfield *et al.*, 2008). The relationship between bodyweight and serum creatinine has been studied in 34 dogs (van den Brom and Biewenga, 1981); this has led to the development of a formula to predict creatinine concentration from bodyweight (BW). The derived formula was utilized in some European countries for many years:

Expected creatinine (μmol/l) = 70 μmol/l + 1.2 x BW

Expected creatinine is the predicted mean value in a population of a given body size; BW is bodyweight in kg. This formula gained popularity because it fitted with clinicians' experience of the need to relate plasma creatinine concentration to body size, as opposed to most other biochemical parameters. While the formula did not take into account the spread in data and therefore could not provide upper and lower reference limits, it represented a useful adjunct to established reference ranges. Measured plasma creatinine concentration was compared with the concentration predicted by the formula. If the value was close to the value predicted it would support the notion of normal kidney function. If the value was substantially higher or lower than predicted it would support a notion of normal or abnormal kidney function in the dog. Though a useful conceptual approach, the formula did not obtain worldwide recognition, possibly owing to the limited number of dogs involved in its derivation (n = 34) and the difficulty with variability in reference ranges of creatinine.

Data from 567 dogs with BW ranging from 1.8 to 75.8 kg are shown in Figure 10.2. There is a clear trend towards higher plasma creatinine concentrations in large dogs compared with small dogs. There is also very wide inter-individual variation in plasma creatinine concentration in dogs of similar body size, and overlap between smaller and larger dogs. The lower plasma creatinine resulting from higher GFR and lower muscle mass in small individuals, as observed in dogs, is not apparent in other species such as cats and humans, possibly because cats and humans do not have as wide a variation in body size.

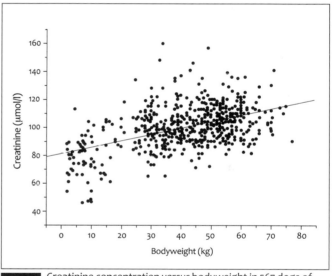

10.2 Creatinine concentration *versus* bodyweight in 567 dogs of various sizes.
(Courtesy of R Heiene, J Aasen, C Trangerud and E Teske)

There can also be differences between laboratories in the interpretation of the measured plasma creatinine concentration. A recent study in Europe explored variation among commercial and academic laboratories offering creatinine analysis for veterinary patients (Ulleberg *et al.*, 2011). Inter- and intra-laboratory variation were clinically acceptable because the plasma creatinine concentration for most samples was generally similar. Laboratory sample means above or below the overall sample mean did not unequivocally reflect high or low reference intervals in that laboratory. The data are presented from 10 laboratories that received samples divided over three batches from the same group of dogs with 'borderline' creatinine concentrations (Figure 10.3). A variable number of samples were classified as normal or abnormal by different laboratories, whereas the actual measured value was nearly identical. In the laboratories with the lowest and

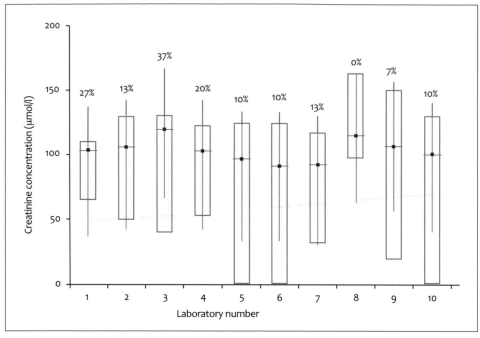

10.3 Analytical values and reference ranges in plasma/serum creatinine in 10 healthy dogs (plotted on x-axis). Three aliquots from each of the dogs were analysed at 10 European referral laboratories. While the analytical variability was low, the percentage of samples classified as abnormal varied from 0 to 37%, based upon the variability in reference ranges between laboratories.
(Reproduced from Ulleberg *et al.*, 2011 with permission from *Acta Veterinaria Scandinavica*)

highest upper reference limits (laboratories 1 and 8), 27% and 0% of the healthy dogs were classified as abnormal, respectively. The discrepant reference intervals largely reflect the different populations used to establish the reference intervals, rather than analytical variation due to different laboratory methods.

Methodological differences in creatinine measurement have been shown to be of greater importance if small bench-top analysers are used to measure creatinine concentration. The bench-top (point of care) laboratory analysers used by many clinics have very different reference intervals. Such bench-top analysers have been examined, and the measured value showed great variation from clinic to clinic (Braun *et al.*, 2008). In human medicine, there is much focus upon standardization of creatinine analysis to ensure that International Organization for Standardization (ISO) standards are met. The use of formula-based estimations for predicting GFR, the so-called 'eGFR formulae', has prompted demands for stringent accuracy in creatinine assays.

There are several important conclusions when evaluating plasma creatinine concentration in a patient:

- Serum or plasma creatinine concentration is the most widely used marker of renal function for diagnosing early CKD and is important for use in the International Renal Interest Society (IRIS) staging system (see below and Chapter 12)
- Clinicians should take into consideration body size and muscle mass when interpreting plasma creatinine concentration
- A small dog should have lower creatinine concentration than a larger dog. This should be considered when interpreting creatinine concentration
- It may be more useful to monitor an animal by evaluating the trend in plasma creatinine concentration, i.e. monitoring plasma creatinine concentration over time with each animal serving as its own baseline, rather than using defined reference intervals. Increase in plasma creatinine concentration with time, even within the laboratory reference interval, is consistent with the presence of early stage CKD (as long as

pre- and post-renal causes of azotaemia have been ruled out), and such patients should be classified as having IRIS CKD Stage 1
- Variation in reference intervals between laboratories may be due to variability in the population used by the laboratory to derive the reference interval. The ages of the animals in the reference population should be taken into account when considering the reference interval
- The utility of creatinine in diagnosing early CKD is increased by also considering urea concentration and urine specific gravity (USG). A relatively high urea compared with creatinine points to a pre-renal component, for instance dehydration. A dehydrated animal should have concentrated urine unless concentrating capacity is lost, such as in early CKD, although there are other reasons for reduced concentrating capacity (see Chapter 2).

Urea

Urea is synthesized in the liver from ammonia; it is freely filtered at the glomeruli and partially reabsorbed by the renal tubules. The rate of urea reabsorption depends on the tubular flow rate and the presence of antidiuretic hormone; thus, in dehydrated animals or patients with poor cardiac output, more urea is reabsorbed. Urea formation is also enhanced by increased protein intake such as following a meal, or in pathological conditions such as gastrointestinal haemorrhage, pyrexia, catabolic disease states or therapy with glucocorticoids, presumably due to their catabolic effect. Lower urea concentration can be seen in malnourished patients or those fed a low protein diet. Urea generation is also reduced in patients with liver failure or a portosystemic shunt.

The considerable influence of non-renal factors is important to recognize when interpreting plasma urea concentration and, therefore, urea is considered a less reliable marker of renal function than creatinine. The plasma urea to creatinine ratio may be helpful in identifying a non-renal component to the azotaemia, although the data to support cut-off values for clinical use of this ratio are limited.

Calcium and phosphate

Changes in calcium and phosphate concentrations are unusual in early CKD. Total calcium may be decreased if a patient is hypoalbuminaemic and total calcium concentration should be interpreted in light of the albumin concentration. A decrease in ionized calcium concentration and increase in phosphate concentration, both remaining within the reference interval, may be indicative of the development of bone and mineral disturbances in early stage CKD (see Chapter 11 and the section on further diagnostic indicators of CKD, below). As the number of functioning nephrons, and consequently GFR, decreases in patients with CKD, there is reduced ability to excrete phosphate ions in the urine and phosphate retention occurs. The increased circulating phosphate within the blood forms complexes with ionized calcium, causing a decrease in ionized calcium concentration and subsequent stimulation of parathyroid hormone (PTH) production. In the early stages of kidney disease the increased PTH concentration can compensate for the phosphate retention and maintain normophosphataemia and normal ionized calcium concentrations. However, as the number of nephrons with the ability to respond to PTH and excrete phosphate declines further, hyperphosphataemia becomes apparent. Even later in the disease, ionized hypocalcaemia may occur. Therefore, concentrations of phosphate and ionized calcium are insensitive markers in early kidney disease and changes in concentration will not be seen until later stages.

Electrolytes

The kidneys are essential for maintaining normal body fluid volume and electrolyte homeostasis, and therefore loss of function may result in disruption. However, in early CKD it is likely that sufficient renal function exists to maintain normal electrolyte concentrations (Figure 10.4), and decreased extracellular fluid volume does not seem to be a feature of early CKD in cats (Finch et al., 2015). Hypokalaemia can develop in CKD and is considered more common in cats than in dogs. As can be seen from Figure 10.4, 15% of cats with 'compensated CKD', which may be considered equivalent to IRIS CKD Stage 2, had hypokalaemia (Elliott and Barber, 1998). Factors that can contribute to its development include urinary losses, renin–angiotensin–aldosterone system (RAAS) activation, increased aldosterone production, reduced intake through poor appetite and vomiting. Low plasma potassium concentration was shown to be a risk factor for hypertension in cats with CKD (Syme et al., 2002). Hypernatraemia may develop if a patient becomes dehydrated owing to lack of water intake in a polyuric state.

Thus, abnormalities in plasma electrolyte concentrations would not be expected to be sensitive indicators of early kidney disease. The presence of persistent hypokalaemia in the absence of azotaemia in cats should be further investigated with measurement of systemic arterial blood pressure and plasma aldosterone concentration, as this may be suggestive of hyperaldosteronism (Conn's syndrome).

Urinalysis

The glomerular barrier functions to allow the filtration of water and small solutes from plasma to the renal tubules in the process of urine formation. The principal components of the barrier are the glomerular endothelial cells, glomerular basement membrane and podocytes. Disruption at any of these levels can contribute to altered permeability. The normal glomerular filtration barrier is poorly permeable to large ionic molecules such as albumin; however, in glomerulopathies the barrier becomes disrupted and proteinuria can develop. In addition, if there is renal tubular damage there can be altered handling of protein in the tubules, which contributes to proteinuria and altered urine concentrating ability. Thus persistent proteinuria can be an indicator of pathological and functional damage to the glomeruli and/or tubules (see Chapter 5).

Measuring proteinuria

Before interpreting urine protein concentration it is important to undertake microscopic examination of the urine sediment and rule out inflammatory disease of the urinary tract (see Chapters 5 and 6). Urinary dipsticks are a quick and simple method for detecting proteinuria, however they are unable to detect urine albumin concentration <30 mg/dl (microalbuminuria). Microalbuminuria may be an early marker of kidney disease and is important in the early detection of CKD in human patients. A study in cats found that urine albumin to creatinine ratio predicted the development of azotaemic CKD within 12 months; however, this offered no advantage over the measurement of urine protein to creatinine ratio (UPC) (Jepson et al., 2009). Species-specific assays are required to measure albumin in the urine and are not routinely available at commercial laboratories. Proteinuria can be quantified by measuring UPC. Spot urine samples are considered to correlate with 24-hour urine collection for determining proteinuria. When evaluating a patient, persistence of proteinuria is demonstrated by repeat UPC measurements at least 2 weeks apart, each time ensuring the urine sediment is benign.

| Electrolyte | | Normal µmol/l (n=42) | Chronic kidney disease | | |
			Compensated (mean creatinine concentration 229 µmol/l) (n=15)	Uraemic (mean creatinine concentration 316 µmol/l) (n=23)	End-stage (mean creatinine concentration 909 µmol/l) (n=26)
Sodium	Mean ± SEM	150.8 ± 0.6	152.1 ± 0.9	151.8 ± 0.8	151.8 ± 1.7
	% Hypernatraemic	2	13	15	26
	% Hyponatraemic	0	0	0	4
Potassium	Mean ± SEM	4.22 ± 0.1	4.08 ± 0.2	4.08 ± 0.1	4.86 ± 2.1
	% Hyperkalaemic	2	7	3	22
	% Hypokalaemic	2	20	18	9
Chloride	Mean ± SEM	118.8 ± 0.5	116.8 ± 0.9	116.2 ± 0.6	110.8 ± 2.1
	% Hyperchloraemic	0	0	0	4
	% Hypochloraemic	0	0	3	35

10.4 Electrolyte findings in normal cats and in cats with chronic kidney disease (CKD) at various stages. The reference intervals for sodium, potassium and chloride were 140–156 mmol/l, 3.5–5.5 mmol/l and 110–130 mmol/l, respectively. SEM = standard error of the mean.
(Adapted from Elliott and Barber, 1998)

There can also be large day-to-day variability in UPC, with a minimum change of 80% required to demonstrate a significant difference in mildly proteinuric patients (UPC approximately 0.5) (Nabity *et al.*, 2007).

In conclusion, persistent renal proteinuria in a non-azotaemic patient is indicative of early kidney disease and merits thorough investigation, monitoring and treatment. Borderline renal proteinuria is predictive of the development of azotaemic CKD in cats and so also warrants careful monitoring and investigation in both cats and dogs. A more comprehensive discussion of proteinuria can be found in Chapter 5.

Urine specific gravity and urine osmolality

Urine specific gravity (USG) is considered an insensitive marker of kidney function. As discussed in Chapter 2, the kidney is responsible for water balance, ensuring that the amount by which water intake exceeds insensible water losses is matched by urine output. The amount of water excreted per day by the kidney will be influenced by a number of factors (water intake, diet, medications; see Chapter 2) and USG in a normal animal can vary from 1.001 to 1.060 (dog) or 1.080 (cat). Therefore, the terms normal or abnormal USG should be avoided and, rather, a USG should be assessed as appropriate or inappropriate in the light of historical and clinical findings. Cats that have undergone partial surgical ablation of the kidneys retain significant concentrating ability and their capacity to concentrate urine appears to be greater than that of dogs or humans. The utility of USG alone in predicting the future development of CKD is poor for the reasons discussed above. This was found to be the case when ageing cats were screened and followed over time to determine which became azotaemic (Jepson *et al.*, 2009). Its usefulness may improve if USG is used in combination with changes in other markers, such as urea and creatinine.

Fractional excretion of electrolytes

Non-protein-bound electrolytes can be filtered at the glomerulus and reabsorbed in the renal tubules. The rate at which this occurs depends on factors such as renal function, fluid volume status, dietary intake and hormonal influences. Urine is required to be collected over 24 hours for electrolyte measurement, because spot samples do not show good correlation with 24-hour samples, particularly in cats (Finco *et al.*, 1997). However, the clinical use of fractional excretion in the diagnosis of early CKD is limited owing to the influence of dietary intake, in particular, which is highly variable across the patient population at risk.

Urine culture and sensitivity

Urine culture should be performed in patients with suspected CKD. Subclinical bacterial infections can occur, and therefore clinical signs or other findings suggestive of a urinary tract infection may not be present. Urine to be submitted for culture should be obtained by cystocentesis.

Diagnostic imaging within the practice setting

A full discussion of imaging of the kidneys can be found in Chapter 7. Structural abnormalities within the kidneys may precede evidence of changes in renal function. Abdominal radiographs can be helpful in identifying radiopaque urinary tract calculi and for assessing renal size. Renal size is generally considered to be 2.5–3.0 times the length of the second lumbar vertebra (L2) in cats and 2.5–3.5 times L2 in dogs (see Chapters 4 and 7). In CKD, the kidneys are often small; however, unilateral renomegaly may be identified if a kidney has become hypertrophied in response to loss of function in the contralateral kidney.

Ultrasonography is the diagnostic imaging modality of choice for evaluating the kidneys. An experienced ultrasonographer will be able to identify changes in renal architecture, pyelectasia or hydronephrosis. A less experienced ultrasonographer may observe changes in renal size or a grossly irregular appearance to the kidneys. Ultrasonographic changes suggestive of lymphoma include a generalized diffuse increase in echogenicity in the cortex and medulla, reduced corticomedullary definition and renomegaly. If renal lymphoma is suspected then fine needle aspirates of the kidney may be helpful in confirming this.

IRIS staging system for CKD

A full discussion of the IRIS staging system for CKD is presented in Chapter 12. It is applied to cats and dogs with confirmed CKD where there are historical or clinical findings of CKD (i.e. the diagnosis of CKD has to be made before staging). Staging is based upon fasting plasma creatinine concentration (in a well hydrated patient), with substaging based on UPC and systolic blood pressure. Plasma creatinine concentration, in this context, is a biomarker for GFR. Substaging for proteinuria and hypertension takes into account two important parameters which are amenable to therapeutic interventions aimed to slow progression of kidney disease. The IRIS classification system makes use of measured plasma creatinine concentration without reference to which laboratory is used, nor to the animal's age or body size. It pertains to the plasma creatinine concentration when an animal is clinically stable. The plasma creatinine concentration should not be used for staging if a patient is dehydrated, experiencing an acute-on-chronic episode or CKD is part of a generalized disease such as systemic lupus erythematosus. The IRIS CKD staging system provides a tool for veterinary surgeons (veterinarians) to communicate about patients without depending on the reference interval for healthy animals set by any particular laboratory, which may vary according to the reference population, as explained above. It is widely used in clinical and research work to promote standardization, aid in diagnosis and management and predict prognosis.

The IRIS staging system is based upon plasma creatinine and clinicians must be aware of the limitations when using this marker. It remains a fact that creatinine is among the most studied and well known biomarkers available to veterinary clinicians. Just as individual variation in body size or hair colour is recognized, there is individual variation in muscle mass and in GFR.

Glomerular filtration rate

Glomerular filtration is a selective pressure-driven filtration process through the glomerulus and into the Bowman's space, with the passage of solutes determined by their molecular size, charge and conformation. Fluid that is filtered through the glomerulus and into the Bowman's space and then renal tubules is known as the ultrafiltrate. Within the renal tubules the ultrafiltrate is modified by processes of selective reabsorption of solutes and water and active secretion of substances from the peritubular interstitial fluid into the tubular fluid. These processes ultimately influence the final composition of urine (Figures 10.5 and 10.6).

Measurement of GFR is regarded as the most sensitive index of functioning renal mass. It is defined as the amount of glomerular ultrafiltrate formed in the nephrons of both kidneys per unit of time. The ultrafiltrate entering the Bowman's space cannot be measured directly and, therefore, the clearance of a filtration marker is measured. Single-nephron GFR is the product of the effective

ultrafiltration pressure and ultrafiltration coefficient. The effective ultrafiltration pressure is governed by hydraulic and oncotic pressures in the glomerular capillaries and Bowman's capsule. Therefore, marked hypotension may decrease GFR as a result of reduced hydraulic pressure in the glomerular capillaries for which renal haemodynamic regulatory mechanisms cannot compensate. A lower urinary tract obstruction will increase hydraulic pressure in the Bowman's space and decrease GFR. The ultrafiltration coefficient is determined by glomerular conductivity and capillary surface area.

Measurement of GFR can be based on plasma or urinary clearance of endogenous or exogenously administered filtration markers. An ideal filtration marker should:

1. Not be protein bound.
2. Be freely filtered at the glomerulus.
3. Not undergo any metabolism within the body.
4. Be renally cleared only or have negligible non-renal clearance.
5. Not undergo tubular secretion or reabsorption.
6. Be non-toxic.
7. Not alter GFR following administration.

If the marker meets these criteria the plasma clearance of that substance will equal its urinary clearance and both will equate to GFR.

Urinary clearance methods

Urinary clearance (also referred to as renal clearance) is defined as the hypothetical volume of plasma from which the marker is completely removed by the kidneys to provide the amount of marker appearing in urine per unit of time. It is calculated as:

Urinary clearance =
$$\frac{\text{concentration of marker in urine} \times \text{urine flow rate}}{\text{concentration of marker in plasma}}$$

Inulin is considered the gold standard filtration marker for this purpose. Measurement of urinary clearance requires infusion of the marker at a constant rate to achieve a steady

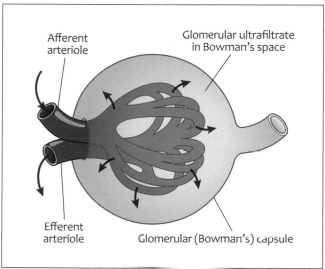

10.5 Structure of the glomerulus.
(Reproduced from Finch, 2014 with permission from the *Journal of Feline Medicine and Surgery*)

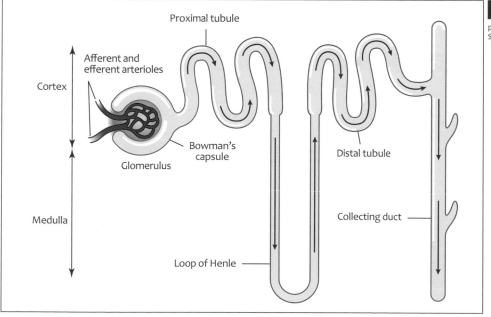

10.6 Structure of the nephron.
(Reproduced from Finch, 2014 with permission from the *Journal of Feline Medicine and Surgery*)

state plasma concentration, as well as accurately timed and completed urine collection. This necessitates urinary catheterization and bladder emptying. Consequently, these methods are impractical for clinical use and remain largely a research tool.

Plasma clearance methods

Plasma clearance methods involve the administration of a bolus dose of filtration marker and timed collection of blood samples. The term plasma clearance is used despite determination of the concentration of filtration marker in serum because it is plasma that is presented to the filtration barrier and GFR is dependent on renal plasma flow.

Radiolabelled markers such as ^{99}Tc-DTPA and ^{51}Cr-EDTA can be used and offer the advantage of assessment of individual kidney function through scintigraphy. This may be helpful in determining contralateral renal function if nephrectomy is to be performed. However, use of these markers requires nuclear medicine facilities, and therefore they are not widely available.

Creatinine can be administered exogenously as a filtration marker, however the lack of availability of a medical grade formulation for intravenous injection is a significant disadvantage for this marker. Owing to the larger volume of distribution of creatinine when compared with other filtration markers, this is a much lengthier test to perform. Furthermore, in dogs, extra-renal clearance of creatinine has been identified, which may be important in patients with CKD where GFR is low (Steinbach *et al.*, 2010).

Inulin

Although urinary clearance of inulin is considered the gold standard of GFR measurement techniques, assessment of plasma clearance of inulin is not recommended. In a study using plasma clearance of inulin in dogs, approximately 40% of the administered inulin was unaccounted for in urine recovery. This was considered to be the result of biliary clearance.

Iohexol

Iohexol is readily available for clinical use as the radiographic contrast marker Omnipaque®. In human patients there are concerns regarding nephrotoxicity with contrast agents; however, development of nephropathy secondary to iohexol has not been reported in cats and dogs. Furthermore, iohexol was not found to be cytotoxic to canine renal cells (Schick and Haller, 1999). Iohexol demonstrates endo- and exo-isomerism and certain laboratories are able to provide concentrations of both isomers. It has been suggested that the clearance of the two isomers may differ in cats (Le Garreres *et al.*, 2007; van Hoek *et al.*, 2007; 2008; 2009), which may lead to inaccuracies in measurement of GFR if only total iohexol concentration is determined. However, a more recent study clearly demonstrated that there is no difference in clearance between the two isomers in cats and that, following administration, there is no conversion of one isomer to the other (Finch *et al.*, 2011). This is true also for dogs, rats and humans. Therefore, the isomers can be considered as one pharmacological entity (i.e. total iohexol concentration is measured) when performing analysis. Details of laboratories and method of analysis of iohexol in plasma can be found in Figure 10.7.

Pharmacokinetic concepts in plasma clearance

Accurate plasma clearance methods rely on collection of blood samples at multiple time points to create a plasma concentration *versus* time curve. The clearance (Cl) is then calculated as:

Cl = dose/AUC

where AUC is the area under the plasma concentration *versus* time curve. Filtration markers are distributed throughout a number of compartments within the body. This allows a pharmacokinetic model to be constructed which can be used to calculate the AUC. Such compartments should be considered more as mathematical tools than as defined physiological spaces (Figure 10.8).

Limited sampling methods for clinical practice

Techniques that require collection of only a limited number of samples have become an important goal for clinicians when measuring clearance. This is important for making GFR measurement more practical in the clinical situation by reducing stress in a patient associated with repeated

Laboratory	Contact details	Method of analysis
deltaDOT	deltaDOT Ltd London BioScience Innovation Centre, 2 Royal College Street, London NW1 0NH, UK Tel: 0044 207 6912075 info@deltaDOT.com www.deltadot.com	High performance capillary electrophoresis (HPCE)
Laboratory of Pharmacology and Toxicology	Laboratory of Pharmacology and Toxicology Faculty of Veterinary Medicine, Ghent University, Salisburylaan 133, 9820 Merelbeke, Belgium Tel: 0032 9 264 73 47 veterinaire.farmacotoxico@ugent.be www.vetftb.ugent.be	High performance liquid chromatography – ultraviolet (HPLC-UV)
Diagnostic Center for Population and Animal Health	Diagnostic Center for Population and Animal Health, Michigan State University, 4125 Beaumont Rd, Lansing, MI 48910-8104, US Tel: 001 517 3531683 www.dcpah.msu.edu	Inductively coupled plasma – mass spectrometry (ICP-MS)

10.7 Details of laboratories and the methods of analysis for measuring iohexol employed by the laboratory.

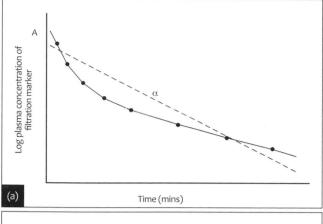

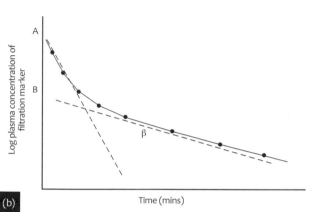

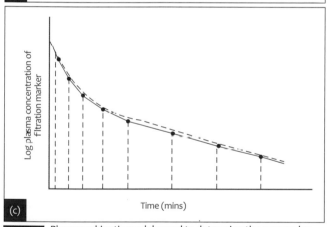

10.8 Pharmacokinetic models used to determine the area under the plasma concentration *versus* time curve. (a) One-compartment; minimum number of samples = 2. (b) Two-compartment; minimum number of samples = 4. (c) Non-compartment; minimum number of samples is unknown, however, the use of three gives inaccurate glomerular filtration rate estimation.

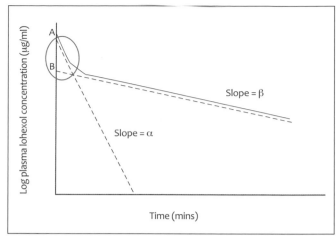

10.9 Plasma concentration *versus* time curve indicating the missing area under the curve (AUC) associated with the slope–intercept method. The slope–intercept method of determining plasma clearance relies on a limited number of samples (generally three) collected during the elimination phase of the clearance curve (usually starting 60 minutes after administration of the filtration marker). As the initial distribution exponential is ignored, this creates a 'missing area under the curve' (blue circle), leading to an underestimation in the calculated AUC and hence overestimation of the glomerular filtration rate (GFR) (because GFR is calculated as dose/AUC).

sampling technique. Calculation of clearance from a limited number of samples collected during the elimination phase is referred to as the slope–intercept technique.

Formulae that correct for the distribution exponential (the missing AUC) when using a slope–intercept method have been developed for human patients (Brochner-Mortensen, 1972), dogs (Heiene and Moe, 1999) and more recently cats (Finch *et al.*, 2011). Figure 10.10 presents reported formulae for correcting for the one-compartment assumption. The human and feline correction formulae were developed by forcing the regression through the origin to ensure that a constant is not generated. Hence, when the uncorrected clearance is 0 ml/min/kg the corrected clearance is 0 ml/min/kg, which makes biological sense. The canine formula does include a constant (-0.03) and may therefore underestimate clearance at very low clearance rates. Iohexol and nuclear medicine markers such as ^{51}Cr-EDTA are considered to distribute throughout the extracellular fluid volume (ECFV) and will require similar corrections for the one-compartment assumption. Therefore, the

Parameter	Species	Correction/prediction formula
Slope–intercept GFR (ml/min/kg)	Cat	$1.036 \times GFR_{uncorrected} - 0.062 \times [GFR_{uncorrected}]^2$
	Dog	$-0.03 + 1.06 \times GFR_{uncorrected} - 0.07012 \times [GFR_{uncorrected}]^2$
Single-sample formula for GFR (ml/min/kg)	Cat	$((1.027 \times \beta_1) \times ECFV) / BW$ $\beta_1 = ((1/t) \times \ln(Vt/ECFV)) \times 0.93$
ECFV (ml)	Cat	$313.68 + (119.81 \times BW)$

10.10 Formulae for determining glomerular filtration rate (GFR) using limited sampling plasma clearance methods in cats. The slope–intercept formula corrects for the missing area under the curve when collecting only a limited number of samples (generally three) during the elimination phase of the clearance curve (samples collected at 120, 180 and 240 min). The uncorrected clearance ($GFR_{uncorrected}$), which is standardized to bodyweight (BW), is inserted into the formula to obtain the corrected clearance (in ml/min/kg). Single-sample GFR is determined from a single sample collected at time t (180 min) and the volume of distribution of iohexol at time t (Vt), which is calculated as the dose of iohexol administered/serum concentration at time (t). An estimate of extracellular fluid volume (ECFV) is also required, which can be obtained from BW (kg) using a second formula.

sampling and also reducing the costs associated with analysis. Based on data in human patients, it is assumed that the initial rate of distribution phase of a marker is independent of renal clearance (GFR) and an estimate of GFR may, without significant loss of accuracy, be based on the second elimination exponential (collection of samples after 60 minutes). Exclusion of the distribution exponential leads to an overestimation of GFR because the AUC is underestimated (Figure 10.9). The error becomes particularly important in patients with normal or near normal renal function where the initial rapid distribution exponential contributes to a relatively larger proportion of the AUC than in patients with a low GFR. Hence, when measuring GFR to detect early kidney disease it is important to correct for distribution (see below) if using a limited correction formulae, although not formally validated, may be accurate for use with nuclear medicine markers. It is unlikely that the formulae will be appropriate for use with exogenous creatinine used as a clearance marker because of its much larger volume of distribution, considered to approximate total body water rather than ECFV, and therefore this requires a three-compartment model. All of these correction formulae are second-order polynomials which, as quadratic equations, have a maximum value for the parabolic curve. This may result in underestimation of clearance at high GFR (Finch *et al.*, 2014). It is unclear at what level this underestimation becomes important in cats and dogs; however, it may have most significance in hyperthyroid cats where GFR is markedly increased.

Measuring plasma iohexol clearance using the slope–intercept technique in the practice setting

1. Administer a bolus of iohexol (Omnipaque® 300) intravenously at a dose of 0.5–1.0 ml/kg over approximately 30 seconds.
2. Collect blood samples at 120, 180 and 240 minutes following administration of iohexol and transfer to serum tubes. Ensure the exact time of sample collection is recorded for plotting the plasma concentration *versus* time curve.
3. Harvest the serum and submit to a commercial laboratory (see Figure 10.7) for iohexol analysis.

Calculation of clearance from plasma iohexol concentrations

Most laboratories will calculate plasma iohexol clearance and report the GFR. It is important that they indicate their method of calculation to allow you to check that they are correcting the slope–intercept result for the distribution exponential (missing AUC). When calculating the GFR, plot the log-transformed iohexol concentrations to create a plasma concentration versus time curve using a standard computer software program such as Microsoft® Excel®, or manually using graph paper. The slope–intercept method involves calculation of the AUC using a one-compartment model. The AUC for a one-compartment model is calculated as A/α (mg/ml × min). The intercept (A; mg/ml) is determined by extrapolating the line back to the time 0 intercept and the slope (α; (mg/ml)/min) is determined using a standard mathematical approach ($y_2 - y_1/x_2 - x_1$). Clearance is then calculated as the total dose of iohexol administered (mg)/AUC (mg/ml × min). It is clear from inspection of the units that GFR must therefore be in units of ml/min.

The clearance measurement is then standardized to BW (e.g. 12.27 ml/min ÷ 4.23 kg = 2.9 ml/min/kg). This result is the uncorrected clearance and requires correction with one of the species-specific correction formulae for the one-compartment assumption. For example, if the patient is a cat the corrected clearance is obtained by inputting the uncorrected clearance into the formula: $(1.036 \times \text{GFR}_{uncorrected}) - (0.062 \times \text{GFR}_{uncorrected}^2)$. This would give a corrected clearance result for the above example of $(1.036 \times 2.9) - (0.062 \times [2.9]^2) = 2.48$ ml/min/kg.

Single-sample clearance

A further simplification of the limited sampling technique is to determine GFR from a single plasma sample. Some approaches in dogs and cats have applied linear or non-linear regression analysis to derive equations for single-sample methods from multi-sample methods and to select the best sampling time. These empirical methods have limitations because the clearance determined from a single sample and the clearance determined from multiple samples are not independent measurements. Theoretically, this approach would be valid in a patient where the distribution volume is equal to the average distribution volume of the patients studied and renal function is similar to that of the population used to generate the formula. In normal healthy patients this error may be small; however, in patients with abnormal renal function the range of the volume of distribution may be greater and therefore the error larger.

There are two prerequisites for single-sample methods. The first is knowledge of the volume of distribution of the filtration marker. For example, for iohexol the volume of distribution is considered to approximate ECFV. The second is that the sample is collected at a time point when GFR is transiently independent of ECFV. This is considered to be when there is complete mixing of marker throughout the ECFV (i.e. the distribution phase can be considered to have reached completion). As renal function declines this time point is further from the time of administration of the marker. This is because of the influence of renal function on ECFV and the clearance (elimination phase) of the marker at this time. This is in contrast to the initial phase of the distribution exponential, which is relatively independent of clearance.

A single-sample method of determining GFR based on these theoretical methods has been developed for cats (Finch *et al.*, 2013b). The formula required for this is presented in Figure 10.10. A measurement of ECFV is required, and a formula based on BW can be used for this (see Figure 10.10). The optimal sampling time for single-sample clearance in cats was found to be 180 minutes. It is recommended that, in patients with a very low GFR, sampling time be delayed. Studies from human patients have suggested delays of up to 24 hours. If sampling is performed too early in patients with very low GFR, single-sample clearance will overestimate true clearance. The single-sample formula remains poorly validated for cats with very low GFR; however, given that the clinical indication for GFR determination is often in patients with normal or near normal renal function, this method can be considered to be appropriate for most cats. A similar approach has not been validated for dogs. At the time of writing, however, commercial laboratories are recommending that GFR be measured using a three-sample method because this allows assessment of the plasma concentration *versus* time curve to ensure complete intravenous administration of the filtration marker (iohexol).

Standardization of GFR measurements

The most common method for standardizing GFR measurements in dogs and cats is to use the BW in kg. In humans, GFR measurements are standardized to body surface area (BSA), which is considered to reflect basal metabolic rate and kidney size more closely than BW. A further method is to standardize to ECFV. All three methods have been shown to be appropriate for cats (Finch, 2014) whereas in dogs the optimal standardization remains unclear.

Reference interval for GFR

Despite several published studies measuring GFR in dogs and cats, reference intervals remain poorly defined. Variations in the filtration marker used, method followed and study population are likely to influence GFR measurement. Therefore, it is important for each clearance protocol that a separate reference interval is established. The reference interval derived in 25 healthy non-azotaemic (plasma creatinine concentration <140 μmol/l) cats using corrected slope–intercept iohexol clearance was 0.92–2.88 ml/min/kg (Finch, 2014). An effect of BW was found to be important in a study of 118 healthy dogs and, therefore, different reference intervals were derived for dogs of different BW (Bexfield *et al.*, 2008) (Figure 10.11). The method used to determine GFR in this study was also a corrected slope–intercept iohexol clearance technique.

In conclusion, theoretically the measurement of GFR using a three-sample plasma clearance method (analysed by the corrected slope–intercept method) should be the gold standard for assessing kidney function. The published reference intervals are wide and based on relatively small numbers of animals. Experience of measuring GFR in patients seen in general practice is limited but growing as the number of laboratories offering iohexol measurement increases. Prospective studies are warranted to determine the predictive value of measuring GFR in the diagnosis of early stage CKD.

Weight quartile (kg)	Number of dogs	Reference interval (ml/min/kg)
1.8–12.4	29	1.54–4.25
13.2–25.5	30	1.29–3.5
25.7–31.6	30	0.95–3.36
32–70	29	1.12–3.39

10.11 Reference intervals for glomerular filtration rate (GFR) for dogs in different weight quartiles.
(Adapted from Bexfield *et al.*, 2008)

Further diagnostic indicators of early kidney disease

Bone and mineral disturbances

Bone and mineral disturbances have been documented to occur in the early stages of CKD in both the dog (Cortadellas *et al.*, 2010) and the cat (Finch *et al.*, 2012) when assessed by measuring the hormones that regulate calcium and phosphate such as parathyroid hormone (PTH), calcitriol and fibroblast growth factor (FGF)-23. A full discussion of the physiology of calcium and phosphorus balance and the pathophysiology of bone and mineral disturbances associated with CKD can be found in Chapter 11. Currently measurement of these hormones is not used clinically to identify CKD at an early stage. Both parathyroid hormone and calcitriol assays are available through selected diagnostic laboratories. However, the hormone which seems to increase in the plasma earliest in CKD and to have the greatest potential as an early marker is FGF-23 although there is currently no commercial laboratory offering an assay.

Fibroblast growth factor-23

FGF-23 is produced by osteoblasts and osteocytes. It is a 'phosphatonin' with similar actions to PTH in increasing phosphate excretion from the renal tubules in response to increased phosphate or calcitriol concentrations. FGF-23 has an inhibitory action on calcitriol production and, hence, can also indirectly decrease intestinal phosphate absorption. The FGF-23 mediated decrease in calcitriol is thought to play a role in the development of bone mineral disturbances in CKD. Further supporting evidence for its role is that clinical patients with early stage CKD have decreased 1-alpha-hydroxylase activity associated with loss of renal tubular cells but not decreased erythropoietin concentrations. This suggests that renal mass reduction alone cannot explain the decreased calcitriol concentrations.

Concentrations of FGF-23 are increased in human patients with CKD prior to phosphate increase. This has now also been demonstrated in cats (Finch *et al.*, 2013a). In this study it was found that FGF-23 concentrations were increased in non-azotaemic cats which subsequently developed azotaemic CKD within a 12-month period. Worthy of note is the fact that FGF-23 undergoes renal clearance and, hence, as renal function declines, increases in FGF-23 concentration can be expected. Indeed, this has been demonstrated in cats, in which there was an inverse relationship with GFR (Finch *et al.*, 2013a). However, further work in cats with matched IRIS CKD stages found that cats with higher phosphate concentrations had significantly higher FGF-23 concentrations (Geddes *et al.*, 2013), suggesting that reduced renal clearance alone does not explain the elevation. Based on this evidence, FGF-23 measurement may in the future provide useful diagnostic information for feline patients with early CKD, not only by identifying the presence of CKD at an early stage but also perhaps by indicating those patients that would benefit from dietary phosphate restriction as part of their management. Further research is warranted to determine the diagnostic utility of FGF-23 in detecting early CKD in cats. Early reports of FGF-23 measurement in dogs with CKD suggest similar findings to those reported in cats and people (Kogika *et al.*, 2016).

Other surrogate plasma markers of reduced GFR

As discussed above, plasma creatinine concentration has been used for many years as the diagnostic indicator of reduced kidney function despite a number of limitations. Other by-products of cell metabolism rely on the kidney for their excretion from the body and meet the criteria of a suitable surrogate biomarker for GFR (freely filtered, not reabsorbed, not secreted by the renal tubule and lacking other routes of metabolism and elimination from the body). All surrogate markers of GFR have the same problem as creatinine when used as an early marker of reduced kidney function – that is, that the relationship between plasma concentration of the marker and GFR is an exponential one, with plasma concentration increasing only a small amount with early reductions in GFR. The advantages that new biomarkers of GFR may offer over creatinine are in the rate of production of the marker and the effect of extra-renal factors influencing the marker. For creatinine, muscle mass is the major factor affecting the rate of production and this varies between individual animals (affecting the reference intervals) and reduces with age, limiting the ability to detect loss of kidney function in animals as they become older. The two other biomarkers of GFR that have received most attention in veterinary medicine are symmetric dimethylarginine (SDMA) and cystatin C.

Symmetric dimethylarginine

SDMA is a product of the metabolism of cellular proteins, with the arginine residues being methylated at the post-translational modification stage. SDMA is released from cellular proteins by proteolysis and meets the criteria for a GFR marker discussed above. Serum SDMA concentrations in humans (Kielstein *et al.*, 2006), dogs (Nabity *et al.*, 2015) and cats (Braff *et al.*, 2014) correlate well with GFR. These studies also demonstrate a strong relationship between serum SDMA and creatinine concentrations. Furthermore, longitudinal studies in dogs with X-linked hereditary nephropathy suggest that use of SDMA with a cut-off value of 14 µg/dl was able to detect abnormal kidney function in affected dogs before serum creatinine was increased (Nabity *et al.*, 2015). In a colony of ageing cats, longitudinal studies also suggested that serum SDMA (with a cut-off value of 14 µg/dl) was able to detect the onset of CKD at an earlier stage than plasma creatinine and was not affected by muscle mass (Hall *et al.*, 2014). The promise shown by these studies suggests that SDMA is likely to prove a useful addition to the diagnostic panels veterinary surgeons have access to when investigating patients with suspected kidney disease.

These data have prompted the IRIS group to recommend considering measurement of serum SDMA, owing to its utility as an indicator of IRIS CKD Stage 1 (see Chapter 12) and in the assessment of the treatment needs of patients with low muscle mass in IRIS CKD Stages 2 and 3. Nevertheless, at this point it is important to caution that these are preliminary data on small well defined groups of patients. Once SDMA is used in general practice alongside the tried and tested renal biomarker, plasma creatinine, to screen large populations of heterogeneous patients, its utility will be further characterized. With experience it should be possible to determine what, if any, extra-renal factors complicate the use of SDMA in the assessment of renal function in dogs and cats. This is particularly important if its routine use in the diagnosis of kidney disease is to be recommended.

Cystatin C

Cystatin C is a small non-glycosylated cysteine proteinase inhibitor produced by all nucleated cells which can be measured by immunoturbidometric methods (Ghys *et al.*, 2014). Cystatin C is considered a better marker of GFR than serum creatinine in human patients, but there are also studies identifying situations in which it is not reliable, and in human medicine serum cystatin C has not replaced serum creatinine but is used as an additional marker of GFR. In dogs, it has not shown any systematic advantage above creatinine as a marker of GFR (Almy *et al.*, 2002) although studies using an enzyme-linked immunosorbent assay (ELISA) have suggested that serum cystatin C may be a superior marker for detecting early CKD in dogs (Miyagawa *et al.*, 2009). Studies in cats have defined a reference interval for healthy individuals but currently do not suggest that serum cystatin C is likely to be an earlier biomarker of CKD than plasma creatinine (Ghys *et al.*, 2015). In conclusion, lack of standardization of methods for measurement of serum cystatin C currently complicate its use in clinical practice alongside creatinine in the early diagnosis of CKD.

Urinary enzymes and other urinary biomarkers

There is great interest in biomarkers of kidney disease which may provide more accurate assessment of kidney function than the use of routine biomarkers such as creatinine and urea. These include urinary enzymes (Figure 10.12). However, overlap between groups tested or lack of inclusion of important control groups, such as lack of a CKD group in studies evaluating biomarkers for AKI, limit their diagnostic usefulness. Although these biomarkers may be potentially useful adjuncts to traditional tests, further research is needed.

Urinary biomarker	Nephron segment from which the molecule originates	Selected clinical conditions in which the biomarker has been studied in dogs and cats
High-molecular weight proteins (should not have been filtered)		
Albumin	Glomerulus and proximal tubule	Chronic kidney disease (CKD), acute kidney injury, hypercortisolism, diabetes mellitus, pyometra
Immunoglobulins (IgG and IgA)	Glomerulus	Leishmaniosis, leptospirosis, pyometra, hypercortisolism, diabetes mellitus
C-reactive protein (CRP)	Glomerulus	CKD, pyometra
Low-molecular weight proteins (should have been reabsorbed)		
Retinol-binding protein (RBP)	Proximal tubule	CKD, X-linked hereditary nephropathy (XLHN), pyometra, hypercortisolism, diabetes mellitus, hyperthyroidism
Beta-2-microglobulin (β2m)	Proximal tubule	XLHN
Cystatin C (cys C)	Proximal tubule	More commonly evaluated in plasma
Tubular enzymes (released from damaged tubule cells)		
N-acetyl-beta-D-glucosaminidase (NAG) cytosolic enzyme	Proximal > distal tubule	Aminoglycoside nephrotoxicosis, maleate administration, pyometra, hypercortisolism, diabetes mellitus, CKD, acute kidney injury, leishmaniosis, urinary tract inflammation, evaluated as predictor for development of azotaemia in healthy cats or cats treated for hyperthyroidism
Gamma-glutamyltransferase (GGT) brush border enzyme	Proximal tubule	
Alanine aminopeptidase (AAP) cytosolic enzyme	Proximal tubule	
Alkaline phosphatase (AP) brush border enzyme	Proximal > distal tubule	
Glutathione S-transferase π (GST)	Distal tubule	

10.12 Selected urinary biomarkers and urinary enzymes. (continues) ▶

Urinary biomarker	Nephron segment from which the molecule originates	Selected clinical conditions in which the biomarker has been studied in dogs and cats
Tubular proteins (leakage from damaged tubule cells)		
Kidney injury molecule-1 (KIM-1)	Proximal tubule	Considered one of the most useful enzymes for acute kidney injury in human medicine. Pilot data available in cats
Na⁺/H⁺ exchanger isoform 3 (NHE–3)	Proximal tubule and ascending limb	
Inflammatory markers (release from damaged tubule cells)		
Neutrophil gelatinase-associated lipocalin (NGAL)	Proximal tubule	To distinguish acute from CKD
Interleukin-18 (IL-18)	Proximal tubule	

10.12 (continued) Selected urinary biomarkers and urinary enzymes.

The greatest clinical utility for urinary enzymes currently appears to be in identifying AKI in clinical toxicity or in an intensive care unit (ICU) setting, however. This topic is covered in depth in Chapter 21. There are some studies that have sought to evaluate the same biomarkers in patients with CKD. Urinary retinol-binding protein (RBP) and urinary *N*-acetyl glucosaminidase (NAG) have been shown to be significantly higher in dogs with CKD than in healthy dogs (Smets *et al.*, 2010). NAG is also reported to be increased in cats with CKD (Jepson *et al.*, 2010). The largest studies to date evaluating biomarkers for CKD have measured urinary neutrophil gelatinase-associated lipocalin (NGAL) (Segev *et al.*, 2013; Steinbach *et al.*, 2014). In these studies, urinary NGAL was significantly higher in dogs with AKI than in dogs with CKD and also significantly higher in dogs with CKD when compared with healthy dogs.

Release of urinary enzymes may occur in a variety of situations where cellular stress is present (including hypoxia due to poor renal circulation). This makes urinary enzymes an indicator of cellular damage, but it is also unlikely that urinary enzymes will reliably distinguish between acute and chronic kidney disease or identify acute-on-chronic episodes. In the future, as research progresses, however, panels of urinary enzymes may indicate ongoing renal damage which is likely to be happening in patients with early CKD. Thus they may become very useful in identifying high-risk patients or patients with early CKD.

From a pathophysiological point of view, carbamylated haemoglobin provides a unique diagnostic tool with the potential reliably to distinguish AKI from CKD in dogs (Heiene *et al.*, 2001). It appears more promising for that purpose than the urinary enzymes. The degree of carbamylation is directly related to the exposure of haemoglobin to urea over the preceding 3 months, as opposed to enzyme leakage that may or may not occur from injured cells. This is similar to the rationale behind the measurement of fructosamine or glycosylated haemoglobin in diabetic patients. The laboratory method requires further validation and establishment of reference intervals is needed before its clinical use can be recommended.

For some biomarkers (NAG, RBP, NGAL) species-specific tests are available and are currently marketed for research rather than clinical diagnostic purposes. Other biomarkers (e.g. gamma-glutamyltransferase (GGT)) may be analysed using routine methods for plasma samples, provided the laboratory validates its work in unusual concentration ranges because urine levels will be higher than plasma levels. Carbamylated haemoglobin can be analysed in canine blood using a kit that is commercially available and marketed for human medical diagnostic laboratories, provided the laboratory has access to capillary electrophoresis (Heiene *et al.*, 2001). Therefore, most of these tests are not commercially offered by a laboratory for clinical patients, but can be set up with reasonable effort in a scientific laboratory.

Conclusion

Routine diagnosis of CKD currently relies on plasma creatinine concentration, often in combination with urea concentration and USG. The relatively low sensitivity and specificity of these markers in early stage CKD limits their use for screening in such patients, although serial measurements of plasma creatinine in an individual patient will increase the sensitivity with which early CKD can be detected for those practices whose annual health screens include routine plasma biochemistry. Measurement of GFR is considered the gold standard for assessment of renal function, but the limited sampling strategies and poor accessibility of commercial laboratories offering analysis of some filtration markers (particularly iohexol) inhibit its measurement in clinical practice. Additional plasma and urinary biomarkers may become very useful tools in the future when used alongside plasma creatinine concentration in the early diagnosis of CKD, but require further research before firm recommendations regarding their interpretation and prognostic significance can be made. The availability of serum SDMA as a commercial test should facilitate this research on large populations of dogs and cats.

Preservation of renal function should be actively pursued, and early identification of patients with CKD is considered important for implementing therapeutic interventions aimed at slowing further progression of disease. However, prospective randomized controlled clinical trials are urgently needed to demonstrate the clinical benefits of these interventions at the early disease stage. Research is also required to identify reliable predictors for individual patients with early stage CKD that will have progressive disease.

References and further reading

Almy FS, Christopher MM, King DP and Brown SA (2002) Evaluation of cystatin C as an endogenous marker of glomerular filtration rate in dogs. *Journal of Veterinary Internal Medicine* **16(1)**, 45–51

Bexfield NH, Heiene R, Gerritsen RJ *et al.* (2008) Glomerular filtration rate estimated by 3-sample plasma clearance of iohexol in 118 healthy dogs. *Journal of Veterinary Internal Medicine* **22**, 66–73

Braff J, Obare E, Yerramilli M, Elliott J and Yerramilli M (2014) Relationship between serum symmetric dimethylarginine concentration and glomerular filtration rate in cats. *Journal of Veterinary Internal Medicine* **28**, 1699–1701

Braun JP, Cabe E, Geffre A, Lefebvre HP and Trumel C (2008) Comparison of plasma creatinine values measured by different veterinary practices. *Veterinary Record* **162**, 215–216

Brochner-Mortensen J (1972) A simple method for the determination of glomerular filtration rate. *Scandinavian Journal of Clinical and Laboratory Investigation* **30**, 271–274

Cortadellas O, Fernandez del Palacio MJ, Talavera J and Bayon A (2010) Calcium and phosphorus homeostasis in dogs with spontaneous chronic kidney disease at different stages of severity. *Journal of Veterinary Internal Medicine* **24**, 73–79

Elliott J and Barber PJ (1998) Feline chronic renal failure: clinical findings in 80 cases diagnosed between 1992 and 1995. *Journal of Small Animal Practice* **39**, 78–85

Finch NC (2014) Measurement of glomerular filtration rate in cats: methods and advantages over routine markers of renal function. *Journal of Feline Medicine and Surgery* **16**, 736–748

Finch NC, Geddes RF, Syme HM and Elliott J (2013a) Fibroblast growth factor 23 (FGF-23) concentrations in cats with early nonazotemic chronic kidney disease (CKD) and in healthy geriatric cats. *Journal of Veterinary Internal Medicine* **27**, 227–233

Finch NC, Heiene R, Bird NJ, Elliott J and Peters AM (2014) Evaluation of non-polynomial equations for one-compartment correction of slope-intercept GFR: theoretical prediction and experimental measurement. *Scandinavian Journal of Clinical and Laboratory Investigation* **74**, 611–619

Finch NC, Heiene R, Elliott J, Syme HM and Peters AM (2013b) A single sample method for estimating glomerular filtration rate in cats. *Journal of Veterinary Internal Medicine* **27**, 782–790

Finch NC, Heiene R, Elliott J, Syme HM and Peters AM (2015) Determination of extracellular fluid volume in healthy and azotemic cats. *Journal of Veterinary Internal Medicine* **29**, 35–42

Finch NC, Syme HM and Elliott J (2012) Parathyroid hormone concentration in geriatric cats with various degrees of renal function. *Journal of the American Veterinary Medical Association* **241**, 1326–1335

Finch NC, Syme HM, Elliott J *et al.* (2011) Glomerular filtration rate estimation by use of a correction formula for slope-intercept plasma iohexol clearance in cats. *American Journal of Veterinary Research* **72**, 1652–1659

Finco DR, Brown SA, Barsanti JA, Bartges JW and Cooper TA (1997) Reliability of using random urine samples for "spot" determination of fractional excretion of electrolytes in cats. *American Journal of Veterinary Research* **58**, 1184–1187

Geddes RF, Finch NC, Elliott J and Syme HM (2013) Fibroblast growth factor 23 in feline chronic kidney disease. *Journal of Veterinary Internal Medicine* **27**, 234–241

Ghys LF, Paepe D, Duchateau L *et al.* (2015) Biological validation of feline serum cystatin C: The effect of breed, age and sex and establishment of a reference interval. *Veterinary Journal* **204(2)**, 168–173

Ghys LF, Paepe D, Smets P *et al.* (2014) Cystatin C: a new renal marker and its potential use in small animal medicine. *Journal of Veterinary Internal Medicine* **28(4)**, 1152–1164

Hall JA, Yerramilli M, Obare E, Yerramilli M and Jewell DE (2014) Comparison of serum concentrations of symmetric dimethylarginine and creatinine as kidney function biomarkers in cats with chronic kidney disease. *Journal of Veterinary Internal Medicine* **28**, 1676–1683

Heiene R and Moe L (1999) The relationship between some plasma clearance methods for estimation of glomerular filtration rate in dogs with pyometra. *Journal of Veterinary Internal Medicine* **13**, 587–596

Heiene R, Vulliet PR, Williams RL and Cowgill LD (2001) Use of capillary electrophoresis to quantitate carbamylated hemoglobin concentrations in dogs with renal failure. *American Journal of Veterinary Research* **62**, 1302–1306

Jepson RE, Brodbelt D, Vallance C, Syme HM and Elliott J (2009) Evaluation of predictors of the development of azotemia in cats. *Journal of Veterinary Internal Medicine* **23**, 806–813

Jepson RE, Vallance C, Syme HM and Elliott J (2010) Assessment of urinary *N*-acetyl-beta-D-glucosaminidase activity in geriatric cats with variable plasma creatinine concentrations with and without azotemia. *American Journal of Veterinary Research* **71**, 241–247

Kielstein JT, Salpeter SR, Bode-Boeger SM, Cooke JP and Fisher D (2006) Symmetric dimethylarginine (SDMA) as endogenous marker of renal failure – a meta-analysis. *Nephrology Dialysis Transplantation* **21(9)**, 2446–2451

Kogika M, Martorelli C, Caragelasco D *et al.* (2016) Fibroblast growth factor 23 (FGF-23) in dogs with chronic kidney disease. *Journal of Veterinary Internal Medicine* **30**, 1491–1492

Le Garreres A, Laroute V, de la Farge F, Boudet KG and Lefebvre HP (2007) Disposition of plasma creatinine in non-azotaemic and moderately azotaemic cats. *Journal of Feline Medicine and Surgery* **9**, 89–96

Miyagawa Y, Takemura N and Hirose H (2009) Evaluation of the measurement of serum cystatin C by an enzyme-linked immunosorbent assay for humans as a marker of the glomerular filtration rate in dogs. *Journal of Veterinary Medical Science* **71(9)**, 1169–1176

Nabity MB, Boggess MM, Kashtan CE and Lees GE (2007) Day-to-day variation of the urine protein:creatinine ratio in female dogs with stable glomerular proteinuria caused by X-linked hereditary nephropathy. *Journal of Veterinary Internal Medicine* **21**, 425–430

Nabity MB, Lees GE, Boggess MM *et al.* (2015) Symmetric dimethylarginine assay validation, stability, and evaluation as a marker for the early detection of chronic kidney disease in dogs. *Journal of Veterinary Internal Medicine* **29(4)**, 1036–1044

Paltrinieri S, Rossi G and Giordano A (2014) Relationship between rate of infection and markers of inflammation/immunity in Holy Birman cats with feline coronavirus. *Research in Veterinary Science* **97**, 263–270

Schick CS and Haller C (1999) Comparative cytotoxicity of ionic and non-ionic radiocontrast agents on MDCK cell monolayers *in vitro*. *Nephrology Dialysis Transplant* **14**, 342–347

Segev G, Palm C, Leroy B, Cowgill LD and Westropp JL (2013) Evaluation of neutrophil gelatinase-associated lipocalin as a marker of kidney injury in dogs. *Journal of Veterinary Internal Medicine* **27**, 1362–1367

Smets PM, Meyer E, Maddens BE, Duchateau L and Daminet S (2010) Urinary markers in healthy young and aged dogs and dogs with chronic kidney disease. *Journal of Veterinary Internal Medicine* **24**, 65–72

Steinbach S, Binkert B, Schweighauser A *et al.* (2010) Quantitative assessment of urea generation and elimination in healthy dogs and in dogs with chronic kidney disease. *Journal of Veterinary Internal Medicine* **24**, 1283–1289

Steinbach S, Weis J, Schweighauser A, Francey T and Neiger R (2014) Plasma and urine neutrophil gelatinase-associated lipocalin (NGAL) in dogs with acute kidney injury or chronic kidney disease. *Journal of Veterinary Internal Medicine* **28**, 264–269

Syme HM, Barber PJ, Markwell PJ and Elliott J (2002) Prevention of systolic hypertension in cats with chronic renal failure at initial evaluation. *Journal of the American Veterinary Medical Association* **220(12)**, 1799–1804

Ulleberg T, Robben J, Nordahl KM, Ulleberg T and Heiene R (2011) Plasma creatinine in dogs: intra- and inter-laboratory variation in 10 European veterinary laboratories. *Acta Veterinaria Scandinavica* **53**, 25

van den Brom WE and Biewenga WJ (1981) Assessment of glomerular filtration rate in normal dogs: analysis of the ^{51}Cr-EDTA clearance and its relation to several endogenous parameters of glomerular filtration. *Research in Veterinary Science* **30**, 152–157

Van Hoek IM, Lefebvre HP, Kooistra HS *et al.* (2008) Plasma clearance of exogenous creatinine, exo-iohexol, and endo-iohexol in hyperthyroid cats before and after treatment with radioiodine. *Journal of Veterinary Internal Medicine* **22**, 879–885

Van Hoek IM, Lefebvre HP, Paepe D *et al.* (2009) Comparison of plasma clearance of exogenous creatinine, exo-iohexol, and endo-iohexol over a range of glomerular filtration rates expected in cats. *Journal of Feline Medicine and Surgery* **11**, 1028–1030

Van Hoek IM, Vandermeulen E, Duchateau L *et al.* (2007) Comparison and reproducibility of plasma clearance of exogenous creatinine, exo-iohexol, endo-iohexol, and ^{51}Cr-EDTA in young adult and aged healthy cats. *Journal of Veterinary Internal Medicine* **21**, 950–958

Chapter 11

Assessment of calcium and phosphate homeostasis in chronic kidney disease

Rebecca Geddes and Jonathan Elliott

The reduction in the number of functioning nephrons associated with chronic kidney disease (CKD) affects the homeostasis of a number of solutes excreted in the urine, including phosphate and calcium. Adaptive changes in hormones that regulate calcium and phosphate (Ca-P) homeostasis occur in the early stages of CKD, maintaining normal plasma levels of phosphate and calcium but only through elevated fibroblast growth factor-23 (FGF-23) and/or parathyroid hormone (PTH) concentrations. Elevation in plasma phosphate concentration to outside the laboratory reference range (hyperphosphataemia) and ionized hypocalcaemia are relatively late stage events in CKD, whereas increased plasma concentrations of FGF-23 and PTH are recognized as early indicators of mineral and bone disorders (MBD) associated with CKD. CKD-MBD has replaced the previous terminology of secondary renal hyperparathyroidism (SRHP) as understanding of the multiple players involved in this complex process has developed. This chapter will review the physiology of phosphate homeostasis, the pathophysiology of CKD-MBD at different stages of CKD and discuss the potential utility of the hormones involved as prognostic markers and indicators of response to treatment.

Phosphate (and calcium) homeostasis

Homeostasis of phosphate requires a balance between dietary intake, exchange of phosphate between extracellular and bone storage pools, and renal excretion. It is not yet completely understood how this physiological regulation is achieved. Both phosphate and calcium are subject to control by the calcitropic hormones, PTH and calcitriol (1,25-dihydroxycholecalciferol or active vitamin D3), therefore their regulation should be considered together. Figure 11.1 illustrates the actions of PTH and calcitriol on their target tissues (bone, intestine and kidney) in response to a decrease in extracellular ionized calcium concentration. PTH is the primary player in the regulation of extracellular fluid (ECF) ionized calcium, which is sensed by the calcium sensing receptor (CaSR) in the plasma membrane of the parathyroid gland chief cells. Low ionized calcium (below the set point), activates the CaSR and triggers increased PTH release, the acute actions of which on bone and the kidney increase ionized calcium back towards the set point. PTH increases resorption of calcium (and phosphate) from bone, and causes a decrease in calcium excretion by the kidney (and an increase in phosphate excretion). In effect, reserves of calcium held in bone are used to defend against hypocalcaemia in the short term and the effect of PTH on the kidney ensures that calcium is retained in the plasma and phosphate is excreted. PTH also increases the synthesis of calcitriol by the kidney, by upregulating the activity of the vitamin D synthesis enzyme (25-hydroxy-vitamin D 1-alpha-hydroxylase). Calcitriol increases calcium and phosphate absorption from the intestine, inhibits PTH synthesis and secretion and has a permissive action on formation of bone when PTH concentrations are reduced. This system ensures that when bone stores of calcium (and phosphate) are released to maintain the concentration of ionized calcium in the ECF, the body activates mechanisms that restore the bone reserves to normal when the acute need for calcium is over.

Phosphate ions are freely filtered at the glomerulus and their excretion is controlled by an overflow mechanism. Phosphate ions are reabsorbed via sodium–phosphate co-transporters up to a certain threshold and remaining phosphate ions are then excreted in the urine. Above the threshold, the rate of phosphate loss in the urine (overflow) is directly proportional to the plasma phosphate concentration, but GFR controls the steepness of this relationship as illustrated in Figure 11.2. PTH reduces proximal tubular capacity to reabsorb phosphate ions by reducing the number of transporters in the proximal tubular apical membranes, which reduces the threshold plasma phosphate concentration at which phosphate ions spill over into the urine and thereby increases phosphate loss in the urine (Figure 11.2). As shown in Figure 11.1, however, PTH also increases resorption of phosphate from bone, therefore the ability of PTH to reduce ECF phosphate concentration is hampered by these competing effects on bone and kidney and works best in animals with normal renal function. As the capacity of the kidney to increase phosphate excretion in response to PTH is dependent on GFR (Figure 11.2), in patients with markedly reduced kidney function, secretion of PTH may lead to phosphate accumulation in the body outside the bone stores. The primary purpose of PTH is to regulate ECF calcium concentration.

As indicated, the mechanisms of phosphate and calcium homeostasis are intrinsically linked. An increase in plasma phosphate concentration causes a reciprocal decrease in ionized calcium concentration (law of mass action). Calcitriol increases gastrointestinal (GI) absorption

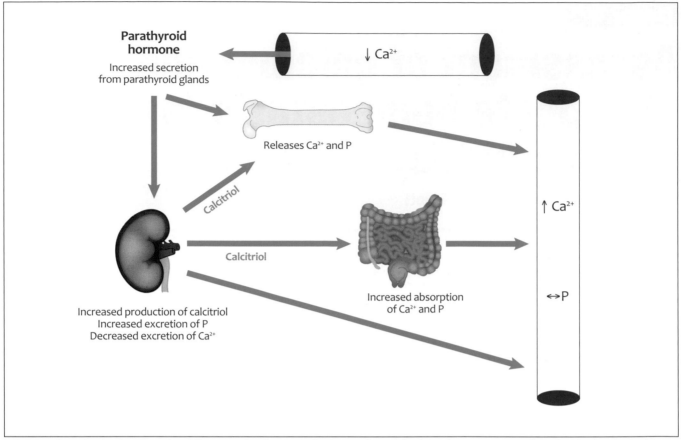

11.1 The main stimulus of parathyroid hormone (PTH) secretion by the parathyroid glands is a decrease in extracellular fluid (ECF) ionized calcium (Ca^{2+}). PTH acts to increase ionized calcium concentration, but also has effects on phosphate (P) concentration. PTH decreases excretion of calcium and increases excretion of phosphate by the kidney. It also increases production of calcitriol by the kidney, and both calcitriol and PTH stimulate release of calcium and phosphate from bone. Calcitriol also increases absorption of calcium and phosphate in the intestines. Overall, therefore, ECF calcium concentrations are increased and phosphate concentrations are kept approximately stable. Once ECF calcium is normalized, secretion of PTH is inhibited, forming a homeostatic feedback loop.

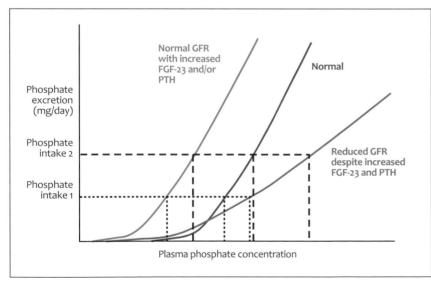

11.2 Renal function curves for phosphate excretion. In the normal situation, phosphate ions appear in the urine once plasma phosphate exceeds the reabsorptive transport maximum for phosphate. Above the threshold, if dietary intake of phosphate increases, phosphate excretion increases. The slope of the curve is dependent on glomerular filtration rate (GFR), although its position is shifted to the left by increases in parathyroid hormone (PTH) and fibroblast growth factor (FGF)-23, both of which reduce the number of sodium–phosphate co-transporters in the proximal tubules, thereby increasing phosphate excretion. In CKD, as GFR falls the gradient of this renal excretion curve becomes less steep and the plasma phosphate concentration for a given dietary intake will increase, despite increases in plasma PTH and FGF-23. (Modified after Geddes *et al.*, 2013c with permission from the *Journal of Veterinary Emergency and Critical Care*)

of calcium and phosphate and PTH increases their resorption from bone. However, in the kidney PTH acts to increase calcium reabsorption and decrease phosphate reabsorption from the glomerular filtrate in the renal tubules. Raised plasma phosphate concentration stimulates PTH secretion and inhibits calcitriol formation in the kidney, forming homeostatic feedback loops (see 'Phosphate and PTH' for further discussion of feedback processes). However, it always seemed odd that there was no hormone whose primary function was to regulate phosphate. Understanding of phosphate regulation has been enhanced over the last 10 years by the discovery of phosphate-regulating hormones, termed the 'phosphatonins', which are now well characterized in human medicine.

The phosphatonins

A 'phosphatonin' was postulated to exist because human patients with tumour-induced osteomalacia had profound hypophosphataemia and hyperphosphaturia, which was rectified following tumour removal, suggesting that the tumour was secreting a substance causing phosphate wasting. FGF-23 was proposed as the possible candidate for 'phosphatonin' (White *et al.*, 2000). A number of findings established that FGF-23 is biologically relevant; recombinant FGF-23 was shown to cause hypophosphataemia and increase renal phosphate clearance when injected into mice, and biologically active FGF-23 was shown to circulate in healthy humans, suggesting that it had a role in phosphate homeostasis. Other candidate phosphatonins were found but most seem to work indirectly through FGF-23.

FGF-23 is secreted mostly from bone in response to raised plasma phosphate and calcitriol concentrations. FGF-23 has a cofactor, Klotho, which allows it to activate the FGF receptor. In the kidney, FGF-23 downregulates the sodium–phosphate co-transporters (it has the same action as PTH on the co-transporters) and the vitamin D synthesizing enzyme (25-hydroxyvitamin D 1-alpha-hydroxylase), increasing phosphate excretion and reducing calcitriol formation. In the parathyroid gland, it acts to decrease PTH production and secretion. The main actions of FGF-23 are illustrated in Figure 11.3.

Mice lacking the gene for FGF-23 have shortened lifespans and are hyperphosphataemic and hypercalcaemic, with high serum calcitriol and suppressed PTH concentrations, demonstrating how important FGF-23 is in normal phosphate (and calcium) homeostasis. The mechanisms by which increased dietary phosphate intake leads to raised circulating FGF-23 concentrations are poorly understood. However, the discovery of FGF-23 is a major advance in understanding Ca-P homeostasis, because FGF-23 is a hormone whose secretion is governed primarily by increased phosphate and whose actions lead to lowering of ECF phosphate through increased renal excretion, reduced intestinal uptake (via inhibition of calcitriol) and reduced release from bone (via inhibition of PTH). Inevitably, discovery of FGF-23 has altered our understanding of mineral and bone disorders that accompany CKD.

Prevalence of mineral and bone disorders in CKD

Phosphate and PTH

Hyperphosphataemia and hyperparathyroidism are common findings in both feline and canine patients with CKD. A study by Barber and Elliott estimated an overall prevalence for hyperparathyroidism of 84% in cats with CKD (Barber and Elliott, 1998). This study preceded the International Renal Interest Society (IRIS) staging system for CKD, and the 80 cats with naturally occurring azotaemic CKD included were subjectively categorized as 'compensated' (no clinical signs, approximating to IRIS Stage 2), 'uraemic' (signs of the uraemic syndrome, approximating to IRIS Stage 3) and 'end-stage' (approximating to

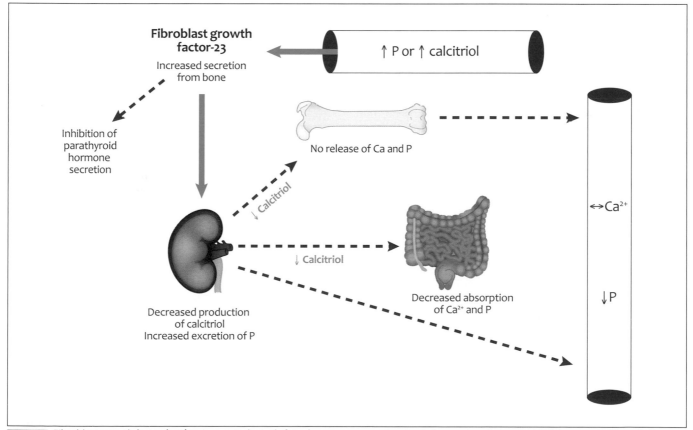

11.3 Fibroblast growth factor (FGF)-23 is secreted mostly from bone in response to raised plasma phosphate or calcitriol concentrations. In the kidney, FGF-23 increases phosphate excretion using the same mechanism as parathyroid hormone (PTH), but it also inhibits calcitriol formation. FGF-23 also inhibits PTH secretion. Therefore, there is no drive to resorb calcium (Ca²⁺) or phosphate (P) from bone and no increase in absorption of calcium or phosphate from the intestines in response to FGF-23 (this contrasts with PTH; see Figure 11.1). Overall, extracellular fluid (ECF) phosphate concentrations decrease and calcium concentrations remain approximately stable in response to increased secretion of FGF-23. Once ECF phosphate is normalized, secretion of FGF-23 is inhibited, forming a homeostatic feedback loop.

IRIS Stage 4). The prevalence of both hyperphosphataemia and hyperparathyroidism increased with the severity of disease, but 47% of the compensated cases already had elevated PTH, and 20% had phosphate above the reference range. Hyperparathyroidism was noted in cases with normal ionized calcium and plasma phosphate concentrations. Ionized hypocalcaemia (and low circulating calcitriol) was documented primarily in the 'end-stage' cats (IRIS Stage 4).

In addition, a prospective longitudinal study of non-azotaemic cats by Finch *et al.* (2012) demonstrated that plasma PTH concentrations are significantly increased in cats that develop azotaemia within 12 months, when compared with cats which remain non-azotaemic (plasma creatinine concentration ≤140 μmol/l (≤1.6 mg/dl)) over the same time period. Of the cats that went on to develop azotaemia, 19% had elevated plasma PTH concentrations at entry to the study (i.e. before they became azotaemic), despite none of the cats being hyperphosphataemic. The Ca-P product also increased significantly over the 12-month study period in these cats. In agreement with the previous study, at the 12-month time point, a greater proportion of the azotaemic cats (30 cats in IRIS Stage 2 and one cat in IRIS Stage 4) had hyperparathyroidism (35%) than were hyperphosphataemic (16%).

Similar findings have been published for canine CKD. Cortedellas *et al.* (2010) studied 54 dogs with CKD, diagnosed on the basis of persistent proteinuria (urine protein to creatinine ratio (UPC) ≥0.5) or azotaemia (plasma creatinine ≥125 μmol/l (≥1.4 mg/dl)), and classified the cases according to the IRIS staging system. As in the cat, hyperparathyroidism was the most common abnormality of Ca-P homeostasis, occurring in 75.9% of cases overall and increasing in prevalence with IRIS stage: 36.4% of Stage 1, 50% of Stage 2, 96% of Stage 3 and 100% of Stage 4 cases. The prevalence of hyperphosphataemia (plasma phosphate >1.78 mmol/l) was lower at Stages 1 and 2. Calcitriol concentrations were below the reference range in only 10 cases, which were all in the later stages (5/25 (20%) in IRIS CKD Stage 3 and 5/8 (62.5%) in IRIS CKD Stage 4).

These data suggest that, for both cats and dogs, the elevation in PTH concentration associated with CKD precedes the development of hyperphosphataemia, ionized hypocalcaemia and low plasma calcitriol concentrations. These findings are consistent with the situation in human patients and laboratory animal models of CKD. This has led to significant recent modifications to the classical and modified 'trade-off hypotheses' proposed in the 1980s and 1990s, respectively (summarized in the first edition of this manual; Barber and Elliott, 1996) to explain the pathophysiology of SRHP, which is now more commonly referred to as CKD mineral and bone disorders (CKD-MBD). The updated modified trade-off hypothesis, discussed below, explains why overt hyperphosphataemia is one of the last derangements of Ca-P homeostasis to occur.

Calcium

Calcium derangements are much less common in CKD than phosphate derangements. Hypercalcaemia based on total calcium measurement has been reported to be present in 10–11.5% of cats at diagnosis of CKD. The prevalence of ionized hypercalcaemia in feline CKD is difficult to assess, because many cross-sectional studies of cats at diagnosis of CKD have measured only total calcium. Interestingly, however, it has previously been demonstrated in both dogs and cats with CKD that ionized calcium can be normal to decreased in the face of

total hypercalcaemia. The pathogenesis of total hypercalcaemia in CKD is thought to be multifactorial; postulated mechanisms include PTH-mediated bone resorption of calcium, decreased renal calcium excretion, increased intestinal absorption due to enhanced sensitivity to calcitriol and increased complexing of calcium with anions. The pathogenesis of ionized hypercalcaemia in CKD is thought to be a consequence of autonomous hypersecretion of PTH, termed tertiary hyperparathyroidism.

FGF-23 and CKD

As might be expected, there are few data on FGF-23 in veterinary species. The human medical literature suggests that FGF-23 serum levels increase early in CKD, possibly prior to the increase in PTH concentration. The concentrations continue to rise, exceeding laboratory reference values by 1000-fold in predialysis CKD. Two publications support the fact that this situation also applies to the cat. In a subset of cases enrolled in the above study by Finch and colleagues, plasma FGF-23 concentrations at baseline were increased in cats that went on to develop azotaemia when compared with the group that remained non-azotaemic (Finch *et al.*, 2013). This study found a significant positive relationship between plasma FGF-23 and PTH concentrations and a negative relationship between plasma FGF-23 and GFR measured by plasma iohexol clearance. It is possible that elevated plasma FGF-23 concentration is more prevalent than CKD-MBD in the non-azotaemic and mild azotaemic stages of CKD in cats, as is the case in humans, and further studies are now required to measure both hormones concurrently.

A further study examined a group of 100 cats with and without azotaemic CKD (Geddes *et al.*, 2013b). Plasma FGF-23 measurements were found to be significantly different among the modified IRIS stages, increasing with declining renal function (Figure 11.4). Furthermore, plasma phosphate, creatinine, total calcium, PTH and packed cell volume (PCV) were all independent predictors of plasma FGF-23 concentration. Within a given IRIS CKD stage (Stage 2 or 3), if cats were classified according to the IRIS plasma phosphate target concentrations (discussed further below) as being above or below the target for that stage (IRIS CKD Stage 2: 1.45 mmol/l; IRIS CKD Stage 3: 1.61 mmol/l), those with phosphate concentrations above the target levels had significantly higher plasma FGF-23 concentrations than those with plasma phosphate below the target, despite the fact that their plasma creatinine concentrations were not significantly different.

Further evidence for the influence of phosphate on the circulating level of FGF-23 comes from a retrospective study showing that restricting phosphate intake in cats with azotaemic CKD reduces plasma FGF-23 concentration (Geddes *et al.*, 2013a). In this study cats were similarly classified as hyperphosphataemic if their plasma phosphate concentration was above the IRIS target level for their stage or normophosphataemic if their plasma phosphate concentration was equal to or below the IRIS target for their stage. Feeding a renal diet to the hyperphosphataemic cats (n=15) was associated with a significant decrease in plasma phosphate, PTH and FGF-23, but not creatinine concentrations. In the normophosphataemic group (n=18), feeding a renal diet was associated with a significant decrease in plasma FGF-23, but not phosphate, PTH or creatinine concentrations. This study was limited by its retrospective nature and lack of a randomized control group. A comparator group was included that did not receive a change in diet and was followed

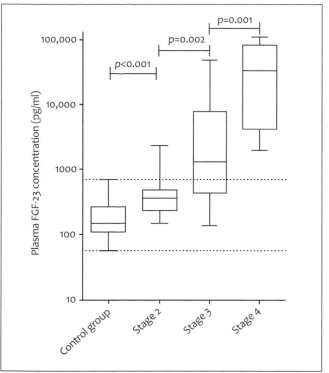

11.4 Cats were divided into four groups according to a modified IRIS staging system: control group: plasma creatinine concentration ≤177 μmol/l (n = 44); Stage 2: plasma creatinine concentration 177–250 μmol/l (n = 20); Stage 3: plasma creatinine concentration 250–440 μmol/l (n = 22); and Stage 4: plasma creatinine concentration >440 μmol/l (n = 14). The boxes represent the 25th and 75th percentiles and the central lines in the boxes represent the median values. The whiskers represent the range of concentrations. The scale for fibroblast growth factor (FGF)-23 is logarithmic. The dotted lines represent the upper and lower limits of the 95% reference interval for FGF-23 in geriatric cats. The Kruskal–Wallis test and Mann–Whitney U tests with Bonferroni correction found that FGF-23 concentrations were significantly different among all four groups (Kruskal–Wallis test: P <0.001, Mann–Whitney U tests all P <0.002).
(Modified after Geddes et al., 2013b with permission from the Journal of Veterinary Internal Medicine)

over an equivalent period, but these cats were not recruited contemporaneously nor was their diet controlled, although none was fed a renal diet. Nevertheless, these findings support the fact that FGF-23 is regulated by dietary phosphate intake and that FGF-23 may be the earliest indicator of ongoing CKD-MBD in normophosphataemic azotaemic cats.

Plasma FGF-23 is cleared by the kidney and is therefore liable to increase with a reduction in GFR. However, it has also been demonstrated that, in hyperphosphataemic human patients with CKD, phosphate is the most important predictor of FGF-23 when GFR is <30 ml/min/1.73 m² (Westerberg et al., 2007). As discussed above this seems also to apply to the cat. Preliminary data suggest that FGF-23 increases with IRIS CKD stage in dogs (Kogika et al., 2016). It is difficult to tease apart these factors in the patient with CKD, however, because GFR also influences plasma phosphate concentration, as discussed above.

Updated pathophysiology of CKD-MBD

Although the role of FGF-23 is only beginning to be unravelled in companion animals, it is appropriate to update the working hypothesis for the pathophysiology of CKD-MBD

(formerly secondary renal hyperparathyroidism) on the basis of the human literature.

An updated 'trade-off' hypothesis still begins with phosphate retention developing as GFR starts to decline in the failing kidney, but the mechanisms involved in early CKD and late stage CKD should be considered separately. In early CKD, phosphate retention will drive increases in FGF-23 concentration (via a currently unknown sensor), which has a number of effects:

- Inhibition of the sodium–phosphate co-transporters in the kidney, which will act to increase fractional excretion of phosphate in the remaining nephrons
- Inhibition of 1-alpha-hydroxlyase, by increased phosphate and FGF-23, will result in lower concentrations of calcitriol, thereby decreasing phosphate absorption from the GI tract
- FGF-23 will directly inhibit PTH secretion via activation of the FGF receptor in the parathyroid gland. The inhibition of PTH will prevent the drive to increase ionized calcium concentration by releasing calcium (and phosphate) from bone.

In patients with early CKD this increase in FGF-23, and consequent increase in urinary phosphate excretion, will therefore be sufficient to restore phosphate homeostasis and prevent the development of CKD-MBD (Figure 11.5).

In more severe CKD, there will be three reasons why FGF-23 will continue to increase:

- As GFR decreases, intact FGF-23 will also increase because it is renally cleared
- Once GFR drops to below a critical rate (which has shown to be 30 ml/min/1.73 m² in human patients), plasma phosphate concentrations start to increase and will stimulate further FGF-23 secretion
- End-organ resistance to FGF-23 will develop as a result of downregulation of its receptors, resulting in FGF-23 losing its direct inhibition of PTH.

At this point FGF-23 might be considered a uraemic toxin, because it will continue to decrease calcitriol concentrations without being effective as a hyperphosphaturic factor owing to the decline in renal function. Reduced calcitriol will both reduce inhibition of PTH secretion in the parathyroid gland and indirectly increase PTH secretion via reduced GI uptake of ionized calcium, leading to reduced plasma ionized calcium. Low plasma ionized calcium concentration then becomes a major driving force for a rise in PTH; additionally, hyperphosphataemia will stimulate PTH secretion directly. Resistance to FGF-23 at the level of the parathyroid gland means that PTH secretion is no longer inhibited despite the presence of high concentrations of FGF-23.

The development of overt hyperphosphataemia tends to occur late in the progression of CKD-MBD in this model because PTH and FGF-23 are both phosphaturic, and the fractional excretion of phosphate is at its highest in patients with both high FGF-23 and high PTH. Therefore, the increases in both of these hormones will compensate for the reduction in nephron mass until GFR falls below a critical rate. In very late stage CKD (IRIS CKD Stage 4) there is end-organ resistance to both of these hormones, resulting in hyperphosphataemia and calcitriol deficiency despite vastly increased plasma concentrations of FGF-23 and PTH (Figure 11.5).

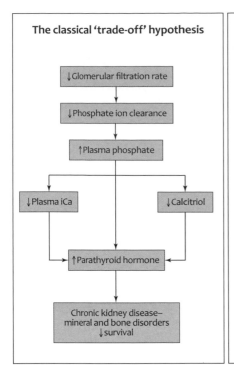

The classical 'trade-off' hypothesis

↓ Glomerular filtration rate

↓ Phosphate ion clearance

↑ Plasma phosphate

↓ Plasma iCa

↓ Calcitriol

↑ Parathyroid hormone

Chronic kidney disease–mineral and bone disorders ↓ survival

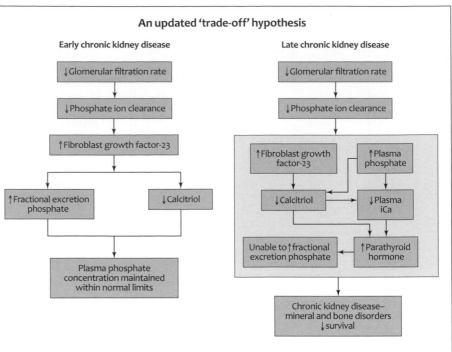

An updated 'trade-off' hypothesis

Early chronic kidney disease

↓ Glomerular filtration rate

↓ Phosphate ion clearance

↑ Fibroblast growth factor-23

↑ Fractional excretion phosphate

↓ Calcitriol

Plasma phosphate concentration maintained within normal limits

Late chronic kidney disease

↓ Glomerular filtration rate

↓ Phosphate ion clearance

↑ Fibroblast growth factor-23

↑ Plasma phosphate

↓ Calcitriol

↓ Plasma iCa

Unable to ↑ fractional excretion phosphate

↑ Parathyroid hormone

Chronic kidney disease–mineral and bone disorders ↓ survival

11.5 The traditional *versus* recently updated views of the 'trade-off' hypothesis. Under the classical explanation of the 'trade-off' hypothesis, the reduction in glomerular filtration rate (GFR) leads to reduced phosphate ion clearance in the kidney and therefore to an increase in plasma phosphate concentration. Increasing plasma phosphate stimulates parathyroid hormone (PTH) secretion directly, and indirectly via inhibition of calcitriol production in the kidney and by reducing plasma ionized calcium (iCa) concentration via the law of mass action. The 'trade-off' for an increase in phosphate ion excretion is an increase in plasma PTH concentration, leading to a number of deleterious effects. In the updated hypothesis, the decrease in phosphate ion clearance stimulates fibroblast growth factor (FGF)-23 secretion, which increases the fractional excretion (FE) of phosphate ions and inhibits calcitriol production in the kidney in early CKD. This maintains plasma phosphate concentration within normal limits. In late stage CKD, the kidney is unable to increase the FE of phosphate ions any further owing to low nephron mass, and hyperphosphataemia develops. Increased plasma phosphate, reduced calcitriol and reduced ionized calcium all drive the increase in PTH concentration, and the clinical manifestations of chronic kidney disease mineral and bone disorders (CKD-MBD) develop.

(Modified after Geddes *et al.*, 2013c with permission from the *Journal of Veterinary Emergency and Critical Care*)

Clinical consequences of CKD-MBD in cats and dogs

CKD-MBD is associated with decreased survival and significant morbidity. Clinical manifestations of CKD-MBD include soft tissue mineralization (Figure 11.6) and renal osteodystrophy (Figure 11.7). Cats with CKD can develop pathological fractures, loose teeth and 'rubber jaw' syndrome as a consequence of bone demineralization. In one study of 74 cats with CKD, 9.8% had generalized osteoporosis, 7.3% had nephrocalcinosis and 9.5% had soft tissue mineralization (DiBartola *et al.*, 1987). Soft tissue structures that may show mineralization in feline CKD include the kidneys, thoracic and abdominal aorta, the gastric wall and pulmonary arteries and capillaries (see Figure 11.6). Metastatic calcifications in the paws can also form in cats and dogs, which can cause lameness. Soft tissue mineralization is considered more likely to occur when the calcium–phosphate product (Ca x P) exceeds 5.65 mmol²/l² (70 mg²/dl²). Additionally, having a Ca x P >5.65 mmol²/l² has recently been demonstrated to be a negative prognostic indicator in dogs with CKD. In this study, dogs with CKD and a Ca x P >5.65 mmol²/l² had a median survival time of only 30 days, whereas 50% of the dogs with a Ca x P ≤5.65 mmol²/l² were still alive at the end of the 455-day follow-up period (Lippi *et al.*, 2014).

In dogs with experimentally induced CKD, hyperphosphataemia has been associated with a more rapid progression of CKD and with decreased survival (Brown *et al.*, 1991; Finco *et al.*, 1992). Hyperphosphataemia is also associated with shorter survival times in feline patients with naturally occurring CKD (King *et al.*, 2007; Boyd *et al.*, 2008), and plasma phosphate has been documented to predict progression of feline CKD (Chakrabarti *et al.*, 2012). Plasma FGF-23 concentration at diagnosis of feline CKD is an independent predictor of both survival time and CKD

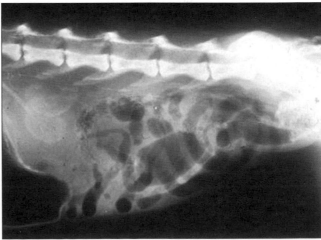

11.6 Soft tissue calcification affecting the kidneys and gastric wall, with some metastatic calcification evident in the abdominal vasculature, due to chronic kidney disease mineral and bone disorder (CKD-MBD) in an 11-year-old male Domestic Shorthaired Cat. Radiograph taken post mortem.

(Reproduced from Barber, 1998)

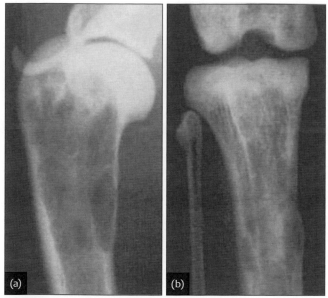

| 11.7 | Post-mortem (a) lateral radiograph of the proximal humerus and (b) cranial–caudal radiograph of the proximal tibia of a cat with severe chronic kidney disease (CKD) and marked CKD-mineral and bone disorder (CKD-MBD). Note the cystic lesions in both long bones leading to thinning of the cortices. (Reproduced from Barber, 1998) |

concentration is widely and cheaply available. To aid in the use of plasma phosphate as a biomarker of CKD-MBD, the IRIS targets for plasma phosphate concentration were devised. These targets (Figure 11.8) are well within the laboratory reference range and should be used for all azotaemic patients when assessing Ca-P homeostasis to try and prevent or reverse increases in the phosphaturic hormones, PTH and FGF-23. The aim should be to maintain plasma phosphate concentrations towards the lower end of (or at least within) the target range for that patient's stage of CKD. Measurement of plasma phosphate concentration should be performed in stable patients that have been fasted for the blood sample, because circulating phosphate is elevated following a recent meal.

Stage	Plasma creatinine (μmol/l)		Target plasma phosphate for dogs and cats	
	Dogs	Cats	mmol/l	mg/dl
1	<125	<140	0.81–1.45	2.5–4.5
2	125–179	140–249	0.81–1.45	2.5–4.5
3	180–439	250–439	0.81–1.61	2.5–5
4	>440	>440	0.81–1.94	2.5–6

| 11.8 | The International Renal Interest Society targets for plasma phosphate concentration. |

progression over 12 months (where progression was defined as an increase in plasma creatinine of >25%) (Geddes et al., 2015). In these studies, inclusion of FGF-23 removed both PTH and phosphate from the statistical models. This may be explained by the fact that FGF-23 seems to be the earliest biochemical derangement of Ca-P homeostasis to develop, therefore it may be a useful biomarker of CKD-MBD. Whether FGF-23 is itself a uraemic toxin, or a marker of other causes of uraemic toxicity, is currently under investigation. Recent evidence suggests that, in humans, FGF-23 can induce left ventricular hypertrophy (Faul et al., 2011), and is an independent predictor of myocardial infarction, stroke and cardiovascular mortality in patients with CKD (Bouma-de Krijger et al., 2014). However, although these findings may shed some light on how FGF-23 may act as a uraemic toxin in human patients, cardiovascular incidents are not a commonly recognized cause of death or euthanasia in feline or canine patients with CKD.

Reducing phosphate intake by feeding a clinical renal diet has been shown prospectively to improve survival time in both dogs and cats with naturally occurring azotaemic CKD (Elliott et al., 2000; Jacob et al., 2002; Ross et al., 2006). This indicates the importance of assessing patients for the presence of CKD-MBD so that management strategies can be employed to limit the deleterious effect these derangements have on disease progression and therefore patient survival time.

Assessment of CKD-MBD

Radiographic identification of soft tissue mineralization is also only evident in late stages of CKD, yet CKD-MBD begins in the pre-azotaemic stage. Additionally, from the above discussion it is clear that hyperphosphataemia occurs late in the development of CKD-MBD. This is particularly true if laboratory reference ranges for plasma phosphate are used, and yet measurement of plasma phosphate

Although the IRIS phosphate targets are useful, it is clear from the studies by Geddes et al. (2013ab) that plasma FGF-23 concentration may be elevated in cats in IRIS Stages 2 and 3 that have plasma phosphate concentrations within the target range. Ideally, full assessment of Ca-P homeostasis would include direct measurement of the most significant variables involved, primarily PTH and FGF-23. Measurement of calcium and calcitriol may also be useful, but data suggest that derangements in these are again more prevalent in the later stages of CKD.

If calcium concentration is being assessed for calculation of the Ca-P product then measurement of total calcium is required. This is readily available in clinical practice. However, ionized calcium is the biologically active calcium fraction and has been shown to correlate poorly with total calcium in cats with CKD (Schenck and Chew, 2010). Therefore, ideally, ionized calcium measurements should be made if any concerns arise regarding total calcium concentrations in patients with CKD (e.g. the presence of concurrent hypercalcaemia). Ionized calcium measurement is less readily available, subject to change with pH and temperature and influenced by many anticoagulants used in routine blood sample collection. Calcitriol is very expensive to measure and there are very few laboratories that offer the assay.

Measurement of plasma PTH concentrations is possible and many different PTH assays are commercially available. Their availability is, however, limited to a few diagnostic laboratories. It is important to measure intact (biologically active) PTH in the patient with CKD because C-terminal fragments of PTH which are not biologically active accumulate as a result of reduced renal clearance. The original intact PTH assay (Allegro Intact PTH; manufactured by Nichols Institute) which was validated for the dog (Torrance and Nachreiner, 1989) and cat (Barber et al., 1993) is no longer manufactured commercially. Data recently published by the authors are based on a different intact PTH assay (Total Intact PTH Immunoradiometric Assay – coated bead version, manufactured by Scantibodies) which has been independently validated for use in the cat (Pineda et al., 2012; Williams et al., 2012). The results seem very similar to those of the original Allegro Intact PTH assay. Additional issues with measuring PTH in clinical patients include:

- The hormone is labile; samples need to be handled carefully and transported to the laboratory on ice or treated with protease inhibitors
- It is difficult to distinguish low PTH concentrations from normal PTH in the cat owing to problems with sensitivity, thus monitoring response to treatment will not reveal changes in PTH within the reference range
- The assay is expensive to run.

At the time of writing there are no commercial laboratories offering FGF-23 assays. The authors have validated a sandwich enzyme-linked immunosorbent assay (ELISA) for use in the cat (Geddes *et al.*, 2013b), which is sold in kit form (manufactured by Kainos). The reference range published for the cat (56–700 pg/ml) is higher than for humans (8–54 pg/ml) (Yamazaki *et al.*, 2002), therefore problems of lack of sensitivity at the low end of the reference range encountered for PTH do not occur with FGF-23. Because the assay is a sandwich ELISA with antibodies against both C- and N-termini, it detects intact FGF-23 molecules which are physiologically active. However, to activate its receptor *in vivo*, FGF-23 requires its co-ligand Klotho and it may be that, in the future, measurement of Klotho alongside FGF-23 will provide more information about CKD-MBD. In the cat, FGF-23 appears to be very stable in plasma or serum, and post-sample degradation does not seem to be a problem (Geddes *et al.*, 2013b). In the future, if this assay becomes commercially available it might be used to diagnose:

- The presence of CKD-MBD in patients that are normophosphataemic, and therefore the need for dietary phosphate restriction in these patients
- The response to dietary phosphate restriction in the above patients and those that have become normophosphataemic.

In addition, it is possible that FGF-23 could be used as a prognostic marker at the initial diagnosis of CKD. There is significantly more work required in the cat to develop target FGF-23 levels that should be achieved following phosphate restriction as a treatment for CKD-MBD. However, it seems likely that, as a biomarker, FGF-23 will have significant utility and advantages over the measurement of plasma phosphate concentration for the assessment of CKD-MBD in cats and possibly in dogs. Clinical research has not addressed FGF-23 and its utility in the dog to date. For further information on the utility of biomarkers for CKD-MBD in human patients see Evenepoel *et al.* (2014). At present, therefore, assessment of CKD-MBD in both cats and dogs with CKD is primarily reliant on measurement of plasma phosphate concentration in stable, fasted patients and interpretation of these measurements in line with the IRIS phosphate targets.

References and further reading

Barber PJ (1998) *Parathyroid gland function in the ageing cat* [thesis]. University of London, London, UK

Barber PJ and Elliott J (1996) Assessment of parathyroid function in renal function. In: *BSAVA Manual of Canine and Feline Nephrology and Urology*, ed. J Elliott and J Bainbridge. BSAVA Publications, Gloucester

Barber PJ and Elliott J (1998) Feline chronic renal failure: calcium homeostasis in 80 cases diagnosed between 1992 and 1995. *Journal of Small Animal Practice* **39**, 108–116

Barber PJ, Elliott J and Torrance AG (1993) Measurement of feline intact parathyroid-hormone – assay validation and sample handling studies. *Journal of Small Animal Practice* **34**, 614–620

Bouma-de Krijger A, Bots ML, Vervloet MG et al. (2014) Time-averaged level of fibroblast growth factor-23 and clinical events in chronic kidney disease. *Nephrology Dialysis Transplant* **29**, 88–97

Boyd LM, Langston C, Thompson K, Zivin K and Imanishi M (2008) Survival in cats with naturally occurring chronic kidney disease (2000–2002). *Journal of Veterinary Internal Medicine* **22**, 1111–1117

Brown SA, Crowell WA, Barsanti JA, White JV and Finco DR (1991) Beneficial effects of dietary mineral restriction in dogs with marked reduction of functional renal mass. *Journal of the American Society of Nephrology* **1**, 1169–1179

Chakrabarti S, Syme HM and Elliott J (2012) Clinicopathological variables predicting progression of azotemia in cats with chronic kidney disease. *Journal of Veterinary Internal Medicine* **26(2)**, 275–281

Cortadellas O, del Palacio MJF, Talavera J and Bayon A (2010) Calcium and phosphorus homeostasis in dogs with spontaneous chronic kidney disease at different stages of severity. *Journal of Veterinary Internal Medicine* **24**, 73–79

DiBartola SP, Rutgers HC, Zack PM and Tarr MJ (1987) Clinicopathologic findings associated with chronic renal disease in cats: 74 cases (1973–1984). *Journal of the American Veterinary Medical Association* **190**, 1196–1202

Elliott J, Rawlings JM, Markwell PJ and Barber PJ (2000) Survival of cats with naturally occurring chronic renal failure: effect of dietary management. *Journal of Small Animal Practice* **41**, 235–242

Evenepoel P, Rodriguez M and Ketteler M (2014) Laboratory abnormalities in CKD-MBD: markers, predictors, or mediators of disease? *Seminars in Nephrology* **34**, 151–163

Faul C, Amaral AP, Oskouei B et al. (2011) FGF23 induces left ventricular hypertrophy. *Journal of Clinical Investigation* **121**, 4393–4408

Finch NC, Geddes RF, Syme HM and Elliott J (2013) Fibroblast growth factor 23 (FGF-23) concentrations in cats with early nonazotemic chronic kidney disease (CKD) and in healthy geriatric cats. *Journal of Veterinary Internal Medicine* **27**, 227–233

Finch NC, Syme HM and Elliott J (2012) Parathyroid hormone concentration in geriatric cats with various degrees of renal function. *Journal of the American Veterinary Medical Association* **241**, 1326–1335

Finco DR, Brown SA, Crowell WA et al. (1992) Effects of dietary phosphorus and protein in dogs with chronic renal failure. *American Journal of Veterinary Research* **53**, 2264–2271

Geddes RF, Elliott J and Syme HM (2013a) The effect of feeding a renal diet on plasma fibroblast growth factor 23 concentrations in cats with stable azotemic chronic kidney disease. *Journal of Veterinary Internal Medicine* **27**, 1354–1361

Geddes RF, Elliott J and Syme HM (2015) Relationship between plasma fibroblast growth factor 23 concentration and survival time in cats with chronic kidney disease. *Journal of Veterinary Internal Medicine* **29**, 1494–1501

Geddes RF, Finch NC, Elliott J and Syme HM (2013b) Fibroblast growth factor 23 in feline chronic kidney disease. *Journal of Veterinary Internal Medicine* **27**, 234–241

Geddes RF, Finch NC, Syme HM and Elliott J (2013c) The role of phosphorus in the pathophysiology of chronic kidney disease. *Journal of Veterinary Emergency and Critical Care* **23**, 122–133

Jacob F, Polzin DJ, Osborne CA et al. (2002) Clinical evaluation of dietary modification for treatment of spontaneous chronic renal failure in dogs. *Journal of the American Veterinary Medical Association* **220**, 1163–1170

King JN, Tasker S, Gunn-Moore DA and Strehlau G (2007) Prognostic factors in cats with chronic kidney disease. *Journal of Veterinary Internal Medicine* **21**, 906–916

Kogika M, Martorelli C, Caragelasco D et al. (2016) Fibroblast growth factor 23 (FGF-23) in dogs with chronic kidney disease. *Journal of Veterinary Internal Medicine* **30**, 1491–1492

Lippi I, Guidi G, Marchetti V, Tognetti R and Meucci V (2014) Prognostic role of the product of serum calcium and phosphorus concentrations in dogs with chronic kidney disease: 31 cases (2008–2010). *Journal of the American Veterinary Medical Association* **245**, 1135–1140

Pineda C, Aguilera-Tejero E, Raya AI et al. (2012) Feline parathyroid hormone: validation of hormonal assays and dynamics of secretion. *Domestic Animal Endocrinology* **42**, 256–264

Ross SJ, Osborne CA Kirk CA et al. (2006) Clinical evaluation of dietary modification for treatment of spontaneous chronic kidney disease in cats. *Journal of the American Veterinary Medical Association* **229**, 949–957

Schenck PA and Chew DJ (2010) Prediction of serum ionized calcium concentration by serum total calcium measurement in cats. *Canadian Journal of Veterinary Research* **74**, 209–213

Torrance AG and Nachreiner R (1989) Human-parathormone assay for use in dogs: validation, sample handling studies, and parathyroid function testing. *American Journal of Veterinary Research* **50**, 1123–1127

Westerberg PA, Linde T, Wikstrom B et al. (2007) Regulation of fibroblast growth factor-23 in chronic kidney disease. *Nephrology Dialysis Transplant* **22**, 3202–3207

White KE, Evans WE, O'Riordan JLH et al. (2000) Autosomal dominant hypophosphataemic rickets is associated with mutations in FGF23. *Nature Genetics* **26**, 345–348

Williams TL, Elliott J and Syme HM (2012) Calcium and phosphate homeostasis in hyperthyroid cats: associations with development of azotaemia and survival time. *Journal of Small Animal Practice* **53**, 561–571

Yamazaki Y, Okazaki R, Shibata M et al. (2002) Increased circulatory level of biologically active full-length FGF-23 in patients with hypophosphatemic rickets/osteomalacia. *Journal of Clinical Endocrinology and Metabolism* **87**, 4957–4960

Diagnostic algorithms for grading acute kidney injury and staging the chronic kidney disease patient

Jonathan Elliott and Larry D. Cowgill

The terminology in current use to describe the different severities of chronic kidney disease (CKD) and acute kidney injury (AKI) is confusing and is applied in different ways by different authorities. In 1998, the International Renal Interest Society (IRIS) was formed and one of its main purposes was to devise, through consensus and debate, a staging system for CKD to allow better communication of the concepts underlying the diagnosis and management of this complex disease syndrome to general veterinary practitioners and veterinary students throughout the world. This consensus has now been extended to a new IRIS grading system for AKI. The IRIS group now has representation from 11 different countries. The staging system first proposed for CKD has been utilized by members of the IRIS Board and refined on the basis of this use. In addition, feedback has been obtained from the American and European Societies of Veterinary Nephrology and Urology and modifications made according to this feedback. The grading system for AKI has been proposed by IRIS and it is in the process of gaining feedback from the American and European societies to ensure wide acceptance of the concepts on which it is built.

In veterinary medicine, staging systems have been used for defining heart failure where a modification of a system used in human medicine is routinely applied. Likewise, the IRIS system for staging CKD is based on similar systems used in human medicine. It should be viewed as work in progress. As more information is published in the form of original studies involving the diagnosis, prognosis and management of CKD and AKI in dogs and cats, modifications to these staging and grading systems and the treatment recommendations that go with them will be made. The concepts upon which staging and grading are based are presented in Squires (2007) and the application of the IRIS staging system to the management of CKD is presented in Chapter 23. Chapter 21 describes the current approach to the management of AKI. Since the IRIS group launched the concept of the CKD staging system, there have been an increasing number of publications using it in case classification for observational and interventional studies, growing the evidence for its application in this way. In the future, the authors expect a consensus to be reached on linking the management of AKI to the IRIS AKI grading system. The purpose of this chapter is to define the staging and grading systems precisely, and to explain the reasoning that underlies them and their appropriate application.

Selecting dogs and cats to be staged or graded

The IRIS CKD staging system only applies to dogs and cats with stable CKD, where stable CKD may be defined as a patient with a serum creatinine which changes by <25 μmol/l (0.3 mg/dl) over a period of 2–4 weeks. In other forms of disease affecting kidney function, the plasma creatinine concentration (upon which the staging system is based) can change dramatically over a short period of time. Hence, staging is not appropriate under these circumstances and AKI grading may be appropriate (see below). In Squires (2007), the approach to the azotaemic animal is outlined. In summary, if the recognized azotaemia is stable yet persistent over weeks to months, the kidney disease is chronic and not reversible. If, on the other hand, the recognized azotaemia is sudden in onset and/or progressive within or above the reference interval over a short interval of time, it is important to:

- First, recognize the patient has an AKI
- Second, determine the cause of the azotaemia as:
  - Volume-responsive (pre-renal)
  - Primary intrinsic renal
  - Post-renal
- If the cause of the AKI is primary intrinsic kidney disease, the veterinary surgeon (veterinarian) needs to determine whether the kidney disease is:
  - Purely acute
  - Decompensated chronic (sometimes termed 'acute on chronic').

The acutely ill patient with unstable kidney disease is a patient that should have its kidney disease graded. It may go on to have stable CKD after 4–8 weeks of management of its kidney disease (either as a result of AKI or because it was a patient with acutely decompensated CKD), whereupon staging of its CKD may be appropriate (see Figure 12.1). The important point for the purposes of staging is that only short-term stable CKD can be staged accurately by the IRIS CKD staging system. This does not mean that kidney function in the CKD patient never changes. It may remain stable for very long periods of time, it may gradually progress with serial serum creatinine slowly increasing with time or there may be sudden decrements in kidney function associated with deterioration in the patient's clinical status (decompensated CKD, see above). However, CKD staging is most informative when undertaken during a period of stability. To check for evidence of progression, re-staging the apparently stable case approximately every 6 months or sooner if clinically indicated would be informative. In those cases that decompensate, if stability is re-established following treatment of the acute episode, re-staging should also be undertaken at that point.

IRIS grading system for the patient with AKI

Acute kidney injury represents a spectrum of dysfunction associated with a sudden onset of renal parenchymal injury, most typically recognized by generalized failure of the kidneys to meet the excretory, metabolic and endocrine demands of the body, i.e. acute renal failure (ARF) (Cowgill and Langston, 2011). In contrast to CKD (see below), AKI is characterized by short-term loss of kidney function that is anticipated to change over time. Veterinary surgeons recognize acute kidney disease by its advanced and most overt manifestation, ARF, but this convention blinds the clinician to identifying the early and most subtle forms of disease when therapeutic options to minimize its progression and severity are greatest.

ARF is characterized by sudden haemodynamic, filtration, tubulointerstitial or outflow injury to the kidneys, subsequent accumulation of metabolic toxins (uraemic toxins) and dysregulation of fluid, electrolyte and acid–base balance. However, ARF reflects only a subset of patients with AKI who have the highest morbidity and mortality (Figure 12.1). The term 'acute kidney injury' (versus acute renal failure) better reflects the broad spectrum of acute diseases of the kidney from its least to its most severe manifestations and has become the preferred terminology for this condition (Hoste and Kellum, 2007; Kellum and Lameire, 2013). AKI may be imperceptible to the clinician at early stages or be so advanced as to require dialysis support for overt failure of kidney function, or may culminate in death (Figure 12.1).

As an additional departure from historical perceptions, the clinical presentation of AKI encompasses the conventional categories of pre-renal and post-renal conditions which may be independent of, or coexistent with, intrinsic kidney disease. Consequently, small animal patients should be diagnosed with AKI regardless of the pre-renal, intrinsic renal parenchymal and/or post-renal components of the disease, and then assessed for grading, diagnostic evaluation and management. AKI typically affects intrinsically normal kidneys, but events predisposing to AKI are frequently superimposed on pre-existing CKD to produce clinical features that mimic AKI (acute-on-chronic kidney disease). Currently, there are no markers to define or stratify the spectrum of injury that constitutes AKI, although some novel biomarkers are showing promise, and, until recently, precise definitions for AKI had not been established in veterinary medicine (De Loor et al., 2013; Segev et al., 2013; Palm et al., 2016). In addition, there has been no formal categorization of the spectrum of the functional or clinical abnormalities to standardize its classification, severity, grade, clinical course, response to therapy or prognosis for recovery.

To better emphasize the concept that AKI represents a continuum of renal injury, several 'staging' schemes (RIFLE, AKIN, KDIGO) have been proposed for human patients to stratify the extent and duration of kidney injury and predict clinical outcomes (Bellomo et al., 2004; Hoste and Kellum, 2007; Mehta et al., 2007; Molitoris et al., 2007; Kellum and Lameire, 2012). There is considerable overlap between these systems for human patients, and criteria for each staging category are based ostensibly on insensitive markers of kidney injury including relative changes in glomerular filtration rate (GFR) and serum creatinine, or urine output, and duration of signs. Unfortunately, the criteria that define these staging schemes in human patients are not consistently applicable in companion animal patients with naturally occurring disease. In human patients, AKI is a condition that manifests typically within the hospital setting. There is an emerging recognition of AKI in veterinary emergency and critical care medicine; however, in contrast to human patients, small animal

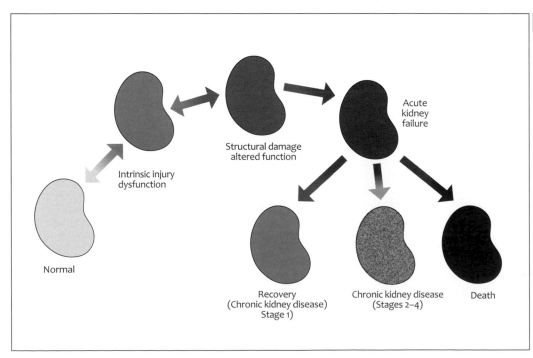

12.1 The spectrum of acute kidney injury (AKI) from early kidney injury/dysfunction to kidney failure. Acute kidney failure is the most recognizable presentation of AKI, but identification of earlier stages of injury is critical for timely diagnosis and to facilitate more effective management.

Normal

Intrinsic injury dysfunction

Structural damage altered function

Acute kidney failure

Recovery (Chronic kidney disease) Stage 1

Chronic kidney disease (Stages 2–4)

Death

patients most commonly develop AKI outside the hospital setting. As a consequence, the abruptness of the disease and the magnitude of changes in GFR, azotaemia and/or urine production are imprecisely known or quantified for comparable categorization.

Progressive (and often subtle) azotaemia as measured by plasma creatinine concentration is the hallmark of AKI, but is observed inconsistently in small animals because the azotaemia has not developed or become fully established at the time of presentation for the disease, or because serial observations are not performed consistently on animals exposed to medications, subjected to therapeutic procedures, or hospitalized for illnesses that can compromise kidney function. Plasma creatinine increases progressively with the duration and severity of the kidney injury or the completeness of urinary outflow obstruction; however, reductions in lean body mass, decreased creatinine generation, and overhydration can lower the plasma creatinine concentration and mask sequential changes. Despite its insensitivity and limitations as a biomarker of kidney injury, plasma creatinine currently stands as the best, most time-tested and most familiar marker of decreased renal excretory function.

To date, no formally adopted classification system has been established for small animals with AKI to stratify or characterize the severity of the renal impairment as has been established recently for CKD in dogs and cats and AKI in humans (Cowgill and Langston, 2011; Lee et al., 2011; Thoen and Kerl, 2011; Harison et al., 2012). IRIS CKD staging was developed as a consensus scheme to promote more uniform characterization and recognition of CKD in small animals, with the goals to promote understanding of its pathophysiology and better facilitate its evaluation and rational management. Recently, IRIS has adapted this same schematic approach to the classification and grading of AKI in dogs and cats (IRIS, 2013). Unlike IRIS CKD staging, grading of AKI does not imply that the kidney disease is stable over the short-term or at steady state. To the contrary, the 'grade' represents a moment in the observed course of the disease and is predicted to change as the condition worsens, improves or transitions to CKD (see Figure 12.1). This caveat also implies that serial assessment and sequential grading should be used to monitor the immediate and ongoing course of the disease and update therapeutic decisions and outcomes. Figure 12.2 outlines the IRIS AKI grading scheme for dogs and cats based on plasma creatinine, urine formation and the requirement for renal replacement therapy (RRT). It is intended to facilitate classification, functional stratification and therapeutic decision-making for animals with AKI. IRIS has purposefully adopted the term 'grading' to help prevent confusion and mis-application of the respective CKD and AKI classification approaches to categorize kidney diseases with disparate diagnostic and management requirements. It is fundamentally important that the clinician understand their differences, appropriate applications and proper terminologies.

IRIS AKI Grade I defines non-azotaemic animals with historical, clinical, laboratory (biomarkers such as glucosuria, cylinduria, proteinuria, inflammatory sediment, microalbuminuria or emerging novel biomarkers, e.g. neutrophil gelatinase-associated lipocalin (NGAL), serum symmetric dimethylarginine (SDMA), clusterin, cystatin C) or imaging evidence of AKI, and/or those with clinical oliguria or anuria. Historical features which define AKI might include exposure to plant or chemical toxins, infectious or acquired diseases or environmental

AKI grade	Plasma creatinine	Clinical description
Grade I	<140 µmol/l (<1.6 mg/dl)	**Non-azotaemic AKI:** • Documented AKI (historical, clinical, laboratory or imaging evidence of AKI, clinical oliguria/anuria, volume responsiveness[a]) and/or • Progressive *non-azotaemic* increase in plasma creatinine; ≥26.4 µmol/l (≥0.3 mg/dl) within 48 hours • Measured oliguria (<1 ml/kg/h, dogs) or anuria over 6 hours[b]
Grade II	140–220 µmol/l (1.6–2.5 mg/dl)	**Mild AKI:** • Documented AKI and static or progressive azotaemia • Progressive azotaemic increase in plasma creatinine, ≥26.4 µmol/l (≥0.3 mg/dl) within 48 hours, or volume responsiveness[a] • Measured oliguria (<1 ml/kg/h, dogs) or anuria over 6 hours[b]
Grade III	221–439 µmol/l (2.6–5 mg/dl)	**Moderate to severe AKI:** • Documented AKI and increasing severity of azotaemia and functional renal failure
Grade IV	440–880 µmol/l (5.1–10 mg/dl)	
Grade V	>880 µmol/l (>10 mg/dl)	

12.2 International Renal Interest Society (IRIS) acute kidney injury (AKI) grading criteria for both dogs and cats. [a] Volume-responsive indicates an increase in urine production to >1 ml/kg/h over 6 hours, and/or decrease in plasma creatinine to baseline over 48 hours in response to fluid administration. [b] Normal euvolaemic cats may produce a urine volume <1 ml/kg/h; however, cats producing <1 ml/kg/h of urine in response to fluid supplementation should be considered to have physiological oliguria.

exposure (e.g. heat stroke). Clinical features include physical examination findings or abnormal urine. IRIS AKI Grade I includes animals with progressive (hourly or daily) increases in plasma creatinine of ≥26.4 µmol/l (≥0.3 mg/dl) within the non-azotaemic range during a 48-hour interval. IRIS AKI Grade I also includes animals whose decreased urine production is readily fluid volume responsive (presumably pre-renal in aetiology). Fluid volume responsiveness represents an increase in urine production to >1 ml/kg/h within 6 hours, and/or a decrease in plasma creatinine to baseline over 48 hours in response to fluid administration.

IRIS AKI Grade II defines animals with documented AKI characterized by mild azotaemia in addition to other historical, biochemical, anatomical or urine production characteristics of AKI (as indicated above for Grade I), and similarly includes those whose oliguria and/or azotaemia is readily fluid volume responsive (pre-renal). Fluid volume responsiveness is as defined under IRIS AKI Grade I. IRIS AKI Grade II also includes animals that have an increase from their baseline creatinine concentration of ≥0.3 mg/dl (≥26.4 µmol/l) during a 48-hour interval associated with pre-existing CKD: so-called 'acute-on-chronic' disease (see Figure 12.2).

IRIS AKI Grades III, IV and V define animals with documented AKI and progressively greater degrees of parenchymal damage and functional failure (uraemia) as predicted by plasma creatinine.

Each grade of AKI is further subgraded on the basis of current urine production as oligo/anuric (O; oliguria, <1 ml/kg/h, or anuria, no urine produced, over 6 hours) or non-oliguric (NO; >1 ml/kg/h), and on the requirement for renal replacement therapy (RRT). The inclusion of subgrading by urine production is based on the important interrelationship of urine production to the pathological or functional contributions to the renal injury, and its influence on the clinical presentation, therapeutic options and outcome of AKI. The classification of oliguria as a urine production of <1 ml/kg/h recognizes that this rate of urine production might be identified in some cats with normal kidney function and highly concentrated urine. It nevertheless serves as a relevant cut-off for the majority of hydrated animals receiving parenteral fluids, and those animals with decreased urine concentrating ability associated with the kidney injury.

Subgrading on the requirement for RRT is established on the need to correct life-threatening iatrogenic or clinical consequences of AKI including severe azotaemia, hyperkalaemia, acid–base disorders, overhydration, oliguria or anuria, or the need to eliminate exogenous nephrotoxins. The requirement for RRT could occur at any AKI grade. Subgrading based on the requirement for RRT has similar clinical, therapeutic and prognostic implications to those of urine production when used to categorize the severity of the renal injury as well as its influence on outcome.

Figure 12.3 illustrates the concept of IRIS AKI grading in a dog receiving gentamicin at 8 mg/kg by subcutaneous injection twice daily as part of an experimental study of AKI. The dog has an AKI, based on the history of receiving a nephrotoxic medication. For the first 16 days the designation is IRIS AKI Grade I, NO, but it changes transiently to AKI Grade II then progresses on day 17 to AKI Grade III. The figure also illustrates the recovery from the AKI and downgrading of the injury beyond day 35. Following recovery, the dog should be categorized as an IRIS CKD Stage 1 owing to the history of non-azotaemic kidney damage over the past 2 weeks.

The IRIS AKI grading scheme deviates from classification systems proposed or adapted from human medicine, because it is not based solely on identified changes in kidney function or predetermined knowledge of baseline kidney function as predicted by GFR or plasma creatinine. The IRIS scheme necessarily incorporates these features as sensitive predictors of kidney injury for hospital-based patient assessment. However, more appropriately for veterinary medicine, the diagnosis of the AKI is founded on historical and diagnostic assessments of the patient at presentation from the community, where there is often no documentation of baseline kidney function or progressive changes in kidney function. The AKI is subsequently stratified (graded) on assessment of the absolute plasma creatinine and urine production at the time of presentation. Sequential grading throughout the course of the disease provides a standardized assessment and documentation of the patient's clinical course, the efficacy of therapy and outcome. Animals recognized and managed early with IRIS AKI Grades I and II may regain adequate renal function within 2–5 days, forestalling progressive life-threatening azotaemia and electrolyte disorders, and usually need only short-term support. Those with higher IRIS AKI grades at presentation or whose IRIS AKI grade progresses during hospitalization may require weeks of supportive care before the onset of kidney repair. Animals with severe kidney failure, IRIS AKI Grades IV or V, may die within 5–10 days despite appropriate conventional management unless supported with RRT for an indefinite time. This disparity between the window of survival with conventional supportive therapy and the extended time required to repair severe AKI underlies, in part, the poor prognosis and outcomes associated with severe stages of AKI which may be better predicted with stratified grading.

As has been demonstrated in human nephrology, AKI classification has the potential to better discriminate the pathophysiological and therapeutic spectrum of AKI (Kellum and Lameire, 2013). Very importantly, it has the potential to sensitize the clinical evaluation of patients to promote earlier recognition of AKI. Like IRIS CKD staging, grading of AKI should promote better comparative assessment of clinical status and therapeutic strategies. The IRIS AKI grading scheme should be considered preliminary. It remains subject to consensus revision and modification as appropriate biomarkers are validated to provide greater specificity and sensitivity to the grading of AKI, and as evidence-based observations warrant its modification with systematic review. Finally, AKI grading may facilitate more accurate analyses of the prognosis and treatment outcomes for AKI in dogs and cats.

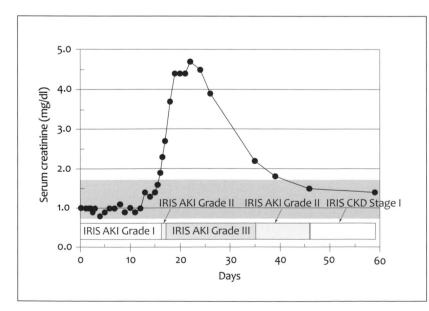

12.3 Serial changes in serum creatinine concentration and International Renal Interest Society (IRIS) acute kidney injury (AKI) grading in a dog with gentamicin-induced AKI as part of an experimental study. The IRIS AKI grading effectively categorized the sequential course of the AKI from inapparent to failure and subsequent recovery. The shaded area reflects the reference range for serum creatinine.
(Data from Palm et al., 2016)

IRIS CKD staging system

Plasma creatinine (PCr) is utilized as the major factor for staging because this is the most readily available test of kidney function for veterinary practitioners. The limitations of PCr are well recognized and are outlined in Chapter 10. The staging system would undoubtedly be improved should a practical method of adjusting plasma creatinine concentration to take account of body condition score in general, and muscle mass in particular, be devised, because these govern the rate of production of creatinine, or by identification of an alternative fully validated surrogate marker for GFR unaffected by muscle mass or age. Correction factors for PCr are available in human medicine but the complexity of devising appropriate systems for veterinary practice should not be underestimated.

In addition, at the inception of the IRIS CKD staging system, the IRIS group expected that measurement of GFR by a plasma clearance method would eventually replace PCr concentration as the major criterion for staging. To date there is no internationally accepted standard method of measuring GFR in dogs and cats that can be used in veterinary practice, and variation within and between methods and between breeds within a species makes it difficult to use GFR in the IRIS CKD staging system at present. In the future, additional surrogate markers of GFR may add value to the IRIS staging system. One such marker, SDMA (see Chapter 10), is starting to be used in veterinary practice and appears to be a more sensitive biomarker than PCr for early CKD. The IRIS Board has made some preliminary suggestions as to how SDMA might be used alongside PCr. These additions to the guidelines are preliminary, and are based on early data derived from the use of SDMA in veterinary patients

(see Chapter 10). The IRIS Board fully expects them to be updated as the veterinary profession gains further experience using SDMA alongside the long-established marker, PCr, in the diagnosis and therapeutic monitoring of canine and feline CKD.

Figure 12.4 presents the staging system based on plasma creatinine.

This staging system recognizes that a large proportion of kidney tissue has to be damaged before a rise in plasma creatinine concentration is detectable. Hence Stage 1 and early Stage 2 encompass plasma creatinine concentrations which are well within or in the upper end of the reference ranges for most laboratories. For an animal to be classified in Stage 1, therefore, some other abnormality has to have been detected which makes the clinician suspect that a disease process is ongoing within the kidney. This could include:

- Inadequate urinary concentrating ability in the absence of an extra-renal cause
- The detection of persistent renal proteinuria (see Chapter 5)
- Abnormal size, shape or tissue architecture of the kidneys detected on palpation and confirmed by diagnostic imaging
- Abnormal findings on kidney biopsy
- Increasing PCr concentrations (even though they remain within the laboratory reference range) noted on serial plasma samples
- A persistent elevation in plasma (serum) SDMA above 14 µg/dl.

Having more than one of these findings increases the certainty of the diagnosis of CKD. It is important to remember that diagnosis of CKD is a prerequisite for going on to apply the IRIS CKD staging system.

Stage	Creatinine (µmol/l)*	Comments
At risk	Dogs: <125 µmol/l (<1.4 mg/dl) Cats: <140 µmol/l (<1.6 mg/dl)	• History suggests that the animal is at increased risk of developing chronic kidney disease (CKD) in the future because of a number of factors (e.g. exposure to nephrotoxic drugs, breed, high prevalence of infectious disease in the area or old age)
1	Dogs: <125 µmol/l (<1.4 mg/dl) Cats: <140 µmol/l (<1.6 mg/dl)	• Non-azotaemic • Some other renal abnormality present, e.g. inadequate concentrating ability without identifiable non-renal cause; abnormal renal palpation and/or abnormal renal imaging findings; proteinuria of renal origin; abnormal renal biopsy results; increasing plasma creatinine concentrations noted on serial samples over weeks or months • A persistent elevation in plasma symmetric dimethylarginine (SDMA) above 14 µg/dl would indicate reduced renal function and may be a reason to categorize a dog or cat (with plasma creatinine <125 or <140 µmol/l respectively) in Stage 1 CKD
2	Dogs: 125–179 µmol/l (1.4–2 mg/dl) Cats: 140–249 µmol/l (1.6–2.8 mg/dl)	• Mild renal azotaemia (lower end of the range lies within the reference range for many laboratories but the insensitivity of creatinine as a screening test means that animals with creatinine values close to the upper reference limit often have excretory failure) • Clinical signs usually mild or absent • In Stage 2 patients with low body condition scores, if SDMA is ≥25 µg/dl this may indicate that the degree of renal dysfunction has been underestimated. Consider some of the treatment recommendations listed under Stage 3 for these patients (see Chapter 23)
3	Dogs: 1810–439 µmol/l (2–5 mg/dl) Cats: 250–439 µmol/l (2.8–5 mg/dl)	• Moderate renal azotaemia • Many extra-renal clinical signs may be present • In Stage 3 patients with low body condition scores, if SDMA is ≥45 µg/dl this may indicate that the degree of renal dysfunction has been underestimated. Consider some of the treatment recommendations listed under Stage 4 for these patients (see Chapter 23)
4	>440 µmol/l (>5 mg/dl)	• Severe renal azotaemia • Many extra-renal clinical signs are usually present • Increasing risk of systemic clinical signs and uraemic crises

12.4 The IRIS staging system based on plasma creatinine. *To convert to mg/dl, divide by 88.4; note that these blood creatinine levels apply to average-sized dogs – those of extreme size may vary.

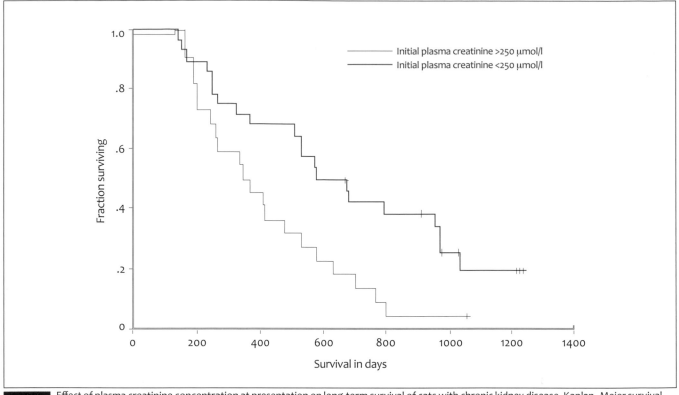

12.5 Effect of plasma creatinine concentration at presentation on long-term survival of cats with chronic kidney disease. Kaplan–Meier survival curves from 50 cats entered into a prospective study (Elliott *et al.*, 2000). The cats have been divided into two groups on the basis of their initial plasma creatinine concentration at entry to the study as either Stage 2 (creatinine <250 μmol/l; all cats in this study had plasma creatinine concentrations >177 μmol/l) or Stage 3 (creatinine >250 μmol/l; all cats in this study had plasma creatinine concentrations <440 μmol/l).

The IRIS Board has also decided that practitioners should be aware that some of their patients may be at higher risk of developing CKD and so warrant closer (serial) monitoring of their kidney function. Some of these factors will depend on geographical location and the prevalence of infectious diseases leading to CKD, and may depend on the use of nephrotoxic drugs to treat infections or cancer (see Roura (2016), for a brief review).

The precise PCr concentrations used to divide the different stages outlined in Figure 12.4 were reached by consensus and debate. They were based on clinical experience of the Board members and from data derived from longitudinal studies. For example, Figure 12.5 shows survival curves for cats presenting to first-opinion veterinary practice in IRIS CKD Stage 2 or Stage 3. As can be seen, there is a significant difference between the survival times of these two groups of cats. PCr has repeatedly been identified as a risk factor affecting survival (all-cause mortality) in cats with CKD (Syme *et al.*, 2006). The examination of plasma SDMA concentrations alongside PCr may help to identify those patients where PCr may have underestimated their stage of CKD because of loss of muscle mass. SDMA does not appear to be affected by muscle mass in the same way as PCr (Hall *et al.*, 2014).

It is likely that some animals with CKD pass through all these stages if their kidney disease progresses. Some animals, however, will remain stable within one stage and die of some other disease before their kidney disease has had chance to progress (Chakrabarti *et al.*, 2012). Cases may be presented to the veterinary surgeon at any stage, depending on how observant their owner is and how open they are to routine health screening.

The staging system is useful in providing practitioners with helpful prognostic information and allowing them to determine the likely consequences of the kidney disease

which will need to be addressed by management protocols at different stages. For example, Figures 12.6 and 12.7 show the prevalence and severity of metabolic acidosis and hyperparathyroidism across IRIS CKD Stages 2 to 4. This has implications for management recommendations at the different stages. Chapter 23 uses the IRIS CKD staging system to make recommendations for the management of CKD in dogs and cats.

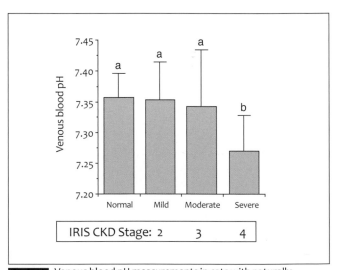

12.6 Venous blood pH measurements in cats with naturally occurring chronic kidney disease (CKD). Blood pH measurements were made using a patient-side monitor (iSTAT machine; SDI Devices Ltd, USA). The reference range devised from 28 aged normal cats was 7.27–7.44. None of the cats in Stage 2, 3 of 20 (15%) in Stage 3 and 10 of 19 (52.4%) in Stage 4 had venous blood pH below 7.27 and therefore were considered to be acidaemic. IRIS = International Renal Interest Society.
(Data from Elliott *et al.*, 2003)

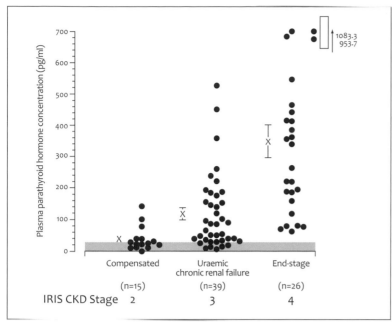

The distribution of plasma parathyroid hormone (PTH) concentrations in cats at different stages of chronic kidney disease (CKD). representing a cross-sectional study of 80 cats presenting to first-opinion practices at initial diagnosis of CKD. Plasma PTH concentrations were measured using an intact immunoradiometric assay (Allegro Intact PTH Assay, Nichol's Institute Diagnostics, UK). The classification system was based on clinical presentation rather than plasma creatinine concentration. Nevertheless, plasma creatinine concentrations in the three groups were for the majority of cases equivalent to IRIS Stages 2, 3 and 4. PTH concentrations outside of the laboratory reference range were found in 47% of cats in Stage 2, 87% of cats in Stage 3 and 100% of cats in Stage 4. IRIS = International Renal Interest Society.
(Reproduced with permission from Barber and Elliott, 1998)

Substaging of CKD

In addition to staging cases of CKD on the basis of plasma creatinine, the IRIS group recommends that cases are substaged on the basis of two other diagnostic factors, namely:

- The quantity of protein excreted in urine (see Chapter 5)
- The systemic arterial blood pressure (see Chapter 15).

Assessment of both of these parameters is important because proteinuria and systemic hypertension can occur at any of the four stages of CKD and, in human medicine, each is an independent risk factor for progressive renal injury and as such warrants specific treatment protocols. Epidemiological evidence in veterinary medicine supports the concept that CKD progresses more rapidly the more proteinuric the dog (see below) and strong associations between proteinuria and CKD progression and all-cause mortality have been found in feline patients with CKD. The evidence that systemic hypertension is an independent risk factor for progressive renal injury in the CKD patient (rather than a factor that influences proteinuria) is less convincing, although as a complicating problem related to CKD that causes significant morbidity and mortality through effects on other organ systems (brain, heart and eye) it certainly remains an important part of the staging system.

Substaging based on protein in the urine

Chapter 5 discusses in detail the diagnostic approach to identifying protein in the urine and classifying proteinuria as:

- Pre-renal
- Renal
- Post-renal.

The substaging of cases on the basis of proteinuria refers only to renal proteinuria. Pre-renal and post-renal

causes should be ruled out if the substaging system recommended below is to be utilized. Figure 12.8 presents the substaging system to be adopted.

UPC value[a]	Interpretation
<0.2, dogs and cats	Non-proteinuric (NP)
0.2–0.4, cats 0.2–0.5, dogs	Borderline proteinuric (BP)
>0.4, cats >0.5, dogs	Proteinuric (P)

12.8 Substaging on urine protein to creatinine ratio (UPC). [a]Calculated using mass units.

The above recommendations have been modified in light of the American College of Veterinary Internal Medicine (ACVIM) Consensus Statement on Proteinuria (Lees *et al.*, 2005). It is important to recognize that persistent proteinuria is more likely to be pathological than transient proteinuria. As discussed in Chapter 5, therefore, substaging on the basis of urine protein to creatinine ratio (UPC) should demonstrate persistence, ideally by collecting at least three urine samples over at least a 2-week period.

The action required having identified an animal as being either proteinuric or borderline proteinuric depends on the stage of CKD according to its PCr. A UPC >0.5 in a dog with a PCr of 350 μmol/l (Stage 3) is far more significant than in a dog with a PCr of 100 μmol/l (Stage 1). The reason for this is that, as the mass of functioning nephrons declines so the filtered load of protein presented to the tubules is reduced. Hence, the appearance of lower amounts of protein in the urine attains higher significance. Chapter 21 recommends how animals presenting at different stages of CKD should be treated.

As mentioned above, a further reason that proteinuria is singled out for special attention in animals with CKD is that there is good evidence that it is a prognostic indicator in dogs and cats with CKD. A longitudinal study in dogs with naturally occurring CKD has demonstrated that animals with UPC >1.0 have a three-fold higher risk of suffering a uraemic crisis when compared with dogs presented with

UPC <1.0 (Jacob *et al.*, 2005). In cats with CKD, proteinuria is an independent risk factor for all-cause mortality (Syme *et al.*, 2006), it is a risk factor for the onset of azotaemia in clinically healthy cats (Jepson *et al.*, 2009) and for a 25% increase in plasma creatinine concentration within 1 year of the diagnosis of CKD in cats (Chakrabarti *et al.*, 2012).

Substaging based on systemic arterial blood pressure

The application of indirect blood pressure measurement techniques to clinical practice (see Chapter 15) means that this important physiological parameter can and should be assessed in dogs and cats with CKD. Systemic hypertension can be damaging to the kidneys, and kidney disease can give rise to problems with blood pressure regulation, leading to inappropriately high blood pressure. In addition, high blood pressure can cause damage to other target organs such as the heart (left ventricular hypertrophy), the eye (hypertensive retinopathy) and the brain, leading to extra-renal signs and morbidity in the CKD patient. For these reasons the IRIS Board recommends that all patients with CKD have their blood pressure measured regardless of the stage of their kidney disease. Anti-hypertensive treatment may be appropriate, depending on the level of risk and/or the presence of evidence of target-organ damage. Hence, blood pressure is used to substage dogs and cats according to the risk of target-organ damage and whether there is evidence of extra-renal target-organ damage. This substaging system is presented in Figure 12.9.

Systolic (mmHg)	Diastolic (mmHg)	Classification	Risk of future target-organ damage
<150	<95	Normotensive	Minimal or no risk (Highly unlikely to see evidence of extra-renal damage at this level)
150–159	95–99	Borderline hypertensive	Low risk
160–179	100–119	Hypertensive	Moderate risk
≥180	≥120	Severely hypertensive	High risk

12.9 Substaging on blood pressure. Extra-renal complications might include: left ventricular concentric hypertrophy in the absence of structural/valvular heart problems identified; ocular abnormalities compatible with damage by high blood pressure such as hyphaema or hypertensive retinopathy; neurological signs such as dullness and lethargy or seizures. At each classification of blood pressure it is helpful to note whether extra-renal complications of hypertension are present or not.

The IRIS Board recognizes that there are a number of different methods available for measuring blood pressure and the veterinary profession has not agreed on a standardized approach. These blood pressure recommendations are therefore a guide for applying whatever blood pressure measuring technique is chosen but will be useful provided practitioners standardize their approach within their own practice and ensure that the technique used remains the same for a given animal from one visit to the next. Details concerning the measurement technique, which are important to standardize, are discussed in Chapter 15. It is also recognized that among dog breeds there are some differences in blood pressure reference ranges. If dealing with a breed known to have higher blood pressure than average (e.g. sight hounds), the following adaptation of the staging system can be adopted:

- Normotensive category: <10 mmHg above the breed reference range
- Borderline hypertensive to hypertensive category: 10–40 mmHg above the breed reference range
- Severely hypertensive category: >40 mmHg above the breed reference range.

In the same way that proteinuria was categorized on the basis of persistence, the blood pressure risk should also be based on multiple sequential measurements to document persistence of risk. This recommendation applies when there is no evidence of extra-renal target-organ damage. If extra-renal target-organ damage (e.g. hypertensive retinopathy) is identified, then treatment (see Chapters 15 and 23) should begin immediately these signs are recognized. If no evidence of extra-renal target-organ damage is recognized, the following actions are recommended:

- For patients found persistently to be in the borderline hypertensive category: re-evaluate every 2 months to determine whether blood pressure is increasing
- For patients found persistently to be in the hypertensive category without systemic signs of target-organ damage: re-evaluate, and if blood pressure remains persistently in this category based on multiple measurements made over 2 months, institute treatment
- For patients in the severely hypertensive category without systemic signs of target-organ damage, re-evaluate over 7 days and if blood pressure remains persistently in this category based on multiple measurements made over this time, institute treatment.

Conclusions

The IRIS scheme thus allows CKD in dogs and cats to be staged on the basis of the fasting plasma or serum creatinine concentration and further characterized according to urine protein content and systemic blood pressure. Figure 12.10 presents an algorithm for the complete staging system applied to a feline patient. A similar algorithm can be produced for the canine patient. The following examples serve to illustrate the entire staging system:

- A proteinuric (UPC 1.2) dog with systolic blood pressure of 154 mmHg (but no evidence of extra-renal damage) and PCr of 260 µmol/l (2.95 mg/dl) would be classified as Stage 3-P-borderline hypertensive (no extra-renal complications)
- A dog with borderline proteinuria (UPC 0.3), PCr of 550 µmol/l (6.22 mg/dl) and blood pressure of 130 mmHg (with no evidence of extra-renal damage) would be classified as Stage 4-BP-normotensive
- A non-proteinuric (UPC 0.12) cat with systolic blood pressure of 210 mmHg having bilateral retinal detachment and PCr of 180 µmol/l (2.03 mg/dl) would be classified as Stage 2-NP-severely hypertensive (with extra-renal complications).

The IRIS CKD staging system reflects current knowledge and opinion about CKD in dogs and cats and will continue to develop as the results of new research are published. Consistent and widespread use of such staging should aid practitioners with diagnosis and prognosis in CKD, providing a framework for logical treatment plans (see Chapter 23), and facilitate communication between veterinary surgeons about this complex disease syndrome.

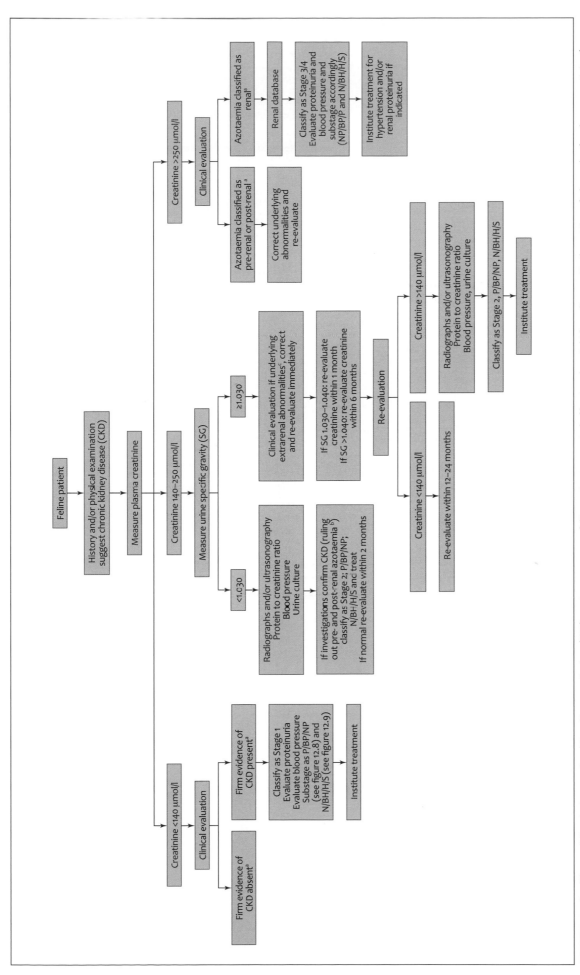

12.10 An algorithm applying the International Renal Interest Society (IRIS) staging system to a feline patient suspected of having chronic kidney disease. [a] In the setting of a low value for plasma creatinine (<125 μmol/l in dogs or <140 μmol/l in cats), firm evidence of kidney disease would usually be morphological, such as abnormal renal architecture on survey radiographs, abnormal renal ultrasound findings, or biopsy diagnosis of renal disease. [b] The classification of pre-renal azotaemia (generally due to dehydration or renal ischaemia) or post-renal azotaemia (generally due to ureteral or urethral obstruction, or rupture of part of the urinary tract) will depend on careful evaluation of history, physical examination and other clinical findings. This determination may require additional tests, based on clinical judgement. For example, radiographic studies and/or abdominal paracentesis (with analysis of ascitic fluid creatinine concentration) may be required to establish a diagnosis of ruptured urinary bladder in an azotaemic cat with a history of blunt abdominal trauma. The classification of azotaemia as renal is based on the presence of azotaemia with no identifiable pre-renal or post-renal causes. As a general guide, dogs and cats with renal azotaemia usually have a urine specific gravity <1.030. [c] These abnormalities may include any pre-renal factor that leads to dehydration or systemic arterial hypotension or post-renal factors such as ureteral or urethral obstruction, or urinary tract rupture. RI = renal insufficiency; SG = urine specific gravity. Proteinuria substaging (see Figure 12.8): NP = non-proteinuric; BP = borderline proteinuric; P = proteinuric. Blood pressure substaging on risk of extra-renal damage (see Figure 12.9): N = normotensive; BH = borderline hypertensive; H = hypertensive; S = severely hypertensive.

Acknowledgements

The authors wish to acknowledge all the IRIS board members who, since its inception in 1998, have contributed to the generation of these staging and grading systems, which are reviewed on an annual basis. They are: S Brown* (USA), C Brovida* (Italy), J-P Cotard (France), L Cowgill* (USA), J Elliott* (UK), M-J Fernandez del Palacio (Spain), S Gnass (Germany), G Grauer* (USA), R Heiene* (Norway), A Huttig* (Germany), A Kosztolich (Austria), H Lefebvre* (France), AR Michell (UK), R Mitten (Australia), D Polzin* (USA), J-L Pouchelon (France), X Roura* (Spain), R Santilli (Italy), G Segev* (Israel), H Syme* (UK), A Van Dongen* (Netherlands), T Watanabe* (Japan) and D Watson* (Australia).

* Indicates current IRIS Board members

References and further reading

Barber PJ and Elliott J (1998) Feline chronic renal failure: calcium homeostasis in 80 cases diagnosed between 1992 and 1995. *Journal of Small Animal Practice* **39**, 108–116

Bellomo R, Ronco C, Kellum JA *et al.* (2004) Acute renal failure – definition, outcome measures, animal models, fluid therapy and information technology needs: the Second International Consensus Conference of the Acute Dialysis Quality Initiative (ADQI) Group. *Critical Care* **8**, R204–R212

Chakrabarti S, Syme HM and Elliott J (2012) Clinicopathological variables predicting progression of azotemia in cats with chronic kidney disease. *Journal of Veterinary Internal Medicine* **26**, 275–281

Cowgill LD and Langston CE (2011) Acute kidney insufficiency. In: *Nephrology and Urology of Small Animals*, ed. J Bartges and D Polzin, pp. 472–516. Wiley-Blackwell, Hoboken, NJ

De Loor J, Daminet S, Smets P *et al.* (2013) Urinary biomarkers for acute kidney injury in dogs. *Journal of Veterinary Internal Medicine* **27**, 998–1010

Elliott J, Rawlings JM, Markwell PJ and Barber PJ (2000) Survival of cats with naturally occurring renal failure: effect of conventional dietary management. *Journal of Small Animal Practice* **41**, 235–242

Elliott J, Syme HM, Reubens E and Markwell PJ (2003) Assessment of acid–base status of cats with naturally occurring chronic renal failure. *Journal of Small Animal Practice* **44**, 65–70

Hall JA, Yerramilli M, Obare E, Yerramilli M, Yu S and Jewell DE (2014) Comparison of serum concentrations of symmetric dimethylarginine and creatinine as kidney function biomarkers in healthy geriatric cats fed reduced protein foods enriched with fish oil, L-carnitine, and medium-chain triglycerides. *Veterinary Journal* **202**, 588–596

Harison E, Langston C, Palma D *et al.* (2012) Acute azotemia as a predictor of mortality in dogs and cats. *Journal of Veterinary Internal Medicine* **26(5)**, 1093–1098

Hoste EA and Kellum JA (2007) Incidence, classification, and outcomes of acute kidney injury. *Contributions to Nephrology* **156**, 32–38

IRIS (2013) *International Renal Interest Society Grading of Acute Kidney Injury.* Available from: www.iris-kidney.com/pdf/grading-of-acute-kidney-injury.pdf

Kellum JA and Lameire N (2013) KDIGO AKI Guideline Work Group. Diagnosis, evaluation, and management of acute kidney injury: a KDIGO summary (Part 1). *Critical Care* **4**, 204–218

Jacob F, Polzin DJ, Osborne CA *et al.* (2003) Association between initial systolic blood pressure and risk of developing a uremic crisis or of dying in dogs with chronic renal failure. *Journal of the American Veterinary Medical Association* **222**, 322–329

Jacob F, Polzin DJ, Osborne CA *et al.* (2005) Evaluation of the association between initial proteinuria and morbidity rate or death in dogs with naturally occurring chronic renal failure. *Journal of the American Veterinary Medical Association* **226**, 393–400

Jepson RE, Brodbelt D, Vallance C, Syme HM and Elliott J (2009) Evaluation of predictors of the development of azotemia in cats. *Journal of Veterinary Internal Medicine* **23**, 806–813

Lee YJ, Chang CC, Chan JP *et al.* (2011) Prognosis of acute kidney injury in dogs using RIFLE (Risk, Injury, Failure, Loss and End-stage renal failure)-like criteria. *Veterinary Record* **168**, 264–269

Lees GE, Brown SA, Elliott J *et al.* (2005) Assessment and management of proteinuria in dogs and cats: 2004 ACVIM Forum Consensus Statement (small animal). *Journal of Veterinary Internal Medicine* **19**, 377–385

Mehta RL, Kellum JA, Shah SV *et al.* (2007) Acute Kidney Injury Network: report of an initiative to improve outcomes in acute kidney injury. *Critical Care* **11**, R31

Molitoris BA, Levin A, Warnock DG *et al.* (2007) Improving outcomes of acute kidney injury: report of an initiative. *Nature Clinical Practice Nephrology* **3**, 439–442

Palm CA, Segev G, Cowgill LC *et al.*, (2016) Urinary neutrophil gelatinase-associated lipocalin as a marker for identification of acute kidney injury in dogs with gentamicin-induced nephrotoxicity. *Journal of Veterinary Internal Medicine* **30(1)**, 200–203

Roura X (2016) *Risk factors in dogs ad cats for development of chronic kidney disease.* Available from: www.iris-kidney.com/education/risk_factors.html

Segev G, Palm C, Leroy B *et al.* (2013) Evaluation of neutrophil gelatinase-associated lipocalin as a marker of kidney injury in dogs. *Journal of Veterinary Internal Medicine* **27**, 1362–1367

Squires RA (2007) Uraemia. In: *BSAVA Manual of Canine and Feline Nephrology and Urology, 2nd edn*, ed. J Elliott and G Grauer. pp. 54–68. BSAVA Publications, Gloucester

Syme HM, Markwell PJ, Pfeiffer D and Elliott J (2006) Survival of cats with naturally occurring chronic renal failure is related to severity of proteinuria. *Journal of Veterinary Internal Medicine* **20**, 528–535

Thoen ME and Kerl ME (2011) Characterization of acute kidney injury in hospitalized dogs and evaluation of a veterinary acute kidney injury staging system. *Journal of Veterinary Emergency and Critical Care* **2**, 648–657

Chapter 13

Renal biopsy

Shelly L. Vaden and Cathy Brown

Dogs and cats with renal diseases can often be described as having acute kidney injury (AKI), chronic kidney disease (CKD) or a glomerulopathy on the basis of the patient history and the results of physical examination and clinical laboratory tests. However, renal biopsy may be required in order to establish a definitive diagnosis, determine the severity of the lesion and formulate an optimal treatment plan. Despite the need for renal biopsy, veterinary surgeons (veterinarians) may be reluctant to perform one on their patients because of concerns over expense and potential complications, as well as the belief that the diagnoses rendered may lack consistency. The expense and complication rate can be minimized by correct patient selection and use of the proper technique. Consistent and accurate diagnoses are more likely to be obtained when renal biopsy specimens are appropriately processed and evaluated. This chapter summarizes the indications, contraindications, techniques and complications of renal biopsy, as well as the appropriate processing and evaluation of the renal biopsy specimen.

Indications

Renal biopsy is indicated only when having an accurate histological diagnosis is likely to alter patient management (Figure 13.1). Patients whose management is most likely to be altered by results of a renal biopsy include those with protein-losing nephropathy (i.e. glomerular disease) or AKI. Client factors that need to be considered include the willingness to pay for the procedure and proper evaluation

of the specimen, as well as the desire to pursue additional treatment of their dog or cat, as may be indicated by the histological diagnosis.

Renal biopsy is generally not indicated in patients with CKD (Stage 4 and possibly Stage 3). The results are unlikely to alter the prognosis, therapy or outcome in these patients. Furthermore, an increased risk of complications from renal biopsy in humans with CKD has been observed (Parrish, 1992).

Renal biopsy results may also aid in the formulation of an accurate prognosis (e.g. whether or not there is evidence of tubular cell regeneration in AKI).

Contraindications and other considerations

A thorough evaluation of the patient prior to renal biopsy should identify any existing contraindications to the procedure (Figure 13.2). This evaluation process should include obtaining a current history, performing a complete physical examination, measuring systemic blood pressure, analysing the results of a biochemical profile, complete blood count, urinalysis and coagulation profile, and assessing the size, shape, contour and internal architecture of the kidney via abdominal ultrasonography (see Chapter 7).

Dogs and cats with moderate to severe thrombocytopenia (platelet counts <80,000 per µl), dogs with prolonged one-stage prothrombin time (OSPT >1.5 x normal) and cats with prolonged activated partial thromboplastin

Protein-losing nephropathy
• Biopsy may be one of the more important steps in successful management of specific glomerular disease (see Chapter 24)
• Identify and treat potential underlying diseases before biopsy. Biopsy may not be needed if proteinuria resolves after effective treatment of an underlying disease
• Appropriate evaluation may require light, electron and immunofluorescent microscopy

Acute kidney injury
• Biopsy may be indicated in patients with persistently severe uraemia or non-obstructive oliguria, or those that deteriorate during appropriate medical management
• May help determine an aetiological diagnosis that may lead to specific therapeutic measures
• May facilitate prognostication
• Light microscopic evaluation may be sufficient. However, samples should be collected for electron and immunofluorescent microscopy in the event that the primary disease is glomerular

Mass lesions
• Biopsy may be needed if mass aspiration cytology is non-diagnostic

13.1 Indications for renal biopsy.

• Chronic kidney disease (CKD) late Stage 3 and Stage 4
• Severe azotaemia (serum creatinine >440 µmol/l (5 mg/dl))
• Severe anaemia
• Uncorrectable coagulopathy
• Administration of non-steroidal anti-inflammatory drugs (NSAIDs) within previous 5 days
• Uncontrolled hypertension
• Severe hydronephrosis
• Large or multiple renal cysts
• Peri-renal abscess
• Extensive pyelonephritis
• Inexperienced operator
• Incomplete patient immobilization

13.2 Contraindications for renal biopsy.

Percutaneous
- Ultrasound guidance – preferred method for dogs >5 kg and all cats
- Blind or palpation technique – better suited for cats; rarely performed in dogs
- Keyhole technique – used in dogs when ultrasound guidance is not available
- Laparoscopy – requires specialized equipment and expertise; preferred method of some clinicians

Surgical
- Wedge biopsy – preferred method for dogs <5 kg, animals with isolated areas of kidney that need to be avoided or animals undergoing laparotomy for another reason

13.3 Methods used to obtain renal biopsy specimens.

time (aPTT >1.5 x normal) had a greater risk of haemorrhage from ultrasound-guided biopsy procedures in one study (Bigge *et al.*, 2001). Severe azotaemia (serum creatinine >440 µmol/l (5 mg/dl)), uncontrolled systemic hypertension, administration of a non-steroidal anti-inflammatory drug (NSAID) within the previous 5 days and operator inexperience also may increase the risk of haemorrhage. These factors may not be absolute contraindications to renal biopsy; however, the clinician should be prepared to monitor such patients for severe haemorrhage following the biopsy and have suitable blood products from a compatible donor available to administer to the patient if needed.

Severe hydronephrosis is a contraindication to renal biopsy because of the possibility that the needle might penetrate a distended renal pelvis that is under increased pressure, and the increased risk of transecting the larger arteries located in the corticomedullary junction and the medulla. Kidney biopsy is generally not recommended when there are large or multiple renal cysts because biopsy might induce renal pain or renal cyst infection, and a specimen that contains large cysts may have limited diagnostic value. Renal pain develops after rupture of the cyst because of release of cystic fluid into the peri-renal tissues. While the risk of inducing cyst infections through renal biopsy is low, poor antibacterial drug penetration into the cyst fluid makes these infections particularly difficult to treat.

Peri-renal abscessation and extensive pyelonephritis are contraindications to renal biopsy because of the possibility of seeding the abdomen with bacteria or other infectious agents. Ideally, lower urinary tract infections should be eliminated prior to renal biopsy. Some authors have included a solitary kidney as a contraindication to biopsy; however, biopsy may be performed if proper technique is used and other contraindications are absent.

Procurement of the specimen

Renal biopsy samples can be obtained using one of several techniques (Figure 13.3). Regardless of the method selected, only cortical tissue should be obtained. In most cases, evaluation of cortical tissue alone is diagnostic. When the kidney is penetrated more deeply, the risk of serious haemorrhage increases if the corticomedullary junction, medulla or pelvis is penetrated because renal vessels progressively increase in size from the surface of the kidney towards the renal pelvis. Furthermore, biopsy of the medulla has been reported to cause large areas of infarction and fibrosis (Osborne *et al.*, 1972; Nash *et al.*, 1983).

If possible, the biopsy specimen should be taken from either the cranial or the caudal pole of the kidney because it is easier to stay in a larger portion of cortex in these locations. In the dog with generalized kidney disease, the right kidney is often preferred over the left kidney for renal biopsy because it is more stable, as the caudate lobe of the liver provides resistance to movement during the biopsy procedure. Conversely, the left kidney is more movable during the procedure but can be found in a more caudal position, providing easier access in some deep-chested dogs. Feline kidneys are located more caudally in the abdomen compared with canine kidneys. Both feline kidneys can be easily localized and immobilized, making both equally suitable for renal biopsy.

Once collected, renal biopsy specimens should be divided into three pieces, each of which contains glomeruli. The largest piece should be placed in formalin, a smaller piece should go into a fixative suitable for electron microscopy (e.g. 4% formalin plus 1% glutaraldehyde in sodium phosphate buffer) and another small piece should either be frozen or placed in a fixative suitable for immunofluorescent microscopy (e.g. ammonium sulphate-*N*-ethylmaleimide fixative, also known as Michel's solution). While light microscopy findings may be highly suggestive of a particular glomerular disease, particularly with more advanced disease, electron microscopy is required to verify the presence of deposits, to detect small deposits not evident on light microscopy, to identify the location of the deposits in the glomerulus (subendothelial, subepithelial, intramembranous, mesangial) and to detect basement membrane or podocyte abnormalities. Immunofluorescent microscopy is used to determine the specific nature of the immune deposits (immunoglobulin (Ig)G, IgA, IgM, complement) and further define the disease process (Cianciolo *et al.*, 2013).

Patient sedation or anaesthesia

The patient must be immobilized if a proper renal biopsy technique is to be used. The likelihood that serious complications will develop may increase if the patient is not properly immobilized. Providing general anaesthesia to the patient also allows for the procurement of a higher quality biopsy specimen (Vaden *et al.*, 2005). General anaesthesia is most likely to produce complete immobilization of the patient. Although some very ill patients may be immobilized by sedatives alone, incomplete anaesthesia of the peritoneum may result in sudden abdominal movement during the biopsy procedure, which must be avoided.

Percutaneous renal biopsy

Percutaneous renal biopsy can be performed using one of several techniques, all of which use a needle to obtain the biopsy specimens. Many needles are available in various gauges and lengths that theoretically could be used for renal biopsy. The authors prefer either a 16 or 18 G needle that is 9 cm in length for renal biopsy. Use of a 14 G biopsy needle was associated with a greater likelihood that biopsy specimens contained medulla in one study (Vaden *et al.*, 2005). The selected needle should be one in which the cannula does not move deeper into the tissue during activation. Needles that have throw mechanisms that go beyond where the tip of the needle is placed at the beginning of the procedure allow limited control of the depth of the biopsy and may be associated with an increased risk of penetration of the needle into the medulla.

While the Tru-cut biopsy needle was once the needle of choice for renal biopsy, it is no longer recommended because it can be difficult to use, and improper technique can yield poor-quality specimens and result in unnecessary trauma to the kidney. Likewise, the Vim-Silverman needle is no longer routinely used for renal biopsy. The authors prefer disposable spring-loaded biopsy needles. These needles can easily be operated using only one hand. The spring-loaded stylet of the needle, which is visible by ultrasonography, is advanced first. The cutting cannula is activated when the operator fully depresses the plunger. The specimen is retrieved from the specimen notch when the needle is removed from the animal. Alternatively, automatic spring-loaded biopsy guns can be used. These guns are loaded with disposable needles of appropriate gauges and lengths that are available from a variety of manufacturers. The weight and size of the gun can make its use more difficult when compared with the spring-loaded biopsy needle. The operator needs to have large, strong hands and experience with the needle to use the gun single-handedly with ease.

Obtaining a good quality biopsy specimen with limited damage to the kidney requires the use of a sharp biopsy needle. A small stab incision through the skin at the entry site for the biopsy needle keeps the needle sharp as it passes through the skin. Because needles become dull after several biopsies have been performed, and the needles are relatively inexpensive, reuse of these disposable needles is not recommended. Prior to activation of the cutting mechanism, the tip of the needle should be placed through the renal capsule to prevent sliding of the needle along the capsule and to avoid tearing the capsule. However, care should be taken not to penetrate too deeply beyond the renal capsule prior to activation as this may limit the amount of cortex in the sample. Alternatively, samples taken from the most peripheral parts of the kidney (pericapsular) may contain too few glomeruli and be inadequate for histopathologic evaluation (Zatelli *et al.*, 2003). In most cases, at least two quality cortical samples should be obtained when a percutaneous method is used. After biopsy, digital pressure should be applied to the kidney transabdominally for approximately 5 minutes to minimize haemorrhage.

Percutaneous biopsy using ultrasound guidance

Percutaneous renal biopsy using ultrasound guidance (Figure 13.4) is the renal biopsy method of choice for dogs that are larger than 5 kg and for all cats that do not have other contraindications for renal biopsy. Ultrasonography is used to identify and examine the kidneys, establish that many of the contraindications for renal biopsy are not present, and guide correct placement of the biopsy needle through the cortex. While the

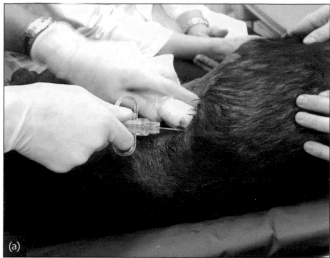
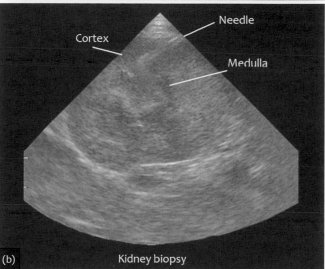

13.4 (a) Ultrasound-guided renal biopsy in a dog. Note that the probe is held in one hand while the needle is held in the other hand. (b) The ultrasonographic image of the dog in (a). This image is used to guide the needle to the kidney and through the cortex.
(Reproduced from Vaden (2004) with permission from Elsevier)

relative hyperechogenicity of the normal renal cortex allows for easy differentiation from the medulla, differentiation may be more difficult in diseased kidneys.

The patient is placed in left lateral recumbency for biopsy of the right kidney or in right lateral recumbency for biopsy of the left kidney. The hair over the biopsy site is removed, the skin is aseptically prepared and sterile coupling gel is applied. A sterile sleeve is placed over the ultrasound probe. The kidneys are scanned for general examination of the renal architecture and for selection of the biopsy site. The tip of the needle is guided through the stab incision in the skin and to and through the renal capsule with one hand while the probe is held with the other (see Figure 13.4). The biopsy specimen is taken using the method that is appropriate for the selected needle, making sure that the needle remains in the renal cortex (Figure 13.5). Although some clinicians prefer to use the needle guides that are available for the ultrasound probe, the authors do not use these. The guides are probe-specific and not available for all probes. Some ultrasonographers find the guides are too confining. Furthermore, the requirement for specific computer software for operation of the guides can make their use rather expensive.

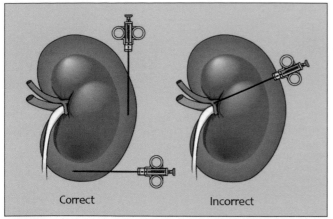

Correct   Incorrect

13.5 Schematic demonstrating correct and incorrect methods of directing the renal biopsy needle. Note that the needle should remain in the renal cortex, preferably in either the cranial or caudal pole. The needle should not cross the corticomedullary junction nor enter either the renal medulla or pelvis.

(Reproduced from Vaden (2004) with permission from Elsevier)

In a study of 229 dogs undergoing ultrasound-guided renal biopsy, a single biopsy was considered adequate for light microscopic evaluation in 207 (90.4%) of the dogs. Only nine (3.9%) of the dogs had biopsy specimens that contained fewer than five glomeruli (Zatelli *et al.*, 2003).

Blind or palpation technique

Performing renal biopsy with guidance by palpation is rarely done in dogs because their kidneys are more cranially located and can be difficult to immobilize by palpation. Blind biopsy is more frequently performed with feline kidneys, which are relatively more caudal in position and more easily immobilized. With the cat in lateral recumbency, the uppermost kidney is localized by palpation. The hair is clipped from the area over the kidney and the skin is aseptically prepared. A small stab incision is made through the skin. While one hand immobilizes the kidney, the other hand advances the needle through the stab incision and directs it towards the cranial or caudal pole of the kidney. The tip of the needle is stabbed just through the capsule, making sure the angle is such that the needle will pass only through renal cortex. The cutting mechanism of the needle is then activated.

Keyhole technique

The keyhole technique can be used in dogs if ultrasound guidance is not available. The dog is placed in left lateral recumbency for biopsy of the right kidney. The dog's back should be facing the surgeon. The hair in the lumbar fossa is clipped and the skin is aseptically prepared. An oblique paralumbar 7.5–10 cm skin incision is made on a line that bisects the angle between the last rib and the edge of the lumbar musculature. If the incision is made too far caudal or ventral, it may be impossible to palpate the kidney. If the incision is made too far dorsal, a large vascular muscle mass will need to be dissected. An incision that is too cranial may lead to puncture of the intercostal artery. The muscle fibres are separated along muscle planes and the peritoneum is incised. The peritoneal incision must be large enough to allow for easy insertion of the surgeon's index finger over the caudal pole of the kidney. The index finger holds the kidney against the edge of the lumbar musculature. The other hand inserts the biopsy needle through a separate small stab incision in the lateral body wall. The biopsy needle is guided into the peritoneal cavity and the tip of the needle is stabbed just through the capsule, making sure the angle is such that the needle will pass only through renal cortex. The needle cutting mechanism is activated as appropriate for the selected needle.

The need to displace the kidney a considerable distance prior to biopsy when the keyhole technique is used may be the cause of artefacts that are sometimes reported in samples obtained with this method (e.g. peritubular and glomerular capillary congestion and extravasation of erythrocytes into the tubular lumina and Bowman's space).

Laparoscopic biopsy

Laparoscopy is a rigid endoscopic procedure performed under sterile conditions that is used to examine the peritoneal cavity after establishment of a pneumoperitoneum. Laparoscopy offers an advantage over the other percutaneous biopsy techniques in that direct visualization and inspection of the kidneys through insertion of the laparoscope allows for visual control of the biopsy. Visualization of the kidneys increases the chance that biopsy will yield diagnostic tissue, particularly if focal lesions are present. When compared with surgery, laparoscopy is less invasive and can be performed more quickly, allowing for comparatively less patient morbidity. As with surgery, other abdominal organs can be inspected and biopsy specimens collected, if necessary, although complete abdominal exploration is not possible. Haemorrhage following biopsy can be monitored during laparoscopy and direct pressure can be applied with the laparoscope or laparoscopic tools if needed. Laparoscopy requires appropriate equipment and operator expertise.

Contraindications specific to laparoscopy include peritonitis, extensive abdominal adhesions, hernias, obesity, coagulopathies and operator inexperience. Creation of air emboli, pneumothorax or subcutaneous emphysema, the introduction of gas into a hollow viscus, damage to internal organs with the Verres needle or trocar and cardiac arrest are reported complications of laparoscopy. Evacuation of the urinary bladder and colon prior to penetration into the abdomen will reduce the chance that these organs are punctured. Operator experience and attention to detail, as well as the use of a surgically placed port instead of the Verres needle, may reduce the risk of these complications. None of these complications was reported in either of two studies of laparoscopic renal biopsy performed in dogs and cats (Grauer *et al.*, 1983; Vaden *et al.*, 2005).

Laparoscopy can be performed through a right lateral, left lateral or midline incision. The right kidney is readily visible in dogs in left lateral recumbency. To separate the abdominal wall from the organs, a pneumoperitoneum is created via injection of carbon dioxide through the Verres needle or a surgically placed trocar and cannula unit. If the Verres needle technique is used, the trocar and cannula unit for the laparoscope are then inserted through a small (1 cm) skin incision. Once the assembly is in the abdomen, the trocar is removed from the cannula and replaced by the laparoscope. The abdominal organs can be systematically inspected. A biopsy needle can then be introduced into the abdomen through a separate site. The renal biopsy is performed while observing the procedure through the laparoscope.

Surgical biopsy

Surgical biopsy may be the preferred method in dogs that are small (<5 kg) or in animals that either have isolated areas in the kidney (e.g. large cysts) that need to be avoided during the biopsy procedure or are undergoing laparotomy for another reason. Likewise, surgical biopsy may be safer in animals that have other listed contraindications to biopsy. A surgical wedge biopsy is preferred over a surgical needle biopsy because of better control over the depth of biopsy and the volume of tissue collected with a wedge biopsy. Surgical wedge biopsy specimens were five times more likely to be of good quality than were surgical needle biopsy specimens in one study (Vaden *et al.*, 2005).

The surgical biopsy can be obtained through a paracostal incision, if only one kidney is to be examined and a biopsy performed, or a cranial midline abdominal incision if other intra-abdominal procedures are to be performed or both kidneys need to be examined prior to biopsy. The paracostal incision is made with the patient in lateral recumbency. The incision is parallel and 2 cm caudal to the last rib. The oblique muscles are divided between fibres and retracted. The kidney is located after separating the transverse abdominal muscle.

The kidney can be elevated through the incision by placing umbilical tape around both poles. Exposure of the kidney may be difficult through the paracostal incision if the animal is obese. Following exposure, the kidney is immobilized with the thumb and forefinger prior to biopsy. A wedge-shaped incision is made through the capsule and into the cortex. Tissue forceps are used to gently lift the biopsy wedge while the scalpel blade is used to sever any remaining attachments. Monofilament absorbable suture material (e.g. 1.5 metric (4/0 USP)) in a simple continuous pattern is used to close the renal capsule. Pressure is applied with thumb and forefinger to appose the edges during suturing.

Care of the patient following renal biopsy

For several hours after renal biopsy, isotonic fluids should be given intravenously in amounts needed to produce diuresis. Theoretically, this will decrease the chance that blood clots will form in the renal pelvis or ureter and cause obstruction to urine flow. The patient should be kept relatively quiet and in the hospital for 24 hours after biopsy to reduce the risk of serious haemorrhage that may occur if the blood clot becomes dislodged from the biopsy site. The patient's packed cell volume should be evaluated 24 hours after biopsy, or sooner if a concern arises that major bleeding is occurring. Dogs should be walked only on a leash for 72 hours after biopsy. The colour of the urine should be monitored for several days after renal biopsy. Gross haematuria is common after renal biopsy and usually resolves within 24 hours. Persistent gross haematuria warrants re-evaluation of the kidneys and biopsy site.

Complications

Renal biopsy minimally affects renal function and the frequency of severe complications is relatively low when proper technique is employed (Osborne, 1971; Jeraj *et al.*, 1982; Grauer *et al.*, 1983; Hager *et al.*, 1985; Wise *et al.*, 1989; Leveille *et al.*, 1993; Minkus *et al.*, 1994; Groman *et al.*, 2004; Vaden *et al.*, 2005). While complications following renal biopsy are limited, the reported frequency

has varied between 1% and 18% (Figure 13.6). Differences in biopsy technique and patient status at the time of biopsy undoubtedly contribute to this wide range of reported complication rates. Patient factors that are reported in association with the development of complications in dogs include age (>4 years), bodyweight (<5 kg) and the presence of severe azotaemia (serum creatinine >440 μmol/l (5 mg/dl)) (Vaden *et al.*, 2005). In one study, having a radiologist or internist perform the biopsy appeared to be associated with the development of complications (Vaden *et al.*, 2005). The use of percutaneous methods to collect the renal biopsy samples, or sedation and local anaesthesia instead of general anaesthesia, may have led to this association.

- Arteriovenous fistula formation
- Biopsy of non-renal tissue (e.g. liver, adrenal gland, fat, muscle, connective tissue, spleen)
- Cyst formation
- Death
- Haemorrhage:
  - Microscopic haematuria
  - Macroscopic haematuria
  - Peri-renal haematoma
  - Intra-renal haematoma
  - Intra-abdominal haemorrhage due to laceration of vessel or other organ or vessel
- Hydronephrosis
- Infarction and thrombosis
- Infection
- Scar formation and fibrosis

13.6 Reported complications of renal biopsy.

Between 20% and 70% of dogs and cats are reported to develop microscopic haematuria after renal biopsy (Minkus *et al.*, 1994; Vaden *et al.*, 2005). Microscopic haematuria is self-limiting, generally resolving within 48–72 hours. Macroscopic haematuria is less common, developing in approximately 1–4% of dogs and cats after renal biopsy. If the kidneys are examined carefully by ultrasonography after biopsy, small peri-renal haematomas are commonly identified. Severe haemorrhage, often severe enough to require blood transfusion, was the most commonly reported complication in one study, occurring in 9.9% of dogs and 16.9% of cats (Vaden *et al.*, 2005). Hydronephrosis developing secondary to obstruction of the renal pelvis or ureter by a blood clot is an uncommon complication of renal biopsy. Death resulting from renal biopsy is also uncommon, occurring in 3% or fewer dogs and cats.

Histological changes following renal biopsy have been well documented. Linear infarcts representing needle tracts associated with varying amounts of atrophy and fibrosis appear to be common after renal biopsy. Retention cysts can also be found in association with the needle tract and probably form secondary to tubular obstruction (Sweet *et al.*, 1969). Severe renal parenchymal changes of haemorrhage, thrombosis, infarction and fibrosis correlate with the presence of major renal vessels or medulla in the biopsy specimen (Osborne *et al.*, 1972; Nash *et al.*, 1983). Performing multiple kidney biopsies does not appear to produce more damage than a single biopsy, providing the biopsy needle remains in cortical tissue (Nash *et al.*, 1986).

Despite renal histological changes, renal biopsy had minimal effect on kidney function in one study (Drost *et al.*, 2000). However, the effect of renal biopsy on the kidney should not be taken lightly. It is possible that renal biopsy in an animal with pre-existing renal disease could contribute to progressive loss of renal function in association with some of these major histological changes.

Morphological classification of renal disease

The normal renal cortex contains scattered glomeruli and numerous tubules within a scant interstitium (Figure 13.7). Most of the tubules in the cortex are proximal because the proximal tubule is much longer than the distal tubule. Proximal tubules have microvilli, have a larger diameter, contain fewer cells and are more numerous in cross-section owing to their longer length. Distal tubules have more closely packed cells, the cells are cuboidal and they have a sharper luminal border.

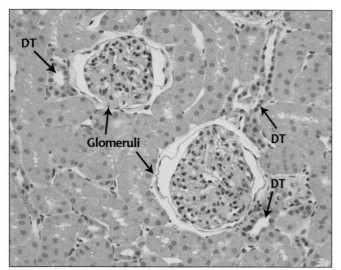

13.7 Normal renal cortex containing glomeruli, tubule cross-sections and scant interstitium. Most tubular profiles are proximal in origin, with fewer distal tubules (DT) present. (H&E stain; original magnification X100)

Tubules are normally in close apposition, because the normal cortical interstitium contains only peritubular capillaries, scant matrix and scattered interstitial cells. All of these renal components are initially evaluated in slides stained with haematoxylin and eosin (H&E) in order to determine lesion distribution, severity and the primary site of renal disease (interstitial or glomerular).

Non-glomerular causes of AKI, such as acute tubular necrosis (ATN) and acute tubulointerstitial nephritis, may be diagnosed using routine H&E stains (Figure 13.8). ATN may be caused by ischaemic or toxic insults. Ischaemic ATN is difficult to detect histologically, because the morphological lesions are focal and mild. The injury usually results in sublethal cell injury, seen as cell swelling, brush border loss and tubular dilatation. This type of injury is due to decreased renal blood flow associated with hypotension, shock, blood loss, hypovolaemia or sepsis. While ischaemic ATN is a common cause of AKI in humans, it is rarely documented in animals. Dogs with acute septicaemic leptospirosis, prior to the development of serum antibody titres and interstitial nephritis, may develop icterus and severe AKI with only mild acute tubular degeneration histologically (Figure 13.8); this ATN is attributed to both ischaemia and toxic factors released by the spirochaetes (Davila de Arriaga et al., 1982).

Nephrotoxic ATN is more commonly recognized in dogs and cats. Tubular epithelial necrosis primarily affects the proximal tubule, with the severity of the necrosis dependent on the offending toxin/toxicant (Figure 13.9). The susceptibility of the proximal tubule cells to toxic

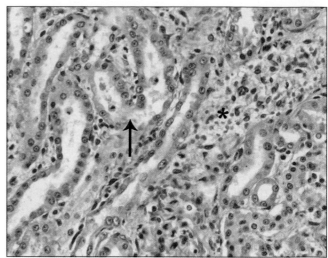

13.8 Acute tubular necrosis in a dog with acute leptospirosis. Proximal tubules are dilated with attenuation of the epithelium, brush border loss and occasional sloughing of necrotic epithelial cells into the lumen (arrowed). The tubules are no longer touching due to expansion of the interstitium with oedema and erythrocytes (*). (H&E stain; original magnification X200)

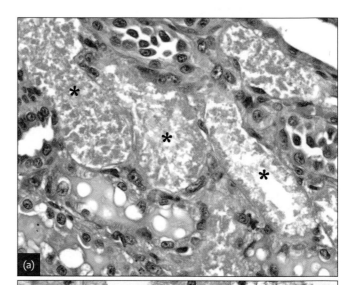

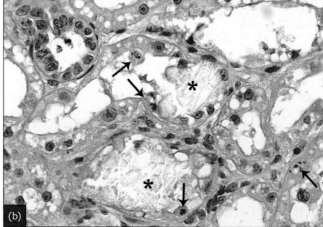

13.9 (a) Toxic acute tubular necrosis in a cat with Easter lily toxicosis. Segments of the proximal tubule are devoid of viable epithelium, and are lined or filled with necrotic cellular debris (*). (b) Toxic acute tubular necrosis in a cat with ethylene glycol toxicosis. Tubules are mildly dilated and the epithelium is attenuated, with individual cell necrosis and karyorrhexis (arrowed). Histological diagnosis is dependent on the finding of large numbers of oxalate crystals (*) within tubules. (H&E stain; original magnification X400)

injury is a reflection of their large microvillus surface area, their high oxygen requirements and their normal absorptive and excretory function, which may actually lead to excretion of toxins/toxicants into this segment.

The cortical interstitium is inconspicuous in the normal kidney and tubules are in close apposition. The cortical interstitial compartment may be expanded by oedema, blood (see Figure 13.8), inflammatory (Figure 13.10a) or neoplastic cells, or fibrous connective tissue, resulting in separation of the tubules. Tubulointerstitial diseases in cats and dogs are often infectious in aetiology, and some of these infectious diseases, such as feline infectious peritonitis and subacute leptospirosis, may be confirmed with immunohistochemical staining (Figure 13.10b). Interstitial fibrosis, recognizable with H&E stains, is better appreciated with a Masson's trichrome stain. Fibrosis is indicative of chronic disease, and the severity of fibrosis is positively correlated with the degree of renal dysfunction. Interstitial fibrosis is a poor prognostic indicator because it is associated with irreversible renal injury and nephron loss.

The glomerulus is a tuft of highly branched capillaries that invaginate into an extension of the proximal tubule. The afferent arteriole enters and arborizes to form the glomerular capillary tuft and exits as the efferent arteriole; these arterioles enter and exit at the vascular pole (Figure 13.11). Scaffolding, made up of mesangial cells and their surrounding extracellular mesangial matrix, supports the capillary loops. The capillary tuft is draped by glomerular basement membrane (GBM), and is covered by a layer of interdigitating visceral epithelial cells (podocytes). The glomerular filtration barrier consists of endothelium, GBM and podocytes (Figure 13.12). Proteinuria results when there is disruption of the filtration barrier, which may be caused by the deposition of immune complexes, complement or amyloid, by a change (either acquired or congenital) in the composition of the GBM, or by injury to the endothelial cells or podocytes. Glomerular injury may also affect mesangial cells, resulting in mesangial cell proliferation and/or increased production of mesangial matrix.

Glomerular involvement seen by light microscopy may be focal (<50% of glomeruli involved) or generalized (all or almost all glomeruli involved). Within an affected glomerulus, the lesion may be segmental (only part of the capillary tuft affected) or global (the entire tuft involved).

The goal of renal biopsy in glomerular diseases is to identify accurately the specific changes occurring in the glomerulus in order to determine the prognosis and potential treatment options for the identified glomerular disease. Human renal biopsy samples are routinely evaluated with light microscopy (LM), transmission electron microscopy (TEM) and immunofluorescence (IF) in order to obtain an accurate and therapeutically useful diagnosis. In contrast, specimens from small animals with proteinuric diseases have historically been evaluated with LM alone, leading to inaccurate diagnoses which limited the utility of the renal biopsy. More recently, renal biopsy samples from a large number of proteinuric dogs have been evaluated by veterinary nephropathologists using all three diagnostic modalities (Cianciolo et al., 2013; Schneider et al., 2013). Based on the diagnostic evaluation of a large number of cases, the routine use of LM, TEM and IF is feasible and necessary for making accurate morphological diagnoses of glomerular disease which can then be used to guide treatment options.

The number of glomeruli present in the biopsy specimens should be recorded as a measure of the adequacy of the biopsy; a minimum of five glomeruli should be present.

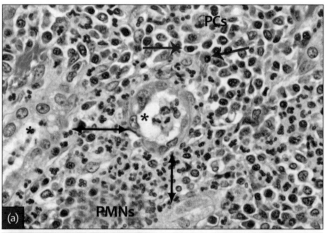

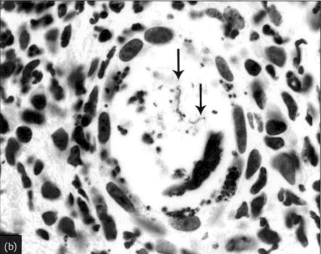

13.10 (a) Subacute puruloplasmacytic tubulointerstitial nephritis in a dog with leptospirosis. Tubules are separated (double arrows) by large numbers of neutrophils (PMNs) and plasma cells (PCs, arrowed), and fewer macrophages. Neutrophils are also present within tubules (*). (H&E stain; original magnification X200). (b) Typical positive leptospiral immunohistochemistry, showing clumps of positive staining material in interstitial macrophages, tubular epithelial cells and the tubular lumen. Intact spirochaetes (arrowed) are also present within the tubular lumen. (Avidin–biotin–peroxidase method, haematoxylin counterstain; original magnification X400)

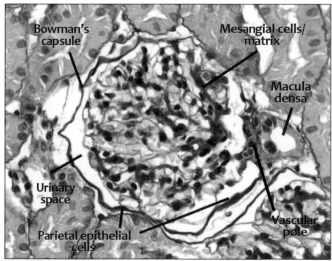

13.11 Normal canine glomerulus stained with periodic acid–Schiff haematoxylin (PASH). The basement membranes of Bowman's capsule, tubules and the glomerular capillaries, and the mesangial matrix stain dark pink. (PASH stain; original magnification X400)

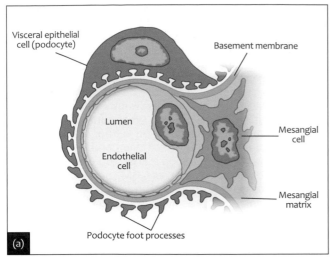

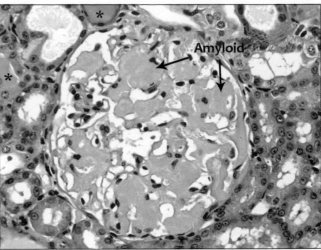

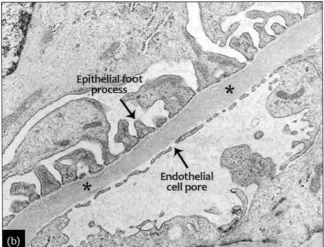

13.13 Glomerular amyloidosis in a dog. Large nodular accumulations of eosinophilic homogeneous material (amyloid, arrowed) displace nuclei to the periphery. Glassy eosinophilic casts (*), indicative of proteinuria, are present in distal tubules. (H&E stain; original magnification X400)

13.12 (a) Normal glomerular capillary. (b) Electron micrograph of the normal glomerular capillary wall. Note the fenestrated capillary endothelium that results in endothelial cell pores, the glomerular basement membrane (*) and the podocyte foot processes.
(b Reproduced from Vaden (2005) with permission from Elsevier. Original image courtesy of JC Jennette, Chapel Hill, NC, School of Medicine, University of North Carolina)

On LM, glomeruli should be evaluated for histological features such as endocapillary or mesangial hypercellularity, evidence of GBM remodelling or thickening, matrix increase, amyloid deposition, segmental sclerosis, hyalinosis and synechiae. As thicker sections will appear more cellular, have more mesangial matrix and have thicker capillary loops, renal biopsy specimens should be routinely sectioned and evaluated at 2–3 μm. Biopsy samples with glomerular deposits suggestive of amyloid (Figure 13.13) should be cut at 8–10 μm, stained with Congo red or standard toluidine blue, and viewed with polarized light to confirm this diagnosis.

While routine H&E stains are useful for identifying tubulointerstitial and vascular changes, additional stains are required to demonstrate glomerular lesions. Periodic acid–Schiff haematoxylin (PASH), Jones methenamine silver (JMS), or periodic acid–methenamine silver stains highlight the GBM and are used to detect remodelling changes, such as GBM spikes, holes or double contours. Masson's trichrome is used to identify immune deposits and to evaluate collagen deposition. While the presence of GBM remodelling and/or immune deposits seen via light microscopy is suggestive of immune-complex glomerulonephritis (ICGN), IF and TEM are required for definitive diagnosis. In the normal glomerulus stained with PASH

(see Figure 13.11), the thickness and contour of the capillary walls should be assessed in peripheral capillary loops, and when cut at a right angle the normal loops will be thin, uniform and crisp. The mesangial matrix can be seen as disconnected branches containing mesangial cells. Matrix typically surrounds one or two mesangial cell nuclei; mesangial matrix expansion is present if matrix extends to encircle more cells. More than three mesangial cell nuclei in close proximity are indicative of mesangial hyperplasia.

In a recent study, renal biopsy samples from 501 dogs with proteinuria were evaluated using LM, IF and TEM and classified morphologically (Schneider et al., 2013). In that report, amyloidosis was present in only 76 (15.2%) of proteinuric dogs. The most common diagnosis was ICGN, occurring in 241 dogs (48.1%). ICGN in dogs may be further classified via LM and TEM as membranous glomerulonephropathy (MGN) (Figure 13.14) or membranoproliferative glomerulonephritis (MPGN) (Figure 13.15). MGN and MPGN are immune-mediated diseases associated with the deposition of immune complexes and complement in the glomerulus. With IF, cases of ICGN exhibit granular staining along capillary loops with antibodies against IgG, lambda light chains (LLC) and C3. The detection of electron-dense deposits (immune complexes) via TEM is the gold standard for demonstrating immune complexes. Given that positive IF staining may occur as a result of non-specific trapping of immunoreactants in injured portions of the capillary tuft in non-ICGN diseases, TEM is generally required to substantiate the diagnosis of ICGN. Immune complexes may localize on either side of the GBM, in the mesangium, or in a combination of these sites (see Figure 13.12). Immune complexes are thought to occur in these areas primarily via in situ formation – the antigen is filtered across the endothelium, but then 'sticks' or implants within the glomerulus owing to characteristics of the antigen (i.e. size, charge). The implanted antigen then combines with antibody, forming antigen–antibody complexes. Alternatively, there may be trapping of preformed circulating immune complexes. Changes in the filtration barrier and consequent proteinuria are the result of the response, particularly of the podocyte, to these immune complexes.

In MGN, immune complexes are present on the subepithelial aspect of the GBM; immune complexes are also present in the mesangium in some cases. In the sub-epithelial location, complement is activated and injures podocytes, resulting in foot process effacement and disruption of the normal filtration barrier. The glomerulus may be normocellular or exhibit mild mesangial hypercellularity, but endocapillary hypercellularity is not present. With light microscopy, spikes may be evident with PASH as the basement membrane extends between the unstained immune deposits (Figure 13.14). Evidence of GBM remodelling will not be present in more acute cases of MGN. Ultrastructurally, there are subepithelial electron-dense deposits (immune complexes) with or without deposits in the mesangium; GBM remodelling or resorption of electron-dense deposits in chronic lesions may be present. Podocyte foot process effacement with or without other evidence of podocyte injury is evident in all cases of ICGN.

In MPGN, the immune complexes are present predominantly on the subendothelial aspect of the glomerular basement membrane, and in this location they activate circulating inflammatory mediators, resulting in more severe glomerular injury and endocapillary hypercellularity. This glomerular endocapillary hypercellularity is a hallmark of MPGN and is comprised of inflammatory cells, increased numbers of endothelial cells, and mesangial cells interposed in the peripheral capillary loops (Figure 13.15a). With trichrome stain, magenta immune deposits may be observed. Double contours of the GBM ('tram-tracks' or GBM reduplication) are best appreciated with JMS or PASH, and are indicative of mesangial cell interposition, a common but not unique finding in MPGN (Figure 13.15b). Mesangial interposition is defined as the extension or movement of the mesangial cell between

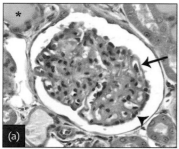
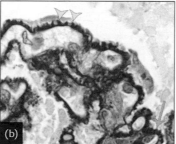
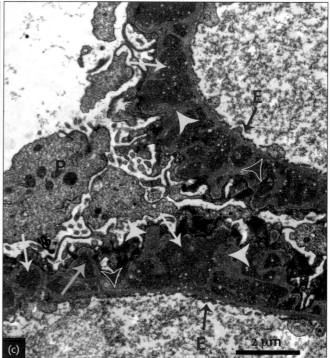

13.14 Membranous glomerulonephropathy (MGN). (a) MGN is characterized by normal glomerular cellularity or mild mesangial cell hyperplasia; endocapillary hypercellularity is absent. Global diffuse capillary wall thickening may be appreciated in more chronic cases (arrowed) due to remodelling; special stains are required to visualize these changes. Podocytes are hypertrophied (arrowhead), which is a non-specific indication of podocyte injury. Protein in a renal tubule (*) is also seen here.(H&E stain; original magnification X400) (b) Well developed spikes (yellow arrowheads) of remodelled glomerular basement membrane (GBM) extending from the abluminal aspect of the capillary wall. Occasional holes, representing immune complexes surrounded by GBM, are also present (light blue arrow). (PASH stain; original magnification X600) (c) Peripheral capillary loops in chronic MGN. Numerous large electron-dense deposits are present on the subepithelial aspect of the GBM (yellow arrows), with new GBM present as spikes on either side (yellow arrowheads) or encircling them (holes) (light blue arrow). Note diffuse podocyte foot process effacement and mild microvillus transformation. E = endothelium; P = podocyte; red arrowheads = native GBM. (Electron micrograph; original magnification X4000)

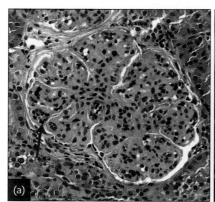
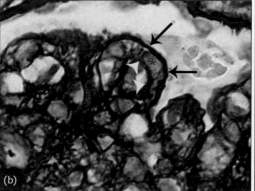
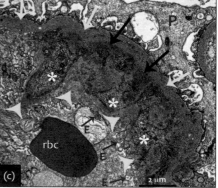

13.15 Membranoproliferative glomerulonephritis (MPGN). (a) MPGN is characterized by global diffuse glomerular endocapillary hypercellularity, extending to the peripheral capillary loops (arrowed), and variable thickening of the capillary walls. (H&E stain; original magnification X400) (b) Capillary wall thickening in MPGN is due to the formation of GBM double contours, demonstrated with special stains. In contrast to MGN, remodelling occurs on the vascular side of the GBM, associated with mesangial cell (*) interposition. Yellow arrowheads = new remodelled GBM; arrows = native GBM. (JMS stain; original magnification X400) (c) Electron micrograph of a peripheral capillary loop from a dog with MPGN. Large granular electron-dense deposits (immune complexes, black arrows) are present on the subendothelial aspect of the GBM (yellow arrows). Mesangial cell processes (*) are interposed between the native GBM and the overlying endothelial cells (E), with production of new GBM (arrowheads, double contours). There is multifocal podocyte foot process effacement. P = podocyte; rbc = intracapillary red blood cell. (Original magnification X4000)

the endothelium and the GBM to the peripheral aspect of the capillary loop. New GBM is produced between the transposed mesangial cell and the overlying endothelial cell, resulting in the double contour appearance on LM. In MPGN, mesangial interposition is typically seen in association with subendothelial electron dense deposits (Figure 13.15c). Glomerular crescents occur in some cases of MPGN, and are indicative of severe injury to the capillary wall. Breaks or gaps in the GBM allow the passage of fibrinogen, and later macrophages, into the urinary space. Fibrin and macrophages induce parietal epithelial cell proliferation, and glomerular crescents form. Glomerular diseases with significant crescent formation are typically more severe and have a rapidly progressive clinical course.

While the LM findings may be highly suggestive of MGN or MPGN, particularly with more advanced disease, electron microscopy is required to verify the presence of deposits, to detect small deposits not evident by light microscopy, and to identify the location (subendothelial, subepithelial, intramembranous and/or mesangial) of the deposits in the glomerulus. Immunofluorescence further defines the disease process, by determining the specific nature of the immune deposits (IgG, IgA, IgM and/or complement).

Primary focal segmental glomerulosclerosis (FSGS) is the most common cause of the nephrotic syndrome in adult humans but has only recently been recognized as occurring in dogs (Aresu *et al.*, 2010; Schneider *et al.*, 2013). Using LM, IF and TEM, it is apparent that primary FSGS is a relatively common pattern of glomerular disease in dogs (Schneider *et al.*, 2013). In that report, primary FSGS (accounting for 20.6% of all diagnoses) was more common than amyloidosis. FSGS is the result of injury/degeneration of podocytes (podocytopathy). In primary FSGS, the cause of this injury is idiopathic or due to genetic podocyte abnormalities. A familial form of protein-losing nephropathy resembling FSGS has been described in Soft Coated Wheaten Terriers (see Chapter 14) that have a specific mutation in genes encoding podocyte slit diaphragm proteins. Familial FSGS has also been reported in Miniature Schnauzers, although the genetic basis of the defect in this breed has not been determined.

Secondary forms of FSGS may occur in association with ICGN, toxins, viral infections or nephron paucity. Secondary FSGS is well recognized in dogs with CKD and nephron loss. The morphological changes in primary and secondary FSGS are similar. FSGS differs from amyloidosis and ICGN in that initially only some glomeruli are affected (i.e. it is focal) and the lesion affects only a portion of the capillary tuft (i.e. it is segmental). On light microscopy, FSGS is characterized by solidification of a portion (a segment) of the capillary tuft by extracellular matrix and mesangial cells, with obliteration of the capillary lumen (Figure 13.16). Secondary changes, such as hyalinosis and adhesions of the sclerotic portion of the tuft to Bowman's capsule (synechiae), are common. With PASH stain, hyalinosis appears as glassy eosinophilic material in the capillary wall; this material comprises serum lipoproteins which have leaked across the damaged portion of the GBM. Synechiae result from podocyte loss with denuding of the GBM; this is followed by adhesion to parietal epithelial cells and Bowman's capsule. Ultrastructurally, FSGS is characterized by extensive podocyte foot process effacement without TEM or IF evidence of immune-complex deposition.

Some glomerular diseases are associated with no or only non-specific changes on LM, further underscoring the importance of electron microscopy in the diagnosis of

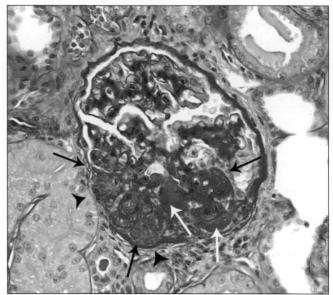

13.16 Focal segmental glomerulosclerosis in a dog, involving solidification of a portion of the capillary tuft by extracellular matrix and mesangial cells (black arrows). The sclerotic segment is adhered to Bowman's capsule (synechiae, arrowheads) and there are areas of hyalinosis (white arrows). (PASH stain; original magnification X400)

glomerular disease. Minimal change disease is a disease of podocytes characterized by essentially normal glomeruli on LM and diffuse podocyte foot process effacement on TEM. Minimal change disease is the most common cause of the nephrotic syndrome in children, and accounts for 15–20% of cases in human adults. This disease is steroid-responsive in humans; without treatment, it may progress and become non-steroid-responsive. In dogs and cats, drug-induced minimal change disease has been reported, with resolution of proteinuria after drug withdrawal in some patients (Sum *et al.*, 2010). Inherited defects in the structure of the GBM, (hereditary nephritis) involving mutations in type IV (basement membrane) collagen, have been described in several purebred and mixed breeds of dog (see Chapter 14). The light microscopic lesions are non-specific, consisting predominantly of glomerulosclerosis. Diagnosis of this disease is dependent on the ultrastructural finding of diffuse irregular splitting of the GBM (Figure 13.17).

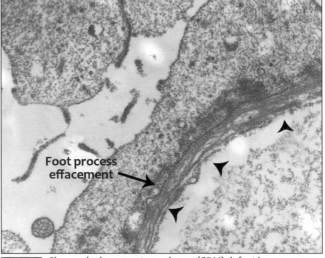

Foot process effacement

13.17 Glomerular basement membrane (GBM) defect in a young dog. Ultrastructurally, the GBM shows diffuse splitting with a multilayered appearance (arrowheads) and spreading (effacement) of the podocyte foot processes.

Summary

The widespread accessibility of ultrasonography makes percutaneous biopsy using ultrasound guidance available for many veterinary patients. When this is not available or not suitable for a given patient, the other techniques can be used. Most importantly, it has now been clearly established that the routine use of LM, TEM and IF in diagnostic evaluation of biopsy specimens is not only necessary but also feasible. These advances mean that optimal therapeutic plans can be developed in individual patients, using the histological diagnosis as a guide (see Chapter 24).

References and further reading

Aresu L, Zanatta R, Luciani L, Trez D and Castagnaro M (2010) Severe renal failure in a dog resembling human focal segmental glomerulosclerosis. *Journal of Comparative Pathology* **143(2–3)**, 190–194

Bigge LA, Brown DJ and Pennick DG (2001) Correlation between coagulation profile findings and bleeding complications after ultrasound-guided biopsies: 434 cases (1993–1996). *Journal of the American Animal Hospital Association* **37(3)**, 228–233

Cianciolo RE, Brown CA, Mohr FC *et al.* (2013) Pathologic evaluation of canine renal biopsies: methods for identifying features that differentiate immune-mediated glomerulonephritides from other categories of glomerular diseases. *Journal of Veterinary Internal Medicine* **27**, S10–S18

Davila de Arriaga AJ, Rocha AS, Yasuda PH and De Brito T (1982) Morpho-functional patterns of kidney injury in the experimental leptospirosis of the guinea-pig (*L. icterohaemorrhagiae*). *Journal of Pathology* **138(2)**, 145–161

Drost WT, Henry GA, Meinkoth JH *et al.* (2000) The effects of a unilateral ultrasound-guided renal biopsy on renal function in healthy sedated cats. *Veterinary Radiology and Ultrasound* **41**, 57–62

Grauer GF, Twedt DC and Mero KN (1983) Evaluation of laparoscopy for obtaining renal biopsy specimens from dogs and cats. *Journal of the American Veterinary Medical Association* **183(6)**, 677–679

Groman RP, Bahr A, Berridge BR and Lees GE (2004) Effects of serial ultrasound-guided renal biopsies on kidneys of healthy adolescent dogs. *Veterinary Radiology and Ultrasound* **45(1)**, 62–69

Hager DA, Nyland TG and Fisher P (1985) Ultrasound-guided biopsy of the canine liver, kidney and prostate. *Veterinary Radiology* **26**, 82–88

Jeraj K, Osborne CA and Stevens JB (1982) Evaluation of renal biopsy in 197 dogs and cats. *Journal of the American Veterinary Medical Association* **181(4)**, 367–369

Leveille R, Partington BP, Biller DS and Miyabayashi T (1993) Complications after ultrasound-guided biopsy of abdominal structures in dogs and cats: 246 cases (1984–1991). *Journal of the American Veterinary Medical Association* **203(3)**, 413–415

Minkus G, Reusch C, Horauf A *et al.* (1994) Evaluation of renal biopsies in cats and dogs – histopathology in comparison with clinical data. *Journal of Small Animal Practice* **35**, 465–472

Nash AS, Boyd JS, Minto AW and Wright NG (1983) Renal biopsy in the normal cat: an examination of the effects of a single needle biopsy. *Research in Veterinary Science* **34(3)**, 347–356

Nash AS, Boyd JS, Minto AW and Wright NG (1986) Renal biopsy in the normal cat: examination of the effects of repeated needle biopsy. *Research in Veterinary Science* **40(1)**, 112–117

Osborne CA (1971) Clinical evaluation of needle biopsy of the kidney and its complications in the dog and cat. *Journal of the American Veterinary Medical Association* **158(7)**, 1213–1228

Osborne CA, Low DG and Jessen CR (1972) Renal parenchymal response to needle biopsy. *Investigative Urology* **9**, 463–469

Parrish AE (1992) Complications of percutaneous renal biopsy: a review of 37 years' experience. *Clinical Nephrology* **38(3)**, 135–141

Schneider SM, Cianciolo RE, Nabity MB *et al.* (2013) Prevalence of immune-complex glomerulonephritides in dogs biopsied for suspected glomerular disease: 501 cases (2007–2012). *Journal of Veterinary Internal Medicine* **27**, S67–S75

Sum SO, Hensel P, Rios L *et al.* (2010) Drug-induced minimal change nephropathy in a dog. *Journal of Veterinary Internal Medicine* **24**, 431–435

Sweet EI, Davidson AJ and Hayslett JP (1969) Complications of needle biopsy of the kidney in the dog. A radiological and pathological correlation. *Radiology* **92(4)**, 849–854

Vaden SL (2004) Renal biopsy: methods and interpretation. *Veterinary Clinics of North America: Small Animal Practice* **34**, 887–908

Vaden SL (2005) Glomerular diseases. In: *Textbook of Veterinary Internal Medicine, 2nd edn*, ed. SJ Ettinger and EC Feldman, pp. 1787–1789. Elsevier, St. Louis

Vaden SL, Levine JF, Lees GE *et al.* (2005) Renal biopsy: a retrospective study of 283 dogs and 65 cats. *Journal of Veterinary Internal Medicine* **19(6)**, 794–801

Wise LA, Allen TA and Cartwright M (1989) Comparison of renal biopsy techniques in dogs. *Journal of the American Veterinary Medical Association* **195(7)**, 935–939

Zatelli A, Bonfanti U, Santilli R, Borgarelli M and Bussadori C (2003) Echo-assisted percutaneous renal biopsy in dogs. A retrospective study of 229 cases. *The Veterinary Journal* **166**, 257–264

Chapter 14

Genetic basis for urinary tract diseases

Meryl P. Littman

An inherited illness, based on genotype, is suspected when multiple family members are affected or a breed predisposition is noted beyond its popularity or what is seen in the general population. Alternatively, a trait (phenotype), whether present at birth (congenital) or of later onset, could be due to an acquired environmental insult, *in utero* or thereafter, which affects development or function. Additional test matings may reveal a genetic basis for the trait. Pedigree analysis may indicate the mode of inheritance, for example, simple Mendelian (sex-linked, sex-limited, autosomal, recessive or dominant) or complex (involving multiple genes, with possible modifiers, variable expression, incomplete penetrance, environmental triggers, and/or epigenetic and acquired factors that may influence gene expression/transcription via deoxyribonucleic acid (DNA) methylation or histone modification that may be vertically transmitted to offspring).

New genetic tools, including maps of the human, canine and feline genomes, the Online Mendelian Inheritance in Man (OMIM) compendium (www.ncbi.nlm.nih.gov/pubmed/) resource of candidate genes involved with illness, single nucleotide polymorphism (SNP)-chip technology, genome-wide association studies (GWAS), fine sequencing (mapping) techniques for candidate genes, and specialized computer software to analyse millions of datasets, have allowed geneticists to enter an exciting era of discovery. DNA can be extracted from whole blood, buccal swabs (epithelial cells), semen or other cellular tissue, and DNA genotypes from affected cases can be compared with properly chosen control cases, to locate a genetic marker linked to a particular phenotypic trait or, better yet, a mutation (variant allele, e.g. a deletion, addition or a non-synonymous SNP) in one or more causative genes, which then elucidates the underlying molecular basis for the abnormality. Accurate phenotypic characterization is paramount, for both the affected and valid control cases selected for such investigations. Sophisticated diagnostic tests to characterize the phenotype and exclude non-genetic causes include serology/polymerase chain reaction (PCR), imaging, and renal biopsy examination by trained personnel using transmission electron microscopy (TEM), immunofluorescence (IF), and thin section (3 µm) light microscopy (LM) with special stains (Cianciolo *et al.*, 2013) (see Chapter 13).

Once a specific DNA test is developed, individuals can be screened for the at-risk variant alleles, indicating which animals may benefit from monitoring and early intervention. Prevalence studies showing the frequency of the variant alleles in the population will help guide whether carriers can be swiftly excluded from the breeding population, or whether loss of genetic diversity would ensue (inbreeding of a small population, producing new genetic problems). Genetic counselling is important, to choose mates carefully with attention to all the traits in the breed to perpetuate or prevent, while maintaining genetic diversity in the population. The same phenotype in different breeds may be caused by identical mutations (e.g. hyperuricosuria) or a variety of alterations in the same candidate gene or in different genes, ultimately requiring different genetic tests to detect carrier status (e.g. cystinuria). The development of dog and cat breeds, with small foundation stock and popular sires, led to long haplotypes and extensive linkage disequilibrium, so that relatively small numbers of cases may yield statistically robust results. Although only some of the many inherited diseases currently have genotype characterization, many more will be investigated and solved in the near future. Now is a good time to bank blood, semen or cellular tissue DNA samples from animals with well characterized affected and control phenotypes. The best control cases are related to the affected population, but well past the age of onset, with documented absence of the criteria for the condition.

Inherited glomerulopathies

Signs of glomerular disease such as protein-losing nephropathy (PLN) may be dramatic and due to systemic hypertension, thromboembolic events and/or oedema, effusions and nephrotic syndrome; eventually signs of secondary whole nephron damage and Stage 3 or 4 chronic kidney disease (CKD) are seen (e.g. lethargy, anorexia, weight loss, vomiting/diarrhoea, polyuria/polydipsia (PU/PD) and anaemia). Isosthenuria is a relatively late finding of primary glomerular disease, as secondary tubular disease ensues. The hallmark of glomerular disease is proteinuria, due to a defect in the permselective barrier involving the capillary endothelium, glomerular basement membrane, and slit diaphragm between the podocyte foot processes, allowing protein to leak into the urine. Tubular cells are damaged by trying to reabsorb protein. The earliest laboratory sign of glomerular disease is persistent proteinuria, detected by urine protein to creatinine ratio (UPC), microalbuminuria test, sulphosalicylic acid (SSA) turbidometric test, or by finding ≥+2 dipstick protein readings (or ≥+1 with low urine specific gravity: USG ≤1.012) (see Chapters 5 and 6). It is important to consider other sources and causes of proteinuria, such as infection or inflammation of the lower urinary tract (bladder, urethra, prostate), and to be certain that the proteinuria is due to glomerular disease (see Chapter 5 for a discussion of proteinuria). Sodium dodecyl sulphate polyacrylamide gel electrophoresis (SDS-PAGE) may help to determine whether the proteinuria is of low molecular weight, associated with tubular disease, or higher molecular weight, associated with albuminuria from glomerular leakage. In addition to proteinuria, common blood test abnormalities may include hypoalbuminaemia, hypercholesterolaemia and possibly azotaemia, hyperphosphataemia and/or anaemia. As azotaemia worsens, proteinuria may decline as a result of decreased filtering units, and hypoalbuminaemia may wane or be masked by dehydration, thus the glomerular cause of disease may be difficult to ascertain at the time of Stage 3 or 4 CKD.

For only a few of the more than two dozen breeds predisposed to PLN is the underlying molecular basis defined. Diagnostic tools have been published to help characterize the phenotype more accurately (blood profiles, serology/PCR tests to rule out infectious diseases, imaging and renal biopsy samples examined to visualize ultrastructural details by TEM, IF, LM and special stains; Littman *et al.*, 2013a).

A full discussion of the diagnosis and treatment of PLN is covered elsewhere (see Chapters 5, 13, 24, and ACVIM, 2013).

Glomerular basement membrane defects

Glomerulosclerosis (GS), glomerulonephritis (GN), glomerular basement membrane (GBM) defects and other types of glomerular thickening may look similar by LM alone, but with TEM examination ultrastructural detail better defines accurate phenotypic characterization. Some forms of inherited canine PLN show GBM laminar splitting, as in human Alport syndrome (also referred to as hereditary nephritis, HN), narrowing the field of candidate genes to study. Collagen IV, the backbone of the GBM, forms heterotrimers of six possible chains, named alpha-1–alpha-6, which are encoded by genes *COL4A1*–*COL4A6* (*COL4A1* and *COL4A2* are on chromosome 22, *COL4A3* and *COL4A4*

are on chromosome 25, and *COL4A5* and *COL4A6* are on the X chromosome). Adult mammalian GBM is mostly made up of alpha-3-alpha-4-alpha-5 heterotrimers. Immuno fluorescent techniques using antibodies directed against specific alpha chains identify the presence or absence of these chains as well as their location. Breeds that show an X-linked mode of inheritance for HN (XLHN) have had their *COL4A5* gene completely sequenced. In Samoyed dogs with XLHN, a SNP in exon 35 changes a G to a T (c.3079G>T), which causes a premature stop codon and a truncated alpha-5 chain which cannot cross-link properly in the nanostructure of collagen IV. Carrier male Samoyeds show proteinuria at 3–6 months of age and CKD by 6–24 months, while carrier females (mosaics) are also proteinuric but do not show CKD until >5 years of age. An allele-specific PCR test (DNA test) now identifies carriers before they are bred (Figure 14.1), curtailing PLN among pet Samoyeds. Another model of XLHN, in mixed-breed dogs from Navasota, Texas, shows a dominant mode of inheritance, with carriers of both sexes showing proteinuria by 6 months and CKD at 6–18 months. Sequencing of the candidate gene *COL4A5* showed a 10 base-pair (bp) deletion in exon 9 (c.689_699delTAATCCAGGA), causing a frame shift and a premature stop codon in exon 10 (see also Lees, 2013).

Familial nephropathy in English Cocker Spaniels at 10–24 months), with an autosomal mode of inheritance, was difficult to eradicate for many decades until the identification by TEM of ultrastructural changes led to suspicion of an autosomal recessive form of HN. Sequencing the candidate gene *COL4A4* showed a non-synonymous SNP in exon 3, changing an A to a T (c.115A>T), causing a premature stop codon. A DNA (PCR) test for the variant allele is now available. In Europe, the current mutation frequency in the breed is down to 6% (www.antagene.com).

Two female littermate English Springer Spaniels, presenting at 7 months and progressing to CKD over 2–3 months, were identified with HN by TEM; the *COL4A4* defect found was a non-synonymous SNP in exon 30, changing C to T (c.2712C>T), causing a premature stop codon.

Other breeds with ultrastructural changes in the GBM but for which the genetic defect has not yet been defined

Breed	Phenotype	Site	Mode of Inheritance	Genotype (test available)*
Dogs				
Airedale Terrier	Podocytopathy/GS ± ICGN (as in Soft Coated Wheaten Terriers)	G	Complex	*NPHS1* c.3067G>A and *KIRREL2* c.1877C>G (PennGen, Laboklin)
Akita	Possibly amyloidosis	K		
Alaskan Malamute	JRD	K		
American Foxhound	ICGN (leishmaniosis)	G		
American Staffordshire Terrier	Cystinuria	T		
	Hyperuricosuria	T	AR	*SLC2A9* c.616G>T (many labs)
Australian Cattle Dog, Australian Stumpy Tail Cattle Dog	Cystinuria, Type II-A	T	AD (incomplete penetrance)	*SLC3A1* c.1095_1100del (PennGen, Orivet, Paw Print Genetics)
Australian Labradoodle	Cystinuria, Type I-A	T	AR	*SLC3A1* c.350delG (PennGen, Orivet, VetGen)
Australian Shepherd	Cobalamin malabsorption and mild proteinuria	GI, K	AR	*AMN* c.3G>A (PennGen)
	Cystinuria	T		
	Hyperuricosuria	T	AR	*SLC2A9* c.616G>T (many labs)

14.1 Inherited urinary tract abnormalities in dogs and cats. AD = autosomal dominant; AR = autosomal recessive; FSGS = focal segmental glomerulosclerosis; G = glomerular; GBMD = glomerular basement membrane defect; GI = gastrointestinal; GN = glomerulonephritis; GS = glomerulosclerosis; HN = hereditary nephritis; ICGN = immune-complex glomerulonephritis; JRD = juvenile renal disease; K = kidney; LUT = lower urinary tract; MPGN = membranoproliferative glomerulonephritis; PCKD = polycystic kidney disease; T = tubular; TCC = transitional cell carcinoma *See www.wsava.org/HereditaryDefects.htm for available laboratories. (continues) ▶

Breed	Phenotype	Site	Mode of Inheritance	Genotype (test available)*
Basenji	GN (with small intestinal immunoproliferative disease)	G		
	Fanconi syndrome	T	AR	Fanconi: *FAN1* 321bp deletion (Animal Molecular Genetics Lab, University of Missouri; Paw Print Genetics; Urine metabolic screening at PennGen)
	Cystinuria	T		
Bassett Hound	Cystinuria	T		
Beagle	Renal agenesis	K		
	Amyloidosis	K		
	Glomerulopathy (HN?)	G		
	Cobalamin malabsorption and mild proteinuria	GI, K	AR	*CUBN* c.786delC (Laboklin, Michigan State University)
	TCC	LUT		
Bernese Mountain Dog	MPGN	G	AR, possible sex-linked modifier	
Black Russian Terrier	Hyperuricosuria	T	AR	*SLC2A9* c.616G>T (many labs)
Border Collie	Cobalamin malabsorption and mild proteinuria	GI, K	AR	*CUBN* c.8392delC (Michigan State University, VetGen)
Border Terrier	JRD/Fanconi syndrome	K, T		
	Ectopic ureter	LUT		
Boston Terrier	Urethral prolapse	LUT		
	Hypospadias	LUT		
Boxer	JRD/reflux nephropathy	K		
Briard	Ectopic ureter	LUT		
Brittany Spaniel	MPGN Complement deficiency	G	AR	C3 c.2136delC (Paw Print Genetics)
Bullmastiff	Glomerulopathy/FSGS	G	AR	
Bull Terrier, English Bull Terrier	GBMD	G	AD	
	PCKD	K	AD	*PKD1* c.9772G>A (Antagene, Paw Print Genetics)
Cairn	PCKD (infantile)	K	AR	
Cavalier King Charles Spaniel	Renal agenesis	K		
	Xanthinuria	T		
Chihuahua	Cystinuria	T		
Chow Chow	JRD, cystic glomeruli	K		
Coton de Tulear	Hyperoxaluria (infantile)	T	AR	*AGXT* c.996G>A (Paw Print Genetics, VetGen)
Dachshund	Cystinuria	T		
Dalmatian	GBMD	G	AD	
	Hyperuricosuria	T	AR	*SLC2A9* c.616G>T (many labs) Test LUA (low uric acid) dogs; http://luadalmatians-world.com/wordpress/about-lua/
	Hypospadias	LUT		
Dobermann	Renal agenesis	K		
	JRD/glomerulopathy/HN?	K, G		
	GN (sulphonamides)	G		
	Urinary incontinence/intrapelvic bladder?	LUT		
Dutch Kooiker	JRD	K		
English Bulldog	Renal/ureteral duplication	K		
	Cystinuria, Type III	T	Sex-limited	*SLC3A1* c.574A>G, c.2091A>G also *SLC7A9* c.649G>A (linked) (PennGen, Orivet, Laboratorio Genefast, Vetogene)
	Hyperuricosuria	T	AR	*SLC2A9* c.616G>T (many labs)
	Ectopic ureter, urethrorectal fistula, urethral prolapse, urethral duplication	LUT		
English Cocker Spaniel	GBMD	G	AR	*COL4A4* c.115A>T (Antagene, Genetic Technologies, Genindexe, Genomia, Laboklin, Optigen, Orivet, Van Haeringen)

14.1 (continued) Inherited urinary tract abnormalities in dogs and cats. AD = autosomal dominant; AR = autosomal recessive; FSGS = focal segmental glomerulosclerosis; G = glomerular; GBMD = glomerular basement membrane defect; GI = gastrointestinal; GN = glomerulonephritis; GS = glomerulosclerosis; HN = hereditary nephritis; ICGN = immune-complex glomerulonephritis; JRD = juvenile renal disease; K = kidney; LUT = lower urinary tract; MPGN = membranoproliferative glomerulonephritis; PCKD = polycystic kidney disease; T = tubular; TCC = transitional cell carcinoma. *See www.wsava.org/HereditaryDefects.htm for available laboratories. (continues) ▶

Breed	Phenotype	Site	Mode of Inheritance	Genotype (test available)*
English Foxhound	Amyloidosis	K		
English Springer Spaniel	GBMD	G	AR	COL4A4 c.2712C>T (Orivet, Paw Print Genetics)
Entlebucher Mountain Dog (Swiss Dog)	Ectopic ureter	LUT	Complex	
Finnish Harrier	JRD(Davidson)	K		
Fox Terrier	Ectopic ureter	LUT		
French Bulldog	Cystinuria, Type III	T	Sex-limited	SLC3A1 c.574A>G, c.2091A>G also SLC7A9 c.649G>A (linked) (PennGen, Orivet, Laboratorio Genefast, Vetogene)
	Hyperuricosuria	T	AR	SLC2A9 c.616G>T (many labs)
French Mastiff (Dogue de Bordeaux)	Juvenile glomerulopathy	G	AR	
German Shepherd Dog	ICGN (Ehrlichia canis)	G		
	Cystadenocarcinomas (with nodular dermatofibrosis, uterine leiomyomas)	K	AD (homozygous lethal in embryo)	FLCN c.764A>G (Laboratorio Genefast, Paw Print Genetics, VetGen, Vetnostic)
	Hyperuricosuria	T	AR	SLC2A9 c.616G>T (many labs)
German Spitz	Hyperuricosuria	T	AR	SLC2A9 c.616G>T (many labs)
Giant Schnauzer	Cobalamin malabsorption and mild proteinuria	GI, K	AR	AMN c.1113_1145del (PennGen, VetGen)
	Hyperuricosuria	T	AR	SLC2A9 c.616G>T (many labs)
Golden Retriever	ICGN (Lyme nephritis)	G		
	JRD	K		
	Ectopic ureter	LUT		
Gordon Setter	JRD/reflux nephropathy	K		
Greyhound	Vasculopathy (skin, renal)	G		
Griffon	Ectopic ureter	LUT		
Irish Terrier	Cystinuria, Type III	T	Sex-limited	
Jack and Parson Russell Terrier	Hyperuricosuria	T	AR	SLC2A9 c.616G>T (many labs)
Keeshond	JRD	K		
Labradoodle	Cystinuria, Type I-A	T	AR	SLC3A1 c.350delG (PennGen, Orivet, VetGen)
Labrador Retriever	ICGN (Lyme nephritis)	G		
	Liver disease/Fanconi	T		
	Cystinuria, Type I-A	T	AR	SLC3A1 c.350delG (PennGen, Orivet, VetGen)
	Ectopic ureter	LUT		
Landseer	Cystinuria, Type I-A	T	AR	SLC3A1 c.586C>T (16 labs)
Large Munsterlander	Hyperuricosuria	T	AR	SLC2A9 c.616G>T (many labs)
Lhasa Apso	JRD	K		See text
Mastiff	Cystinuria, Type III	T	Sex-limited	Linked test (PennGen)
Miniature Pinscher	Cystinuria, Type II-B	T	AD	SLC7A9 c.964G>A (PennGen, Orivet) Homozygous not seen (may be lethal)
Miniature Poodle	Urethrorectal fistula, urethroperineal fistula, urethral duplication	LUT		
Miniature and Toy Poodle	Ectopic ureter	LUT		
Miniature Schnauzer	GS or possibly HN	G		
	JRD	K		
	Persistent Muellerian duct syndrome	LUT	AR (sex-limited)	AMHR2 c.238C>T, i.e. anti-Muellerian hormone receptor 2, aka MISRII, Muellerian Inhibiting Substance Type II receptor (Baker Institute for Animal Health, Optigen, Paw Print Genetics)

14.1 (continued) Inherited urinary tract abnormalities in dogs and cats. AD = autosomal dominant; AR = autosomal recessive; FSGS = focal segmental glomerulosclerosis; G = glomerular; GBMD = glomerular basement membrane defect; GI = gastrointestinal; GN = glomerulonephritis; GS = glomerulosclerosis; HN = hereditary nephritis; ICGN = immune-complex glomerulonephritis; JRD = juvenile renal disease; K = kidney; LUT = lower urinary tract; MPGN = membranoproliferative glomerulonephritis; PCKD = polycystic kidney disease; T = tubular; TCC = transitional cell carcinoma. *See www.wsava.org/HereditaryDefects.htm for available laboratories. (continues) ▶

Breed	Phenotype	Site	Mode of Inheritance	Genotype (test available)*
Native American Indian Dog	2-8 dihydroxyadenine urolithiasis	LUT	AR	APRT c.260G>A (no matching laboratories)
Navasota mixed-breed	GBMD	G	X-linked dominant	COL4A5 c.689_699delTAATCCAGGA (Paw Print Genetics)
Newfoundland	Juvenile collagenofibrotic glomerulopathy	G	AR	
	Cystinuria, Type I-A	T	AR	SLC3A1 c.586C>T (16 labs)
	Ectopic ureter	LUT		
Norwegian Elkhound	Periglomerular fibrosis	G		
	Glucosuria	T		
Pekingese	Renal agenesis	K		
Pembroke Welsh Corgi	Glomerulopathy	G		
	Renal telangiectasia	K		
	Cystinuria	T		
Rottweiler	Glomerulopathy (HN?)	G		
Samoyed	GBMD	G	X-linked recessive HN Females are mosaics	COL4A5 c.3079G>T (Laboklin, Paw Print Genetics, VetGen)
Scottish Deerhound	Cystinuria, Type III, as in Irish Terriers	T	Sex-limited	
Scottish Terrier	Cystinuria, Type III	T	AR	
	Glucosuria	T		
	TCC	LUT		
Shar Pei (Chinese)	Amyloidosis	G		HAS2 g.23,746,089_23,762,189dup16.1kb (no matching laboratories)
Shetland Sheepdog	ICGN (Lyme nephritis)	G		
	Renal agenesis	K		
	TCC	LUT		
Shih Tzu	JRD	K	AD (incomplete penetrance)	See text
Siberian Husky	Ectopic ureter	LUT		
Skye Terrier	Ectopic ureter	LUT		
Soft Coated Wheaten Terrier	Podocytopathy/GS ± ICGN See text	G	Complex	NPHS1 c.3067G>A, KIRREL2 c.1877C>G (PennGen, Laboklin)
	JRD	K		
South African Boerboel	Hyperuricosuria	T	AR	SLC2A9 c.616G>T (many labs)
Standard Poodle	JRD	K		
Weimaraner	Hyperuricosuria	T	AR	SLC2A9 c.616G>T (many labs)
West Highland White Terrier	PCKD (infantile)	K	AR	
	Ectopic ureter	LUT		
	TCC	LUT		
Wire-Haired Fox Terrier	TCC	LUT		
Cats				
Abyssinian	Amyloidosis (T>G)	K	AD (incomplete penetrance)	
	Proliferative glomerulopathy	G	AR	
British Longhaired; British Shorthaired	PCKD	K	AD	PKD1 c.10063C>A (many labs)
Burmilla	PCKD	K	AD	PKD1 c.10063C>A (many labs)

14.1 (continued) Inherited urinary tract abnormalities in dogs and cats. AD = autosomal dominant; AR = autosomal recessive; FSGS = focal segmental glomerulosclerosis; G = glomerular; GBMD = glomerular basement membrane defect; GI = gastrointestinal; GN = glomerulonephritis; GS = glomerulosclerosis; HN = hereditary nephritis; ICGN = immune-complex glomerulonephritis; JRD = juvenile renal disease; K = kidney; LUT = lower urinary tract; MPGN = membranoproliferative glomerulonephritis; PCKD = polycystic kidney disease; T = tubular; TCC = transitional cell carcinoma. *See www.wsava.org/HereditaryDefects.htm for available laboratories. (continues)

Breed	Phenotype	Site	Mode of Inheritance	Genotype (test available)*
Domestic Shorthaired	Hyperoxaluria (infantile)	T	AR	*GRHPR* Intron 4 acceptor site G>A; no matching laboratories
	Cystinuria	T		*SLC3A1* c.1342C>T (no matching laboratories)
Exotic Shorthaired	PCKD	K	AD	*PKD1* c.10063C>A (many labs)
Himalayan	PCKD	K	AD	*PKD1* c.10063C>A (many labs)
Maine Coon	PCKD (different)	K		See text
Persian	PCKD	K	AD	*PKD1* c.10063C>A (many labs)
Ragdoll	PCKD	K	AD	*PKD1* c.10063C>A (many labs)
Scottish Fold	PCKD	K	AD	*PKD1* c.10063C>A (many labs)
Selkirk Rex	PCKD	K	AD	*PKD1* c.10063C>A (many labs)
Siamese	Amyloidosis (T>G)	K		

14.1 (continued) Inherited urinary tract abnormalities in dogs and cats. AD = autosomal dominant; AR = autosomal recessive; FSGS = focal segmental glomerulosclerosis; G = glomerular; GBMD = glomerular basement membrane defect; GI = gastrointestinal; GN = glomerulonephritis; GS = glomerulosclerosis; HN = hereditary nephritis; ICGN = immune-complex glomerulonephritis; JRD = juvenile renal disease; K = kidney; LUT = lower urinary tract; MPGN = membranoproliferative glomerulonephritis; PCKD = polycystic kidney disease; T = tubular; TCC = transitional cell carcinoma. *See www.wsava.org/HereditaryDefects.htm for available laboratories.

include Bull Terriers (average onset 3.5 years, range 11 months to 8 years) and Dalmatians (average onset 18 months, range 8 months to 7 years), both of which appear to have autosomal dominant forms of HN, with clinical variability and adult onset of CKD later in life, noted up to 10 years of age. Beagles, Dobermanns and Rottweilers with familial PLN are also described with GBM changes suggestive of HN.

Podocytopathy

Mutations in the proteins of the glomerular slit diaphragm are called podocytopathies (Littman *et al.*, 2013c; Vaden *et al.*, 2013); they cause PLN and focal segmental glomerulosclerosis (FSGS or GS). A myriad of slit diaphragm molecules interact and eventually connect to the actin cytoskeleton of podocyte foot processes, causing dynamic three-dimensional changes in the shape and size of the slit diaphragm, which responds to its nano-milieu. There are many podocytopathies in humans causing PLN with various modes of inheritance and varied onset (infantile, juvenile or adult). The first podocytopathy in dogs was discovered recently (Littman *et al.*, 2013c) and there are likely to be many others identified in the future.

For several decades Soft Coated Wheaten Terriers (SCWT) in North America were known to have a predisposition for PLN (10–15% incidence), often combined with protein-losing enteropathy (PLE), but the underlying defects were unknown. There was no age limit, with many dogs bred before showing illness with PLE (average age of onset 4.7 ± 2.6 years), comorbid PLE/PLN (5.9 ± 2.2 years) or PLN (6.3 ± 2 years) (Littman *et al.*, 2000). Renal histopathology was described as GS and/or GN. An immunodysregulation was theorized, and possibly immune-complex GN (ICGN), because SCWT have a predisposition for PLE with inflammatory bowel disease (IBD) and food allergies; pANCA antibodies; Addison's disease (possibly immune-mediated); and female predisposition (F:M ratio = 1.4–1.9 for PLE and/or PLN), which suggests immunodysregulation (however, sexual bias may exist because breeders own more females). Other theories involved structural/developmental defects, considering the breed's predisposition for GS, intestinal lymphangiectasia/PLE, and juvenile renal disease (JRD) with fetal glomeruli (renal dysplasia). Since there are a myriad of candidate genes involved with structure and function of the immune system, gastrointestinal tract and kidney, a genome-wide association study (GWAS) was done to narrow the focus of investigation. Using only 62 DNA samples from related SCWT dogs with well-characterized phenotypes (42 affected dogs and 20 geriatric controls) based on blood, urine and histopathology results, a GWAS showed highly statistically significant differences in dogs with PLN *versus* controls on chromosome 1 in a region containing 65 genes, including four genes deemed 'candidate genes' (related to renal structure or function). No such interval was found in this pilot GWAS study for PLE or JRD, which appear to be inherited separately from PLN. Fine mapping (gene sequencing) showed a single non-synonymous SNP in each of two genes (*NPHS1* and *KIRREL2*) that are next to each other on chromosome 1 and encode the slit diaphragm proteins, nephrin and Neph3/filtrin. In exon 22 of *NPHS1*, G is changed to A (c.3067G>A), altering a conserved glycine residue to an arginine (G1023R) in the fibronectin type 3 domain of nephrin, a change that is 'probably damaging' to the protein structure, the highest rating given by PolyPhen-2 analysis. In exon 15 of *KIRREL2*, C is changed to G (c.1877C>G), changing a proline residue in a conserved proline-rich interval to an arginine (P626R), rated as 'possibly damaging' to the structure/function of Neph3/filtrin. In humans, there are at least 176 different mutations defined in *NPHS1* associated with PLN in different families. No mutations are known yet in *KIRREL2* in humans, however decreased expression of Neph3/filtrin is associated with PLN.

A customized Taqman assay for these PLN-associated variant alleles was produced and 145 SCWT with known phenotypes tested. Since the variant alleles in these two genes are in linkage disequilibrium, they can be thought of as one unit (i.e. if *NPHS1* is mutated, so is *KIRREL2* in that SCWT, and if *NPHS1* is wildtype/normal, so is *KIRREL2*). Homozygous positive dogs for the variant alleles showed highest risk, heterozygous dogs showed intermediate risk, and homozygous negative dogs showed lowest risk for development of PLN in their lifetimes ($p = 7.78 \times 10^{-10}$). When non-SCWT breeds were tested for the *NPHS1* ($n = 747$ dogs of 114 breeds) and *KIRREL2* ($n = 550$ dogs of 105 breeds) variant alleles, only three dogs had these SNPs, including two Airedale Terriers (one was homozygous positive and had PLN, and the other was heterozygous) and one Bloodhound, uniquely heterozygous for the *KIRREL2* SNP only.

The DNA test for these PLN-associated variant alleles found in SCWT and Airedale Terriers is available at the University of Pennsylvania (www.scwtca.org/health/dna-test.htm; PennGen, http://research.vet.upenn.edu/penngen) and in Europe (Laboklin, www.laboklin.de). Prevalence studies on SCWT samples from North America, Europe and Australia (Littman *et al.*, 2013b) of 1208 SCWT samples show the variant alleles to occur worldwide: 38% (42% most recently with *n* = 2166) were homozygous negative, 45% (43%, *n* = 2166) were heterozygous, and 17% (15%, n = 2166) were homozygous positive, with a variant allele frequency of 40% (37%, *n* = 2166). Prevalence studies with 297 North American Airedale Terriers (Littman *et al.*, 2014) showed that 47% were homozygous negative, 44% were heterozygous and 9% were homozygous positive. The variant allele frequency among 221 Airedale Terriers was 28%; however, among 24 dogs closely related to Airedale Terriers that died with kidney disease, the allele frequency was 42%.

With such high variant allele frequencies, it is unwise to remove all carriers too quickly from the breeding pool, because of the negative effects of loss of genetic diversity. The SCWT breed also has other genetic predispositions to consider when choosing mates, not just the risk of PLN (e.g. allergies, IBD, PLE, JRD, Addison's disease, poor temperament, poor conformation). The current recommendation is to test dogs to determine an individual's risk for developing PLN in its lifetime, to monitor and initiate intervention early, and to choose mates that will avoid producing homozygous positive puppies. It would be wise to breed healthy homozygous positive or heterozygous dogs to homozygous negative dogs, to reduce the variant allele frequency over time and decrease the risk of PLN.

The retrospective studies show a highly statistically significant relationship of the PLN-associated variant alleles with disease, but not all homozygous positive dogs become affected. A complex mode of inheritance, possibly with multiple genes, variable expression, incomplete penetrance and/or environmental triggers is suggested. Prospective studies need to be done to follow heterozygous and homozygous positive dogs throughout their lives to check for disease, comorbidities, environmental triggers and so forth. The predominant histopathological lesion due to genetic podocytopathy is varying degrees of FSGS, but affected podocytes may be susceptible to further damage by inflammation or circulating immune complexes that normal dogs would be able to process (Vaden *et al.*, 2013). It is interesting that SCWT dogs with comorbid PLE/PLN manifest higher UPC values and have earlier onset than SCWT dogs with PLN alone (Littman *et al.*, 2000).

Abnormal glomerular deposition

Amyloidosis

Up to 23% of adult Chinese Shar Peis (median age 4.8 years, range 3.6–17 years) may show renal amyloidosis with amyloid AA deposition affecting the renal medulla, progressing to CKD. Glomerular deposition is also seen in 79% of cases, and 65% of cases show proteinuria with hypoalbuminaemia. The renal amyloidosis is most likely reactive, due to chronic inflammation associated with recurrent fever/hock syndrome from hyaluronidosis (cutaneous mucinosis). Shar Peis are homozygous for an unstable duplication of the hyaluronic acid synthase 2 (*HAS2*) gene that causes their prized wrinkles but also causes periodic fever and possibly renal amyloidosis

(Olsson *et al.*, 2011). Other organs (liver, spleen, adrenals, etc.) may also be affected. Hepatic amyloidosis causes a friable liver which may rupture and cause haemo-abdomen. In addition to signs of progressive CKD with or without PLN, Shar Peis may present with pain in the hocks, muzzle and abdomen, or with diarrhoea and anorexia (Segev *et al.*, 2012).

Other canine breeds which have familial amyloidosis include the Beagle, English Foxhound, and possibly Akitas, but their genetic defects need study. In cats, Abyssinian and Siamese cats are predisposed to renal and possibly hepatic amyloidosis (with risk of rupture), but their renal amyloid deposition is mostly medullary (not glomerular) so proteinuria is not as commonly seen.

Collagen III deposition

A mixed-breed colony used for study of German Shepherd Dogs with renal cystadenocarcinoma were found to have familial abnormal collagen III deposition in the glomerulus, known as collagenofibrotic glomerulonephropathy, with an autosomal mode of inheritance (Rørtveit *et al.*, 2012; 2013). This non-amyloid fibrillary deposition was seen ultrastructurally, and immunohistochemistry documented the fibrils as collagen III. The *COL3A1* gene itself appears uninvolved. As in humans, high serum levels of the aminoterminal propeptide of type III procollagen (PIIINP) can be used as a marker, however the canine model is without hypocomplementaemia. A similar collagen III fibrillary deposition in glomeruli was described in juvenile Newfoundlands (Littman, 2011).

Immune-complex deposition

Labrador and Golden Retrievers, and possibly Shetland Sheepdogs, have a predisposition for 'Lyme nephritis' (Littman, 2013), i.e. ICGN with Lyme-specific immune-complex deposition. Most seropositive dogs do not show Lyme nephritis, even among Lyme-seropositive retrievers, therefore there may be a genetic predisposition for PLN that is triggered by Lyme antigen–antibody complexes which are an added insult (e.g. with genetically abnormal glomeruli, an underlying unidentified podocytopathy, or immunodysregulation).

Bernese Mountain Dogs are very often Lyme-seropositive compared with other breeds and were originally thought to have a predisposition for Lyme nephritis; however, their Lyme-seropositive status is not associated with proteinuria or lameness. It appears that this breed has a familial form of membranoproliferative GN (MPGN), usually presenting at 2–7 years old, with an autosomal recessive mode of inheritance, possibly with an X-linked modifier gene, because it affects mostly females (F:M = 4) (Littman, 2011).

A Brittany Spaniel colony was found to have type 1 MPGN secondary to complement C3 deficiency, with a deletion mutation in the gene that encodes C3. Other breeds predisposed to ICGN triggers are German Shepherd Dogs (*Ehrlichia canis*, or this may be minimal change disease), American Foxhounds (leishmaniosis), Basenjis (IBD), and Dobermanns (sulphonamides) (Littman, 2011). It is possible that SCWT with IBD/PLE have ICGN (dogs with PLE/PLN had higher UPC and earlier onset on average than SCWT with PLN but without PLE). It is theorized that inflammatory disease or immune complexes from food or flora may contribute to incite PLN in SCWT dogs that are heterozygous for the PLN-associated variant alleles, but this needs more study (Vaden *et al.*, 2013).

Other inherited glomerulopathies

There are many other breeds with glomerulopathies (see Figure 14.1), including Beagle, Bullmastiff, Dobermann, French Mastiff, Miniature Schnauzer, Greyhound and others (Littman, 2011), that need more research to understand the inheritance, genetic basis and/or environmental triggers. In the future, a variety of mutations may be found in candidate genes (which cause PLN in humans), such as *NPHS1*, *NPHS2* (podocin), *NPHS3*, *Neph1-3* complex, *ACTN4* (alpha-actinin 4), *ADCK4*, *CD2AP*, *INF2*, *TRPC6*, *MYO1E*, *WT1*, *LAMB2*, *MYH9* and *CUBN* (cubilin). Recently cubilin (*CUBN*) defects (AR) were found in Border Collies and Beagles, associated with a selective intestinal cobalamin malabsorption and chronic mild non-progressive proteinuria (Owczarek-Lipska *et al.*, 2013; Drögemüller *et al.*, 2014; Fyfe *et al.*, 2014). Young related Abyssinian cats in Australia were found to have a proliferative glomerulopathy with haematuria, proteinuria and possible nephrotic syndrome (White *et al.*, 2008).

Inherited nephropathies (whole kidney/whole nephron)

Depending on the severity of diminished renal reserve, inherited whole nephron abnormalities may present with isosthenuria (PU/PD is the earliest sign) and, if progressive, with further changes of CKD (e.g. lethargy, anorexia, weight loss, vomiting/diarrhoea, possible hypertension, azotaemia, non-regenerative anaemia, hyperphosphataemia) (see Chapters 4, 10–12, 23 and www.iris-kidney.com/ for staging and treatments for CKD). Proteinuria (if present) is usually not severe. The kidneys may be small (e.g. with JRD), enlarged (e.g. polycystic) or missing (unilateral renal agenesis).

Renal agenesis

Breeds predisposed to congenital unilateral renal agenesis include the Beagle, King Charles Cavalier Spaniel, Dobermann, Pekingese and Shetland Sheepdog. Of course, bilateral renal agenesis is lethal. Dogs born with one kidney may live a full life, however with 50% renal reserve they are more vulnerable if additional insults occur, such as infection, trauma or ureteral obstruction.

Juvenile renal disease

Inherited defects as well as acquired insults (e.g. toxin, infection, dehydration) may interfere with normal development of the kidney, *in utero* or during the first 3 months of life, causing juvenile renal disease (JRD) (also referred to as renal dysplasia) in one or more puppies in a litter, which may progress eventually to CKD with similar clinical signs and changes on blood, urine and histopathological results. Abnormal differentiation is seen microscopically as persistent fetal (immature) glomeruli, persistent metanephric ducts, and fetal mesenchyme, often distributed within radial bands near more normal tissue. Secondary changes include cystic glomerular atrophy, compensatory hypertrophy and tubulointerstitial nephritis/fibrosis, among other findings. Dogs with JRD are predisposed to pyelonephritis. A severely affected puppy shows PU/PD, poor growth, signs of CKD, and possibly 'rubber jaw' due to renal hyperparathyroidism during growth and lack of mandibular ossification. A wedge biopsy of renal cortical tissue is preferred, so as not to miss the radial band distribution, and in order to count enough glomeruli (100) to get a sense of the true percentage of immature glomeruli present (see Chapter 13 for information on obtaining renal biopsy samples). Specimens obtained after 16 weeks of age normally do not show persistent fetal glomeruli. Familial JRD is mostly seen in the Lhasa Apso, Shih Tzu and SCWT breeds but has also been described in the Alaskan Malamute, Chow Chow, Dutch Kooiker (Dutch Decoy) Dog, Golden Retriever, Miniature Schnauzer, Standard Poodle and others. The mode of inheritance in the Shih Tzu appears to be autosomal dominant with incomplete penetrance, or complex. Dogs are variably affected, so that some puppies present in ESRD at <6 months of age (with fetal glomeruli of 25% or more), while others present at <1–3 years (10–25%), and still others may live well past 5 years (fetal glomeruli 10% or less). Among 74 random Shih Tzu renal biopsy samples, 52% had 1–5% fetal glomeruli, 20% had 6–15% fetal glomeruli, 12% had >15% fetal glomeruli and only 16% were free of any histological evidence of the disease (Bovee, 2003). The kidneys may be small radiographically, with thin cortical areas ultrasonographically. Although a variant allele of a COX-2 promoter was proposed as the cause of JRD in (all) dogs, the study design and conclusions were later questioned (Whiteley *et al.*, 2011) and ultimately refuted in a later study (Safra *et al.*, 2015). Another theory is that the variant allele influences phenotypic expression when accompanied by epigenetic hypermethylation effects (Whiteley, 2014). A DNA test (www.dogenes.com) is available for the variant allele (for multiple breeds) but is not widely accepted or recommended at this time. When the puzzle of JRD is unravelled, there may be one or more causes, with dogs of common ancestry having a similar defect (e.g. Lhasa Apso and Shih Tzu), while other breeds may have different mutations causing the same phenotype, requiring a specific DNA test for each.

Familial JRD in Boxer and Gordon Setter dogs (Littman, 2011) appears to be due to segmental renal hypoplasia, reflux nephropathy during development, and chronic atrophic non-obstructive pyelonephritis caused by vesicoureteral reflux. Presentation is generally at ≤5 years of age with signs of CKD and possibly mild to moderate proteinuria.

Polycystic kidney disease

Feline autosomal dominant forms of polycystic kidney disease (PCKD) are seen mostly in Persian, Himalayan, British Longhaired, British Shorthaired, Exotic Shorthaired and Scottish Fold cats, and their crossbreeds. Breeds with lower (moderate) risk include Asian, Birman, Mombay, Burmilla, Cornish Rex, Devon Rex, Ragdoll, Snowshoe and Tiffanie cats; those with still lower risk include Abyssinian, Angora, Balinese, Bengal, Burmese, Chartreux, Egyptian Mau, Korat, Maine Coon, Norwegian Forest, Ocicat, Oriental Longhaired, Oriental Shorthaired, Russian Blue, Siamese, Singapura, Somali, Tonkinese and Turkish Van cats. In Europe, mutation frequencies in each breed have declined since 2006 (Exotic Shorthaired 17% and Persian 15%, down from 37–50%; Selkirk Rex 5%, Ragdoll 3% and Scottish Fold 1%, down from 12%) (www.antagen.com). The underlying mutation in most affected cats is a non-synonymous SNP in the *PKD1* gene, changing C to A in exon 29 (c.10063C>A), which leads to a stop codon (Lyons *et al.*, 2004). Maine Coon cats appear to have a different, as yet unknown, mutation (Gendron *et al.*, 2013).

In dogs, PCKD is seen in Bull Terriers, Cairn Terriers and West Highland White Terriers (WHWT). In affected Bull

Terriers, a non-synonymous SNP in the *PKD1* gene (c. 9772G>A) changes just one highly conserved amino acid in the encoded protein polycystin-1 (from glycine to lysine), which is predicted to be pathogenic by PolyPhen 2 analysis, altering binding or localization of the protein (Gharahkhani *et al.*, 2011). Polycystin-1 is a renal tubule membrane glycoprotein, necessary for epithelial cell proliferation and differentiation. With abnormal or absent polycystin-1, tubules remodel, forming cysts in the kidney, and 6–68% of affected dogs also have hepatic cysts.

Cats with PCKD may have few or many renal cysts and may give rise to offspring with a variable number of cysts (variable penetrance, homozygous lethal). Clinical severity is also variable, with onset of CKD in early to late adulthood (mean 7 years, range 2–10 years). Multiple large renal cysts cause compression of the parenchyma and progressive loss of renal reserve. Affected cats and Bull Terriers usually present with signs of CKD in middle to old age, while Cairn Terriers and WHWT forms of PCKD are autosomal recessive, presenting early (5–6 weeks of age), and also show hepatic cysts (Lees, 2011).

Ultrasonography may allow visualization of renal cysts at 10 months of age (before breeding), but the technique is expensive, requires experience, and is only 91% sensitive (not a guarantee of normality if cysts are not seen; Scherk, 2014). For Bull Terriers and for most affected cat breeds (except Maine Coon cats) there are DNA tests available (see Figure 14.1). If the allele frequency is high in a breed, it may be unwise to remove all carriers too fast. A negative registry helps breeders to choose mates carefully (International Cat Care PKD Negative Register at icatcare.org/breeders/registers/PKD).

Other whole kidney defects

An autosomal dominant form of neoplasia, multiple renal cystadenocarcinomas and nodular dermatofibrosis, was identified in German Shepherd Dogs, due to a mutation in exon 7 of the canine *BHD* gene (Birt–Hogg–Dubé locus), changing a highly conserved amino acid in the encoded protein folliculin: *FLCN* c.764A>G (Lingaas *et al.*, 2003). Homozygous positive status is lethal in the embryo. Renal telangiectasia in Pembroke Welsh Corgis (presenting at 2–8 years of age) is associated with haematuria, abdominal pain, dysuria, and sometimes ureteral obstruction with clots or calculi. Renal and ureteral duplication have been seen in English Bulldogs.

Inherited tubular disorders

Tubular diseases, whether inherited or acquired, often present with PU/PD because of osmotic diuresis due to a decreased ability to reabsorb solute, for example bicarbonate, glucose or amino acids. Decreased ability to concentrate the urine may or may not be a sign of decreased renal reserve. Other presentations which may have a genetic basis include urolithiasis due to cystinuria, hyperuricosuria, xanthinuria and hyperoxaluria, among others. Stones may cause clinical signs depending on their location (kidney, ureter, bladder, urethra). See Chapters 26 and 27 for management protocols of metabolic urolithiasis.

Fanconi syndrome

Approximately 10% of Basenji dogs are affected with Fanconi syndrome, with multiple renal tubular reabsorptive abnormalities for sodium bicarbonate, phosphate, uric acid, glucose, amino acids and small molecular weight proteins. Metabolic acidosis, wasting from nutrient loss and eventually CKD lead to signs of illness. Dogs treated according to the Gonto protocol with aggressive bicarbonate therapy and other supplements often survive into geriatric years (Yearley *et al.*, 2004; www.basenji.org/ClubDocs/Fanconi-Protocol-2015.pdf). Urine metabolic screening is helpful for acquired or genetic Fanconi syndrome. Fanconi syndrome may also be seen with JRD, e.g. in Border Terriers, or may be acquired, for example from jerky treat renal toxicity (Thompson *et al.*, 2013). A DNA test is available for Basenjis, which have an autosomal recessive form of Fanconi syndrome, due to a 321 bp deletion in the gene *FAN1* (Farias, 2011; Johnson *et al.*, 2012). Lack of function of the *FAN1*-encoded protein causes subnormal mitochondrial DNA repair so that proximal tubular cells may be hypersensitive to low levels of heavy metals such as cadmium. The variable age of onset may be due to differential exposure to environmental toxins (Farias, 2011). In Labrador Retrievers, and perhaps other breeds that are predisposed to chronic active hepatitis, a renal tubular transport defect may be associated with copper-associated hepatitis (Langlois *et al.*, 2013) and heavy metal (copper) effects on the tubules.

Cystinuria

A genetic defect that causes decreased tubular reabsorption of cysteine and the dibasic amino acids ornithine, lysine, and arginine (COLA) often results in cystine urolithiasis because of its low solubility (Bannasch and Henthorn, 2009; Brons *et al.*, 2013). More than 70 breeds have been identified with cystinuria, including the Australian Cattle Dog, Australian Shepherd, Basenji, Bassett Hound, Bullmastiff, Chihuahua, Dachshund, English Bulldog, French Bulldog, Irish Terrier, Mastiff, Miniature Pinscher, Newfoundland, Scottish Deerhound, Scottish Terrier, Staffordshire Terrier and Welsh Corgi. Different mutations causing this phenotype have been found in different breeds, mostly involving the same candidate genes that cause cystinuria in humans, i.e. *SLC3A1* or *SLC7A9*. In humans, >170 mutations in *SLC3A1* alone have been identified. Labrador and Newfoundland/Landseer male dogs may show uroliths as early as 6 months of age, whereas bitches only occasionally present because of stones. Autosomal recessive inheritance is seen in Newfoundland/Landseer dogs with a point mutation in *SLC3A1* (c.586C>T) and in Labrador Retrievers with a frame-shift mutation in *SLC3A1* (c.350delG) causing a nonsense mutation in exon 2, a premature stop codon, and a severely truncated protein of 197 instead of the normal 700 amino acids. The current mutation frequency in Europe for Landseers is 26% (www.antagene.com). Autosomal dominant inheritance is seen in the Australian Cattle Dog with a 6 bp deletion (c.1095_1100del) which removes two threonines in *SLC3A1*, with a more severe phenotype in homozygous than in heterozygous dogs, and in Miniature Pinschers with a missense mutation in *SLC7A9* (c.964G>A), with only heterozygotes presented (homozygous status is lethal). Some breed-specific DNA tests have been developed. The genetic cause for cystinuria has not been found yet for some breeds which show androgen-dependent cystinuria (Mastiff, Scottish Deerhound and Irish Terrier). In this sex-limited inheritance, only intact adult males show cystinuria, and castration is reported to be curative. A linked marker test is available for Mastiffs (Henthorn, personal communication) at the

University of Pennsylvania School of Veterinary Medicine, but more study is needed to find the causative mutation (possibly in *SLC3A1*). The Scottish Deerhound and Irish Terrier defects may or may not be the same as one another, but they do not appear to be the same as that of the Mastiff.

For cystinuric French and English Bulldog breeds, mutations were found in *SLC3A1* (c.574A>G, c.2091A>G) and *SLC7A9* (c.649G>A), affecting non-conserved amino acids, therefore these may be linked markers and not causative (Harnevik *et al.*, 2006). The authors suspect that regulatory or other genes may be involved.

Recently, a cystinuric cat was found to have a missense mutation in *SLC3A1* (c.1342C>T) changing a single highly conserved amino acid (p.Arg448Trp) in the rBAT protein encoded by the *SLC3A1* gene (Mizukami *et al.*, 2015).

Many breeds appear to have mild cystinuria. For breeds without a DNA test, a urine nitroprusside test can be used to assess the dog for increased cystine excretion; however, false-negative results for cystinuria may be due to precipitation, therefore quantitation of urinary ornithine, lysine and arginine, detecting COLA tubular transport abnormalities, is helpful.

Hyperuricosuria

As opposed to inherited cystinuria, where almost every affected breed may have a different mutation and require a specific DNA test, a common variant allele has been associated with a uric acid transporter defect in the liver and kidney, causing hyperuricosuria in many breeds, i.e. *SLC2A9* c.616G>T (Bannasch *et al.*, 2008; Bannasch and Henthorn, 2009; Karmi *et al.*, 2010ab). All Dalmatians are homozygous for this autosomal recessive trait, but not all develop urate urolithiasis. The 'LUA' (low uric acid) Dalmatians, recently recognized by the AKC, were bred by crossing a female Dalmatian with a male Pointer in 1973 (Schaible RS, http://luadalmatians-world.com/word-press/about-lua/), then backcrossing LUA dogs with Dalmatians in each generation. Many laboratories now test for the trait, which appears to be linked to larger spot size.

Many breeds are affected with hyperuricosuria; estimated carrier rates are: Weimaraners 25.4%, Large Munsterlander (Large Munster Spaniel) 23.7%, South African Boerboel 19.75%, Giant Schnauzers 11.2%, Parson Russell Terrier 7.75%, Australian Shepherd 3.46%, American Staffordshire Terrier 3.17%, German Shepherd Dog 2.6%, Pomeranian 1.13% and Labrador Retriever 0.26% (Karmi *et al.*, 2010a). In Europe, the current mutation frequency for Bulldogs and Weimaraners is 35% (www.antagene.com). All types of Bulldog (American, English, French), Black Russian Terrier, German Spitz and Jack Russell Terrier breeds are also recommended for testing if clinically indicated.

Urate urolithiasis may also be seen in breeds predisposed to liver disease (portosystemic shunts, e.g. Yorkshire Terrier, Miniature Schnauzer; chronic active hepatitis, e.g. Dobermann, Labrador Retriever, Cocker Spaniel).

Xanthinuria

Xanthinuria and xanthine urolithiasis may be seen in dogs treated with allopurinol as prevention for urate urolithiasis. Genetic xanthinuria and stone formation in a family of Cavalier King Charles Spaniels showed autosomal recessive inheritance (van Zuilen *et al.*, 1997).

Hyperoxaluria

A DNA test for a point mutation in the alanine glyoxylate aminotransferase gene which changes a conserved amino acid residue (*AGXT* c.996G>A) is available for the autosomal recessively inherited trait that affected seven Coton de Tulear puppies of four unrelated litters with primary hyperoxaluria (PH1), extensive renal oxalate crystal deposition and tubular necrosis at 3–4 weeks of age; the carrier rate among Finnish Coton de Tulear was 8.5% (Vidgren *et al.*, 2012). Autosomal recessive primary hyperoxaluria (PH2) affecting kittens in a colony was associated with a point mutation (G>A) in the acceptor site of intron 4 of the glyoxylate reductase gene *GRHPR*, causing misplicing of exon 5, an abnormally shortened mRNA protein and 119 amino acids missing in glyoxylate reductase (Goldstein *et al.*, 2009).

Breeds predisposed to hyperadrenocorticism are predisposed to calcium oxalate urolithiasis because of hypercalciuria, and to struvite urolithiasis due to predisposition for urinary tract infection, e.g. Miniature Poodles, Bichon Frise, Dachshunds.

Glycosuria

Scottish Terriers and Norwegian Elkhounds may show glycosuria due to a decreased Tm (tubular maximum), i.e. deficient tubular transport for reabsorption of glucose, but the underlying genetic basis is unknown.

Other urolithiasis predispositions

Six dogs with 2,8-dihydroxyadenine urolithiasis (five Native American Indian Dogs and one mixed breed) showed a point mutation in a highly conserved codon in the adenine phosphoribosyltransferase gene (*APRT* c.260G>A) (Furrow *et al.*, 2014).

Lower urinary tract disorders

Inherited lower urinary tract disorders may underlie urinary incontinence, urinary tract infection, or even bladder cancer (Bartges and Kruger, 2011). Breeds predisposed to ectopic ureter include the Border Terrier, Briard, English Bulldog, Entlebucher Mountain Dog (EMD), Fox Terrier, Golden Retriever, Griffon, Labrador Retriever, Miniature and Toy Poodles, Newfoundland, Siberian Husky, Skye Terrier and WHWT (Reichler *et al.*, 2012; Fritsche *et al.*, 2014). In a large study of 552 EMD dogs, only 32.9% were normal; 47.3% had at least one intravesicular and 19.8% had at least one extravesicular ectopic termination. Interestingly, males were more often affected than females. In EMD there appears to be a complex mode of inheritance involving several genes for ectopia as well as a major gene associated with extravesicular termination (Fritsche *et al.*, 2014). Other lower urinary tract disorders have breed predispositions, and include urinary incontinence in large-breed dogs, especially Dobermanns (Lane, 2003), possibly due to intrapelvic bladder/short urethra conformation, urethrorectal fistula (English Bulldog, Miniature Poodle), urethroperineal fistula (Miniature Poodle), male urethral prolapse (Boston Terrier, English Bulldog), urethral duplication (English Bulldog, Miniature Poodle) and hypospadias (Boston Terrier, Dalmatian). Male Miniature Schnauzers with persistent Muellerian duct syndrome (PMDS) have a SNP causing a premature stop codon in the MIS Type II receptor gene, aka *AMHR2* (Wu *et al.*, 2009). The mode of inheritance is autosomal recessive but sex-limited, so only males are affected; about 50% show cryptorchidism and some even develop pyometra in their uterus masculinus. The carrier rate appears high (7/20 samples submitted) and occurs worldwide (www.optigen.com).

Breeds predisposed to transitional cell carcinoma of the bladder include Scottish Terriers, Beagles, Shetland Sheepdogs, Wire-Haired Fox Terriers and WHWT (Mutsaers *et al.*, 2003); in Scottish Terriers the risk may be increased by herbicide exposure or decreased by vegetable consumption (Glickman *et al.*, 2004; Raghaven *et al.*, 2005).

DNA testing and genetic counselling

Samples for DNA testing can be whole blood (0.5–1 ml in EDTA), buccal swabs (cytology brushes), semen or cellular tissue. For buccal swabs, care is needed to avoid oral contamination with another animal's DNA (e.g. dam's milk, saliva, coprophagia, shared bowls, toys, chews), by at least 3 hours' separation. Air-dried swabs are easily mailed to testing laboratories. Blood or semen should arrive at room temperature or chilled, and packaged to prevent leakage or breakage in transit. Cellular tissue should be sent frozen with ice packs overnight. Figure 14.2 lists testing laboratories.

Genetic counselling helps conscientious breeders avoid familial diseases in their lines while perpetuating good qualities and genetic diversity. Because modes of inheritance may be dominant or complex, mixed-breed dogs and their families are also at risk. Recessive traits may appear in backcrosses, for instance in 'doodles'. With new genomic technology, many more specific DNA tests for inherited diseases will become available in the next decade. High-throughput screening tests may someday become available (e.g. for candidate genes of human PLN) but such panels must be developed for each species. Clinicians should monitor websites for continued updates (www.wsava.org/HereditaryDefects.htm) on breed-associated problems for which genetic tests can be used on breeding individuals to choose the best mating pair, in order to avoid producing offspring that will carry at-risk variant alleles. If a trait is dominant and variant allele frequency is low, not breeding from the carriers is advised, whereas if a trait is recessive or complex, or if the variant allele frequency is relatively high, a homozygous positive or heterozygous individual may be bred to a homozygous negative one, thereby decreasing the variant allele frequency over time. If the variant allele frequency is high in the population, excluding all carriers would leave too few animals to breed, and loss of genetic diversity may cause new genetic problems to emerge. Testing individuals for their carrier status not only helps in choosing mating pairs, but may help detect animals at-risk so that early monitoring and interventions can be started at a time when it may be most beneficial.

Animal Genetics Inc. 1336 Timberlane Rd Tallahassee, FL 32312 United States www.animalgenetics.us/ contact@animalgenetics.us	Animal Health Trust (UK) Lanwades Park, Kentford, Newmarket Suffolk CB8 7UU United Kingdom www.aht.org.uk info@aht.org.uk	Animal Molecular Genetics Lab University of Missouri 321 Connaway Hall Columbia, MO 65211-5120 United States www.caninegeneticdiseases.net/ HansenL@missouri.edu
Antagene CS60001 La Tour de Salvagny 69890 France www.antagene.com/ contact@antagene.com	Baker Institute for Animal Health Hungerford Hill Road Ithaca, NY 14853 United States http://bakerinstitute.vet.cornell.edu/faculty/page.php?id=206 vnm1@cornell.edu	Genetic Technologies Ltd 60–66 Hanover Street Fitzroy Vic 3065 Australia www.animalnetwork.com.au/dnatesting/ askus@animalnetwork.com.au
Genindexe 6, rue de sports La Rochelle 17000 France www.genindexe.com/uk/index.php contact@genindexe.com	Genomia s.r.o Janackova 51 32300 Plen, Czech Republic www.genomia.cz/en/ laborator@genomia.cz	HealthGene 2175 Keele Street Toronto, ON M6M 3Z4 Canada www.healthgene.com info@healthgene.com
Laboklin Steubenstraße 4 Post box 1810 Bad Kissingen D-97688 Germany www.laboklin.de/ info@laboklin.de	Laboratorio Genefast Via Castelfranco 17/d Bazzano (BO) 40053 Italy www.genefast.com/ info@genefast.com	Michigan State University – Fyfe 2209 Biomed & Physical Sciences, 567 Wilson Rd. East Lansing, MI 48824 United States www.mmg.msu.edu/fyfe.html fyfe@cvm.msu.edu
Optigen 767 Warren Road, Suite 300 Ithaca, NY 14850 United States www.optigen.com/ genetest@optigen.com	Orivet Genetic Pet Care PO Box 110 St. Kilda 3182 VIC Australia www.orivet.com.au admin@orivet.com.au	Paw Print Genetics 850 E Spokane Falls Blvd, Suite 200 Spokane, WA 99202 United States www.pawprintgenetics.com AskUs@pawprintgenetics.com
PennGen 3900 Delancey Street, Room 4013 Philadelphia, PA 19104 United States http://research.vet.upenn.edu/penngen PennGen@vet.upenn.edu	UC-Davis – Veterinary Genetics Laboratory One Shields Avenue Davis, CA 95617-1102 United States www.vgl.ucdavis.edu custserv@vgl.ucdavis.edu	VetGen 3728 Plaza Drive, Suite 1 Ann Arbor, MI 48108 United States www.vetgen.com/ vetgen@vetgen.com
Vetogene Viale ortles 22/4 Milano 20134 Italy www.vetogene.com info@vetogene.com, michele.polli@unimi.it	Vetnostic Laboratories 2439 Kuser Road Hamilton Township, NJ 08690 United States www.vetnostic.com/index.php?route=common/home rmason@mdlab.com	

14.2 Laboratories offering genetic testing.

Future directions

In humans, next-generation sequencing and targeted exome sequencing are comprehensive panels that can find novel mutations arising in an individual family. At least 37 candidate genes are associated with PLN (Alport syndrome and FSGS) and at least 292 genes are associated with kidney malformations. Such platforms are species-specific so canine/feline platforms need development to capture DNA of exons for full sequencing and evaluation. In addition to helping the individual and the breed, finding genetic bases for disease in dogs and cats may help unravel the mechanisms of complex genetic and environmental interactions. These models are biologically relevant, exposed to similar environments, and prone to the same comorbidities as humans. This is an exciting time for discovery of the underlying molecular basis for diseases, for careful prevention with genetic counselling, and understanding of the underlying pathogenesis so as to choose more specific treatment regimens.

References and further reading

NB: Many classic references are not listed here but are found elsewhere (Lees, 2011; Littman, 2011).

ACVIM (2013) Special Issue: International Renal Interest Society Consensus Clinical Practice Guidelines for Glomerular Disease in Dogs. *Journal of Veterinary Internal Medicine* **27**, S1–75

Bannasch D and Henthorn PS (2009) Changing paradigms in diagnosis of inherited defects associated with urolithiasis. *Veterinary Clinics of North America: Small Animal Practice* **39**, 111–125

Bannasch D, Safra N, Young A *et al.* (2008) Mutations in the *SLC2A9* gene cause hyperuricosuria and hyperuricemia in the dog. *PLoS Genetics* **4**, e1000246

Bartges J and Kruger JM (2011) Congenital diseases of the lower urinary tract. In: *Nephrology and Urology of Small Animals*, ed. J Bartges and DJ Polzin, pp. 809–817. Wiley-Blackwell, Ames

Bovee KC (2003) Renal dysplasia in Shih Tzu dogs. *WSAVA Congress.* Available from www.vin.com/apputil/content/defaultadv1.aspx?meta=Generic&pId=8768&id=3850168

Brons AK, Henthorn PS, Raj K *et al.* (2013) *SLC3A1* and *SLC7A9* mutations in autosomal recessive or dominant canine cystinuria: a new classification system. *Journal of Veterinary Internal Medicine* **27**, 1400–1408

Chew DJ, DiBartola SP and Schenck PA (2011) Familial renal diseases in dogs and cats. In: *Canine and Feline Nephrology and Urology, 2nd edn*, ed. DJ Chew, SP DiBartola and PA Schenck, pp. 197–217. Elsevier, St. Louis

Cianciolo RE, Brown CA, Mohr FC *et al.* (2013) Pathologic evaluation of canine renal biopsies: Methods for identifying features that differentiate immune-mediated glomerulonephritides from other categories of glomerular diseases. *Journal of Veterinary Internal Medicine* **27**, S10–S18

Darrigrand-Haag RA, Center SA, Randolph JF *et al.* (1996) Congenital Fanconi syndrome associated with renal dysplasia in 2 Border Terriers. *Journal of Veterinary Internal Medicine* **10**, 412–419

Davidson AP and Westropp JL (2014) Diagnosis and management of urinary ectopia. *Veterinary Clinics of North America: Small Animal Practice* **44**, 343–353

Drögemüller M, Jagannathan V, Howard J *et al.* (2014) A frameshift mutation in the cubilin gene (*CUBN*) in Beagles with Imerslund–Gräsbeck syndrome (selective cobalamin malabsorption). *Animal Genetics* **45**, 148–150

Farias FHG (2011) Molecular genetic studies of canine inherited diseases [dissertation]. Available from https://mospace.umsystem.edu/xmlui/bitstream/handle/10355/14514/research.pdf?sequence=2

Fritsche R, Dolf G, Schelling C *et al.* (2014) Inheritance of ectopic ureters in Entlebucher Mountain Dogs. *Journal of Animal Breeding and Genetics* **131**, 146–152

Furrow E, Pfeifer RJ, Osborne CA *et al.* (2014) An *APRT* mutation is strongly associated with and likely causative for 2,8-dihydroxyadenine urolithiasis in dogs. *Molecular Genetics and Metabolism* **111**, 399–403

Fyfe JC, Hemker SL, Venta PJ *et al.* (2014) Selective intestinal cobalamin malabsorption with proteinuria (Imerslund–Gräsbeck syndrome) in juvenile Beagles. *Journal of Veterinary Internal Medicine* **28**, 356–362

Gendron K, Owczarek-Lipska M, Lang J *et al.* (2013) Maine Coon renal screening: ultrasonographical characterisation and preliminary genetic analysis for common genes in cats with renal cysts. *Journal of Feline Medicine and Surgery* **15**, 1079–1085

Gharahkhani P, O'Leary CA, Kyaw-Tanner M *et al.* (2011) A non-synonymous mutation in the canine *Pkd1* gene is associated with autosomal dominant polycystic kidney disease in Bull Terriers. *PLoS One* **6**, e22455

Giger U, Brons AK, Fitzgerald CA *et al.* (2014) Updates on cystinuria and Fanconi syndrome: Aminoacidurias in dogs. *Proceedings ACVIM.* Available from www.vin.com/members/proceedings/proceedings.plx?CID=ACVIM2014&PID=92815&O=VIN

Glickman LT, Raghavan M, Knapp DW *et al.* (2004) Herbicide exposure and the risk of transitional cell carcinoma of the urinary bladder in Scottish Terriers. *Journal of the American Veterinary Medicine Association* **224**, 1290–1297

Goldstein R, Narala S, Sabet N *et al.* (2009) Primary hyperoxaluria in cats caused by a mutation in the feline *GRHPR* gene. *Journal of Heredity* **100**, S2–S7

Harnevik L, Hoppe A and Söderkvist P (2006) *SLC7A9* cDNA cloning and mutational analysis of *SLC3A1* and *SLC7A9* in canine cystinuria. *Mammalian Genome* **17**, 769–776

Henthorn PS and Giger U (2013) Unraveling the phenotypic and genetic complexity of canine cystinuria. *Proceedings 6th Tufts' Canine and Feline Breeding and Genetics Conference.* Available from www.vin.com/members/proceedings/proceedings.plx?CID=TUFTSBG2013&PID=90667&O=VIN

Henthorn PS, Liu J, Gidalevich T *et al.* (2000) Canine cystinuria: polymorphism in the canine *SLC3A1* gene and identification of a nonsense mutation in cystinuric Newfoundland dogs. *Human Genetics* **107**, 295–303

Johnson GS, Farias FH, Mhlanga-Mutangadura T *et al.* (2012) Whole genome sequencing reveals a deletion of the last exon of *FAN1* in Basenji dogs with adult-onset Fanconi syndrome [abstract]. *63rd Annual Meeting of the American Society of Human Genetics, San Francisco, California*

Karmi N, Brown EA, Hughes SS *et al.* (2010a) Estimated frequency of the canine hyperuricosuria mutation in different dog breeds. *Journal of Veterinary Internal Medicine* **24**, 1337–1342

Karmi N, Safra N, Young A *et al.* (2010b) Validation of a urine test and characterization of the putative genetic mutation for hyperuricosuria in Bulldogs and Black Russian Terriers. *American Journal of Veterinary Research* **71**, 909–914

Lane IF (2003) Outcomes in urinary incontinence: maximizing response. *ACVIM Forum.* Available from www.vin.com/members/cms/project/defaultadv1.aspx?id=3847900&pid=8874&catid=&

Langlois DK, Smedley RC, Schall WD *et al.* (2013) Acquired proximal renal tubular dysfunction in 9 Labrador Retrievers with copper-associated hepatitis (2006–2012). *Journal of Veterinary Internal Medicine* **27**, 491–499

Lees GE (2011) Congenital kidney diseases. In: *Nephrology and Urology of Small Animals*, ed. J Bartges and DJ Polzin, pp. 568–576. Wiley-Blackwell, Ames

Lees GE (2013) Kidney diseases caused by glomerular basement membrane type IV collagen defects in dogs. *Journal of Veterinary Emergency and Critical Care* **23**, 184–193

Lingaas F, Comstock KE, Kirkness EF *et al.* (2003) A mutation in the canine *BHD* gene is associated with hereditary multifocal renal cystadenocarcinoma and nodular dermatofibrosis in the German Shepherd Dog. *Human Molecular Genetics* **12**, 3043–3053

Littman MP (2011) Protein-losing nephropathy in small animals. *Veterinary Clinics of North America: Small Animal Practice* **41**, 31–62

Littman MP (2013) State-of-the-Art-Review: Lyme nephritis. *Journal of Veterinary Emergency and Critical Care* **23**, 163–173

Littman MP, Dambach DM, Vaden SL *et al.* (2000) Familial protein-losing enteropathy and protein-losing nephropathy in Soft Coated Wheaten Terriers: 222 cases (1983–1997). *Journal of Veterinary Internal Medicine* **14**, 68–80

Littman MP, Daminet S, Grauer GF *et al.* (2013a) Consensus recommendations for the diagnostic investigation of dogs with suspected glomerular disease. *Journal of Veterinary Internal Medicine* **27**, S19–S26

Littman MP, Raducha MG and Henthorn PS (2013b) Prevalence of variant alleles associated with protein-losing nephropathy in Soft Coated Wheaten Terriers [abstract]. *Journal of Veterinary Internal Medicine* **27**, 736

Littman MP, Raducha MG and Henthorn PS (2014) Prevalence of variant alleles associated with protein-losing nephropathy in Airedale Terriers [abstract]. *Journal of Veterinary Internal Medicine* **28**, 1366–1367

Littman MP, Wiley CA, Raducha MG *et al.* (2013c) Glomerulopathy and mutations in *NPHS1* and *KIRREL2* in Soft Coated Wheaten Terrier dogs. *Mammalian Genome* **24**, 119–126

Lyons LA, Biller DS, Erdman CA *et al.* (2004) Feline polycystic kidney disease mutation identified in *PKD1*. *Journal of the American Society of Nephrology* **15**, 2548–2555

Matos AJ, Mascarenhas C, Magalhaes P *et al.* (2006) Efficient screening of the cystinuria-related C663T *Slc3a1* nonsense mutation in Newfoundland dogs by denaturing high-performance liquid chromatography. *Journal of Veterinary Diagnostic Investigation* **18**, 102–105

Mizukami K, Raj K and Giger U (2015) Feline cystinuria caused by a missense mutation in the *SLC3A1* gene. *Journal of Veterinary Internal Medicine* **29**, 120–125

Mutsaers AJ, Widmer WR and Knapp DW (2003) Canine transitional cell carcinoma. *Journal of Veterinary Internal Medicine* **17**, 136–144

Olsson M, Meadows JRS, Truvé K *et al.* (2011) A novel unstable duplication upstream of *HAS2* predisposes to a breed-defining skin phenotype and a periodic fever syndrome in Chinese Shar-Pei dogs. *PLoS Genetics* **7**, e1001332

Owczarek-Lipska M, Jagannathan V, Drögemüller C *et al.* (2013) A frameshift mutation in the cubilin gene (*CUBN*) in Border Collies with Imerslund–Gräsbeck Syndrome (selective cobalamin malabsorption). *PLoS One* **8**, e61144

Raghavan M, Knapp DW, Bonney PL *et al.* (2005) Evaluation of the effect of dietary vegetable consumption on reducing risk of transitional cell carcinoma of the urinary bladder in Scottish Terriers. *Journal of the American Veterinary Medical Association* **227**, 94–100

Reichler IM, Specker CE, Hubler M *et al.* (2012) Ectopic ureters in dogs: Clinical features, surgical techniques and outcome. *Veterinary Surgery* **41**, 515–522

Rørtveit R, Eggertsdóttir AV, Thomassen R *et al.* (2013) A clinical study of canine collagen type III glomerulopathy. *BMC Veterinary Research* **9**, e218

Rørtveit R, Lingaas F, Bønsdorff T *et al.* (2012) A canine autosomal recessive model of collagen type III glomerulopathy. *Laboratory Investigation* **92**, 1483–1491

Safra N, Hayward LJ, Aguilar M *et al.* (2015) DNA sequence variants in the five prime untranslated region of the cyclooxygenase-2 gene are commonly found in healthy dogs and gray wolves. *PLoS One* **10**, e0133127

Scherk M (2014) Feline polycystic kidney disease. *Clinician's Brief* **12**, 79–82

Segev G, Cowgill LD, Jessen S *et al.* (2012) Renal amyloidosis in dogs: a retrospective study of 91 cases with comparison of the disease between Shar-Pei and non-Shar-Pei dogs. *Journal of Veterinary Internal Medicine* **26**, 259–268

Thompson MF, Fleeman LM, Kessell AE *et al.* (2013) Acquired proximal renal tubulopathy in dogs exposed to a common dried chicken treat: retrospective study of 108 cases (2007–2009). *Australian Veterinary Journal* **91**, 368–373

Vaden SL, Littman MP and Cianciolo RE (2013) Familial renal disease in Soft Coated Wheaten Terriers. *Journal of Veterinary Emergency and Critical Care* **23**, 174–183

van Zuilen CD, Nickel RF, van Dijk TH *et al.* (1997) Xanthinuria in a family of Cavalier King Charles Spaniels. *Veterinary Quarterly* **19**, 172–174

Vidgren G, Vainio-Siukola K, Honkasalo S *et al.* (2012) Primary hyperoxaluria in Coton de Tulear. *Animal Genetics* **43**, 356–361

White JD, Norris JM, Bosward KL *et al.* (2008) Persistent haematuria and proteinuria due to glomerular disease in related Abyssinian cats. *Journal of Feline Medicine and Surgery* **10**, 219–229

Whiteley MH (2014) Allelic variation in the canine Cox-2 promoter causes hypermethylation of the canine Cox-2 promoter in clinical cases of renal dysplasia. *Clinical Epigenetics* **6**, 7

Whiteley MH, Bell JS and Rothman DA (2011) Novel allelic variants in the canine cyclooxgenase-2 (cox-2) promoter are associated with renal dysplasia in dogs. *PLoS One* **6**, e16684; see also The *PLoS One* Editors (2012) Expression of concern: novel allelic variants in the canine cyclooxgenase-2 (Cox-2) promoter are associated with renal dysplasia in dogs. *PLoS One* **7(11)**, e49703. doi:10.1371/journal.pone.0049703

Wu X, Wan S, Pujar S *et al.* (2009) A single base pair mutation encoding a premature stop codon in the MIS Type II receptor is responsible for canine persistent Muellerian duct syndrome. *Journal of Andrology* **30**, 46–56

Yearley JH, Hancock DD and Mealey KL (2004) Survival time, lifespan, and quality of life in dogs with idiopathic Fanconi syndrome. *Journal of the American Veterinary Medicine Association* **225**, 377–383

Chapter 15

Measurement of blood pressure

Gilad Segev

The time-averaged systemic blood pressure (over 24 hours) is maintained in healthy individuals within a relatively narrow physiological range, which is necessary for adequate tissue perfusion. Blood pressure provides the driving force for blood flow and, without it, circulation and perfusion would cease.

Blood pressure is determined by the cardiac output (which is a product of stroke volume and heart rate) and the systemic vascular resistances, therefore alterations in blood pressure arise from changes in one or both of these parameters. Small changes in the diameter of the arterioles result in large changes in the total peripheral resistance. Blood pressure is regulated by various mechanisms including the autonomic nervous system, feedback from baroreceptors located in the walls of the carotid sinus and the aortic arch, circulating hormones (e.g. renin, angiotensin II, aldosterone, natriuretic peptides), and locally derived vasoconstrictor and vasodilator metabolites affecting microcirculatory autoregulation. Minute by minute variations in blood pressure mediated by the neuronal control mechanisms can lead to marked fluctuations, making its measurement at the veterinary clinic challenging.

Arterial blood pressure values are expressed in terms of systolic blood pressure (blood pressure during ventricular systole), diastolic blood pressure (blood pressure during ventricular diastole) and mean blood pressure. The difference between the systolic and diastolic blood pressure is termed the 'pulse pressure'. Systolic arterial blood pressure is primarily dependent on stroke volume (which, in turn, depends on arteriolar diameter, left ventricular end-diastolic volume and ventricular systolic force of contraction) and arterial compliance, while diastolic blood pressure is dependent on vasomotor tone and heart rate. For example, a very low heart rate increases the systolic arterial pressure by elevating stroke volume, and decreases the diastolic arterial pressure, thereby increasing pulse pressure in two separate ways (and *vice versa*). This translates into strong, if not bounding arterial pulsation, which should not necessarily be interpreted as proof of an effective capillary perfusion pressure, especially if the heart rate is extremely low.

Systemic hypertension is defined as a persistent increase in arterial blood pressure. In human patients, both the systolic and diastolic blood pressures are of clinical significance (Proia *et al.*, 2014), especially because coronary arterial (and therefore myocardial) perfusion pressure depends mostly on diastolic arterial blood pressure values. However, in veterinary medicine, most studies correlate the risk for target-organ damage (TOD) with the systolic blood pressure. In time, as more evidence accumulates, the importance of the diastolic blood pressure in companion animals will become apparent. In that regard, documentation of blood pressure using devices that measure systolic, diastolic and mean blood pressure (e.g. oscillometry) may carry an advantage.

In recent years, the awareness of hypertension and its clinical significance in dogs and cats has increased dramatically and, currently, blood pressure is being measured frequently in veterinary hospitals and practices worldwide. The American College of Veterinary Internal Medicine (ACVIM) Consensus Statement on Hypertension (Brown *et al.*, 2007) defines this as a persistently elevated blood pressure that causes damage. The International Renal Interest Society (IRIS) chronic kidney disease (CKD) staging system has adopted and adapted these definitions (see Chapter 12).

Underlying causes of hypertension

Essential (primary) hypertension is the most common aetiology of hypertension in human patients. In companion animals, however, hypertension is most commonly associated with an underlying disease, although idiopathic (termed 'essential' in human medicine) hypertension has been described (Brown *et al.*, 2007). Thus, when hypertension is documented, a thorough and systematic search for an underlying cause should be performed. Despite the fact that hypertension in companion animals is most commonly secondary to an underlying disease, TOD may be the first indication of such a disease and of the presence of hypertension (Littman, 1994). This is also supported by the lack of a strong correlation between the severity of kidney dysfunction (the most common cause for secondary systemic hypertension) and the severity of hypertension associated with it (Finco, 2004). For example, hypertension may be severe and lead to TOD even when kidney disease is still in its early and even subclinical stages. This observation (which applies to both dogs and cats) suggests that the underlying disease is just one factor determining the severity of hypertension in the individual patient. Other patient factors (diet, environmental factors such as cadmium exposure (Finch *et al.*, 2012) and genetics) must play a role in determining the severity of hypertension.

Nevertheless, acute kidney injury (AKI) and exposure CKD are the most common diseases associated with hypertension in dogs and cats. Hypertension is documented in 20–60% of cats with kidney disease (Kobayashi *et al.*, 1990; Syme *et al.*, 2002) and in up to 93% of dogs with kidney disease; however, there is high variability among studies (Anderson and Fisher, 1968; Michell *et al.*, 1997; Buranakarl *et al.*, 2007). Despite the wide variation in the prevalence of hypertension in dogs and cats with kidney disease, it is well accepted that a blood pressure measurement should be obtained in any dog or cat with AKI or CKD (especially those with suspected glomerular disease). It is also common for hypertension to develop or worsen throughout the disease course, either during hospitalization in AKI patients or between follow-up examinations in CKD patients. Further considerations of hypertension in kidney disease can be found in Chapters 18, 21 and 23.

Other underlying diseases and conditions associated with systemic hypertension should not be overlooked and include hyperthyroidism, diabetes mellitus, hyperaldosteronism, hyperadrenocorticism and phaeochromocytoma. Iatrogenic causes of hypertension should also be considered and include, but are not limited to, excessive fluid administration in patients with kidney disease or the administration of various medications including erythropoietin and erythropoietin-stimulating agents, phenylpropanolamine (PPA) and other alpha agonists, dopamine, glucocorticoids and mineralocorticoids.

Selection of patients for blood pressure evaluation

Hypertension may persist chronically without necessarily being associated with overt clinical signs. Therefore, systemic hypertension is often referred to, in human medicine, as the 'silent killer'. In humans, early symptoms of hypertension may be subjective and include a headache, flushing, anxiety and other subtle and non-specific clinical signs. It is thus plausible that dogs and cats may be presented with non-specific clinical signs which are associated with, but are not attributed to, systemic hypertension. Despite this, there is currently no recommendation to screen all veterinary patients for hypertension, because this is likely to lead to over-diagnosis and treatment due to the so-called 'white coat hypertension' phenomenon. It is controversial, however, whether this also applies to geriatric patients, as there is evidence to suggest that the prevalence of systemic hypertension increases with age (Bodey and Michell, 1996; Bijsmans *et al.*, 2015). Moreover, many of the underlying conditions that predispose to hypertension (e.g. hyperthyroidism, hyperadrenocorticism, CKD) are more prevalent in older animals, yet may remain clinically occult. Thus, it may be useful to screen geriatric dogs and cats (i.e. from 12 years of age in the cat) for systemic hypertension, as the latter has been shown to increase with age (Bijsmans *et al.*, 2015) and may be an indicator of an underlying subclinical disease (Figure 15.1).

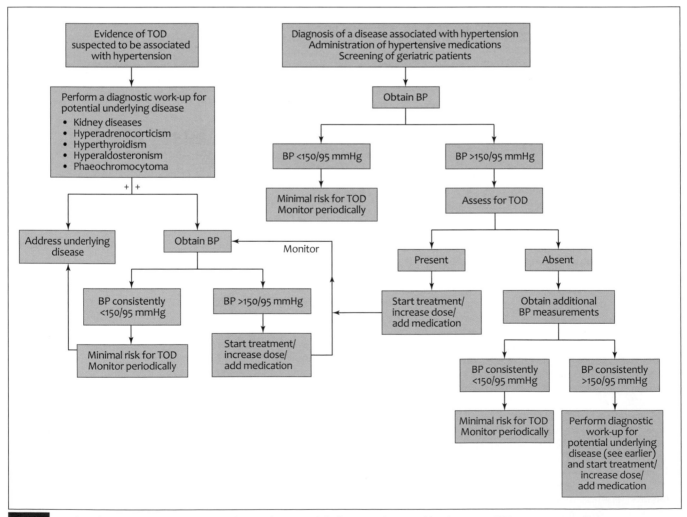

15.1 An algorithm for screening and treating dogs and cats at risk for hypertension. BP = blood pressure; TOD = target-organ damage.

Blood pressure should also be assessed whenever damage to one of the target organs (i.e. kidneys, eyes, brain and heart) is identified, to assess potential association between the damage and hypertension (Figures 15.2 and 15.3). Epistaxis may also be an indicator of an elevated blood pressure. In some cases, the damage to target organs is irreversible and detrimental, therefore it is important to recognize and treat hypertension in a timely manner (see Figure 15.1). There may not be a correlation between the severity of the underlying hypertension-generating disease and the magnitude of hypertension, and TOD (e.g. blindness) is occasionally the first evidence of the underlying disease.

The damage to the heart, as manifested by left ventricular hypertrophy, is presumably the least important clinically, because heart failure secondary to hypertension is rarely documented. Left ventricular hypertrophy is not often severe enough to be readily detected by the traditionally available diagnostic modalities such as electrocardiography, radiography, or even echocardiography. Nonetheless, hypertension may worsen concurrent heart disease. Conversely, ocular lesions are common (Carter *et al.*, 2014), and may frequently lead to blindness. The most prevalent ophthalmological manifestation of hypertension is hypertensive choroidoretinopathy, which may include retinal haemorrhage, oedema and/or detachment (see Figures 15.2 and 15.3). Increased retinal vessel tortuosity, papilloedema, vitreal haemorrhage and hyphaema may also be seen, and glaucoma as well as retinal degeneration are possible secondary complications. Neurological signs may also occur in hypertensive animals when the systemic blood pressure is higher than can be accommodated by autoregulation, especially in patients with AKI (see Figure 15.2). The aetiology of these neurological signs in AKI patients is likely to be multifaceted, including hypertension, uraemia and coagulation disorders due to

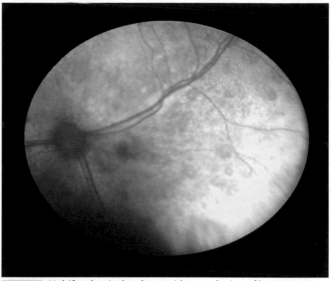

15.3 Multifocal retinal oedema with an early sign of hypertensive retinopathy in a 17-year-old female cat with blood pressure of 215/132 mmHg.
(Courtesy of N Kahane)

decreased platelet function and concurrent disseminated intravascular coagulation. Neurological signs in dogs with AKI have been shown to be negatively associated with the outcome (Segev *et al.*, 2008). The kidneys are not only a possible source for, but also a target organ that is affected by systemic hypertension. The relationship between systemic hypertension and progressive kidney disease is documented in dogs but remains unconfirmed in cats. Nonetheless, systemic hypertension is associated with a more rapid progression of kidney disease, either directly or through worsening of proteinuria, which is a negative prognostic indicator in both dogs and cats (Jacob *et al.* 2003; Jepson *et al.* 2007).

Given that hypertension is secondary in the vast majority of veterinary patients and is age-related, it allows the clinician to focus on a population at risk rather than to screen all patients. Hence, blood pressure should be assessed whenever a disease known to be associated with systemic hypertension is diagnosed (see Figure 15.1) and be offered when geriatric animals are presented for routine health screens. Patients with CKD that are normotensive at initial diagnosis should continue to have their blood pressure monitored (see Chapter 23) as part of their management. This should enable hypertension to be detected before catastrophic ocular lesions have occurred and will limit progressive kidney damage if treatment is started as soon as mild blood pressure elevations are detected.

Finally, blood pressure should be measured in patients that receive medications known to increase it, some of which are prescribed to dogs and cats with kidney disease (e.g. erythropoietin or erythropoietin-simulating agents), thus further increasing the risk of hypertension. While the elevation in blood pressure associated with the administration of some of these medications (e.g. PPA) is considered minimal and clinically insignificant in healthy dogs (Segev *et al.*, 2015), it may pose a risk in patients with pre-existing hypertension, or in patients with underlying disorders that could predispose to hypertension, such as CKD (see Figure 15.1).

Organ	Clinical manifestation
Brain	• Seizures • Behavioural abnormalities • Lethargy • Depression • Disorientation • Ataxia • Altered mentation • Vestibular signs • Variable neurological deficits

Eye	• Acute blindness
	• Hypertensive retinopathy (see Figure 15.3)
	  • Multifocal retinal oedema
	  • Bullous retinal detachment
	  • Retinal haemorrhage (pre-, intra- or subretinal)
	• Increased retinal vessel tortuosity
	• Papilloedema
	• Vitreal haemorrhage
	• Hyphaema
	• Secondary complications
	  • Retinal degeneration
	  • Secondary glaucoma

Kidney	• Progression of kidney disease • Proteinuria
Heart and vasculature	• Left ventricular hypertrophy with potential diastolic heart failure • Arrhythmia • Gallop rhythm • Murmur • Dilatation of the proximal aorta

15.2 End-organ damage potentially associated with systemic hypertension in dogs and cats.

Principles of blood pressure measurement

Blood pressure can be measured using various devices. These are frequently selected on the basis of operator familiarity, cost or convenience, and not necessarily on evidence. A number of studies have evaluated the performance of various blood pressure measuring devices; however, for technical and ethical reasons many of these studies did not compare the tested techniques/device with the gold standard (direct blood pressure measurement). Ideally, however, when a new blood pressure device is introduced, or is considered by a clinician, it is important to evaluate both its precision and its accuracy, compared with the gold standard (see below). The precision and the accuracy should be assessed across a wide range of blood pressures, as these parameters may change among hypotensive, normotensive and hypertensive animals. Ideally, blood pressure should be measured with devices that have been validated against direct blood pressure measurements generated by radiotelemetric devices in healthy animals, in the species of interest, and under the same circumstances in which it is intended to be used (e.g. conscious *versus* unconscious patients). The criteria against which blood pressure devices should ideally be validated for clinical use are set out in the American College of Veterinary Internal Medicine (ACVIM) Consensus Statement on Hypertension (Brown *et al.*, 2007). Whatever the technique used, blood pressure measurement should be performed prior to any other procedure. Adequate time (5–15 minutes) for acclimatization should be allowed, depending on the patient's stress and demeanour.

Direct blood pressure measurement

Direct blood pressure measurement requires arterial catheterization or puncture and is considered the gold standard. This can be achieved using an arterial catheter or a needle, connected to a monitor through a transducer, or by using an implanted radiotelemetric device, which enables continuous monitoring without the bias of inadvertently modifying measured pressure values by the very act of measuring. Although these methods have been shown to be applicable in both dogs and cats, they are mostly reserved for hospitalized patients in intensive care units, in which continuous blood pressure measurement is required, or for research purposes. The interested reader is referred to Stepien and Elliott (2007) for details of direct blood pressure measurement. This approach is not clinically practical for the vast majority of outpatients, and therefore indirect methods are most commonly applied. The majority of these utilize Doppler or oscillometric technologies.

Doppler

Doppler is a widely used technique to measure blood pressure. It utilizes ultrasound to detect blood flow within an artery. A cuff connected to a sphygmomanometer is placed on a limb or on the base of the tail, and a piezoelectric crystal attached to an audio amplifier is placed on the skin over an artery, distal to the cuff (see Figure 15.4bc). Coupling gel is used to facilitate detection of the pulse. When pulse waves are heard clearly, the cuff is inflated to at least 20 mmHg above the point at which the sound of the pulse disappears. The cuff is then manually deflated, gradually and slowly, while the operator carefully observes the pressure on the sphygmomanometer gauge, until pulse waves are heard again. Blood pressure at this point is recorded as the systolic blood pressure. Assessment of diastolic blood pressure using this technique is not possible with any degree of acceptable precision. Doppler machines are considered by many clinicians as the preferred method for blood pressure measurement in cats; however, modern sensitive oscillometric blood pressure devices detect low magnitude oscillations, and can be used to obtain reliable blood pressure readings in cats (Pedersen *et al.*, 2002; Martel *et al.*, 2013). A step-by-step approach to measurement of blood pressure using the Doppler technique is presented below and illustrated in Figure 15.4.

Step-by-step approach to Doppler blood pressure measurement

The equipment needed to undertake Doppler blood pressure measurement is shown in Figure 15.4a.

1. Restrain the patient in a comfortable position and allow time and reassurance for acclimatization. The position of the patient is dependent on temperament and mobility and on the planned position of the cuff:
   - Cuff on forelimb at level of radius: sternal or lateral recumbency or sitting position
   - Cuff on hindlimb proximal to hock (tibial level): lateral recumbency preferred, sternal recumbency may be used if leg is in extension during measurement.
2. Measure the circumference of the limb or tail at the intended cuff site. The width of the cuff selected should be approximately 40% of the circumference of the cuff site (Figure 15.4b). A chart can be prepared in advance to aid rapid cuff selection.
3. Wrap the cuff snugly around the limb and attach to the sphygmomanometer.
4. Clip or dampen hair as needed at the site of Doppler crystal application (palmar or plantar arterial arch), apply coupling gel and hold or tape crystal in position (Figure 15.4c). Verify correct position by listening for clear pulsatile sounds of flow in the artery beneath the crystal. Adjust the crystal position or angle as necessary to improve signal strength if sounds are soft, distant or muffled.
5. Gently position the limb so that the cuff is at the level of the right atrium during readings:
   - Sternum if patient is in lateral position
   - Thoracic inlet level if patient is sternal or sitting.
6. While listening to the sound of flow, inflate the cuff using the bulb manometer to approximately 20 mmHg greater than the pressure needed to cut off flow sounds (Figure 15.4d).
7. Slowly deflate the cuff (1–3 mmHg per second) and note the pressure at which pulsatile sounds of flow recur. This pressure is recorded as the systolic pressure.
8. Completely deflate the cuff and record the heart rate.
9. Record at least six measurements in succession, allowing approximately 30 seconds to 1 minute between measurements to allow for limb reperfusion.
10. Average the readings after excluding outliers to obtain a representative figure for systolic pressure and heart rate. High heart rate may indicate increased levels of patient stress, which may have affected the readings.

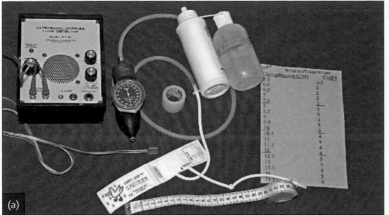

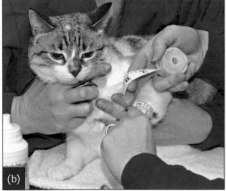

15.4 Doppler blood pressure measurement.
(a) Equipment required for Doppler sphygmomanometric measurement of blood pressure in dogs and cats. The signal amplifier (upper left) is attached to a piezoelectric crystal (lower centre). An inflatable bulb syringe attached to a manometer (upper centre) is used to inflate an appropriately sized cuff. Coupling gel and isopropyl alcohol (upper centre-right) are used to dampen the fur. (b) The cat is held gently in position and a flexible measuring tape is used to measure the circumference of the limb at the level of cuff placement. The cuff size is noted in the patient's record. (c) Coupling gel is applied to the Doppler crystal just before application to the ventral portion of the metacarpal arch of the cat. The patient is held comfortably with the cuff at the level of the right atrium. (d) A bulb syringe attached to the manometer is used to inflate the blood pressure cuff positioned on the distal forelimb of a dog. During measurement, the leg is held gently so that the cuff is at the level of the right atrium.

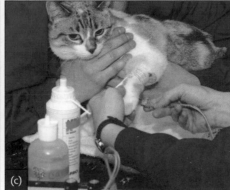

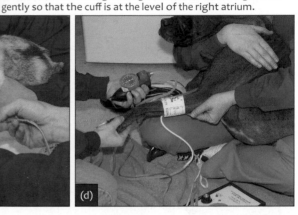

Oscillometry

Indirect oscillometric blood pressure devices employ cuff placement on a limb (Figure 15.5) or on the base of the tail.

Oscillations in the artery wall produced by the arterial blood flow are transmitted to the blood pressure device using a hollow tube. As the cuff deflates, the magnitude of oscillations increases up to a maximum, which corresponds to the mean arterial pressure. The systolic and diastolic blood pressures are then calculated by the machine using a programmed algorithm. Standard oscillometric devices may fail to measure blood pressure values accurately in hypotensive or very small patients owing to the low magnitude of oscillations. The effect of changes in arterial wall compliance in diseased animals (e.g. feline patients with hyperthyroidism, CKD) may also affect the ability of some oscillometric devices to make these measurements.

When using oscillometric blood pressure devices, the heart rate is also displayed and should be compared with the heart rate as measured using electrocardiographic monitoring, auscultation, or palpation of the femoral pulse. When heart rates, as measured by the blood pressure device and by any of these other modalities, do not match, the blood pressure reading is considered unreliable. However, matched heart rates cannot be used as an assurance of the accuracy of blood pressure measurement. Obtaining blood pressure measurements using oscillometry is time consuming and the variability noted among blood pressure readings may, at least partially, be attributed to the variation in blood pressure during the measurement. This is supported by studies using telemetric blood pressure devices that demonstrate that blood pressure is very stable when evaluated over long periods of time, while it may change considerably during a relatively short time period.

A step-by-step approach to this technique is presented below and illustrated in Figure 15.5.

Step-by-step approach to oscillometric blood pressure measurement

The equipment needed to undertake oscillometric blood pressure measurement is shown in Figure 15.5a.

1. Restrain the patient in a comfortable position and allow time and reassurance for acclimatization. The position of the patient is dependent on the patient's temperament and mobility and on the planned position of the cuff (limb cuffs should not be used in standing animals):
   - Cuff on forelimb at level of radius: sternal or lateral recumbency or sitting position (Figure 15.5b)
   - Cuff on proximal forelimb at level of humerus (cats): sternal recumbency
   - Cuff on distal hindlimb at level of metatarsus (median artery): lateral recumbency preferred, sternal recumbency may be used if leg is in gentle extension during measurement (Figure 15.5c)
   - Cuff on proximal tailhead: sternal or lateral recumbency, or standing if relatively immobile.
2. Measure the circumference of the limb or tail at the intended cuff site. The width of the cuff selected should be approximately 40% of the circumference of the cuff site. A chart can be prepared in advance to aid rapid cuff selection (see Figure 15.5a).

▶

Step-by-step approach to oscillometric blood pressure measurement *continued*

3. Wrap the cuff snugly around the limb with the centre of the inflatable bladder of the cuff positioned over the artery, and attach it to the blood pressure monitor.
4. Gently position the limb so that the cuff is at the level of the right atrium during readings (no repositioning required if tail cuff is used):
    *   Sternum if patient is in lateral position
    *   Thoracic inlet level if patient is sternal or sitting.
5. Record at least six measurements in succession, allowing approximately 30 seconds to 1 minute between measurements to allow for limb reperfusion.
6. Discard any readings with clearly spurious results, and average the results of the remaining readings to obtain a representative figure for systolic, diastolic and mean pressures, respectively.
7. Note the heart rate associated with the blood pressure readings. If the heart rate is clearly incorrect, blood pressure measurement may be spurious. In addition, high heart rate during recording may indicate high patient stress levels and possible elevated blood pressure due to the stress of the procedure.

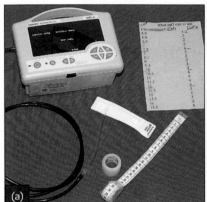 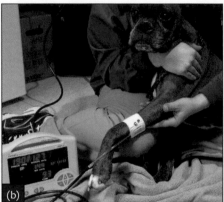 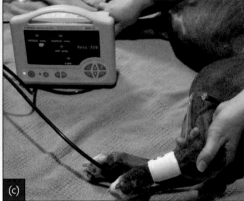

15.5 Blood pressure measurement using an oscillometric blood pressure device. Small dogs and cats may feel more comfortable in their owner's laps, minimizing stress and 'white coat hypertension'. (a) Equipment required for oscillometric blood pressure measurement. A flexible measuring tape (lower right) is used to measure the circumference of the cuff site. A previously devised 'cuff size chart' (upper right) may be useful for rapid choice of cuff size. An automated oscillometric monitor is attached to the appropriately sized cuff, and light tape may be used to secure the cuff in position once it is wrapped around the extremity to be used for measurement. (b) Oscillometric blood pressure measurement. A forelimb cuff is used to measure blood pressure with an automated oscillometric device. Note that, during such measurement, the limb is supported comfortably such that the cuff is at the level of the right atrium (thoracic inlet). The monitor displays systolic/diastolic pressure (e.g. 190/127 mmHg) with mean pressure (144 mmHg) beneath. Heart rate is displayed at the bottom (93 bpm). (c) A hindlimb cuff is positioned distal to the hock, with the dog in lateral recumbency. The limb is gently supported during readings so that the cuff is at the level of the right atrium (the sternum in lateral recumbency). A reading has not yet been obtained for this dog.

High-definition oscillometry

High-definition oscillometry (HDO) is a technology that utilizes a newer generation of oscillometric blood pressure devices. These can be used as a standalone unit, but can also be connected to a computer, which allows visualization of the entire measurement process. Measurement is obtained using a cuff which is inflated to a predetermined pressure. Like other oscillometric blood pressure devices, as the cuff deflates, pulse waves increase to a maximal amplitude, which corresponds to the mean arterial pressure. Systolic and diastolic blood pressures are then calculated using an algorithm from the increase and decrease in amplitude, respectively, as can be simultaneously viewed on the computer screen. HDO provides additional information compared with conventional blood pressure monitors and thus potentially bears several advantages, including a relatively shorter time for obtaining blood pressure readings, real-time visualization of blood pressure data when the device is connected to a computer screen, timely detection of artefacts and errors, and a higher sensitivity at low pressure amplitudes, which improves the ability to measure very low systemic blood pressures (Egner, 2007; Mitchell *et al.*, 2010). HDO can be adjusted to the expected blood pressure range by setting

maximum cuff inflation, linear deflation and the ability to modify the gain to magnify weak blood pressure signals (Egner, 2007; Mitchell *et al.*, 2010). Despite the above potential benefits, some studies have failed to demonstrate the superiority of HDO devices over other techniques, and the results of the currently available studies are still conflicting (Chetboul *et al.*, 2010; Wernick *et al.*, 2010; 2012). Further work is required to assess the performance of the HDO relative to the gold standard of telemetric direct blood pressure measurement, ideally over a wide range of blood pressures under simulated veterinary practice conditions.

Comparison of various technologies for blood pressure measurement

There are a few advantages and disadvantages to each of the aforementioned blood pressure measuring techniques (Figure 15.6). One is not necessarily better than the other, and often these methods can be used in concert and are considered complementary to each other. Based on the current veterinary literature it is impossible to determine whether one method should be considered superior to another in terms of accuracy and precision, because

Technique	Indications	Contraindications	Advantages	Disadvantages
Direct blood pressure measurement (needle/catheter)	Confirm BP; continuous monitoring during anaesthesia/hospitalization; administration of potent hypotensive medications	Caution in patients with bleeding disorders	Accurate over the entire range of BP; continuous measurements (catheter); less affected by arrhythmias	Technically challenging; risk of haemorrhage
Doppler ultrasonography	Single measurement; intermittent monitoring	None	Inexpensive	Signal may not be heard at very low blood pressure; variable underestimation of systolic pressure (5–20 mmHg); requires prolonged manipulation of paws which can be resented by some patients, requires subjective skill of operator to determine pressure; diastolic pressure cannot be measured
Oscillometry	Single measurement; intermittent monitoring	May not be accurate at high heart rates or with arrhythmias	Minimal patient manipulation during measurement; frequent monitoring can be done automatically; alarm at abnormal BP; not reliant on operator to determine pressure	Time-consuming; fails to give pressure readings in some animals; inaccurate at low blood pressures; incorrect cuff size or placement markedly decreases accuracy
High-definition oscillometry	Single measurement, intermittent monitoring	None known	Obtains readings faster than most oscillometric devices; allows visualization of the measurement on computer which can be sent to an expert for interpretation	Expensive; same issues with cuff placement and failure to give blood pressure readings in some animals as for standard oscillometry may apply

15.6 Indications, contraindications, advantages and disadvantages of different blood pressure measurement techniques. BP = blood pressure.

different studies comparing the different techniques have used different oscillometric blood pressure devices and various blood pressure measurement protocols. Thus, each device should be evaluated individually. Regardless of the method used, trained personnel are essential for reproducible results with all devices.

An advantage of oscillometric blood pressure devices is their ability to report systolic, diastolic and mean blood pressure, as opposed to the Doppler technique, in which most clinicians would agree that only the systolic blood pressure can be measured accurately. Another advantage of oscillometric devices is that, once the cuff is placed, blood pressure can be measured without manipulating the patient. This is important in minimizing the stress associated with the measurement and decreasing the likelihood of the white coat hypertension phenomenon. This is in contrast to the Doppler technique, in which there is a need to listen to the audible signal to determine the systolic blood pressure value to be recorded, which may alarm the patient and increase the likelihood of falsely overestimating the true value, owing to the white coat effect (unless the operator uses ear phones to minimize the noise).

Oscillometric devices have an advantage when frequent blood pressure measurements are required at predetermined intervals. These devices can also be programmed to sound an alarm for staff when blood pressure is higher or lower than predetermined values. The time needed to acquire an accurate measurement varies among oscillometric devices and is highly dependent on the operator's experience but, generally speaking, obtaining blood pressure using oscillometric devices is more time-consuming than with the Doppler technique in the hands of an experienced operator. HDO devices may obtain readings substantially faster than most other oscillometric devices (Mitchell *et al.*, 2010). Obtaining a blood pressure

measurement within a short interval is advantageous in animal patients that are often reluctant to remain still for a relatively long period, resulting in motion artefacts.

Comments on blood pressure measurement

Some general comments are worth emphasizing and are relevant to all techniques. Obtaining a blood pressure measurement is relatively easy; however, obtaining an accurate and reliable blood pressure reading requires practice, care and attention to detail. 'White coat hypertension' may result in falsely elevated blood pressure values and is common among animal patients. Stress is not always apparent and cannot be easily predicted by the operator. The experience of the operator is an important factor that influences both the length of time required for measurement and the reliability of the results (Bailey and Bauer, 1993). Owners and veterinary surgeons (veterinarians) should realize that accurate blood pressure measurement is time-consuming, particularly when using oscillometric blood pressure devices, and should therefore plan accordingly and interpret the data appropriately.

To minimize variability, blood pressure measurements should be performed in a consistent manner. Body position and cuff location have an effect on the blood pressure readings (Rondeau *et al.*, 2013), and ideally should remain constant among blood pressure measurements both when continuously monitoring patients and when testing them serially. To ensure proper documentation and consistency among serial measurements, a standard form (Figure 15.7) should be used to record blood pressure readings as well as all the variables during the procedure, including the animal's position, attitude and stress, cuff size and site (in terms of the chosen limb and the cuff location along that specific limb), operator, and use of medications that may influence blood pressure.

Blood Pressure Measurement Form

Clinical signs and underlying disease			BP device		Date	
			Clinician		Time	
Patient details		**Number**	**Systolic**	**Diastolic**	**Mean**	**Pulse**
Case number		1				
Name		2				
Age		3				
Breed		4				
Sex		5				
Demeanour		6				
Patient's position		7				
Cuff site		8				
Cuff size		9				
Limb circumference		10				
Examiner		**Average**				
Relevant medications		**Comments**				

15.7 To ensure proper documentation and consistency among serial measurements, a standard form is used. Blood pressure readings as well as all the variables during the procedure are recorded, including the animal's position, attitude and stress, cuff size and site, operator, and use of medications that may influence blood pressure.

To minimize the effect of white coat hypertension, blood pressure measurement should be performed prior to any other intervention, including physical examination, if the need to measure blood pressure is already known or suspected. A 5–15-minute period of acclimatization to the new environment (based on the patient's anxiety and demeanour) should be allowed before obtaining blood pressure to decrease the effect of stress. It has been shown, using telemetric blood pressure devices implanted in cats, that the mean blood pressure increases an average of 18 mmHg during a clinic visit, and may increase by as much as 75 mmHg from baseline values (Belew *et al.*, 1999). This study also demonstrated that in cats with underlying CKD, blood pressure decreases more slowly with adaptation to the new environment than that of healthy cats. A study in dogs has shown that almost one-third of dogs that were documented to be normotensive in their natural environment were found to be hypertensive in the clinical setting (Kallet *et al.*, 1997). Cats and small dogs may be held by their owners during the measurement if they appear calmer this way. Alternatively, when testing fractious cats, and especially when oscillometry is being used, the cuff can be placed on the limb or the base of the tail when the cat is still within its carrier, and the blood pressure device is then connected to the cat. Measurement should only commence several minutes later when the unhandled cat appears to be calmer and acclimatized.

Based on the guidelines published by the ACVIM, at least five blood pressure measurements should be obtained with <20% difference between the readings, to determine blood pressure accurately and most consistently. With the advances in technology and experience, lower variation is to be expected. When the blood pressure readings are not within a narrow enough range it is recommended to perform additional measurements, to exclude outlier data and, if necessary, to use a different cuff site.

Interpretation of blood pressure measurements

Despite careful standardization of technique as discussed above, blood pressure varies among different breeds, and breed-specific 'normal' blood pressure values for all dog and cat breeds are yet to be determined. This further emphasizes the need for a clinic to standardize their protocols for blood pressure measurement in companion animals. The average systolic, diastolic and mean arterial pressures from 10 studies evaluating normal blood pressure in dogs were 144 mmHg, 83 mmHg and 101 mmHg, respectively. In cats, many of the studies utilize the Doppler technique and thus only the systolic blood pressure is reported, with an average of 140 mmHg. It is plausible that age and sex also have an effect on blood pressure; however, data from dogs and cats in that regard are still conflicting (Brown *et al.*, 2007).

It is helpful to categorize blood pressure on the basis of the level of risk for TOD (see below). A single isolated high blood pressure measurement, unless accompanied by TOD, is not an indication for immediate treatment. Hypertension in the absence of TOD needs to be repeatedly documented (two to three clinic visits) before treatment is initiated.

The risk of TOD is categorized as minimal, low, moderate or severe, based on the severity of hypertension, as outlined below (Brown *et al.*, 2007; see Chapter 12). These proposed cut-off values are a general guide and should be adjusted to reflect the practice's experience when applying their measurement technique and when dealing with a particular breed or type of dog (e.g. a sighthound) where the 'normal' blood pressure appears to be higher than in other breeds. The clinician should always bear in mind that, although the likelihood of 'white coat hypertension' decreases as the blood pressure increases, blood pressure within each of these categories may still be the result of the white coat effect or of a technical error, hence the necessity to document persistence of elevated blood pressure in the absence of TOD prior to decision-making over treatment.

When the systolic and diastolic blood pressure are below 150 and 95 mmHg, respectively, the risk of TOD is considered minimal and the patient is referred to as normotensive. These blood pressure values might logically be the ideal target values for hypertensive dogs and cats that are being managed with anti-hypertensive drugs (see Chapters 18 and 23). Systolic and diastolic blood pressure values of 150–159 mmHg and 95–99 mmHg, respectively, are considered to carry a low risk for TOD. Animals with blood pressure in this range are classified as borderline hypertensive (see Chapter 12). The likelihood of white coat hypertension within this category is relatively high, and in some breeds (e.g. Greyhounds) the reported normal blood pressure values may fall into this range. A moderate risk of TOD is considered when the systolic and diastolic blood pressure values are 160–179 mmHg and 100–119 mmHg, respectively. Animals with blood pressure in this range are classified as moderately hypertensive (see Chapter 12). At this range the likelihood of white coat hypertension is lower compared with previous categories, especially towards the upper range. There is evidence to suggest that blood pressure within these ranges often coexists with TOD such as left ventricular hypertrophy, hypertensive encephalopathy, hypertensive retinopathy and progression of CKD. A severe risk of developing TOD is considered when the systolic and diastolic blood pressure values are higher than 180 mmHg and 120 mmHg, respectively. Animals with blood pressure in this range are classified as severely hypertensive (see Chapter 12).

When systemic hypertension is diagnosed or suspected, an ophthalmological examination is the most commonly applied means to assess for existing secondary TOD in the clinical setting. Kidney diseases are often the cause of hypertension, and the rate of ongoing kidney damage related to hypertension is impossible to assess at the first diagnosis of both problems. The accurate assessment of brain and heart damage is more involved and cost prohibitive, therefore these organs are often not assessed in the initial evaluation of TOD when hypertension has been documented, unless there is a specific indication to do so.

Management of hypertension

Chronic management

The therapeutic goals are to decrease blood pressure while avoiding systemic hypotension, and to minimize TOD, assuming that the lower the blood pressure, the lower the risk of TOD. The target values for systolic and diastolic blood pressure are below 150 mmHg and 95 mmHg, respectively, although this may be difficult to achieve in some patients (particularly dogs). Blood pressure should be decreased gradually to avoid acute-onset hypotension, recognizing that, in the absence of obvious TOD, treatment of hypertension should not be regarded as an emergency, and in most cases hypertension has been chronic prior to presentation to the veterinary clinic. The decision to treat elevated blood pressure is based on the severity and persistence of documented hypertension and on the presence of TOD. Whenever hypertension is documented, a thorough clinical evaluation should be performed to assess for potential underlying diseases

(see above). Identification and elimination of the underlying disease may resolve the hypertension without necessitating pressure-lowering pharmacotherapy. As treatment of hypertension is often life-long, over-diagnosis and over-treatment should be avoided.

Management of hypertension in human patients often requires a combination of several medications. This approach may not be realistic or even justified in veterinary patients because the common aetiologies of hypertension in companion animals are different from those in human patients. Additionally, owners may be reluctant to administer numerous medications (in addition to the medications that are indicated as part of the management of the underlying disease). Once the management of hypertension has commenced, it is important to avoid partially controlling blood pressure with drugs. In health, the autoregulatory mechanism maintains renal blood flow and pressure within the glomerular capillaries almost unchanged throughout a wide range of systemic blood pressures. The autoregulatory capacity of the kidney, however, is compromised by the presence of CKD. Moreover, some anti-hypertensive medications (e.g. dihydropyridine calcium channel blockers) interfere further with this protective mechanism, resulting in translation of the systemic blood pressure (even if lower than the initially untreated blood pressure) to glomerular hypertension. The latter may worsen proteinuria and is associated with progressive glomerular damage and further progression of the kidney disease.

Dietary modification is an important component of the management of hypertension in human patients but is controversial in veterinary medicine. There is no evidence to suggest that severe salt reduction effectively reduces blood pressure. Conversely, there is some evidence to suggest that severe salt reduction may activate the renin–angiotensin–aldosterone system, further aggravating hypertension (Buranakarl et al., 2004); therefore, salt restriction is not recommended as a sole therapy for hypertension, but rather a combination of moderate salt restriction with pharmacotherapy is used, and high salty diets should be avoided in hypertensive animals (see Chapter 18).

Excessive fluid administration and overhydration may promote or worsen hypertension and should also be avoided. In patients with AKI, both the prevalence and the severity of hypertension increase during hospitalization, partially due to inappropriately excessive fluid administration, resulting in hypervolaemia and overhydration. This can be demonstrated by the reduction in blood pressure during the first dialysis treatment when ultrafiltration is performed. In patients with CKD, fluid therapy is often administered subcutaneously, resulting in a high salt load and, when provided in excess, also in hypervolaemia and overhydration, further increasing the risk of hypertension. Therefore, fluid administration should not be regarded as risk free in general, and in the management of hypertension in particular.

Angiotensin-converting enzyme inhibitors (ACEi) and calcium channel blockers are the most commonly used anti-hypertensive drugs. Other medications should be considered in refractory cases, when adverse drug reactions occur, or when specifically indicated by the underlying disease (e.g. phaeochromocytoma, hyperaldosteronism). ACEi decrease the conversion of angiotensin I to angiotensin II, which is a potent vasoconstrictor but also promotes sodium reabsorption from the proximal tubules of the nephrons and stimulates the release of aldosterone, which further promotes renal sodium reabsorption. ACEi, however, are not potent anti-hypertensive drugs and are not expected to control moderate to severe hypertension fully or even sufficiently. ACEi preferentially dilate the efferent glomerular arteriole and therefore decrease pressure within the glomerular capillaries, thereby decreasing glomerular filtration pressure. Consequently, exacerbation of azotaemia may ensue in a subset of treated dogs and cats. This undesired and occasionally life-threatening side effect is more likely to occur in dehydrated patients or patients with severe pretreatment azotaemia. Therefore, in such patients, conservative dosing of ACEi should be exercised initially, while monitoring serum creatinine and urea concentrations, and the dose gradually increased as indicated. Angiotensin receptor blocking drugs are an alternative way of interfering with the renin–angiotensin system which may have some advantages (see Chapter 18).

Dihydropyridine calcium channel blockers (e.g. amlodipine besylate) are potent anti-hypertensive drugs. They are commonly used as first choice drugs, and often as the only anti-hypertensive drugs in cats. Calcium channel blockers interfere with calcium influx needed for vascular smooth muscle contraction. Amlodipine besylate decreases blood pressure in cats by 30–50 mmHg and therefore often completely controls hypertension (Henik et al., 1997; Elliott et al., 2001; Huhtinen et al., 2015). In dogs, however, amlodipine frequently does not completely control hypertension. Moreover, its administration results in preferential dilation of the afferent glomerular arteriole, and consequently systemic blood pressure may be translated to glomerular hypertension, resulting in an elevated filtration pressure with a resultant worsening of proteinuria and further damage to both glomeruli and the nephrons. To minimize the risk of triggering an increase in intraglomerular pressure, in hypertensive dogs, ACEi should be administered concurrently with calcium channel blockers.

Other, less commonly used, anti-hypertensive agents include angiotensin receptor blockers (e.g. telmisartan), beta-blockers, alpha1-adrenoceptor blockers (prazosin), and direct arteriolar dilators (hydralazine). Diuretics, which are commonly used in hypertensive human patients, should be reserved for overhydrated dogs and cats. Diuretics should be avoided in patients with CKD because they are prone to trigger dehydration. Further consideration of the management of hypertension in the CKD patient can be found in Chapters 18 and 23.

Emergency management of hypertension

In a subset of patients, particularly those with AKI, hypertension may be severe and accompanied by severe organ damage, mostly ocular and neurological. In such instances, blood pressure should be lowered over a few hours rather than over a few days. Treatment may be initiated based even on a single, but reliable, high (>180 mmHg) blood pressure reading, accompanied by evidence of end-organ damage.

Medications commonly used in the emergency management of hypertension should be potent. Care should be taken not to decrease the blood pressure extremely quickly because this can lead to significant adverse events (see below). The most commonly used drugs in this group include oral or intrarectal amlodipine besylate, oral or intravenous hydralazine, and intravenous sodium nitroprusside. Less commonly used medications include oral prazosin, intravenous enalaprilat, and oral or intravenous beta-blockers. Given the altered mental status of some of these patients, medications are often used intravenously or intrarectally (e.g. amlodipine). In cats, amlodipine has been shown to be very effective and may be used in such settings to control severe hypertension.

When potent drugs are being used, blood pressure and heart rate should be monitored very closely and frequently. In the most severely affected patients, and particularly in hospitalized patients where potent intravenous drugs are used (e.g. hydralazine and nitroprusside), continuous blood pressure monitoring is recommended to ascertain a gradual decrease in blood pressure values while avoiding the risk of too rapid or too extreme a reduction, leading to life-threatening hypotension. Once blood pressure is stabilized and controlled, management should be continued as for chronic hypertensive patients with very close monitoring in the first few days. Further consideration of the management of the AKI patient can be found in Chapter 21.

Monitoring

Continuous, as well as serial, blood pressure monitoring should be performed using the same blood pressure device (Wernick et al., 2012) and under the same technical, environmental and positional conditions. Timing of monitoring initiation is dependent on the severity of hypertension, TOD and concurrent diseases. Initial assessment should be performed within approximately 7 days after treatment onset. Repeated monitoring should be continued at 7–10-day intervals until blood pressure has reached the target values and remains stable over several consecutive visits. Thereafter, monitoring should be performed quarterly.

References and further reading

Anderson LJ and Fisher EW (1968) The blood pressure in canine interstitial nephritis. Research in Veterinary Science 9, 304–313

Bailey RH and Bauer JH (1993) A review of common errors in the indirect measurement of blood pressure. Sphygmomanometry. Archives of Internal Medicine 153, 2741–2748

Belew AM, Barlett T and Brown A (1999) Evaluation of the white-coat effect in cats. Journal of Veterinary Internal Medicine 13, 134–142

Bijsmans ES, Jepson RE, Chang HM, Syme HM and Elliott J (2015) Changes in systolic blood pressure over time in healthy cats and cats with chronic kidney disease. Journal of Veterinary Internal Medicine 29(3), 855–861

Bodey AR and Michell AR (1996) Epidemiological study of blood pressure in domestic dogs. Journal of Small Animal Practice 37, 116–125

Brown S, Atkins C, Bagley R et al. (2007) Guidelines for the identification, evaluation, and management of systemic hypertension in dogs and cats. Journal of Veterinary Internal Medicine 21, 542–558

Buranakarl C, Ankanaporn K, Thammacharoen S et al. (2007) Relationships between degree of azotaemia and blood pressure, urinary protein:creatinine ratio and fractional excretion of electrolytes in dogs with renal azotaemia. Veterinary Research Communications 31, 245–257

Buranakarl C, Mathur S and Brown SA (2004) Effects of dietary sodium chloride intake on renal function and blood pressure in cats with normal and reduced renal function. American Journal of Veterinary Research 65, 620–627

Carter JM, Irving AC, Bridges JP and Jones BR (2014) The prevalence of ocular lesions associated with hypertension in a population of geriatric cats in Auckland, New Zealand. New Zealand Veterinary Journal 62, 21–29

Chetboul V, Tissier R, Gouni V et al. (2010) Comparison of Doppler ultrasonography and high-definition oscillometry for blood pressure measurements in healthy awake dogs. American Journal of Veterinary Research 71, 766–772

Egner B (2007) Blood pressure measurement. Basic principles and practical application. In: Essential Facts of Blood Pressure in Dogs and Cats, ed. B. Egner, A Carr and S Brown, pp.1–14. VetVerlag, Babenhausen

Elliott J, Barber PJ, Syme HM, Rawlings JM and Markwell PJ (2001) Feline hypertension: clinical findings and response to antihypertensive treatment in 30 cases. Journal of Small Animal Practice 42, 122–129

Finch NC, Syme HM and Elliott J (2012) Association of urinary cadmium excretion with feline hypertension. Veterinary Record 170, 125

Finco DR (2004) Association of systemic hypertension with renal injury in dogs with induced renal failure. Journal of Veterinary Internal Medicine 18, 289–294

Henik RA, Snyder PS and Volk LM (1997) Treatment of systemic hypertension in cats with amlodipine besylate. Journal of the American Animal Hospital Association 33, 226–234

Huhtinen M, Derré G, Renoldi HJ *et al.* (2015) Randomized placebo-controlled clinical trial of a chewable formulation of amlodipine for the treatment of hypertension in client-owned cats. *Journal of Veterinary Internal Medicine* **29(3)**, 786–793

Jacob F, Polzin DJ, Osborne CA *et al.* (2003) Association between initial systolic blood pressure and risk of developing a uremic crisis or of dying in dogs with chronic renal failure. *Journal of the American Veterinary Medical Association* **222**, 322–329

Jepson RE, Elliott J, Brodbelt D and Syme HM (2007) Effect of control of systolic blood pressure on survival in cats with systemic hypertension. *Journal of Veterinary Internal Medicine* **21**, 402–409

Kallet AJ, Cowgill LD and Kass PH (1997) Comparison of blood pressure measurements obtained in dogs by use of indirect oscillometry in a veterinary clinic versus at home. *Journal of the American Veterinary Medical Association* **210**, 651–654

Kobayashi DL, Peterson ME, Graves TK, Lesser M and Nichols CE (1990) Hypertension in cats with chronic renal failure or hyperthyroidism. *Journal of Veterinary Internal Medicine* **4**, 58–62

Littman MP (1994) Spontaneous systemic hypertension in 24 cats. *Journal of Veterinary Internal Medicine* **8**, 79–86

Martel E, Egner B, Brown SA *et al.* (2013) Comparison of high-definition oscillometry – a non-invasive technology for arterial blood pressure measurement – with a direct invasive method using radio-telemetry in awake healthy cats. *Journal of Feline Medicine and Surgery* **15**, 1104–1113

Michell AR, Bodey AR and Gleadhill A (1997) Absence of hypertension in dogs with renal insufficiency. *Renal Failure* **19**, 61–68

Mitchell AZ, McMahon C, Beck TW and Sarazan RD (2010) Sensitivity of two noninvasive blood pressure measurement techniques compared to telemetry in cynomolgus monkeys and beagle dogs. *Journal of Pharmacological and Toxicological Methods* **62**, 54–63

Pedersen KM, Butler MA, Ersboll AK and Pedersen HD (2002) Evaluation of an oscillometric blood pressure monitor for use in anesthetized cats. *Journal of the American Veterinary Medical Association* **221**, 646–650

Proia KK, Thota AB, Njie GJ *et al.* (2014) Team-based care and improved blood pressure control: A community guide systematic review. *American Journal of Preventive Medicine* **47**, 86–99

Rondeau DA, Mackalonis ME and Hess RS (2013) Effect of body position on indirect measurement of systolic arterial blood pressure in dogs. *Journal of the American Veterinary Medical Association* **242**, 1523–1527

Segev G, Kass PH, Francey T and Cowgill LD (2008) A novel clinical scoring system for outcome prediction in dogs with acute kidney injury managed by hemodialysis. *Journal of Veterinary Internal Medicine* **22**, 301–308

Segev G, Westropp JL, Kulik C and Lavy E (2015) Changes in blood pressure following escalating doses of phenylpropanolamine and a suggested protocol for monitoring. *Canadian Veterinary Journal* **56**, 39–43

Stepien RL and Elliott J (2007). Measurement of blood pressure. In: *BSAVA Manual of Canine and Feline Nephrology and Urology, 2nd edn*, ed. J Elliott and GF Grauer, pp.179–186. BSAVA Publications, Gloucester

Syme HM, Barber PJ, Markwell PJ, and Elliott J (2002) Prevalence of systolic hypertension in cats with chronic renal failure at initial evaluation. *Journal of the American Veterinary Medical Association* **15**, 1799–804

Wernick M, Doherr M, Howard J and Francey T (2010) Evaluation of high-definition and conventional oscillometric blood pressure measurement in anaesthetised dogs using ACVIM guidelines. *Journal of Small Animal Practice* **51**, 318–324

Wernick M, Hopfner RM, Francey T and Howard J (2012) Comparison of arterial blood pressure measurements and hypertension scores obtained by use of three indirect measurement devices in hospitalized dogs. *Journal of the American Veterinary Medical Association* **240**, 962–968

Chapter 16

Cardiovascular–renal disorders

Shelly L. Vaden, Clarke Atkins and Mark A. Oyama

There is a complex interaction between the renal and cardiovascular systems, both in health and in disease states. In disease states, this complex interaction can present both diagnostic and therapeutic challenges.

Cardiorenal syndrome is a relatively new term and an evolving field of study in human medicine. The term is used to define a condition in which acute or chronic dysfunction in either the heart or the kidneys causes acute or chronic dysfunction in the other organ system (Ronco et al., 2010). Cardiorenal syndrome is subdivided into the following five types in human patients: type 1, involving acute worsening of heart function leading to kidney injury; type 2, involving chronic disease of the heart leading to kidney injury; type 3, involving acute worsening of kidney function leading to heart injury; type 4, involving chronic kidney disease (CKD) leading to heart injury; and type 5, involving systemic disease(s) leading to simultaneous injury to both the heart and kidney (e.g. sepsis, systemic hypertension, amyloidosis) (Ronco et al., 2010).

Despite this recent focus on cardiorenal syndrome, the clinical relevance and pathophysiological mechanisms of this disorder are incompletely understood in humans. What is known in humans, dogs and cats is that blood volume, vasomotor tone and haemodynamic stability are dependent on the cardiovascular and renal systems and the interactions between the two. The concept of the cardiorenal syndrome combines the cardiovascular system and kidneys as part of a single homeostatic cardiorenal axis, which challenges cardiologists and nephrologists who are treating heart and kidney disease, respectively, to consider this broader perspective.

Kidney and heart diseases are commonly recognized and important sources of morbidity and mortality in dogs and cats. There are clear guidelines for managing diseases of each organ when in isolation. However, when disease exists in both the kidneys and the heart, the situation becomes more challenging. The cornerstone to the management of diseases of either system is maintenance of adequate intravascular fluid volume while avoiding fluid overload; however, heart failure promotes volume overload whereas animals with kidney disease often have trouble maintaining adequate fluid volume. Management of disease in one system is therefore typically diametrically opposed to the management of disease in the other organ system.

While it is clear that there is interplay between the heart and the kidneys in dogs and cats, it is not clear that a true cardiorenal syndrome exists as is assumed to occur in humans. A group of academic and clinical veterinary cardiologists and nephrologists from Europe and North America recently convened with the goal of developing a consensus statement on the pathological interaction between the cardiovascular system and kidneys in dogs and cats (Pouchelon et al., 2015). The goal was to develop a definition of cardiorenal syndrome as it pertains to dogs and cats, to develop diagnostic and therapeutic recommendations for patients that have disease in both organs and to increase awareness of the complex interplay between the two systems. The consensus group chose to refer to the cardiorenal syndrome in veterinary patients as **cardiovascular–renal disorders** (CvRD), thereby acknowledging that the vasculature as well as the heart is involved in this interplay, and that the clinical manifestations of CvRD in the dog and cat are widely varied among individuals and between species and do not present as a single clinical syndrome. The meaning of the term CvRD thereby is different from that of the human CRS.

Cardiac and renal diseases differ between species, limiting our ability to derive information from human data for veterinary applications as well as to make comparisons between dogs and cats. Cardiac disease in humans is primarily a result of hypertension and coronary artery disease. This differs from dogs (mostly primary valvular disease, dilated cardiomyopathy and heartworm disease) and cats (mostly hypertrophic or other cardiomyopathies and, to a lesser degree, systemic hypertension). Likewise, the kidney diseases most often seen in humans are glomerular disease, diabetic nephropathy, hypertensive nephropathy, nephrosclerosis, interstitial nephritis and polycystic kidneys. This does not correlate exactly with what is seen in dogs (glomerular disease, pyelonephritis, acute tubular necrosis) and cats (idiopathic CKD, most often characterized by tubulointerstitial fibrosis of unknown origin).

Nevertheless, there are some aspects of the diseases and their pathophysiology that warrant interspecies comparison and the application of human clinical findings to veterinary medicine. The consensus group developed summary statements that spanned four different subtopics:

- Definition, classification, epidemiology and pathophysiology
- Clinical staging and diagnosis
- Biomarkers, imaging and blood pressure monitoring
- Management.

These subtopics have been selected to form the major sections of this chapter (Pouchelon et al., 2015).

Definition, classification, epidemiology and pathophysiology

Cardiovascular–renal disorders are defined as disease-, toxin- or drug-induced structural and/or functional damage to the cardiovascular system and/or kidneys leading to disruption of the normal interactions between these systems, to the ongoing detriment of one or both. In instances where disease coexists in both organ systems, it can be difficult to determine the directionality of the CvRD or whether concurrent primary diseases are present. Of key concern is the way the kidney and cardiovascular systems interact, including the potential for harm along three different axes, from kidney to cardiovascular system, from cardiovascular system to kidney, and from outside disease processes to both. This led to the formation of three subgroups of CvRD by the consensus group.

- $CvRD_H$ refers to the situation where renal disease has developed secondary to a disease involving the cardiovascular system.
- $CvRD_K$ refers to the situation where cardiovascular disease or dysfunction is secondary to dysfunction of the kidney.
- $CvRD_O$ describes concurrent impairment of both the kidneys and cardiovascular system, due to other disease processes, drugs or toxins that affect both systems, or when a primary disease exists concurrently in both the cardiovascular system and the kidneys.

It is expected that the proposed definition and classification scheme for CvRD in dogs and cats will require reassessment and modification as more veterinary research involving CvRD is performed.

Epidemiology and pathophysiology

In veterinary medicine, the existence and exact nature of CvRD is largely speculative. Nevertheless, there are known pathological conditions in the dog and cat that are characterized by detrimental interactions between the renal and cardiovascular systems (Figure 16.1). In addition to specific disorders, there are limited data that suggest that dogs and cats share some of the same pathophysiological mechanisms in cardiovascular–renal disorders that are found in humans with cardiorenal syndrome, for example the complex interplay of haemodynamic changes, neurohormonal activation and reactive oxygen species. The concept of cardiorenal syndrome, which involves a bidirectional pathway of injury wherein disease of either organ directly contributes to injury of the other (Figure 16.2), presents a broader view of fluid and haemodynamic homeostasis as compared with a more traditional viewpoint, which considers kidney and cardiovascular impairment as separate pathophysiological entities.

Epidemiology and pathophysiology of $CvRD_H$

$CvRD_H$ refers to kidney injury or dysfunction emanating from a primary disease process involving the cardiovascular system. Potential mechanisms of $CvRD_H$ include decreased kidney perfusion secondary to decreased cardiac output, activation of neuroendocrine systems, namely the renin–angiotensin–aldosterone system (RAAS) and sympathetic nervous system (SNS), generation of reactive oxygen species by abnormal or injured endothelial tissue, and passive venous congestion of the kidney. Acute reduction in cardiac output can lead to decreased glomerular filtration rate, increased serum creatinine and urea nitrogen concentrations, and decreased urine output. In both humans and small animals, an increase in serum creatinine by as little as 0.3 mg/dl (26.5 µmol/l) is regarded as indicative of acute kidney injury (AKI; International Renal Interest Society, 2014). The International Renal Interest Society (IRIS) has proposed diagnostic criteria for AKI in dogs and cats (see Chapter 12). Mild AKI, defined as a creatinine concentration >1.6 g/dl (1.7–2.5 g/dl) (>141 µmol/l (142–220 µmol/l)), is detected in dogs or cats treated for heart failure (Goutal et al., 2010). These relatively modest elevations in

CvRD subgroup	Definition and aetiology
$CvRD_H$	*Definition:* Kidney injury or dysfunction developed secondary to a primary disease of the cardiovascular system • Systemic hypertension leading to glomerular injury • Cardiac shock, low cardiac output and systemic hypotension leading to decreased renal perfusion, azotaemia and acute kidney injury • Systemic arterial thromboembolism leading to renal infarction • Heartworm infection leading to glomerulonephritis • Passive congestion of the kidney during heart failure
$CvRD_K$	*Definition:* Cardiovascular disease or dysfunction develops secondary to a primary disease of the kidney • Kidney-mediated systemic hypertension leading to increased afterload, left ventricular hypertrophy, worsening mitral or aortic insufficiency, arrhythmias, vasculopathy and/or retinopathy • Volume overload leading to congestion or systemic hypertension • Hypokalaemia or hyperkalaemia leading to cardiac arrhythmias • Reduced renal clearance of drugs (e.g. digoxin) leading to toxicity • Uraemic hypodipsia, anorexia or emesis leading to volume depletion and reduced cardiac output and perfusion • Uraemic pericarditis • Activation of the renin–angiotensin–aldosterone axis leading to sodium and water retention, cardiac and vascular remodelling or congestion • Anaemia secondary to chronic kidney disease leading to volume overload and reduced cardiac tissue oxygenation
$CvRD_O$	*Definition:* Concurrent impairment of both the kidneys and the cardiovascular systems due to either primary disease of both systems or other disease processes, drugs, toxins or toxicants that affect both systems • Septic or neoplastic emboli leading to renal and cardiac infarction • Gastric dilatation and volvulus leading to cardiac arrhythmias and azotaemia • Infectious disease (e.g. *Trypanosoma cruzi*) • Glycogen storage disease with glycogen deposition in the kidneys and heart • Amyloidosis with amyloid deposition in the kidney and cardiac tissues

16.1 Definitions and suspected cardiovascular–renal disorders (CvRD) in dogs and cats.

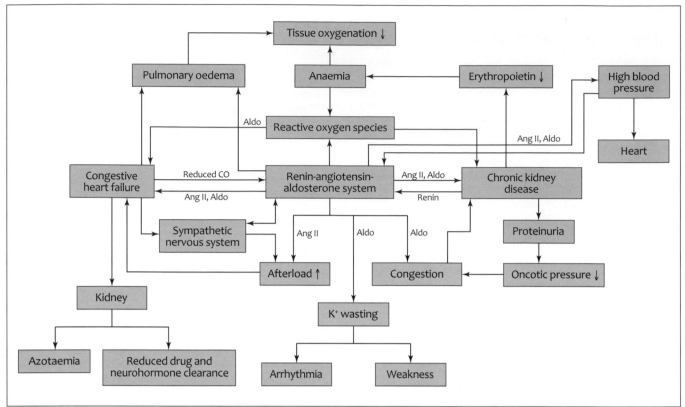

16.2 The complexities of the cardiorenal axis as it relates to cardiovascular–renal disorders (CvRD). The diseased heart (CHF, congestive heart failure) and kidney (CKD, chronic kidney disease) are depicted, as are the renin–angiotensin–aldosterone and sympathetic nervous systems (RAAS and SNS, respectively) and the normal heart and kidney. The failing heart activates the SNS and RAAS via a fall in CO (cardiac output) and blood pressure, while the diseased kidney activates the RAAS via renin release associated with a fall in glomerular filtration rate. The RAAS causes vasoconstriction (with increased afterload), potassium wasting (with resultant cardiac arrhythmias, renal damage and muscular weakness), myocardial and renal remodelling with fibrosis (via angiotensin II [Ang II] and aldosterone [Aldo]). The SNS increases heart rate, contributes to cardiac remodelling and arrhythmias, and causes vasoconstriction, all deleterious to cardiac function. The fall in CO and possibly congestion of the kidney result in azotaemia and reduced drug and hormone clearance via renal excretion. CKD and acute kidney injury both activate the RAAS, damaging the heart, vessels and the kidney itself. If left-sided heart failure and pulmonary oedema exist, tissue oxygenation falls and this is compounded by diminished oxygen-carrying capacity of the blood, which is rendered anaemic in CKD (via reduction in erythropoietin production). In glomerular disease, proteinuria can result in hypoalbuminaemia and reduced plasma oncotic pressure, which contribute to signs of congestion (pulmonary oedema, ascites). RAAS activation by cardiac, vascular (high blood pressure, HBP) or kidney disease and by anaemia increases the presence of reactive oxygen species (ROS) which are generally toxic to living tissues, including the heart, vessels and kidney. HBP, a cardiovascular disease, can be produced by chronic kidney disease, by other (endocrine) disease, or be idiopathic. Therefore HBP is an important lynchpin in the concept of CvRD, because it may produce cardiac disease with left ventricular hypertrophy, diastolic dysfunction and heart failure ($CvRD_K$ or $CvRD_O$, depending on whether there is renal or idiopathic HBP) and kidney disease with glomerular hypertension, glomerulosclerosis and renal failure ($CvRD_H$ or $CvRD_O$, depending on whether the HBP is idiopathic or caused by another disease such as hyperthyroidism). HBP causes vascular hypertrophy and dysfunction, worsening HBP.

renal function indicators, even when they fail to exceed the relevant laboratory reference range, and regardless of whether they are transient or sustained, may lead to permanent structural kidney damage and can worsen clinical outcomes (Harrison *et al.*, 2012). Yet, many practitioners, when managing animals with heart failure, disregard these renal values when elevations are mild.

In animals with acute congestive heart failure the lowest diuretic dosage required to resolve signs of congestion should be prescribed, because overly aggressive diuresis, volume depletion, activation of the RAAS and SNS and decreased kidney perfusion are likely to contribute to kidney injury and $CvRD_H$. It is believed that an additional mechanism, beyond reduced cardiac output, can lead to kidney injury. Venous congestion affects the haemodynamic regulation of glomerular filtration leading to activation of tubuloglomerular feedback mechanisms that cause afferent arteriolar constriction and reduced glomerular filtration rate. Congestion of kidney tissue due to poor cardiac function and elevated systemic venous pressure preferentially increases capsular pressure, decreases glomerular filtration pressure and rate, and substantially decreases kidney function. In humans with heart failure,

incomplete resolution of venous congestion is a primary cause of worsening renal function and is associated with poorer patient outcomes. This creates a clinical dilemma in trying to balance the negative effect of diuretic actions on arterial renal perfusion against the positive effect on venous renal congestion.

The RAAS, and in particular angiotensin II, precipitates and mediates oxidative and cytokine-mediated injury, inflammation and cell death (Mitani *et al.*, 2013). Resulting endothelial dysfunction and formation of ROS provide an important link between kidney and cardiac dysfunction. Congestive heart failure and accompanying elevated cytokine concentrations, reduced iron intake and absorption, and angiotensin-converting enzyme (ACE) suppression (angiotensin II is an erythropoietin secretagogue) contribute to anaemia in humans. Chronic inflammation, seen in some cardiovascular diseases (vegetative endocarditis, vasculitis, myocarditis), may also decrease sensitivity to erythropoietin and, along with kidney injury and diminished erythropoietin production, contribute to anaemia. Diminished or ineffective erythropoietin reduces haemoglobin and its antioxidant properties, and contributes to $CvRD_H$ through increased oxidative stress and apoptosis of kidney and cardiac cells. The importance of haemoglobin in CvRD$_H$ is a subject of debate. When erythropoietin was given therapeutically to increase haemoglobin concentrations in human patients with heart failure, patient outcome did not improve (Jackevicius *et al.*, 2014).

The prevalence of CvRD$_H$ in dogs and cats is unknown. Advances in medical therapy of congestive heart failure have led to improved life expectancy but also have increased the cumulative exposure to potentially nephrotoxic drugs, such as diuretics and ACE inhibitors (ACEi). In dogs and cats, the existence of CvRD$_H$ is indirectly supported by the observation that kidney dysfunction increases with severity of heart disease. In a retrospective study (Nicolle *et al.*, 2007), 50% of 124 dogs with chronic valvular heart disease were azotaemic, but 70% of dogs with the most severe stages of disease were azotaemic. In dogs with severe disease, both serum urea nitrogen and creatinine were higher and glomerular filtration rate was lower (almost a two-field reduction) when compared with dogs with more mild disease. In a retrospective study of cats with hypertrophic cardiomyopathy, azotaemia was present in 59% of the cats (Gouni *et al.*, 2008). An important confounder in these and similar studies is the potential for diuretic-induced pre-renal azotaemia in animals receiving therapy for congestive heart failure. The extent to which heart disease directly induces kidney injury in dogs and cats requires further study.

Diseases of the vasculature are included in the definition of CvRD and include disorders such as systemic hypertension. Hypertension-induced glomerular damage in veterinary patients is well described (IRIS Canine GN Study Group Diagnosis Subgroup *et al.*, 2013) and among the various proposed aetiologies of CvRD, systemic hypertension is one of the most plausible.

Epidemiology and pathophysiology of CvRD$_K$

CvRD$_K$ refers to cardiovascular injury or dysfunction emanating from a primary disease process involving the kidney. In humans, clinical experience and knowledge indicate that CvRD$_H$ is more common than CvRD$_K$ (Ronco *et al.*, 2008). There are both known and suspected negative effects of kidney disease on the cardiovascular system. For example, electrolyte abnormalities that can cause cardiac arrhythmias, such as hyperkalaemia, are associated with AKI and CKD. Various drugs used for the treatment of cardiac disease, such as digoxin, enalapril and atenolol, undergo renal excretion. Primary kidney dysfunction can lead to signs of toxicity of these drugs, including arrhythmias, hypotension and worsening myocardial function. Fluid volume and haemodynamic status in patients with severe kidney disease is generally abnormal. Uraemic patients that are anorexic, hypodipsic and vomiting are even further volume depleted, leading to a reduction in cardiac output. Kidney injury can also lead to systemic volume overload that contributes to congestion, especially in those animals with coexisting valve disease, diastolic dysfunction or kidney-mediated anaemia. Systemic hypertension is a common sequel to CKD and can result in myocardial hypertrophy and dysfunction. Lastly, azotaemia itself may have adverse effects on the cardiac myocytes.

Epidemiology and pathophysiology of CvRD$_O$

CvRD$_O$ refers to kidney and cardiovascular injury or dysfunction emanating from either a primary disease process outside the two systems or instances where primary kidney and cardiovascular diseases coexist. Examples of the former include sepsis or infectious diseases, while an example of the latter is the presence of both primary glomerular disease and myxomatous mitral valve degeneration. It is clear that the incidence of primary kidney disease and primary heart disease increases with age. As medical advances have increased the length of survival of animals with these conditions, the possibility that an animal will develop primary disease in the other organ system has also increased. Once primary kidney and cardiovascular disease are established, CvRD$_O$ pertains to the previously described interactions between the two systems that can accelerate injury to either or both.

Clinical staging and evaluation

The diagnosis of either kidney or cardiovascular disease requires the integration of information obtained from multiple different sources. The presenting complaint, medical history and physical examination can alert the clinician to the kidney, heart or vasculature as deserving of further diagnostic testing. Blood and urine testing, non-invasive blood pressure measurement and radiographic and ultrasonographic imaging are diagnostic tools routinely available for both kidney and cardiovascular disease. Accurate diagnosis and staging are essential to the detection of CvRD and in designing subsequent therapeutic plans.

Staging of heart disease

The International Small Animal Cardiac Health Council (ISACHC) system classifies animals on the basis of limited indices, such as clinical signs of heart failure and the existence or absence of cardiac hypertrophy (International Small Animal Cardiac Health Council, 1999). One weakness of the ISACHC system is its non-specificity regarding anatomical or aetiological diagnosis. Nevertheless, alternative systems, such as the American College of Veterinary Internal Medicine system which was specifically designed for dogs with myxomatous mitral valve degeneration, fail to account for important cardiovascular abnormalities that can develop in CvRD, including systemic hypertension, diastolic and systolic dysfunction, arrhythmias and alterations in biomarkers. For the purposes of CvRD, ISACHC or similar systems are, in isolation, incomplete means to assess involvement of the cardiovascular system. Additional diagnostic and staging tools, such as cardiac imaging and biomarkers, are discussed in later sections.

Staging of acute kidney injury and chronic kidney disease

When considering the potential involvement of the kidney in CvRD, the most appropriate classification system for AKI or CKD is the IRIS classification (see Chapter 12). The term AKI reflects the effects of a broad spectrum of acute insults to the kidney. The IRIS classification systems are useful in assessing potential kidney involvement in CvRD because they encompass a continuum of damage from mild to severe, including several key indices of kidney function. AKI is identified by an acute rise in serum creatinine concentration, oliguria/anuria and/or the sudden appearance of glucosuria, cylinduria or proteinuria. A sudden decrease in the ability to concentrate urine might also be an indication of AKI. Once AKI has been identified, the IRIS system uses the serum creatinine concentration to assign a Grade of I, II, III, IV or V. Each grade of AKI is further subgraded on the basis of non-oliguria (NO) or oli-goanuria (O) and the requirement for 'renal replacement therapy', such as haemodialysis and ultrafiltration. Relatively small changes in serum creatinine concentrations can signal AKI, the severity of which can fluctuate as the patient improves, worsens or transitions to CKD.

A diagnosis of CKD is made using multiple criteria, including history, physical examination, laboratory examination and renal imaging. Once a diagnosis of kidney disease has been made and it has been identified as being chronic and stable (based on at least two assessments of serum creatinine), the IRIS staging system can be used to classify the case as Stage 1, 2, 3 or 4, according to the serum creatinine concentration. The patient is then sub-staged according to the systemic arterial blood pressure (an important pathophysiological mechanism of cardiorenal syndrome; Figure 16.3) and proteinuria (non-proteinuric, borderline proteinuric or proteinuric).

Arterial pressure classification	Risk	Systolic BP (mmHg)
Normotensive	Minimal	<150[a]
Borderline hypertensive	Low	150–159
Hypertensive	Moderate	160–179
Severe hypertensive	High	≥180

16.3 International Renal Interest Society (IRIS) classification of blood pressure (BP). [a] It is preferable to use breed-specific ranges when available, which may differ from the ranges given in the table. Further modifications are: C = evidence of target-organ damage/complications; NC = no evidence of target-organ damage/complications.

Biomarkers, imaging and blood pressure measurement

Biomarkers, typically laboratory results, are objectively measured and evaluated as indicators of normal or pathogenic processes, and as responses to therapeutic interventions. Ideally, biomarkers not only reflect the severity of the pathological process, but also predict outcome, guide therapy and assess the risk of adverse events. In veterinary medicine, biomarkers generally refer to substances that can be measured in either blood or urine. Currently there are no specific biomarkers for any form of CvRD.

The consequence of heart disease or cardiac therapy on the kidneys (CvRD$_H$) is evaluated with traditional tests of kidney function or damage. As newer biomarkers are developed, these may provide additional information regarding renal injury. Biochemical assays for assessment of kidney function are widely used and accepted (Figure 16.4). For example, serum creatinine is used to assess glomerular filtration rate (GFR), and serum and urine albumin and total protein concentrations are used to assess glomerular permselectivity. Urine glucose and amino acid concentrations are used to assess proximal tubular function, while serum electrolyte and bicarbonate concentrations reflect the kidney's ability to maintain electrolyte and acid–base balance. Lastly, urine specific gravity allows assessment of renal concentrating ability. The validity of the traditional markers is well established in the setting of both AKI and CKD. Although their ability to differentiate primary kidney injury from CvRD$_H$ is untested, these traditional markers are probably sufficiently sensitive to detect kidney dysfunction due to CvRD$_H$. There has been a recent surge of interest in the search for novel biomarkers of kidney injury and it is likely that several will become

Parameter	Traditional blood and urine tests	Potential novel markers
Glomerular filtration rate	Serum creatinine Plasma clearance tests	Symmetric dimethylarginine (SDMA)
Glomerular permselectivity	Serum albumin Urine protein to creatinine ratio Microalbuminuria	Urine immunoglobulin G
Tubular damage or dysfunction	Serum creatinine Serum electrolytes Serum bicarbonate Urine glucose Urine amino acids Urine protein to creatinine ratio Urine specific gravity	Urine N-acetyl B-D-glucosaminidase (NAG) Urine retinol binding protein (RBP) Urine gamma-glutamyl transpeptidase (GGT) Urine cystatin-C Urine kidney injury molecule-1 (KIM-1) Urine neutrophil gelatinase-associated lipocalin (NGAL) Urinary clusterin

16.4 Traditional and novel tests of kidney function.

available that will have utility in detecting early renal injury secondary to cardiac disease.

The most common biomarkers used to assess cardiovascular disease are N-terminal pro-B-type natriuretic peptide (NT-proBNP), B-type natriuretic peptide (BNP), N-terminal pro-atrial natriuretic peptide (NT-proANP) and cardiac troponin I (cTnI). While these biomarkers have been well studied in the setting of primary cardiovascular diseases such as cardiomyopathy and valvular disease (Oyama, 2013), their validity is less well established than that of some of the biomarkers used for assessment of kidney function, such as creatinine or urine specific gravity. Cardiac biomarkers currently cannot be used as the sole basis for staging of cardiac disease in dogs and cats.

The natriuretic peptides, including NT-proBNP, BNP and NT-proANP, are constitutively produced by the myocardium and help to regulate plasma volume, sodium excretion and vasomotor tone in both health and disease. Therefore, these peptides are up- or downregulated moment-to-moment, leading to clinically relevant individual and breed variations in both healthy and diseased animals. Few studies of cardiac biomarkers have been performed in small animals with renal disease. Serum or plasma concentrations of NT-proBNP, BNP and cTnI are increased in animals with renal dysfunction because they are excreted in the urine. In the setting of renal dysfunction, it is difficult to know whether increased natriuretic peptide concentrations reflect cardiac injury, decreased excretion or normal variation.

Cardiac troponin is a part of the actin–myosin complex. Studies reveal that cTnI concentrations are increased in dogs and cats with cardiac, as well as extra-cardiac, disease and predict clinical outcomes (Oyama, 2013). This suggests that cTnI measurement may aid in the detection of subclinical cardiac injury due to CvRD$_K$; however, interpretation of the cTnI assay is clouded by lack of information regarding the timecourse and magnitude of cTnI release in most disease conditions.

Imaging

Diagnostic imaging plays an important role in assessment of cardiac anatomy and function. While routinely performed in animals with known cardiac disease, it may be useful if performed in animals with known kidney disease and suspected CvRD$_K$. Radiographic and ultrasound imaging provide morphological expressions of the anatomical and functional changes, and results from these and other diagnostic tools are often complementary, such that the presence, cause, severity and consequences of heart disease are best understood after combining the information derived from these and other sources such as the physical examination and medical history.

Typically, the objective of a cardiothoracic radiographic examination is to detect changes in the cardiac silhouette, vascular structures and lung airway and parenchymal patterns, ultimately determining whether there are signs of cardiac disease or failure. Echocardiography is used to assess cardiac morphology and function, in both early and advanced stages of cardiac disease. Doppler echocardiography, including spectral Doppler, colour-flow Doppler, tissue Doppler and more advanced modalities such as strain, strain rate and two-dimensional (2D) speckle tracking, provides specific information about the velocity and direction of blood flow and the condition of the myocardium. Changes in radiographic and echocardiographic indices, along with biomarkers, can help to assess morbidity, non-cardiac thoracic disease, disease progression and prognosis in dogs and cats with heart disease. Thus, radiographic and echocardiographic imaging techniques are cornerstones of the cardiac diagnostic examination. The reader is referred to several excellent reviews of cardiothoracic radiographic and echocardiographic interpretation for more information (Buchanan and Bucheler, 1995; Litster and Buchanan, 2000; Thomas et al., 1993; Guglielmini et al., 2009; Chetboul, 2010; Chetboul and Tissier, 2012).

Renal imaging is routinely performed in animals with known kidney disease but should also be considered for animals with known cardiovascular disease and suspect CvRD$_H$. Various imaging modalities are available to assess the kidney and urinary system. Evaluation of plain survey radiographs, and in particular the ventrodorsal view, allows determination of kidney number, size, shape and position as well as the detection of radiodense uroliths. Ultrasound examination of the kidney and urinary tract allows visualization of renal parenchymal abnormalities, renal pelvic and ureteral dilatation, infarcts, cysts, tumours, mineralization and uroliths, although small abnormalities may escape detection. Renal ultrasonography is used to help in the diagnosis of specific diseases, such as pyelonephritis, lymphoma, renal aplasia/other congenital renal disease or ethylene glycol intoxication. Colour-flow Doppler ultrasonography, in combination with a renal 2D ultrasound examination, may be used to detect abnormal renal blood flow. Contrast techniques, such as the excretory urogram, or more advanced techniques, such as computed tomography or magnetic resonance imaging, with or without contrast, may provide additional information regarding the patency of the urinary system and the presence of abnormalities (see Chapter 7).

Blood pressure measurement

One of the most well understood interactions between the renal and cardiovascular systems revolves around the fact that both organ systems are intimately involved in regulation of arterial blood pressure. Blood pressure measurement is routinely recommended in patients with kidney or cardiovascular disease and the reader is referred to several excellent reviews on the measurement of blood pressure in dogs and cats (Brown et al., 2007; Syme, 2011; Stepien, 2014; see also Chapter 15). Systemic hypertension (SHT) is commonly associated with other diseases, such as hyperadrenocorticism, hyperaldosteronism, phaeochromocytoma, hyperthyroidism, hypothyroidism, diabetes

mellitus and canine acromegaly (Brown et al., 2007). SHT is also associated with certain therapeutic agents, such as glucocorticoids, mineralocorticoids, erythropoietin and phenylpropanolamine (Brown et al., 2007). SHT may be stress-induced (i.e. 'white coat hypertension') or may occur in the absence of other identifiable disease (i.e. idiopathic, primary or 'essential' hypertension) (Belew et al., 1999; Marino et al., 2011).

As in humans, SHT in dogs and cats is a potential cause of irreversible lesions in cardiac, vascular, renovascular, ocular and central nervous system tissues. Systolic blood pressure >160 mmHg poses a progressive risk of target-organ damage (IRIS, 2014). With regard to the canine kidney, SHT is associated with decreased GFR and an increased rate of renal injury, proteinuria, uraemic crisis and death (Jacob et al., 2003). In the cat, the relationship between hypertension and kidney disease is less clear. It is known that hypertension is a risk factor for proteinuria which is, in turn, a risk factor for worsening kidney disease (Syme et al., 2006; Chakrabarti et al., 2012). In a correlative study of laboratory variables and pathological lesions in the kidneys of cats with CKD, interstitial fibrosis correlated with the severity of azotaemia, hyperphosphataemia and anaemia. Proteinuria was associated with interstitial fibrosis and glomerular hypertrophy, whereas higher time-averaged systolic blood pressure was associated with glomerulosclerosis and hyperplastic arteriolosclerosis (Chakrabarti et al., 2013). Cardiovascular injury secondary to SHT includes left ventricular concentric hypertrophy, arrhythmia, haemorrhage, vascular and myocardial remodelling and fibrosis, and development of aortic insufficiency, diastolic dysfunction and heart failure (Maggio et al., 2000; Snyder et al., 2001; Sampedrano et al., 2006).

The reported prevalence of SHT in dogs and cats with CKD varies considerably, depending on the population selected, the stage of kidney disease and the blood pressure measuring technique employed, but CKD assuredly represents a considerable percentage of the population at risk for SHT (Brown et al., 2007). SHT is estimated to occur in 60–90% of dogs and 20–65% of cats with kidney disease (Stepien, 2014). The relationship of SHT with mitral valve disease is complex, and blood pressure varies by stage of disease. In one study, dogs with milder cardiac disease had higher blood pressure than those with more advanced disease (Petit et al., 2013). This possibly results from diminishing systolic left ventricular function (and the resultant fall in SBP) as cardiac disease progresses. Certainly, hypertension worsens mitral insufficiency and hastens disease progression. The minimum database in animals with SHT should include a complete blood count, serum biochemistry panel, serum total thyroxine concentration, urinalysis and abdominal ultrasonography (Brown et al., 2007). Ruling out endocrine or other causes of SHT may require additional disease-specific assays.

Disorders that cause systemic hypotension can also cause kidney and cardiovascular injury. Hypotension due to severe volume depletion, low cardiac output or collapse of systemic vascular resistance reduces tissue perfusion and GFR and activates maladaptive neurohormonal responses (Morales et al., 2002). Systemic hypotension, defined as systolic pressure <90 mmHg, has been associated with acute heart failure; hypotension occurs in 16% of cases with acute heart failure, during hospitalization (Goutal et al., 2010). In a study of dogs with mitral valve disease, systolic blood pressure was inversely correlated with the clinical severity of disease (Petit et al., 2013). Treatment of SHT is discussed under 'Management of CvRD', below (see also Chapters 15, 18, 21 and 23).

Management of CvRD

Treatment of CvRD is challenging for several reasons. The biggest and most common challenge is the fact that animals with advanced kidney disease frequently require fluid therapy to replace fluid deficits, whereas animals in heart failure commonly need diuretic therapy to alleviate congestion (pulmonary oedema or third-space effusions). There is a tendency for azotaemia to develop in animals prescribed diuretics, and for animals with heart failure to develop congestion when given fluids, thus complicating the assessment and management of animals with CvRD. Nutrition can also present a challenge because dogs and cats with kidney disease often receive a diet modified in protein and phosphorus content, while animals with heart failure, particularly those with cardiac cachexia, are commonly prescribed protein supplementation. It is also important for the practitioner to understand the benefits and risks of ACEi in the setting of concurrent kidney and cardiovascular disease and the potential influence of systemic hypertension on both organ systems. Thus, the heart and kidney are both affected by abnormal intravascular fluid volume, systemic blood pressure and commonly employed treatments such as diuretics, vasodilators and supplemental fluids used to correct these imbalances.

The clinical staging and management of heart failure, and of AKI and CKD, have been extensively described (Borgarelli et al., 2001; Atkins et al., 2009; Ferasin, 2009; Ross, 2011; Polzin, 2013). In brief, heart failure is the condition wherein the diseased heart fails to provide adequate cardiac output or can only do so in the presence of elevated venous filling pressures and the risk of congestion. Treatment of acute and chronic heart failure often involves the use of: diuretics including furosemide; vasodilators, including ACEi (e.g. enalapril, benazepril), amlodipine, nitroglycerin and nitroprusside; neurohormonal blocking agents, including ACEi, spironolactone and beta-blockers; and positive inotropes such as digoxin, dobutamine and pimobendan.

AKI and CKD are conditions wherein the diseased kidney fails adequately to excrete waste products and to maintain fluid volume and electrolyte balance, resulting in azotaemia, and volume and electrolyte abnormalities, with clinical signs of uraemia when the failure is severe. Treatment of AKI or CKD (see Chapters 21 and 23, respectively) often involves the use of parenteral fluids, antihypertensive agents, ACEi, gastrointestinal protectants, alkalizing agents, erythropoiesis-stimulating agents, phosphate binders and dietary modification. Diuretics may be indicated when there is oliguria, volume overload and hyperkalaemia, although 'renal replacement therapy' is the preferred treatment in this setting.

A key aspect to the treatment of both AKI and CKD is maintenance of adequate intravascular volume and pressure to allow sufficient renal perfusion, while avoiding fluid overload and electrolyte imbalance. In contrast, a key aspect of the treatment of congestive heart failure is reduction of intravascular volume and hydrostatic pressure through the use of diuretics and other off-loading therapies. Thus, essential to both cardiac and kidney disease is the need to restore and maintain normal fluid balance, often a particularly difficult aspect of therapy. Excessive reduction in vascular volume in cases of congestive heart failure or excessive increases in vascular volume in cases of oliguric kidney disease can lead to adverse effects in the other organ system. Achieving the correct balance is exponentially more difficult when the heart and kidneys are concomitantly dysfunctional. Treatment of CvRD involves the recognition and simultaneous evaluation of subtle changes in kidney or heart function and an understanding of how the pathophysiology of one disease can interact with and impact the function of the other. An important aspect of managing CvRD is to treat the primary cause of clinical signs while attempting to minimize clinical worsening of the function of the other organ. Management guidelines for CvRD are almost exclusively based on theory and expert opinion because clinical trials specific to CvRD are lacking. It can, however, be said assuredly that careful monitoring is of paramount importance.

Management of CvRD$_H$

In cases of CVRD$_H$, the therapeutic margin is small, because the use of diuretics and ACEi can have adverse effects on renal function, and overly aggressive diuresis with excessive dehydration should be avoided. Strategies to minimize kidney injury during treatment of acute congestive heart failure include reducing the total daily dosage (dosage and/or frequency of administration) of parenteral diuretics and vasodilators and the use of pimobendan or intravenous dobutamine infusion to increase cardiac output and kidney perfusion. A small proportion of clinicians withhold or minimize use of ACEi during in-hospital treatment for acute congestive heart failure, because diuretic-induced volume depletion may increase the risk of ACEi-induced kidney injury (Atkins et al., 2009). If ACEi are withheld or withdrawn during the acute phase, they are typically (re)introduced once the initial episode of acute congestive heart failure is resolved and the animal is discharged to home care. In cases of severe volume depletion, (re)introduction of diuretics or ACEi should only occur after the animal's hydration status has improved or at the recurrence of clinical signs of congestion. One potential therapeutic strategy involving the various ACEi, such as enalapril, benazepril, ramipril and imidapril, is the administration of a dosage at the lower end of the recommended dosage range, followed by evaluation of hydration status and renal function prior to a decision to up-titrate the dosage.

Free-choice water should always be provided to such patients, unless vomiting or diminished mental status dictates otherwise. In severely dehydrated animals or in those with substantial azotaemia or uraemia, intravenous or subcutaneous fluids, with consideration as to a particular fluid's sodium and potassium content, should be carefully administered following diuretic therapy. The use of feeding tubes should be considered in anorexic animals to provide both nutrition and sodium-free hydration. Anti-aldosterone agents, such as spironolactone, are often prescribed in the chronic phases of heart failure (Bernay et al., 2010). The potential for additional (earlier) beneficial effects, such as reduction of cardiac, renal and vascular remodelling in patients with CvRD, merits further investigation (Ovaert et al., 2010). Although rarely a problem, serum potassium concentration should be closely monitored, especially when spironolactone is used in conjunction with ACEi or in the setting of renal dysfunction.

Management of CvRD$_K$

Unstable CvRD$_K$, such as in instances of AKI, acute exacerbations of CKD, or a combination of the two, typically requires hospitalization to restore fluid and electrolyte balance, thereby improving renal function, while simultaneously evaluating the risk of heart failure. Fluid, diuretic and/or anti-hypertensive treatment should be appropriately titrated to the patient on the basis of hydration status and systemic blood pressure measurements, with a goal of restoring and maintaining normal fluid balance and blood pressure, while avoiding sodium and fluid overload. The requirement for and dosages of concurrent cardiac medications need to be reassessed (often with temporary or permanent dosage reduction) during evaluation of patients with unstable CvRD$_K$.

Despite a lack of evidence indicating a reduction in morbidity or improvement in survival, animals with AKI and oligoanuria are often prescribed diuretics. In animals with clinically significant dehydration, parenteral fluid replacement is given to regain fluid and electrolyte balance and to improve urine production in patients without frank heart failure. Even in the absence of clinical signs of heart failure, fluid supplementation should be closely monitored to avoid development of congestion and discontinued if weight gain becomes excessive. In instances where signs of overhydration and congestion occur, fluid administration should be discontinued and the addition of diuretics considered.

A cautious and stepwise approach to fluid replacement or maintenance fluid therapy should be used in dogs and cats with CvRD$_K$. Fluids relatively low in sodium should be chosen when possible (e.g. Normosol M®, 0.18% NaCl in 4% dextrose) along with careful monitoring of bodyweight, respiratory rate and effort, arterial blood pressure, and for development of jugular venous distension or ascites. Resting (i.e. non-panting) respiratory rates >40 breaths per minute are a sensitive indicator of early pulmonary oedema. Fluid overload puts additional stress on the cardiovascular system and heightens the risk of congestion. Except in cases of systemic hypotension, dopamine is not indicated for management of patients with CvRD$_K$ because of the lack of proven efficacy and the potential for adverse side effects, such as arrhythmias and sinus tachycardia. Renal replacement therapies allow better control of the intravascular volume and should be studied further in the management of dogs and cats with CvRD$_K$.

Important aspects of managing all forms of CvRD

There are other aspects to the management of dogs or cats with any form of CvRD. Because of its acute and chronic effects on the heart and kidneys, SHT needs to be identified and treated as per IRIS recommendations. Measuring systemic blood pressure accurately in dogs and cats requires careful attention to equipment and technique. This and a more detailed description of therapy is the subject of several excellent reviews (Brown et al., 2007; Syme, 2011; Stepien, 2014; see also Chapters 15, 18, 21 and 23). Dosages of diuretics, ACEi, inotropes and/or fluids should be carefully tailored to the needs of the individual patient. Ideally, ≤3–5 days following any dosage adjustments, renal function, bodyweight, hydration, electrolyte status and systemic blood pressure should be reassessed. The appetite and nutritional needs of the patient should be monitored, with consideration given to feeding a reduced sodium and phosphate diet, while providing appropriate protein and caloric intake.

In dogs and cats with CvRD, the goal is to maintain normal systolic blood pressure (120–150 mmHg), to avoid hypotension and to prevent or minimize hypertensive target-organ damage (IRIS, 2014). As blood pressure increases above 160 mmHg the risk of target-organ damage increases, and treatment is recommended whether target-organ damage is evident or not. In both dogs and cats, expert opinion advocates dietary sodium restriction with concurrent pharmacological therapy (Brown et al., 2007; IRIS, 2014). In dogs, first-choice therapy in non-emergent SHT is an ACEi, titrated to effect, while monitoring renal function. In cats, first-choice therapy is the calcium channel blocker amlodipine (IRIS, 2014), ideally with an ACEi, in the opinion of the authors. In cases of refractory SHT, combination therapy with ACEi and amlodipine is recommended, with up-titration as needed, in both species.

In animals with any form of CvRD, stepwise changes in diuretics or fluids are performed with concurrent monitoring of hydration, bodyweight, renal function and resting heart and respiratory rates. In both dogs and cats with AKI or CKD, veterinary surgeons (veterinarians) commonly administer intravenous or subcutaneous fluids to patients that are anorexic or have signs of uraemia, and during anaesthesia, in an attempt to maintain hydration and renal perfusion. Fluid administration should be performed with caution, using low-sodium parenteral fluids or sodium-free enteral hydration via a feeding tube, only at amounts needed to achieve therapeutic goals. This is especially true in the face of underlying heart disease or SHT. Any fluid type can precipitate congestive heart failure or a hypertensive crisis if sodium content is high, if administered too rapidly or if administered in excessive volumes. During treatment, the clinician and/or owner should monitor the animal's renal function, respiratory rate and effort, food and water intake, bodyweight and urine output. Changes in these parameters may signal worsening of disease but could also indicate a change in hydration status or the need for medication adjustments. In instances of severe CvRD, in which treatment balance is difficult to achieve, referral to a secondary or tertiary hospital is advised, ideally one where diagnostic and treatment plans are formulated jointly by a cardiologist and internist/nephrologist.

Another important consequence of CvRD is the alteration of drug pharmacokinetics and pharmacodynamics, due to impaired heart or kidney function. For example, furosemide requires active secretion across proximal renal tubule cells in order to reach its active site in the tubular lumen and, therefore, decreased renal perfusion and/or tubular injury decrease the expected diuretic response. Furthermore, drugs that are primarily excreted by the kidneys, such as digoxin, enalapril and atenolol, may require dosage adjustments in animals with AKI or CKD. In patients with CvRD and metabolic acidosis or hypoalbuminaemia, dosages of drugs that are highly protein-bound, such as pimobendan or digoxin, may need to be adjusted. Cardiac cachexia can result in a reduction in dosage requirements, because the drug's volume of distribution or protein binding may be altered. In animals with persistent congestion, the presence of ascites or pleural effusion alters the volume of drug distribution and dosing on lean bodyweight is preferred, being a safer approach. All of these factors necessitate careful monitoring and modification of drug dosages as disease in either system progresses.

Ensuring proper nutrition is an important component of managing CvRD. Moderately sodium-restricted diets are appropriate for animals with either kidney or cardiovascular disease. In addition, animals with kidney disease may benefit from changes in other nutrient content, including but not limited to phosphorus and fatty acids. As previously mentioned, dogs with end-stage heart disease typically lose muscle mass and body condition. Therefore, maintaining adequate protein and caloric intake is an important nutritional goal. In animals with CvRD, this can be very difficult because high protein and phosphorus intakes contribute to azotaemia, kidney disease progression and clinical signs of uraemia. Careful dietary planning, possibly with the support of a veterinary nutritionist, is needed.

Acknowledgements

The authors would like to acknowledge the Cardiorenal Consensus Study Group: Jean-Louis Pouchelon, Clarke E. Atkins, Claudio Bussadori, Mark A. Oyama, Shelly L. Vaden, John D. Bonagura, Valerie Chetboul, Larry D. Cowgill, Jonathan Elliott, Thierry Francey, Virginia Luis Fuentes, Gregory F. Grauer, N. Sydney Moise, David J. Polzin, Astrid M. van Dongen and Nicole van Israël.

References and further reading

Atkins C, Bonagura J and Ettinger S (2009) Guidelines for the diagnosis and treatment of canine valvular heart disease. *Journal of Veterinary Internal Medicine* **23**, 1142–1150

Belew AM, Barlett T and Brown SA (1999) Evaluation of the white-coat effect in cats. *Journal of Veterinary Internal Medicine* **13**, 134–142

Bernay F, Bland JM, Haggstrom J et al. (2010) Efficacy of spironolactone on survival in dogs with naturally occurring mitral regurgitation caused by myxomatous mitral valve disease. *Journal of Veterinary Internal Medicine* **24**, 331–341

Borgarelli M, Tarducci A, Tidholm A et al. (2001) Canine idiopathic dilated cardiomyopathy. Part II: Pathophysiology and therapy. *Veterinary Journal* **162**, 182–195

Brown S, Atkins C, Bagley R et al. (2007) Guidelines for the identification, evaluation, and management of systemic hypertension in dogs and cats. *Journal of Veterinary Internal Medicine* **21**, 542–558

Buchanan JW and Bucheler J (1995) Vertebral scale system to measure canine heart size in radiographs. *Journal of the American Veterinary Medical Association* **206**, 194–199

Chakrabarti S, Syme HM, Brown CA and Elliott J (2013) Histomorphometry of feline chronic kidney disease and correlation with markers of renal dysfunction. *Veterinary Pathology* **50**, 147–155

Chakrabarti S, Syme HM and Elliott J (2012) Clinicopathological variables predicting progression of azotemia in cats with chronic kidney disease. *Journal of Veterinary Internal Medicine* **26**, 275–281

Chetboul V (2010) Advanced techniques in echocardiography in small animals. *Veterinary Clinics of North America: Small Animal Practice* **40**, 529–543

Chetboul V and Tissier R (2012) Echocardiographic assessment of canine degenerative mitral valve disease. *Journal of Veterinary Cardiology* **14**, 127–148

Ferasin L (2009) Feline myocardial disease 2: Diagnosis, prognosis and clinical management. *Journal of Feline Medicine and Surgery* **11**, 183–194

Gouni V, Chetboul V, Pouchelon JL et al. (2008) Azotemia in cats with feline hypertrophic cardiomyopathy: prevalence and relationships with echocardiographic variables. *Journal of Veterinary Cardiology* **10**, 117–123

Goutal CM, Keir I, Kenney S et al. (2010) Evaluation of acute congestive heart failure in dogs and cats: 145 cases (2007–2008). *Journal of Veterinary Emergency and Critical Care* **20**, 330–337

Guglielmini C, Diana A, Pietra M et al. (2009) Use of the vertebral heart score in coughing dogs with chronic degenerative mitral valve disease. *Journal of Veterinary Medical Science* **71**, 9–13

Harrison E, Langston C, Palma D et al. (2012) Acute azotemia as a predictor of mortality in dogs and cats. *Journal of Veterinary Internal Medicine* **26**, 1093–1098

International Renal Interest Society (2014) *IRIS Guidelines*. Available from: www.iris-kidney.com/guidelines

International Small Animal Cardiac Health Council (1999) Recommendations for diagnosis of heart disease and treatment of heart failure in small animals. In: *Textbook of Canine and Feline Cardiology*, ed. PR Fox, DD Sisson and NS Moise, pp. 883–901. WB Saunders, Philadelphia

IRIS Canine GN Study Group Diagnosis Subgroup, Littman MP, Daminet S et al. (2013) Consensus recommendations for the diagnostic investigation of dogs with suspected glomerular disease. *Journal of Veterinary Internal Medicine* **27**, S19–S26

Jackevicius C, Fan CS and Warner A (2014) Clinical outcomes of erythropoietin use in heart failure patients with anemia of chronic kidney disease. *Journal of Cardiac Failure* **20**, 327–333

Jacob F, Polzin DJ, Osborne CA et al. (2003) Association between initial systolic blood pressure and risk of developing a uremic crisis or of dying in dogs with chronic renal failure. *Journal of the American Veterinary Medical Association* **222**, 322–329

Litster A and Buchanan J (2000) Vertebral scale system to measure heart size in radiographs of cats. *Journal of the American Veterinary Medical Association* **216**, 210–214

Maggio F, DeFrancesco T, Atkins CE et al. (2000) Ocular lesions associated with systemic hypertension in cats: 69 cases (1985–1998) *Journal of the American Veterinary Medical Association* **217**, 695–702

Marino CL, Cober RE, Iazbik MC and Couto CG (2011) White-coat effect on systemic blood pressure in retired racing Greyhounds. *Journal of Veterinary Internal Medicine* **25**, 861–865

Mitani S, Yabuki A, Tangiuchi K et al. (2013) Association between the intrarenal renin-angiotensin system and renal injury in chronic kidney diseases of dogs and cats. *Journal of Veterinary Medical Science* **75**, 127–133

Morales DL, Kavarana MN, Helman DN et al. (2002) Restoration of renal function in shock by perfusion of the renal artery with venous blood: a counterintuitive approach. *Critical Care Medicine* **30**, 1297–1300

Nicolle AP, Chetboul V, Allerheiligen T et al. (2007) Azotemia and glomerular filtration rate in dogs with chronic valvular disease. *Journal of Veterinary Internal Medicine* **21**, 943–949

Ovaert P, Elliott J, Bernay F, Guillot E and Bardon T (2010) Aldosterone receptor antagonists – how cardiovascular actions may explain their beneficial effects in heart failure. *Journal of Veterinary Pharmacology and Therapeutics* **33(2)**, 109–117

Oyama MA (2013) Use of cardiac biomarkers in veterinary practice. *Veterinary Clinics of North America: Small Animal Practice* **43**, 1261–1272

Petit AM, Gouni V, Tissier R et al. (2013) Systolic arterial blood pressure in small-breed dogs with degenerative mitral valve disease: a prospective study of 103 cases (2007–2012). *Veterinary Journal* **197**, 830–835

Polzin DJ (2013) Evidence-based step-wise approach to managing chronic kidney disease in dogs and cats. *Journal of Veterinary Emergency and Critical Care* **23**, 205–215

Pouchelon JL, Atkins CE, Bussadori C et al. (2015) Cardiovascular–renal axis disorders in the domestic dog and cat: a veterinary consensus statement. *Journal of Small Animal Practice* **56**, 537–552

Ronco C, Haapio M, House AA et al. (2008) Cardiorenal syndrome. *Journal of the American College of Cardiology* **52**, 1527–1539

Ronco C, McCullough P, Anker SD et al. (2010) Cardio-renal syndromes: Report from the consensus conference of the Acute Dialysis Quality Initiative. *European Heart Journal* **31**, 703–711

Ross L (2011) Acute kidney injury in dogs and cats. *Veterinary Clinics of North America: Small Animal Practice* **41**, 1–14

Sampedrano C, Chetboul V, Gouni V et al. (2006) Systolic and diastolic myocardial dysfunction in cats with hypertrophic cardiomyopathy or systemic hypertension. *Journal of Veterinary Internal Medicine* **20**, 1106–1115

Snyder PS, Sadke D and Jones GL (2001) Effect of amlodipine on echocardiographic variables in cats with systemic hypertension. *Journal of Veterinary Internal Medicine* **15**, 52–56

Stepien RL (2014) Systemic hypertension. In: *Current Veterinary Therapy XV*, ed. JD Bonagura and DC Twedt, pp. 726–730. Elsevier Saunders, St. Louis.

Syme HM (2011) Hypertension in small animal kidney disease. *Veterinary Clinics of North America. Small Animal Practice* **41**, 63–89

Syme HM, Markewell PJ, Pfeiffer D and Elliot J (2006) Survival of cats with naturally occurring chronic renal failure is related to severity of proteinuria. *Journal of Veterinary Internal Medicine* **20**, 528–535

Thomas WP, Gaber CE, Jacobs GJ et al. (1993) Recommendations for standards in transthoracic two-dimensional echocardiography in the dog and cat. Echocardiography Committee of the Specialty of Cardiology, American College of Veterinary Internal Medicine. *Journal of Veterinary Internal Medicine* **7**, 247–252

Chapter 17

Hyperthyroidism and the feline kidney

Tim Williams

Hyperthyroidism and chronic kidney disease in cats

Co-prevalence of hyperthyroidism and chronic kidney disease in cats

Hyperthyroidism is a common condition of senior and geriatric cats that is present in 6% of cats over the age of 9 years old. Similarly, chronic kidney disease (CKD) is common in old cats, hence it is not uncommon for cats with CKD to have concurrent hyperthyroidism, and *vice versa*.

Early studies reported that around 20% of hyperthyroid cats had elevated creatinine concentrations; however, a more recent study of 300 hyperthyroid cats in first-opinion practice reported that 10% of hyperthyroid cats had concurrent azotaemic CKD at the time of the diagnosis of hyperthyroidism (Williams *et al.*, 2010b).

Diagnosis of hyperthyroidism in cats with CKD

The presence of CKD can complicate the diagnosis of hyperthyroidism, because non-thyroidal illness may suppress serum total thyroxine (TT4) concentrations into the laboratory reference interval. It has been suggested that hyperthyroidism should be suspected in a cat with a serum creatinine concentration and serum TT4 concentration in the upper part of the reference interval (TT4 ≥30 nmol/l) (Wakeling *et al.*, 2008). Hyperthyroidism may be confirmed in these cases by utilization of other tests such as the tri-iodothyronine (T3) suppression test, thyroid scintigraphy or documentation of an elevated serum free thyroxine concentration (measured by equilibrium dialysis). Conversely, a diagnosis of concurrent hyperthyroidism can be ruled out by documentation of a detectable serum thyroid-stimulating hormone (TSH) concentration, whereas TSH concentrations below the detection limit of the assay may be observed in both euthyroid cats and cats with hyperthyroidism.

Diagnosis of CKD in cats with hyperthyroidism

The diagnosis of CKD in cats in hyperthyroidism can also be challenging, because excess thyroid hormones cause a range of physiological effects accompanied by biochemical changes, which confound the interpretation of renal function when using standard biochemical and urinalysis testing. These changes can mask underlying CKD in hyperthyroidism, and consequentially renal function in a hyperthyroid cat can only be fully assessed once hyperthyroidism has been treated and euthyroidism is established.

Systemic effects of hyperthyroidism

Effects of hyperthyroidism on biochemical markers of renal function

Serum/plasma creatinine concentrations

Hyperthyroidism is associated with an increase in glomerular filtration rate (GFR), which occurs secondary to increased cardiac output, decreased systemic vascular resistance, increased systemic activation of the renin–angiotensin–aldosterone system (RAAS) and enhanced tubuloglomerular feedback within the kidney. The GFR is inversely proportional to the serum creatinine concentration (see Chapter 10), therefore hyperthyroid cats have lower serum creatinine concentrations as a result of the increased GFR associated with hyperthyroidism. Serum creatinine concentrations are also influenced by muscle mass, which is in turn also reduced in hyperthyroid cats secondary to increased protein breakdown and catabolism. This decreased muscle mass therefore further contributes to a lower serum creatinine concentration in hyperthyroidism. As a result, serum creatinine concentrations in hyperthyroidism are poor indicators of GFR and the presence of concurrent CKD, particularly in cats with low muscle mass and poor body condition scores. Nevertheless, the presence of an elevated serum creatinine concentration in a hyperthyroid cat will reflect the presence of concurrent CKD, provided that pre-renal azotaemia is excluded. These initially azotaemic hyperthyroid cats will have more advanced CKD, the severity of which will be underestimated by the serum creatinine concentrations due to the confounding effects of hyperthyroidism on GFR and body muscle mass.

Serum/plasma urea concentrations

The interpretation of serum urea concentration as a marker of renal function in hyperthyroid cats is also difficult, and up to 70% of hyperthyroid cats have an elevated serum urea concentration. The serum urea concentration is more variable than the serum creatinine concentration in hyperthyroid cats because of the opposing factors of elevated GFR (expected to reduce serum urea concentration) and increased protein catabolism and protein intake (which increase serum urea concentration). Serum urea concentration is therefore not a good marker of renal function in hyperthyroidism.

Serum symmetric dimethylarginine concentrations

Several publications have explored the utility of serum symmetric dimethylarginine (SDMA) concentrations for the diagnosis of CKD in cats (Braff et al., 2014; Hall et al., 2014). Measuring serum SDMA concentrations may be advantageous compared with measurement of serum creatinine concentrations, because creatinine is influenced by changes in body muscle mass, which may accompany the development of CKD, unlike SDMA. However, to date, no publications have explored the effect of hyperthyroidism on serum SDMA concentrations in cats. In humans, hyperthyroidism and hypothyroidism are reported to influence both asymmetric dimethylarginine (ADMA) and SDMA, therefore it is possible that similar influences will also be observed in hyperthyroid cats, which may confound the use of SDMA as a marker of CKD in hyperthyroidism.

Serum and urinary cystatin C concentrations

Cystatin C is another biomarker for CKD, which is produced at a stable rate by all nucleated cells in the body and freely filtered by the glomerulus. Hence, serum cystatin C concentrations should also be less affected than serum creatinine concentrations by the changes in body muscle mass that occur in cats with CKD. However, hyperthyroidism increases cystatin C production by cells, and as a result, serum cystatin C concentrations are increased in hyperthyroid cats (Ghys et al., 2016; Williams et al., 2016), and do not appear to be a reliable marker of renal function in these patients (Williams et al., 2016). Urinary cystatin C to creatinine ratio is also increased in hyperthyroid cats compared with healthy older cats (Ghys et al., 2016), however urinary cystatin C to creatinine ratio was not a reliable marker of concurrent, but masked, azotaemic CKD in one preliminary study (Dillon et al., 2016).

Effects of hyperthyroidism on markers of mineral and bone disorder

Hyperthyroidism has wide-ranging effects on parameters associated with chronic kidney disease-mineral and bone disorder (CKD-MBD) in cats, including serum phosphate and calcium concentrations, plasma parathyroid hormone (PTH), calcitriol and fibroblast growth factor-23 (FGF-23) concentrations. However, it is of interest that the changes in these parameters that are observed in hyperthyroid cats are different from those reported in human patients with Graves' disease (the most common cause of hyperthyroidism in humans). For example, patients with Graves' disease tend to be hypercalcaemic, whereas hyperthyroid cats have a tendency towards hypocalcaemia.

Serum phosphate concentrations

Hyperphosphataemia, which can also be associated with reduced renal function, has been documented in a significant proportion of hyperthyroid cats (between 20 and 43%); however, it is present in hyperthyroid cats with and without concurrent, or masked, CKD (Williams et al., 2012). Hyperphosphataemia in hyperthyroidism is believed to reflect increased renal reabsorption of phosphate, due to a direct effect of thyroid hormone on the kidney. Therefore, assessment of serum phosphate concentrations in hyperthyroidism is not useful for assessing renal function.

Serum total calcium and plasma ionized calcium concentrations

Hyperthyroidism tends to lower the plasma ionized calcium concentration leading to some patients developing hypocalcaemia, an effect which is not associated with the presence of concurrent azotaemia (Williams et al., 2013). The aetiology of the hypocalcaemia associated with hyperthyroidism is still unknown, although the degree of hypocalcaemia is inversely proportional to the serum TT4 concentration.

Plasma PTH, calcitriol and FGF-23 concentrations

Up to 77% of hyperthyroid cats have elevated PTH concentrations, a finding consistent with the MBD observed in CKD (CKD-MBD; see Chapter 11 for a full discussion). However, hyperparathyroidism is present in hyperthyroid cats with and without concurrent, or masked, CKD. Therefore, it is speculated that hyperparathyroidism in hyperthyroidism occurs in response to the hyperphosphataemia and hypocalcaemia that is observed in these cats, rather than reflecting the presence of CKD and CKD-MBD (Williams et al., 2012).

Plasma calcitriol concentrations can also be decreased in cats with CKD, secondary to reduced renal mass and the suppressive effects of hyperphosphataemia and/or FGF-23 on the activity of 1-alpha-hydroxylase in the kidney, which is the enzyme responsible for the production of calcitriol. In hyperthyroid cats, plasma calcitriol concentrations are increased (Williams et al., 2013), which probably reflects increased calcitriol production secondary to stimulation of the 1-alpha-hydroxylase enzyme activity by elevated PTH concentrations associated with hyperthyroidism.

Plasma FGF-23 concentrations appear to be suppressed in hyperthyroid cats with and without concurrent, or masked, CKD (Williams et al., 2012). The decreased serum FGF-23 concentration observed in hyperthyroid cats is thought to be secondary to a combination of increased renal clearance of FGF-23 (due to increased GFR) and hypocalcaemia (which also suppresses FGF-23 secretion).

Effects of hyperthyroidism on urinary parameters influenced by renal function
Urine specific gravity

Urine specific gravity (USG) is reported to be extremely variable in hyperthyroid cats (between 1.009 and ≥1.050). In human patients, hyperthyroidism is associated with reduced urine concentrating ability; however, overt polyuria and polydipsia are uncommon clinical signs. In contrast, polyuria and polydipsia are reported frequently in hyperthyroid cats, which could reflect the high prevalence of CKD in the feline hyperthyroid population when compared with human patients with hyperthyroidism. It is suggested that altered sensitivity of the distal renal tubule to vasopressin in the hyperthyroid state may contribute to reduced urine concentrating ability (see Chapter 2), because treatment of hyperthyroid human patients with vasopressin did not elicit an equivalent antidiuretic response when compared with healthy controls, and this response returned to normal following treatment. It has also been suggested that impaired urine concentrating ability may be due to a reduced medullary sodium concentration in hyperthyroidism (secondary to increased renal blood flow and medullary washout), or may be the result of osmotic diuresis due to the increased filtered solute. The USG is, therefore, not a reliable indicator of renal function in hyperthyroidism. Although USG is generally lower in hyperthyroid cats with concurrent or masked CKD (Williams *et al.*, 2010b), many cats that develop azotaemic CKD following treatment will have USG >1.035 prior to treatment, therefore USG cannot be used reliably to identify hyperthyroid cats with concurrent, but masked, CKD.

Proteinuria

Many hyperthyroid cats are proteinuric, with 64–86% of hyperthyroid cats having a urine protein to creatinine ratio (UPC) >0.4 (van Hoek *et al.*, 2009a; Williams *et al.*, 2010b), the threshold for classification of a patient as proteinuric in the International Renal Interest Society (IRIS) CKD staging system (see Chapter 12). However, the proteinuria associated with hyperthyroidism does not appear to be solely due to increased urinary albumin excretion (Williams *et al.*, 2010b). Proteinuria may be secondary to increased urinary excretion of other proteins, including *N*-acetyl-beta-D-glucosaminidase (NAG), retinol binding protein (RBP) and vascular endothelial growth factor (VEGF) (Lapointe *et al.*, 2008; van Hoek *et al.*, 2009b; Williams *et al.*, 2014a), some of which may also reflect renal tubular injury or dysfunction. However, proteinuria is present in hyperthyroid cats both with and without concurrent, or masked, CKD (Williams *et al.*, 2010b), and the presence of proteinuria is not a useful marker of concurrent renal disease in hyperthyroidism.

Urinary *N*-acetyl-beta-D-glucosaminidase index

N-acetyl-beta-D-glucosaminidase (NAG) is a biomarker of tubular damage in humans, and has been investigated in cats with both CKD and hyperthyroidism. It appears that the urinary NAG index (urinary NAG concentration indexed to urinary creatinine concentration) is increased in hyperthyroidism (regardless of the presence of concurrent CKD) and decreases following treatment (Lapointe *et al.*, 2008). The urinary NAG index is also not a reliable marker of CKD in untreated hyperthyroid cats because it does not predict the development of azotaemia following treatment to establish euthyroidism (Lapointe *et al.*, 2008).

Effect of hyperthyroidism on systolic blood pressure

The diagnosis of systolic hypertension in cats can be problematic because of the 'white coat' effect. It has been suggested that there is a more pronounced white coat effect in hyperthyroid cats if care is not taken to minimize stress, therefore some hyperthyroid cats with elevated systolic blood pressure (SBP) may have white coat hypertension rather than true systolic hypertension.

The prevalence of hypertension in hyperthyroid cats was reported to be high in one early publication, however this study probably overestimated the prevalence of systolic hypertension because a relatively low cut-off point (140 mmHg) was used for the diagnosis of hypertension (Kobayashi *et al.*, 1990). Later studies, in which systolic hypertension was diagnosed as SBP >160 mmHg,

reported the prevalence of hypertension to be 14–23% in hyperthyroid cats (Stiles *et al.*, 1994; Williams *et al.*, 2010b), and this is probably more reflective of the true prevalence of hypertension in hyperthyroid cats in first-opinion practice. Given the high prevalence of white coat hypertension in hyperthyroid cats, the diagnosis of a true hypertensive disorder may be difficult, therefore fundic examination is recommended to try to document the presence of hypertensive retinopathy, which will confirm that a true hypertensive disorder is present. However, it appears that hypertensive hyperthyroid cats generally have a lower incidence of hypertensive retinopathy than hypertensive cats with other comorbid disorders, such as CKD. The decision to treat hypertensive hyperthyroid cats without hypertensive retinopathy requires consideration of the SBP measurement and the presence of comorbid disease such as CKD. Cats with persistently high SBP measurements (>200 mmHg on two or more occasions), or with comorbid diseases such as CKD, may warrant anti-hypertensive therapy prior to, or in conjunction with, anti-thyroid therapy.

Systemic effects of treatment of hyperthyroidism

Effect of treatment of hyperthyroidism on renal function

Treatment of hyperthyroidism results in a decrease in cardiac output, normalization of systemic vascular resistance and a reduction in RAAS activity, all of which contribute to a reduction in GFR. In addition, reversal of hyperthyroidism will lead to reduced muscle catabolism, and increased muscle mass and bodyweight. Together, these factors contribute to an increase in serum creatinine concentration, of approximately 50–100 μmol/l, following treatment to restore euthyroidism. The magnitude of the change in serum creatinine concentration will be dependent on the change in TT4 that occurs following treatment, so that cats with higher initial TT4 concentrations will experience greater increases in serum creatinine concentrations following treatment. It is recommended that the target TT4 for hyperthyroid cats should be within the lower half of the laboratory reference interval, unless the hyperthyroid cat was azotaemic at the time of diagnosis of hyperthyroidism (see 'Hyperthyroid cats with azotaemia at the time of diagnosis of hyperthyroidism', below) (Daminet *et al.*, 2014), although there is currently no evidence in the peer-reviewed literature to support this recommendation.

One study reported that serum creatinine concentrations decreased, rather than increased, when dietary management of hyperthyroidism (Hill's® Prescription Diet® y/d®) was instituted (van der Kooij *et al.*, 2014). Although this could suggest that dietary therapy of hyperthyroidism may preserve renal function, and thus may be advantageous, it should be noted that in this study the TT4 concentrations did not return to within reference intervals in 25% of patients during the study period (8 weeks), and in many cats hyperthyroidism was not well controlled (as defined by a TT4 in the lower half of the laboratory reference interval) (Daminet *et al.*, 2014). It is probable that failure to adequately control hyperthyroidism will have contributed to ongoing loss of body muscle mass and consequentially a decrease in serum creatinine concentrations in cats on dietary therapy. Therefore, dietary therapy may not be beneficial to renal function in treated hyperthyroid cats, although further studies to evaluate this in well controlled hyperthyroid cats are warranted.

As a result of the increase in serum creatinine concentrations that occurs with treatment, some initially non-azotaemic hyperthyroid cats will develop azotaemia following restoration of euthyroidism. Studies in cats treated with radioiodine suggested that up to 49% of initially non-azotaemic hyperthyroid cats develop azotaemia following treatment (Figure 17.1). However, one study of cats treated in first-opinion practice (by anti-thyroid medications and/or thyroidectomy) reported the incidence of post-treatment azotaemia to be lower than this (15–25%; Williams *et al.*, 2010b). Similarly, a questionnaire-based study reported a prevalence of CKD in cats with hyperthyroidism of 27%, although the criteria for diagnosis of CKD were not stated or standardized (Caney, 2013). It is probable that the increased incidence of post-treatment azotaemia in radioiodine-treated cats was, at least in part, attributable to an increased prevalence of iatrogenic hypothyroidism, which we now know will increase the incidence of post-treatment azotaemia (see below).

It should also be noted that, although GFR will stabilize within 1 month of successful treatment of hyperthyroidism, serum creatinine concentrations will continue to increase for up to 3 months following restoration of euthyroidism (Boag *et al.*, 2007). This probably reflects the increase in muscle mass which will occur for several months following treatment of hyperthyroidism. Therefore, it is advisable to check renal function at the time of restoration of euthyroidism and also 3 months later, because serum creatinine concentrations may increase further over this period. As a result, concurrent azotaemic CKD may not be unmasked until up to 3 months following restoration of euthyroidism.

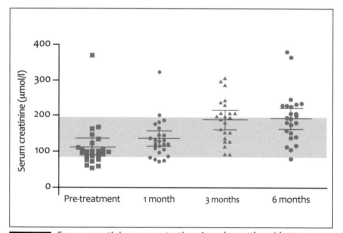

17.1 Serum creatinine concentrations in 24 hyperthyroid cats before and 1, 3 and 6 months after they were treated with radioactive iodine. The horizontal bars show the mean and 95% confidence intervals; the reference interval for creatinine is shown in grey. (Reproduced from Boag *et al.*, 2007 with permission from the *Veterinary Record*)

Effect of treatment of hyperthyroidism on other biochemical parameters

Treatment of hyperthyroidism leads to normalization of serum phosphate and PTH concentrations in cats that do not have concurrent CKD, and a reduction in proteinuria in the majority of cats. In cats suspected of having concomitant CKD, evaluation of these parameters for the assessment of the IRIS CKD substage (for proteinuria) and for evaluation of phosphate restriction (according to IRIS

guidelines) should therefore not be performed until euthyroidism is restored and serum creatinine has stabilized.

Effect of treatment of hyperthyroidism on systolic blood pressure

Treatment of hyperthyroidism also has an influence on SBP in cats. It has been reported that 23% of initially normotensive cats develop persistent systolic hypertension after treatment of hyperthyroidism (Morrow *et al.*, 2009). Therefore, although hypertension is present in 14–23% of hyperthyroid cats at the time of diagnosis, it would appear that hypertension occurs in a similar or greater number of cats following treatment of hyperthyroidism. The development of post-treatment hypertension is not limited to those cats that develop azotaemia; therefore, monitoring of SBP following treatment of hyperthyroidism is important in all cats, because failure to document and treat concurrent hypertension could lead to retinal damage, blindness and possibly further renal injury.

Effect of iatrogenic hypothyroidism on renal function

Iatrogenic hypothyroidism was, until recently, not thought to cause significant morbidity in cats, because cats with low serum TT4 concentrations rarely showed clinical signs of hypothyroidism. However, iatrogenic hypothyroidism is now regarded as an important consequence of overtreatment of hyperthyroidism; it has a range of systemic effects on the renal, haematopoietic and cardiovascular systems, which may in turn increase morbidity and mortality.

The prevalence of iatrogenic hypothyroidism in cats treated with methimazole has been estimated to be approximately 20% (Aldridge *et al.*, 2015). The diagnosis of iatrogenic hypothyroidism can be problematic owing to suppression of serum TT4 concentrations by non-thyroidal illnesses, including CKD, which are common in older cats. Clinical studies have utilized a combination of low serum TT4 concentrations and high serum TSH concentrations (using a canine TSH assay) to diagnose iatrogenic hypothyroidism, and this allows the differentiation of cats with low serum TT4 concentrations secondary to non-thyroidal illness from cats with iatrogenic hypothyroidism (Williams *et al.*, 2010a). However, utilization of this approach in general practice may be limited by the lack of feline-specific reference intervals for TSH in some laboratories and differences in the assay methodology used to measure TSH.

Cats with iatrogenic hypothyroidism have a greater incidence of post-treatment azotaemia than cats that remain euthyroid (with a TT4 within the lower half of the reference interval) following treatment (Williams *et al.*, 2010a). In addition, reversal of iatrogenic hypothyroidism by reduction of the dose of anti-thyroid medication, with the aim of achieving a serum TT4 concentration within the lower half of the laboratory reference interval, will reduce serum creatinine concentrations by approximately 20% and reverse azotaemia in about 50% of azotaemic cats with iatrogenic hypothyroidism (Williams *et al.*, 2014b). Hypothyroidism reduces GFR, which will exacerbate existing azotaemia, therefore reversal of hypothyroidism will cause an increase in GFR and hence a reduction in serum creatinine concentrations.

Predictors of the development of azotaemia following treatment of hyperthyroid cats

Numerous studies have attempted to identify reliable bio-markers of concurrent, but masked, CKD in hyperthyroid cats, but with little success. In general, there is an association between the pre-treatment serum creatinine concentration and the subsequent development of azotaemia, with cats with a serum creatinine concentration in the upper end of the laboratory reference interval being more likely to develop azotaemia following treatment, although a sensitive and specific cut-off point for the prediction of post-treatment azotaemia has not been established. This probably reflects the fact that the change in serum creatinine concentration that occurs following treatment, and thus the development of post-treatment azotaemia, will partly depend on the initial serum TT4 concentration and the muscle mass of the cat.

The utility of other biomarkers of renal function, such as serum urea concentration, USG, UPC and urinary excretion of NAG, RBP and VEGF, to predict which cats will develop post-treatment azotaemia has also been assessed; however, these markers all serve as poor predictors of the development of renal azotaemia following treatment.

The GFR can be measured directly and in a reasonably practical manner using a plasma iohexol clearance test (see Chapter 10), however the GFR of hyperthyroid cats does not appear to be a good predictor of the presence of masked azotaemic CKD (Boag et al., 2007). To date, no GFR value has been shown to be consistently sensitive or specific for the presence of masked CKD in hyperthyroid cats but, because GFR can be measured using a variety of techniques, it is likely that a separate cut-off point for the prediction of post-treatment azotaemia would need to be established for each individual methodology.

Does the development of azotaemia following treatment matter?

The development of azotaemia in hyperthyroid cats following treatment frequently leads to suboptimal treatment of hyperthyroidism (Higgs et al., 2014), the rationale being that maintenance of a mild hyperthyroid state will increase GFR and decrease serum creatinine concentrations. However, this approach is no longer recommended. Overall survival time does not differ between treated hyperthyroid cats that develop azotaemia following treatment and treated hyperthyroid cats that remain non-azotaemic, if euthyroidism is maintained (Figure 17.2; Williams et al., 2010a). Therefore, provided that concurrent azotaemic CKD is managed appropriately, these findings demonstrate that there is no rationale for reducing the dosage of anti-thyroid medication administered to initially non-azotaemic hyperthyroid cats that develop stable mild to moderate (IRIS Stage 2 or 3) azotaemia following treatment.

In contrast, cats with iatrogenic hypothyroidism that develop post-treatment azotaemia have shorter survival times than cats with iatrogenic hypothyroidism that remain non-azotaemic (Figure 17.3; Williams et al., 2010a). This suggests that the composite effect of iatrogenic

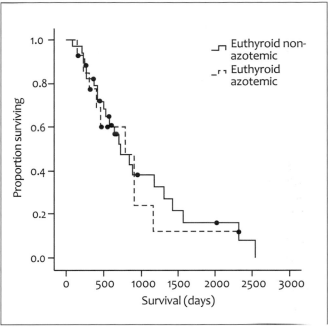

17.2 Kaplan–Meier survival curves for 47 cats treated for hyperthyroidism that were euthyroid after 6 months of treatment. The cats were grouped according to whether or not they were azotaemic at the end of the 6-month follow-up period and survival curves were plotted for each group (azotaemic and non-azotaemic). Circles represent censored individuals. There was no significant difference in the survival time of euthyroid azotaemic and non-azotaemic cats.
(Reproduced from Williams et al., 2010a with permission from the Journal of Veterinary Internal Medicine)

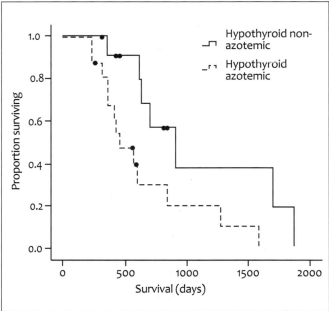

17.3 Kaplan–Meier survival curves for 28 cats treated for hyperthyroidism that were classified as hypothyroid after 6 months of treatment (based on documentation of a low serum total thyroxine (TT4) concentration and high thyroid-stimulating hormone (TSH) concentration). The cats were grouped according to whether or not they were azotaemic at the end of the 6-month follow-up period and survival curves were plotted for each group (azotaemic and non-azotaemic). Circles represent censored individuals. Hypothyroid azotaemic cats had significantly shorter survival times than hypothyroid non-azotaemic cats.
(Reproduced from Williams et al., 2010a with permission from the Journal of Veterinary Internal Medicine)

hypothyroidism and CKD is detrimental and, therefore, that restoration of euthyroidism in cats with iatrogenic hypothyroidism and azotaemia is recommended, because this may improve the overall survival time of these cats.

Partly as a consequence of these clinical findings, treatment trials with reversible therapy (anti-thyroid medication or dietary therapy) in hyperthyroid cats prior to definitive treatment options, such as thyroidectomy or radioiodine, are no longer recommended for all cats (Daminet et al., 2014). Previously, reversible therapy was recommended first because this would allow the presence of concurrent CKD to be unmasked following establishment of euthyroidism. However, because the development of mild to moderate azotaemia following treatment is not associated with a worse outcome for the cat, those cats with concurrent mild to moderate azotaemic CKD are equally good candidates for definitive treatment as hyperthyroid cats without concurrent CKD. Initiation of reversible therapy prior to definitive treatment is, however, still recommended for cats with overt azotaemia at the time of diagnosis of hyperthyroidism (because these cats probably have more severe CKD and a guarded prognosis (see 'Hyperthyroid cats with azotaemia at the time of diagnosis of hyperthyroidism', below)), and in cats awaiting surgical thyroidectomy (in order to reduce anaesthetic risk).

Is hyperthyroidism damaging to the kidney?

Early studies suggested that the overall prevalence of azotaemic CKD in hyperthyroid cats, calculated by summating those cats with azotaemia prior to treatment (20–23%) and those that developed azotaemia following treatment (up to 49%), was higher than the reported prevalence of CKD in the general feline senior and geriatric population. For this reason, it has been postulated that damage occurs to the kidney in the hyperthyroid state, which contributes to the development and/or progression of azotaemic CKD and explains the increased prevalence of CKD in the hyperthyroid population.

There are a number of clinicopathological changes that occur in hyperthyroidism that could be damaging to the kidney. These include: the induction of proteinuria; activation of the RAAS; and derangements in calcium and phosphate homeostasis similar to those associated with CKD-MBD. The association between these clinicopathological changes and the development of azotaemia following treatment has been evaluated in a series of clinical studies of client-owned cats with naturally occurring hyperthyroidism (Williams et al., 2010b; Williams et al., 2012; Williams et al., 2014a). However, the clinical data accumulated to date do not support the hypothesis that these systemic changes are detrimental to renal function in hyperthyroid cats. Hyperthyroid cats with proteinuria, hyperphosphataemia and hyperparathyroidism are no more likely to develop azotaemia following treatment than hyperthyroid cats with less marked clinicopathological changes, which suggests that these changes (when they occur in the hyperthyroid state) may not be damaging to the kidney.

The increased prevalence of azotaemic CKD in the hyperthyroid population, which led to the hypothesis that hyperthyroidism may be damaging to the kidney, may in fact reflect the reduction in GFR which occurs secondary to iatrogenic hypothyroidism, because this was not accounted for in previous studies. It is possible that 50% of cats with iatrogenic hypothyroidism have reversible azotaemia, which may have led to an overestimation of the prevalence of azotaemia in hyperthyroid cats following treatment. More recent data, from hyperthyroid cats treated in first-opinion practice using anti-thyroid medication alone or in combination with thyroidectomy, have suggested that the prevalence of azotaemic CKD in hyperthyroid cats is lower than previously thought, with 10% of hyperthyroid cats having azotaemia prior to treatment and 15–25% of hyperthyroid cats developing azotaemic CKD following treatment. As a result, the prevalence of azotaemic CKD in hyperthyroid cats overall would be around 24–33%, which is consistent with the prevalence of azotaemic CKD in the senior and geriatric feline population (up to 31%). Therefore, at present, there is no evidence to suggest that hyperthyroidism is damaging to the kidney in cats.

Management of hyperthyroid cats with concurrent, or masked, CKD

The recommended approach to the initial management of cats with hyperthyroidism and concurrent or masked CKD (using anti-thyroid medication) is summarized in Figure 17.4.

Hyperthyroid cats with azotaemia at the time of diagnosis of hyperthyroidism

The presence of concurrent CKD in a hyperthyroid cat should not alter the treatment of hyperthyroidism unless the cat has an elevated serum creatinine concentration (azotaemia) with evidence of reduced urine concentrating ability (to exclude pre-renal azotaemia) at the time of diagnosis. In hyperthyroid cats with azotaemia at the time of diagnosis of hyperthyroidism, treatment of hyperthyroidism will be associated with further increases in the serum creatinine concentration, which may result in the cat developing severe azotaemia (IRIS CKD Stage 4). No studies have yet been performed to compare the survival times of hyperthyroid cats with azotaemia prior to treatment that are left untreated with those of hyperthyroid cats that are treated (and therefore develop more severe azotaemia). However, the decision to treat should probably be dependent on the clinical presentation of the individual animal. If the cat has presented because of clinical signs of hyperthyroidism (such as vomiting and diarrhoea), which may compromise the welfare of the animal, then treatment for hyperthyroidism should be initiated. Treatment can also be attempted in cats with mild azotaemia (IRIS CKD Stage 2), although renal function should be monitored closely. However, if the cat has moderate to severe azotaemia (IRIS CKD Stage 3 or 4), then treatment could be deferred if no clinical signs associated with hyperthyroidism are present.

If treatment is initiated in a hyperthyroid cat with azotaemia at the time of diagnosis of hyperthyroidism, it is best to use reversible therapy (anti-thyroid medication or dietary therapy) rather than definitive treatments such as surgical thyroidectomy or radioiodine. When instituting anti-thyroid medication, the lowest available dose (e.g. 1.25 mg methimazole q24h) should be used and serum TT4 concentration and renal parameters monitored closely. The first aim should be to reverse the clinical signs of

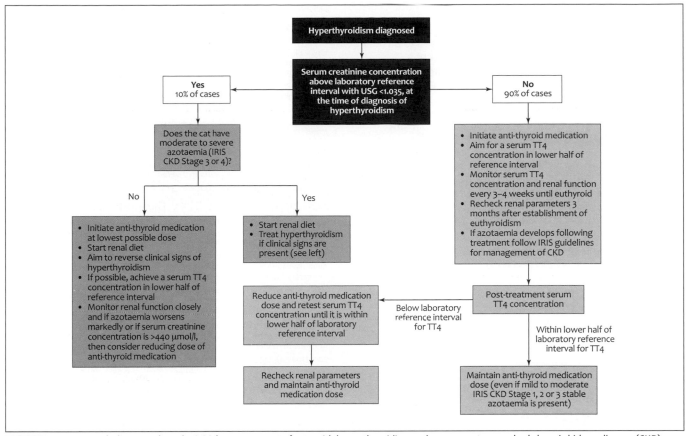

17.4 Recommended approach to the initial management of cats with hyperthyroidism and concurrent or masked chronic kidney disease (CKD). IRIS = International Renal Interest Society; TT4 = total thyroxine; USG = urine specific gravity.

hyperthyroidism and then, if possible, a serum TT4 concentration in the lower half of the reference interval should be attained. If achieving a lower serum TT4 concentration leads to a marked increase in the serum creatinine concentration (particularly if it exceeds 440 µmol/l), then the dose of anti-thyroid medication may have to be reduced. Regardless of whether hyperthyroidism is controlled or not in these cats, a renal diet should be introduced in all cases and the IRIS guidelines for the management of CKD should be followed. Unfortunately, the prognosis in hyperthyroid cats with concomitant azotaemic CKD prior to treatment is generally poor, with a median survival time of 6 months (Williams *et al.*, 2010b). Definitive treatment of hyperthyroidism (by radioiodine or surgery) would therefore not be recommended.

Hyperthyroid cats that are non-azotaemic at the time of diagnosis of hyperthyroidism, but which develop azotaemia following treatment

Initially non-azotaemic hyperthyroid cats should be treated for hyperthyroidism, with the aim of achieving a serum TT4 concentration in the lower half of the laboratory reference interval. Serum TT4 concentrations and renal parameters (serum creatinine concentration and urine specific gravity as a minimum) should be monitored at least every 3–4 weeks until euthyroidism is restored, and then 3 months after restoration of euthyroidism. Azotaemia will develop following treatment in around 15–25% of cases (Williams *et al.*, 2010b), however this should not lead to an alteration in the dose of anti-thyroid medication, and a target TT4

concentration in the lower half of the laboratory reference interval should still be the aim. In cats that develop azotaemic CKD, the IRIS guidelines for the management of feline CKD should also be followed.

If a cat treated with anti-thyroid medication has a serum TT4 concentration below the laboratory reference interval following treatment, the dose of medication may need to be reduced, particularly if the cat is azotaemic or if the TT4 is below the limit of detection. If the TT4 is above the limit of detection but below the laboratory reference interval and the cat is non-azotaemic, then continued monitoring may be appropriate if the cat is clinically well. In cases where dose adjustments are required, the dose should be changed in the smallest possible increments (e.g. 1.25 mg increments of methimazole) and the serum TT4 concentration retested every 3–4 weeks until the TT4 is within the lower half of the reference interval for TT4. Once euthyroidism is restored, renal parameters should also be rechecked, and the IRIS guidelines for the management of CKD followed if renal azotaemia is still present following restoration of euthyroidism.

Following treatment with radioiodine or by surgical thyroidectomy, it may be prudent to monitor cats with a low serum TT4 concentration for up to 6 months. If serum TT4 concentrations remain below the laboratory reference interval for longer than a 6-month period, then thyroxine supplementation should be instituted. In many cases, ectopic thyroid tissue will restore normal thyroid function following definitive treatment of hyperthyroidism (by radioiodine or surgery), however this will not be the case in cats treated with anti-thyroid medications, because these drugs will continue to block thyroxine production within the thyroid gland.

Conclusions

- Hyperthyroidism affects all parameters used to assess renal function, therefore the renal function of a hyperthyroid cat can only be fully assessed once hyperthyroidism has been successfully treated for at least 3 months.
- Many abnormalities associated with hyperthyroidism, such as proteinuria and hyperphosphataemia, are reversed following successful treatment of hyperthyroidism.
- Approximately 15–25% of initially non-azotaemic hyperthyroid cats will develop azotaemia following treatment of hyperthyroidism.
- The development of azotaemia following treatment of hyperthyroidism, in a cat which was not previously azotaemic, is not associated with a worse outcome for the cat. Therefore, hyperthyroidism should continue to be managed effectively (aiming for a serum TT4 concentration in the lower half of the laboratory reference interval), even if stable mild to moderate (IRIS CKD Stage 2 or 3) azotaemia develops following treatment.
- Iatrogenic hypothyroidism will worsen renal function and azotaemia, and may shorten survival time, therefore prolonged iatrogenic hypothyroidism (>6 months) should be avoided.

Acknowledgements

The author would like to acknowledge Harriet Syme for her valuable input when writing this chapter.

References and further reading

Aldridge C, Behrend EN, Martin LG et al. (2015) Evaluation of thyroid-stimulating hormone, total thyroxine, and free thyroxine concentrations in hyperthyroid cats receiving methimazole treatment. *Journal of Veterinary Internal Medicine* **29(3)**, 862–868

Boag AK, Neiger R, Slater L et al. (2007) Changes in the glomerular filtration rate of 27 cats with hyperthyroidism after treatment with radioactive iodine. *Veterinary Record* **161(21)**, 711–715

Braff J, Obare E, Yerramilli M and Elliott J (2014) Relationship between serum symmetric dimethylarginine concentration and glomerular filtration rate in cats. *Journal of Veterinary Internal Medicine* **28(6)**, 1699–1701

Caney SM (2013) An online survey to determine owner experiences and opinions on the management of their hyperthyroid cats using oral anti-thyroid medications. *Journal of Feline Medicine and Surgery* **15(6)**, 494–502

Daminet S, Kooistra HS, Fracassi F et al. (2014) Best practice for the pharmacological management of hyperthyroid cats with antithyroid drugs. *Journal of Small Animal Practice* **55(1)**, 4–13

Dillon H, Archer J, Syme HM, Elliott J and Williams TL (2016) The use of urinary biomarkers to predict the development of azotaemia following treatment of hyperthyroidism in cats. *Proceedings of the British Small Animal Veterinary Association Congress 2016*, p. 510 (abstract)

Ghys LF, Paepe D, Taffin ER et al. (2016) Serum and urinary cystatin C in cats with feline immunodeficiency virus infection and cats with hyperthyroidism. *Journal of Feline Medicine and Surgery* **18(8)**, 658–665

Hall JA, Yerramilli M, Obare E and Jewell DE (2014) Comparison of serum concentrations of symmetric dimethylarginine and creatinine as kidney function biomarkers in cats with chronic kidney disease. *Journal of Veterinary Internal Medicine* **28(6)**, 1676–1683

Higgs P, Murray JK and Hibbert A (2014) Medical management and monitoring of the hyperthyroid cat: a survey of UK general practitioners. *Journal of Feline Medicine and Surgery* **16(10)**, 788–795

Jepson RE, Slater L, Nash S et al. (2006) Evaluation of cystatin C as a marker of GFR in hyperthyroid cats. *Journal of Veterinary Internal Medicine* **20(3)**, 740

Kobayashi DL, Peterson ME, Graves TK et al. (1990) Hypertension in cats with chronic renal failure or hyperthyroidism. *Journal of Veterinary Internal Medicine* **4**, 58–62

Lapointe C, Belanger MC, Dunn M, Moreau M and Bedard C (2008) N-acetyl-beta-D-glucosaminidase index as an early biomarker for chronic kidney disease in cats with hyperthyroidism. *Journal of Veterinary Internal Medicine* **22(5)**, 1103–1110

Morrow L, Adams VJ, Elliott J and Syme H (2009) Hypertension in hyperthyroid cats: prevalence, incidence and predictors of its development. *Journal of Veterinary Internal Medicine* **23**, 700

Stiles J, Polzin D and Bistner S (1994) The prevalence of retinopathy in cats with systemic hypertension and chronic renal failure or hyperthyroidism. *Journal of the American Animal Hospital Association* **26**, 647–651

van der Kooij M, Bečvářová I, Meyer HP, Teske E and Kooistra HS (2014) Effects of an iodine-restricted food on client-owned cats with hyperthyroidism. *Journal of Feline Medicine and Surgery* **16(6)**, 491–498

van Hoek I, Lefebvre HP, Peremans K et al. (2009a) Short- and long-term follow-up of glomerular and tubular renal markers of kidney function in hyperthyroid cats after treatment with radioiodine. *Domestic Animal Endocrinology* **36(1)**, 45–56

van Hoek I, Meyer E, DuchateauL et al. (2009b) Retinol-binding protein in serum and urine of hyperthyroid cats before and after treatment with radioiodine. *Journal of Veterinary Internal Medicine* **23(5)**, 1031–1037

Wakeling J, Moore K, Elliott J and Syme H (2008) Diagnosis of hyperthyroidism in cats with mild chronic kidney disease. *Journal of Small Animal Practice* **49(6)**, 287–294

Williams TL, Dillon H, Elliott J, Syme HM and Archer J (2016) Serum cystatin C concentrations in cats with hyperthyroidism and chronic kidney disease. *Journal of Veterinary Internal Medicine* **30(4)**, 1083–1089

Williams TL, Elliott J, Berry J and Syme HM (2013) Investigation of the pathophysiological mechanism for altered calcium homeostasis in hyperthyroid cats. *Journal of Small Animal Practice* **54(7)**, 367–373

Williams TL, Elliott J and Syme HM (2010a) Association of iatrogenic hypothyroidism with azotemia and reduced survival time in cats treated for hyperthyroidism. *Journal of Veterinary Internal Medicine* **24(5)**, 1086–1092

Williams TL, Elliott J and Syme HM (2012) Calcium and phosphate homeostasis in hyperthyroid cats: associations with development of azotaemia and survival time. *Journal of Small Animal Practice* **53(10)**, 561–571

Williams TL, Elliott J and Syme HM (2014a) Association between urinary vascular endothelial growth factor excretion and chronic kidney disease in hyperthyroid cats. *Research in Veterinary Science* **96(3)**, 436–441

Williams TL, Elliott J and Syme HM (2014b) Effect on renal function of restoration of euthyroidism in hyperthyroid cats with iatrogenic hypothyroidism. *Journal of Veterinary Internal Medicine* **28(4)**, 1251–1255

Williams TL, Peak KJ, Brodbelt D, Elliott J and Syme HM (2010b) Survival and the development of azotemia in hyperthyroid cats. *Journal of Veterinary Internal Medicine* **24(4)**, 863–869

Case example 1: Cat with polydipsia, diarrhoea and weight loss

SIGNALMENT

Sukki, a 15-year-old female neutered Domestic Shorthaired Cat.

HISTORY

Polydipsia, diarrhoea and weight loss.

BIOCHEMISTRY AND ENDOCRINE TESTING AT BASELINE

Parameter	Value	Reference interval
Serum total thyroxine concentration	65 nmol/l	10–55 nmol/l
Serum urea concentration	12.9 mmol/l	3–9.9 nmol/l
Serum creatinine concentration	210 µmol/l	40–177 µmol/l
Urine specific gravity	1.016	Not applicable
Systolic blood pressure	145 mmHg	<160 mmHg
Bodyweight	2.6 kg	Not applicable

Interpretation

Mild hyperthyroidism with concurrent azotaemic chronic kidney disease.

Treatment plan

Given that Sukki has clinical signs attributable to hyperthyroidism, start reversible therapy (anti-thyroid medication) at the lowest possible dose (e.g. 1.25 mg methimazole q24h) and recheck TT4 and renal parameters in 3–4 weeks.

BIOCHEMISTRY AND ENDOCRINE TESTING 3 WEEKS LATER

The diarrhoea has improved; Sukki is still polydipsic but well in herself, according to the owners.

Parameter	Value	Reference interval
Serum total thyroxine concentration	52 nmol/l	10–55 nmol/l
Serum urea concentration	18.9 mmol/l	3–9.9 nmol/l
Serum creatinine concentration	263 µmol/l	40–177 µmol/l
Urine specific gravity	1.017	Not applicable
Systolic blood pressure	150 mmHg	<160 mmHg
Bodyweight	2.6 kg	Not applicable

Interpretation

The TT4 has decreased, although it is not within the lower half of reference interval. The azotaemia has worsened, although clinically Sukki is doing well.

Treatment plan

Increase the dose of anti-thyroid medication (e.g. to methimazole 1.25 mg q12h). Recheck TT4 and renal parameters a further 3–4 weeks later.

BIOCHEMISTRY AND ENDOCRINE TESTING FURTHER 4 WEEKS LATER (7 WEEKS AFTER DIAGNOSIS)

No further diarrhoea, polydipsia is stable. Clinically stable.

Parameter	Value	Reference interval
Serum total thyroxine concentration	31 nmol/l	10–55 nmol/l
Serum urea concentration	24.6 mmol/l	3–9.9 nmol/l
Serum creatinine concentration	320 µmol/l	40–177 µmol/l
Urine specific gravity	1.013	Not applicable
Systolic blood pressure	150 mmHg	<160 mmHg
Bodyweight	2.7 kg	Not applicable

Interpretation

The TT4 is within the lower half of the reference interval. The azotaemia has worsened although it is still consistent with IRIS CKD Stage 3.

Treatment plan

Maintain dose of anti-thyroid medication and recheck renal parameters 3 months later. Follow IRIS guidelines for management of CKD.

Case example 2: Cat with weight loss and polyphagia

SIGNALMENT

Charlie, a 12-year-old male neutered Domestic Shorthaired Cat.

HISTORY

History of weight loss and polyphagia.

BIOCHEMISTRY AND ENDOCRINE TESTING AT BASELINE

Parameter	Value	Reference interval
Serum total thyroxine concentration	120 nmol/l	10–55 nmol/l
Serum urea concentration	11.0 mmol/l	3–9.9 nmol/l
Serum creatinine concentration	126 µmol/l	40–177 µmol/l
Urine specific gravity	1.030	Not applicable
Systolic blood pressure	160 mmHg No evidence of hypertensive retinopathy	<160 mmHg
Bodyweight	3.6 kg	Not applicable

Interpretation

Hyperthyroidism.

Treatment plan

Start anti-thyroid medication (e.g. 5 mg methimazole q12h) and recheck TT4 and renal parameters in 3–4 weeks.

BIOCHEMISTRY AND ENDOCRINE TESTING 3 WEEKS LATER

Polyphagia has resolved, still bright and active.

Parameter	Value	Reference interval
Serum total thyroxine concentration	26 nmol/l	10–55 nmol/l
Serum urea concentration	13.4 mmol/l	3.0–9.9 nmol/l
Serum creatinine concentration	168 µmol/l	40–177 µmol/l
Urine specific gravity	1.026	Not applicable
Systolic blood pressure	180 mmHg No evidence of hypertensive retinopathy	<160 mmHg
Bodyweight	3.9 kg	Not applicable

Interpretation

The TT4 has normalized but renal parameters are within normal limits.

Treatment plan

Continue dose of anti-thyroid medication and recheck a further 3 months later.

BIOCHEMISTRY AND ENDOCRINE TESTING FURTHER 3 MONTHS LATER

Appetite stable, drinking and urinating normally.

Parameter	Value	Reference interval
Serum total thyroxine concentration	30 nmol/l	10–55 nmol/l
Serum urea concentration	13.6 mmol/l	3–9.9 nmol/l
Serum creatinine concentration	190 µmol/l	40–177 µmol/l
Urine specific gravity	1.020	Not applicable
Systolic blood pressure	185 mmHg No evidence of hypertensive retinopathy	<160 mmHg
Bodyweight	4 kg	Not applicable

Interpretation

Well controlled hyperthyroidism with mild azotaemic CKD. Persistent systolic hypertension (and more likely to be a true hypertensive disorder because also has CKD).

Treatment plan

Maintain dose of anti-thyroid medication. Start amlodipine for hypertension, recheck systolic blood pressure in 1–2 weeks. Follow IRIS guidelines for management of CKD.

Case example 3: Cat with polydipsia, polyphagia and diarrhoea

SIGNALMENT

Jessie, a 13-year-old female neutered Domestic Shorthaired Cat.

HISTORY

History of polydipsia, polyphagia and diarrhoea.

BIOCHEMISTRY AND ENDOCRINE TESTING AT BASELINE

Parameter	Value	Reference interval
Serum total thyroxine concentration	70 nmol/l	10–55 nmol/l
Serum urea concentration	7.1 mmol/l	3–9.9 nmol/l
Serum creatinine concentration	100 µmol/l	40–177 µmol/l
Urine specific gravity	1.038	Not applicable
Systolic blood pressure	190 mmHg Evidence of hypertensive retinopathy on retinal examination	<160 mmHg
Bodyweight	2.8 kg	Not applicable

Interpretation

Mild hyperthyroidism and systolic hypertension (with target-organ damage).

Treatment plan

Start anti-thyroid medication (e.g. 2.5 mg methimazole q12h) and amlodipine for hypertension (given the presence of hypertensive retinopathy). Recheck blood pressure in 1–2 weeks and TT4 and renal parameters in 3–4 weeks.

BIOCHEMISTRY AND ENDOCRINE TESTING 3 WEEKS LATER

Diarrhoea has resolved; no further polyphagia and now seeming quiet.

Parameter	Value	Reference interval
Serum total thyroxine concentration	6 nmol/l	10–55 nmol/l
Serum urea concentration	14.5 mmol/l	3–9.9 nmol/l
Serum creatinine concentration	225 µmol/l	40–177 µmol/l
Urine specific gravity	1.017	Not applicable
Systolic blood pressure	140 mmHg	<160 mmHg
Bodyweight	3 kg	Not applicable

Interpretation

TT4 is now below the reference interval. Azotaemic CKD is present.

Treatment plan

Decrease dose of anti-thyroid medication (e.g. to 2.5 mg methimazole in the morning and 1.25 mg methimazole in the evening) with the aim of achieving a serum TT4 within the lower half of the laboratory reference interval. Recheck 3–4 weeks later.

BIOCHEMISTRY AND ENDOCRINE TESTING FURTHER 4 WEEKS LATER (7 WEEKS AFTER DIAGNOSIS)

Clinically doing well, appetite similar to before.

Parameter	Value	Reference interval
Serum total thyroxine concentration	20 nmol/l	10–55 nmol/l
Serum urea concentration	10.4 mmol/l	3–9.9 nmol/l
Serum creatinine concentration	186 µmol/l	40–177 µmol/l
Urine specific gravity	1.026	Not applicable
Systolic blood pressure	135 mmHg	<160 mmHg
Bodyweight	3 kg	Not applicable

Interpretation

The TT4 is now within the lower half of the reference interval. The azotaemia has improved, although azotaemic CKD is still present.

Treatment plan

Maintain anti-thyroid medication at new dose. Follow IRIS guidelines for management of CKD.

Chapter 18

Hypertension and the kidney

Amanda E. Coleman and Scott A. Brown

Systemic arterial hypertension is defined as a sustained elevation in blood pressure (BP). In the majority of veterinary cases that are not considered anxiety-induced ('white coat' hypertension), systemic hypertension is categorized as secondary, occurring in association with a clinical condition or treatment known to cause hypertension. Chronic kidney disease (CKD) is commonly diagnosed in hypertensive cats and dogs. Although definitions of hypertension and methods used for its diagnosis vary among research studies, it is estimated that approximately 20–65% of cats and 30–55% of dogs with CKD are impacted by systemic hypertension, with the greatest estimates of prevalence occurring in association with glomerular diseases.

In keeping with the recommendations of the International Renal Interest Society (IRIS; Figure 18.1), anti-hypertensive treatment is indicated in patients with persistently elevated systemic arterial BP (≥160 mmHg, IRIS BP stages 'hypertensive' or 'severely hypertensive'), because these patients are at increased risk for the development of target-organ damage. The reader is referred to Chapter 15 for information regarding BP measurement and the diagnosis of systemic arterial hypertension and Chapter 12 for a discussion of the IRIS CKD staging system.

Whether systemic hypertension is caused by CKD, occurs in association with a separate condition, or is idiopathic (primary) in origin, its coexistence with CKD signifies an important challenge for the veterinary surgeon (veterinarian), who must maintain a delicate balance between preventing ongoing target-organ damage and avoiding acute deterioration of renal function. The goal of this chapter is to provide guidance for the practitioner with respect to this difficult clinical task.

Systolic BP (mmHg)		Diastolic BP (mmHg)	BP Stage	Risk of future target-organ damage
<150	and	<95	Normotensive	Minimal
150–159	or	95–99	Borderline hypertensive	Low
160–179	or	100–119	Hypertensive	Moderate
≥180	or	≥120	Severely hypertensive	High

18.1 International Renal Interest Society (IRIS) scheme for classification of cats and dogs on the basis of systemic arterial blood pressure (BP).

Pathogenesis of systemic hypertension in patients with kidney disease

The most commonly proposed pathophysiological mechanisms for systemic hypertension in animals with CKD include alterations in renal sodium handling, activation of the renin–angiotensin–aldosterone system (RAAS), and excessive sympathetic nervous system activity. By increasing sodium and water retention and arteriolar vasoconstriction, these mechanisms are thought to contribute to the development of systemic hypertension by increasing blood volume, cardiac output and systemic vascular resistance. A full discourse on this topic is beyond the scope of this chapter; the reader is referred elsewhere for an in-depth review (Syme, 2011).

Impact of systemic hypertension on renal function in kidney disease

It is currently unclear whether chronic systemic hypertension is able to induce *de novo* damage in the normal canine or feline kidney. However, in patients with CKD, glomerular hypertension, an initially beneficial mechanism that enhances the glomerular filtration rate (GFR) by increasing the function of remaining nephrons, is already present. Superimposition of elevated systemic pressure exacerbates glomerular hypertension and contributes to the spontaneous progression of CKD through a final common pathway of progressive glomerulosclerosis and tubulointerstitial fibrosis.

In the normal kidney, renal autoregulation, mediated by myogenic reflexes and tubuloglomerular feedback, maintains renal blood flow and glomerular filtration rate in the face of a wide range of systemic BPs. Beyond a certain upper limit (MAP >150 mmHg in dogs), renal autoregulatory mechanisms are overcome and intraglomerular pressure begins to mirror that of the systemic BP. In normotensive animals, such dramatic increases in BP are rare. However, in CKD, the autoregulatory capabilities of the remaining functional nephrons are impaired even at normal BP, making these structures susceptible to hypertensive injury during any elevation in systemic BP by allowing transmission of the increase in systemic BP directly to the glomerular capillary bed (Figure 18.2).

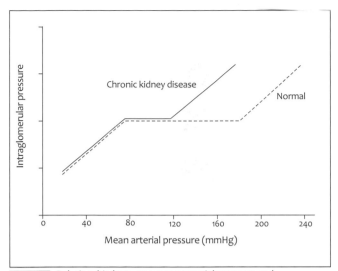

18.2 Relationship between mean arterial pressure and intraglomerular pressure. In the normal kidney (dashed line), renal autoregulation maintains constant glomerular capillary pressure over a relatively wide range of renal arterial 'input' pressures. However, in the diseased kidney (solid line), autoregulatory capabilities are impaired, allowing more direct transmission of systemic pressure to the glomerular capillary. As a result, the pressure in the glomerular capillary increases in a more linear fashion over the same range of arterial pressures, increasing the susceptibility to renal injury.

In animals with CKD, systemic arterial hypertension leads to accelerated loss of renal function associated with mild to moderate levels of renal proteinuria. An increase in proteinuria, specifically an increase in the urine protein to creatinine ratio (UPC), is a negative prognostic indicator in feline and canine CKD. Systolic BP >160 mmHg has been linked to an enhanced rate of deterioration of renal function in dogs. In canine CKD, an association between the initial systolic blood pressure (SBP) and the risk of mortality has been shown, although it is not clear whether this effect is independent of the former's association with the degree of proteinuria.

The rationale for anti-hypertensive treatment is to reverse or limit ongoing target-organ damage and to prevent future target-organ damage. Treatment may reverse some alterations (e.g. hypertensive encephalopathy) or slow the progression of others (e.g. the decline of renal function in animals with CKD). Recognition that the pathophysiology of systemic arterial hypertension and CKD are interrelated has important consequences for treatment. It can be argued that any strategies for the treatment of systemic hypertension must consider the animal as an integrated whole and assign equal importance to the preservation of kidney function and the lowering of BP to reduce target-organ damage.

Treatment strategies for patients with systemic arterial hypertension and kidney disease

In patients affected by both systemic hypertension and CKD, an increase in serum creatinine may be observed as BP control is achieved by the administration of anti-hypertensive medications. While it may be tempting in such a situation to reduce the dose of anti-hypertensive medications in an effort to avoid an acute deterioration of renal function, it is important to remember that this approach is not ideal

for the longer-term goal of renal function preservation. Modest, non-progressive increases in serum creatinine (those of <0.5 mg/dl or 50 μmol/l) often may be tolerable. Greater escalations, or those that progress over the weeks following initiation of therapy, may indicate drug-induced deterioration, necessitating dose reduction of anti-hypertensive medications. One study of humans with mild to moderate CKD reported that an initial anti-hypertensive treatment-induced fall in GFR is predictive of long-term benefit (i.e. preservation of renal function). In other words, a slight rise in creatinine following initiation of therapy may serve as an indirect indicator of a successful, protective reduction in intraglomerular pressure (Apperloo et al., 1997).

In humans with systemic hypertension, monotherapy rarely achieves adequate BP control (particularly for patients requiring a reduction in SBP of ≥15 mmHg), and patient response to individual drugs varies considerably. This is also frequently the case with veterinary patients, and client expectations should be framed accordingly. In general, therapy begins with the administration of anti-hypertensive medications at the low end of their dose ranges, with dose escalation or the addition of a second (or third) drug if BP control is not accomplished (the so-called 'stepped-care' approach). A suggested algorithm for the approach to the treatment of systemic hypertension in patients with CKD is outlined in Figure 18.3, with specific agents discussed in greater detail below.

Therapeutic targets/goals

Unless there is evidence of target-organ damage that is characterized by the potential for rapid progression (i.e. hypertensive retinopathy or encephalopathy), reduction of BP in patients with CKD and hypertension should be considered an intermediate- to long-term target, with a goal of gradual BP reduction over several weeks. The therapeutic goal is to maintain SBP <160 mmHg, which places the patient at low risk for target-organ damage. Drug-induced hypotension (SBP <120 mmHg) is remarkably rare but should also be avoided. The impairment of renal autoregulatory capabilities that renders the kidneys of these patients susceptible to hypertensive injury also confers an increased vulnerability to reductions of renal function or ischaemic injury during bouts of systemic hypotension.

Dietary sodium restriction

Currently, there is no convincing evidence to suggest that dietary sodium restriction is useful for BP reduction in hypertensive dogs and cats. In fact, moderate to severe dietary sodium restriction is associated with activation of the RAAS in normal dogs and in cats with experimentally induced renal insufficiency, with no beneficial reduction in systemic arterial BP, an effect that could potentially do more harm than good in these patients. For this reason, efforts to restrict sodium intake substantially in these patients cannot be recommended at this time.

Avoidance of high-sodium diets is often advised for patients with systemic hypertension. Interestingly, in a study that examined three diets of varying sodium content fed to cats with experimentally-induced renal insufficiency, moderate to high degrees of sodium supplementation were associated with attenuation of RAAS activation without significant increases in BP (Buranakarl et al., 2004). Similar findings have been reported in normal dogs (Krieger et al., 1990). More data are needed to refine recommendations specifically for dietary sodium intake in hypertensive veterinary patients.

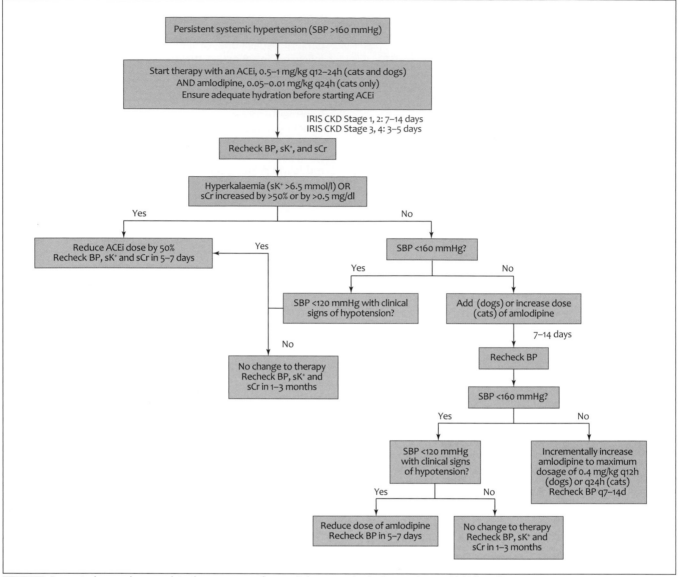

18.3 Suggested general approach to the treatment of systemic hypertension in dogs and cats with kidney disease. ACEi = angiotensin-converting enzyme inhibitor; IRIS = International Renal Interest Society; SBP = systolic arterial blood pressure; sCr = serum creatinine level; sK$^+$ = serum potassium level.

Anti-hypertensive drugs

Pharmacological intervention is the cornerstone of therapy for persistent systemic arterial hypertension. When caring for patients with coexisting systemic arterial hypertension and CKD, anti-hypertensive medications should be considered in the light of each agent's effect on both systemic BP and the renal microcirculation. While the primary goal of therapy is to normalize systemic arterial pressure and, therefore, renal inputs, loss of renal autoregulatory functions in the setting of CKD dictates careful consideration of the impact of therapy on renal haemodynamics and filtration. To this end, it is worthwhile reviewing the factors that influence glomerular capillary hydrostatic pressure (P_{GC}) and GFR. In short, substances that preferentially constrict the afferent arteriole or dilate the efferent arteriole will reduce P_{GC} and GFR, while those that preferentially dilate the afferent arteriole or constrict the efferent arteriole will increase P_{GC} and GFR (Figure 18.4). The effects of individual therapeutic agents (Figure 18.5), which may differentially influence these factors, are considered in greater detail below.

Blockers of the renin–angiotensin–aldosterone system

In both veterinary and human patients with CKD, the development of hypertension is complex and probably multifactorial. Although other causes are likely to exist, derangements of the RAAS have been documented in cats and dogs with naturally occurring and experimental models of CKD. In addition to its potent hypertensive properties, the major effector of this system, angiotensin II, is a critical mediator of renal oxidant stress, which may contribute to the progression of CKD and provide a positive feedback loop for further elevations in BP.

In addition to their anti-hypertensive properties, drugs that block the RAAS also display renoprotective effects by reducing proteinuria and glomerular hypertension. Through a reduction in efferent arteriolar vasoconstriction, P_{GC} is diminished, mitigating intraglomerular hypertension and hyperfiltration. In theory, these drugs may also produce a reduction in total GFR, which can lead to minor increases in serum creatinine, as discussed above. In experimental models of feline and canine CKD, however, GFR reduction

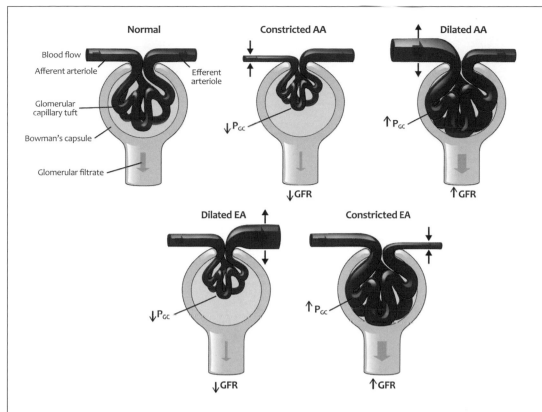

18.4 Effects of changes in renal arteriolar resistance on glomerular capillary pressure and glomerular filtration rate (GFR). Interventions or substances that preferentially constrict the afferent arteriole (AA) (e.g. adenosine) or dilate the efferent arteriole (EA) (e.g. angiotensin-converting enzyme inhibitors) may lead to reductions in glomerular capillary pressure (P_{GC}) and, therefore, GFR. Conversely, interventions or substances that preferentially constrict the efferent arteriole (e.g. angiotensin II via the AT1 receptor, catecholamines via the beta-1-adrenoreceptor) or dilate the afferent arteriole (e.g. L-type calcium channel blockers) lead to increases in P_{GC} and, therefore, GFR. (Courtesy of the University of Georgia)

Drug class	Agents	Recommended oral dosage
Angiotensin-converting enzyme inhibitor	Enalapril	Dogs: 0.5–1 mg/kg q12–24h
		Cats: 0.5 mg/kg q12–24h
	Benazepril	Dogs: 0.5–1 mg/kg q12–24h
		Cats: 0.5 mg/kg q12–24h
Dihydropyridine calcium channel blocker	Amlodipine	Dogs: initial dosage 0.05–0.1 mg/kg q24h Up-titrate to 0.4 mg/kg q12–24h if necessary
		Cats: 0.1–0.4 mg/kg q24h (0.625–1.25 mg/cat q24h)
Angiotensin II, subtype 1, receptor blocker	Telmisartan	Dogs: 1 mg/kg q24h
		Cats: 1 mg/kg q24h
Direct arterial vasodilator	Hydralazine	Dogs: initial dosage 0.5 mg/kg q12h Up-titrate to 2–3 mg/kg q8–12h if necessary
		Cats: 2.5 mg/cat q12–24h
Beta-adrenoreceptor/antagonist	Atenolol	Dogs: 0.5–1 mg/kg q12h (up-titrate over several weeks)
		Cats: 6.25–12.5 mg/cat q12h

18.5 Anti-hypertensive agents used for the treatment of dogs and cats with systemic hypertension and kidney disease.

studied and prescribed with the greatest frequency in cats and dogs. Veterinary reports describe relatively disappointing efficacy of ACEi as monotherapy for the control of hypertension, particularly in cats and when compared with more potent BP-lowering medications such as calcium channel blockers. Average BP reductions of 10–20 mmHg (dogs) and 5–10 mmHg (cats) are expected in animals with kidney disease treated with an ACEi. Changes of this magnitude would be considered clinically significant in humans. However, in part because of the difficulty of measuring small changes in BP in dogs and especially in cats, the importance of such changes may be inappropriately discounted in veterinary medicine.

Although the BP-lowering effects of ACEi are modest, especially in feline hypertension, ACEi administration is associated with a significant reduction in intraglomerular pressure in both dogs and cats. In humans, the renoprotective effects conferred by use of these drugs are independent of their systemic BP-lowering effects. For these reasons, the authors advocate that an inhibitor of the RAAS, such as an ACEi, be co-administered any time a calcium channel blocker is prescribed for patients with systemic hypertension and CKD (see below). This recommendation is even stronger for patients with concurrent proteinuria.

Angiotensin II receptor blockers: ARBs exert their effects on the angiotensin II subtype 1 (AT_1) receptor, which mediates the adverse influences of angiotensin II on both the cardiovascular system and the kidneys (see Figure 18.6). Selectivity for the AT_1 receptor subtype gives drugs of the ARB class a potential advantage over ACEi, because the beneficial effects (e.g. vasodilation) of angiotensin II binding to angiotensin II subtype 2 (AT_2) receptors are preserved. With regard to the intrarenal microcirculation, this may have particularly interesting implications, because vasodilatory AT_2 receptors are found primarily

was not noted after the administration of benazepril or enalapril for approximately 6 months to mildly azotaemic cats or dogs, respectively.

Angiotensin-converting enzyme inhibitors: ACEi interfere with the RAAS by blocking the conversion of angiotensin I to angiotensin II, reducing the amount of the latter that is available to interact with its receptor (Figure 18.6). Of the RAAS-modifying drugs available, ACEi have been

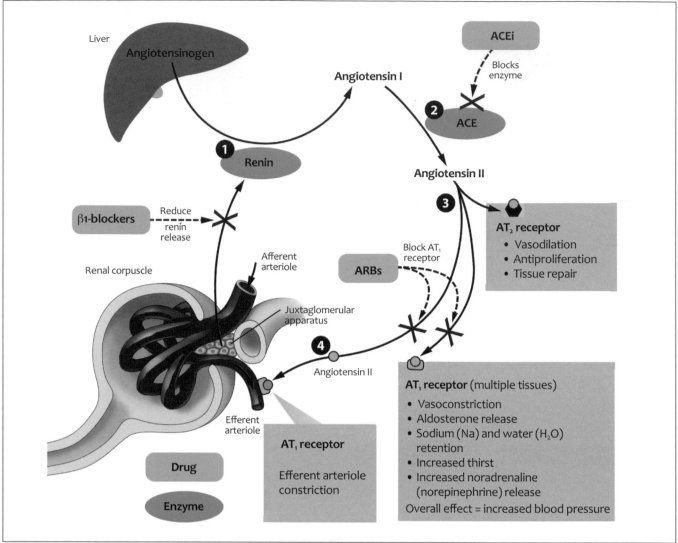

18.6 Overview of the renin–angiotensin–aldosterone system (RAAS) and the site of action of drugs interacting with this system. Renin is released from the juxtaglomerular apparatus in response to a number of physiological stimuli or in certain pathological states. This enzyme cleaves angiotensinogen, produced by the liver, to create the inactive peptide angiotensin I (1). Angiotensin-converting enzyme (ACE) then cleaves angiotensin I to produce the biologically active angiotensin II (2). Angiotensin II is the major effector of the RAAS, and is able to exert its effects by interacting with two receptors, the angiotensin II subtype 1 (AT_1) receptor, and the angiotensin II subtype 2 (AT_2) receptor (3). The AT_1 receptor mediates effects that ultimately result in increased systemic arterial BP, while the AT2 receptor is responsible for beneficial countereffects. Stimulation of AT_1 receptors on the efferent arteriole causes vasoconstriction of this vessel, which increases glomerular capillary pressure and may contribute to the development of glomerular hypertension (4). See text for further details regarding the drugs that interact with this system. ACEi = angiotensin-converting enzyme inhibitor; ARB = angiotensin II type 1 receptor blocker; β1-blocker = beta-1 adrenoreceptor blocking agent.
(Courtesy of the University of Georgia)

on the afferent arteriole. ARBs may therefore preserve GFR better than ACEi, owing to unopposed angiotension II-mediated interaction with the AT_2 receptors and vaso-dilation of both the afferent and efferent arterioles (see Figure 18.4). The clinical importance of this distinction between drug classes is not clear, particularly in light of the fact that ACEi use has not been associated with GFR reduction in models of canine and feline CKD, as discussed above.

Currently, most information regarding the clinical efficacy of ARBs is limited to extrapolation from human studies, anecdotal evidence and the results of a single clinical trial, which examined the effect of telmisartan, as compared with benazepril, on proteinuria in 224 cats (Sent et al., 2015). More work is needed to characterize the potential role of drugs of this class in the treatment of veterinary patients with hypertension and kidney disease. The authors and their colleagues have evaluated the

pharmacodynamics of several ARBs in normal cats and dogs and found the ARB telmisartan to be superior to enalapril (in dogs), benazepril (in cats) and losartan (in dogs and cats) in attenuating the BP response to exogenous angiotensin I administration.

Dihydropyridine calcium channel blockers

The dihydropyridine calcium channel blockers (CCBs) are potent anti-hypertensive agents that directly reduce arteriolar tone by blocking L-type calcium channels of vascular smooth muscle. Of the available orally administered compounds, the second-generation dihydropyridine CCB amlodipine besylate is currently used with the greatest frequency in veterinary patients. Clinically, BP reduction following amlodipine administration is significantly greater than that seen in response to ACEi in both cats and dogs. The BP-lowering effects of amlodipine are, in general, directly related to the pre-treatment BP level. Thus, in normal dogs and cats, amlodipine lowers BP by approximately 10–15 mmHg but, in severely hypertensive cats, amlodipine may lower BP by 50 mmHg or more. On average, reductions of 30–50 mmHg and approximately 25 mmHg have been reported in hypertensive cats and dogs, respectively, when treated with amlodipine (Mathur *et al.*, 2002; Geigy *et al.*, 2011). In a recently published, randomized, double-blinded, placebo-controlled study of moderately hypertensive cats, treatment with a cat-specific oral amlodipine formulation was associated with a mean SBP reduction that was 18 mmHg greater than that observed following placebo administration (Huhtinen *et al.*, 2015). Because of their documented efficacy and relatively long duration of action (24–30 hours), these drugs are frequently selected as first-line agents, particularly in the treatment of feline hypertension.

In addition to its systemic arteriolar vasodilatory effects, amlodipine preferentially dilates the afferent arteriole of canine glomeruli, which may increase P_{GC} and GFR. While less likely to lead to GFR reduction when BP is lowered, this drug effect may aggravate glomerular hypertension, particularly if systemic BP does not decrease adequately when it is used. Further, amlodipine has been shown to impair autoregulation of renal blood flow and GFR, and is associated with RAAS activation in normal dogs and in cats with naturally occurring systemic hypertension (Yue *et al.*, 2001; Atkins *et al.*, 2007; Jepson *et al.*, 2014). The clinical significance of these theoretical and potentially detrimental effects is unclear, and the profound anti-hypertensive properties of these drugs are likely to offset at least some of these effects. Indeed, in one study of cats with naturally occurring systemic hypertension, treatment with amlodipine as monotherapy was associated with a significant reduction in UPC in the majority of cases, particularly when baseline proteinuria was present. In the same study, only 12.8% of all cats experienced an increase in UPC of >0.1 (Jepson *et al.*, 2007). However, it is noteworthy that treatment of high BP with amlodipine was associated with adverse effects in dogs with CKD (Jacob *et al.*, 2003). Many clinicians, including the authors, recommend co-administration of an ACEi or ARB with amlodipine, which may lessen any negative impact on the vulnerable, diseased kidney over the long term.

Other anti-hypertensive agents

For patients in which systemic hypertension persists despite therapy with RAAS-blocking agents, CCB or their combination with additional anti-hypertensive medications may be considered (see Figure 18.5).

Hydralazine: Hydralazine is a potent parenterally or orally administered arteriolar vasodilator that acts via a poorly understood direct mechanism. Following an oral dose, hydralazine has a rapid onset of action, which peaks within 3–5 hours. Significant interindividual variation exists in the response to a given dose of this drug, and hydralazine is often associated with pronounced reflex tachycardia. Because the response to this medication is somewhat unpredictable, starting at the lowest end of the dose range and gradually up-titrating with frequent rechecking of BP is recommended. Furthermore, as the duration of effect is short and unpredictable, use of intermittent intravenous therapy with hydralazine typically results in wide variations in BP over time.

Beta-adrenoreceptor antagonists: In hypertension associated with renal disease, beta-1 adrenoreceptor antagonists (e.g. atenolol) may lower BP by reducing heart rate, cardiac stroke volume and renin release from the juxtaglomerular apparatus. In cats, these drugs have not proven sufficiently effective for BP reduction when used as sole agents (Henik *et al.* 2008). Their use in combination with other anti-hypertensive agents has not been systematically evaluated in hypertensive dogs or cats.

Non-dihydropyridine CCB: These agents, which include the phenylalkylamines (e.g. verapamil) and benzothiazepines (e.g. diltiazem) are less selective for vascular L-type calcium channels than amlodipine, and are therefore associated with negative inotropic and chronotropic myocardial effects. Verapamil, in particular, is a potent arteriolar vasodilator. However, at dosages required to produce clinically significant vasodilation, the negative inotropic effects of this drug limit its usefulness, particularly in patients with concurrent cardiac disease.

Special considerations in the azotaemic patient

Reduction of BP in patients with azotaemia (IRIS CKD Stages 2–4) should be considered an intermediate- to long-term goal, with the aim of gradual BP reduction and avoidance of hypotension (SBP <120 mmHg). Patients with renal azotaemia are unable to produce concentrated urine, and it is important to ensure euvolaemia prior to initiating therapy with medications that reduce efferent arteriolar resistance (e.g. RAAS-blocking agents, particularly ACEi). Likewise, in patients experiencing a decrease in intravascular volume (such as that associated with decreased oral fluid intake or gastrointestinal losses), angiotensin II-mediated constriction of the efferent arteriole may help to maintain GFR, or at least mitigate the drop in GFR that would be expected with these conditions. Therefore, in dehydrated patients, it is reasonable to withhold or delay initiation of therapy with an ACEi until correction of volume status is achieved. However, to prevent progressive target-organ damage, the authors would not hesitate to administer amlodipine concurrently to a hypertensive animal undergoing rehydration.

> **WARNING**
>
> Diuretic medications, which are frequently prescribed as anti-hypertensive agents in humans, should be avoided for this purpose alone in azotaemic dogs and cats, because these drugs can exacerbate volume depletion.

Special considerations in the proteinuric patient

Drugs that lower both intraglomerular and systemic arterial pressure may benefit the proteinuric patient. RAAS-blocking agents, by preferentially dilating the efferent arteriole, lower P_{GC} and, in many cases, reduce urinary protein loss. For this reason, these drugs are particularly attractive for patients with CKD characterized by both hypertension and proteinuria. In these cases, the clinician may consider more aggressive up-titration of an ACEi or initiation of therapy with an ARB (telmisartan). Combination therapy with an ACEi and ARB has not been studied in dogs and cats; in humans, this is commonplace, although there is evidence that the combination may be associated with a higher incidence of complications when compared with monotherapy.

Furthermore, in humans with proteinuria due to CKD, realization of a lower target BP in response to therapy is associated with the greatest long-term benefit in mitigating decline of renal function. In one seminal study, patients with the highest baseline proteinuria experienced the fastest rate of GFR decline when treatment goals were least aggressive, suggesting that the greater an individual's proteinuria prior to initiation of therapy, the greater the potential benefit from strict BP control (Peterson *et al.*, 1995). Similar studies have not been performed in veterinary patients.

Potential impact of subcutaneous fluid administration in patients with CKD and systemic hypertension

Chronic dehydration is a common complication of CKD for which subcutaneous fluid therapy is often indicated, particularly in feline patients. Unnecessary administration of sodium-containing replacement fluids, however, may lead to the development of intravascular volume expansion and fluid overload. In renal insufficiency, a major mechanism for development of hypertension is believed to be hypervolaemia due to an inability to excrete adequate amounts of sodium and water. If necessary for the maintenance of hydration in a patient with CKD and systemic hypertension, maintenance fluids with low sodium content (e.g. 5% dextrose; 0.18% sodium chloride and 4% dextrose; 0.45% sodium chloride and 2.5% dextrose) should be considered.

Dose adjustments of anti-hypertensive drugs in renal disease

In theory, anti-hypertensive medications that are principally (i.e. >50%) eliminated by the kidneys should be used with caution in animals with moderate to severe azotemia (IRIS CKD Stages 3–4), because these drugs may accumulate, leading to an amplified fall in BP. If GFR decreases as a result of hypotension, renal clearance may be further impaired, initiating a vicious cycle. Of the anti-hypertensive drugs used in dogs and cats, the beta-adrenoreceptor antagonists (e.g. atenolol) are those for which this may be most relevant clinically. Although the metabolites of certain ACEi, such as enalapril, are primarily excreted in the urine, the pharmacokinetic characteristics of these drugs are rather complicated, and adverse effects due to drug accumulation are unlikely to be clinically relevant. Indeed, side effects potentially attributable to ACEi accumulation (such as hypotension or significant hyperkalaemia) are uncommon in legitimately hypertensive patients. Nonetheless, some authors recommend the use of benazepril, which is characterized by predominantly hepatic clearance (85% and 55% in cats and dogs, respectively), as the ACEi of choice in patients with renal insufficiency. However, the occurrence of ACEi-induced hypotension or hyperkalaemia in a patient with CKD does not necessitate permanent discontinuation of the drug. Instead, cautious reintroduction at a lower dose is recommended once the drug effects have abated. Amlodipine does not require a similar dose reduction in canine or feline patients with CKD of any stage, because this drug undergoes hepatic metabolism.

Monitoring the patient with systemic hypertension and CKD

Hypertensive patients typically require therapy for the remainder of their lives and, frequently, dosage adjustments are necessary to maintain appropriate BP control. After initiating therapy with anti-hypertensive medications or escalating the doses of these drugs, BP and markers of renal function should be checked within 7–14 days. For animals with moderate or severe renal azotaemia (IRIS CKD Stages 3–4), checking within 3–5 days should be considered. Identification of clinical signs suggestive of hypotension (e.g. lethargy, weakness, syncope) and/or acute exacerbation of azotaemia (e.g. lethargy, vomiting) should also prompt earlier rechecking of these parameters. When an ACEi or ARB is started or if the dose is escalated, checking potassium levels is also advisable, because administration of these drugs may be associated with the development of hyperkalaemia in patients with CKD.

Documentation of one or more of the following indicates the need for dose reduction (i.e. reduction by one half or to the last tolerated dose):

- Systemic hypotension, defined by SBP <120 mmHg with clinical signs of hypotension (e.g. weakness, lethargy and/or syncope)
- Rise in serum creatinine >50 μmol/l (0.5 mg/dl)
- Moderate or severe hyperkalaemia (serum potassium >6.5 mmol/l) for animals receiving RAAS-blocking agents.

Following BP stabilization, BP and serum creatinine should be monitored every 1–3 months, depending on the severity of BP elevation and the degree of concurrent kidney disease. In addition to the parameters outlined above, it is also advisable to quantify urinary protein loss at regular intervals, because proteinuria is a risk factor for animals with CKD and systemic hypertension, and is therefore an important therapeutic target.

References and further reading

Apperloo AJ, de Zeeuw D and de Jong PE (1997) A short-term antihypertensive treatment-induced fall in glomerular filtration rate predicts long-term stability of renal function. *Kidney International* 51(3), 793–797

Atkins CE, Rausch WP, Gardner SY et al. (2007) The effect of amlodipine and the combination of amlodipine and enalapril on the renin-angiotensin-aldosterone system in the dog. *Journal of Veterinary Pharmacology and Therapeutics* 30(5), 394–400

Brown SA, Atkins C, Bagley R et al. (2007) Guidelines for the identification, evaluation, and management of systemic hypertension in dogs and cats. *Journal of Veterinary Internal Medicine* 21, 542–558

Brown SA, Finco DR and Navar LG (1995) Impaired renal autoregulatory ability in dogs with reduced renal mass. *Journal of the American Society of Nephrology* 5, 1768–1774

Buranakarl C, Mathur S and Brown SA (2004) Effects of dietary sodium chloride intake on renal function and blood pressure in cats with normal and reduced renal function. *American Journal of Veterinary Research* 65, 620–627

Geigy CA, Schweighauser A, Doherr M et al. (2011) Occurrence of systemic hypertension in dogs with acute kidney injury and treatment with amlodipine besylate. *Journal of Small Animal Practice* 52(7), 340–346

Henik RA, Stepien RL, Wenholz LJ et al. (2008) Efficacy of atenolol as a single antihypertensive agent in hyperthyroid cats. *Journal of Feline Medicine and Surgery* 10, 577-82

Huhtinen M, Derré G, Renoldi HJ et al. (2015) Randomized placebo-controlled clinical trial of a chewable formulation of amlodipine for the treatment of hypertension in client-owned cats. *Journal of Veterinary Internal Medicine* 29, 786–793

Jacob F, Polzin DJ, Osborne CA et al. (2003) Association between initial systolic blood pressure and risk of developing a uremic crisis or of dying in dogs with chronic renal failure. *Journal of the American Veterinary Medical Association* 222, 322–329

Jepson RE, Syme HM and Elliott J (2014) Plasma renin activity and aldosterone concentrations in hypertensive cats with and without azotemia and in response to treatment with amlodipine besylate. *Journal of Veterinary Internal Medicine* **28**, 144–153

Kjolby MJ, Kompanowska-Jezierska E, Wamberg S and Bie P (2005) Effects of sodium intake on plasma potassium and renin angiotensin aldosterone system in conscious dogs. *Acta Physiologica Scandinavica* **184**, 225–234

Krieger JE, Liard JF and Cowley AW Jr (1990) Hemodynamics, fluid volume, and hormonal responses to chronic high-salt intake in dogs. *American Journal of Physiology* **259**, H1629–H1636

Lefebvre HP and Toutain PL (2004) Angiotensin-converting enzyme inhibitors in the therapy of renal diseases. *Journal of Veterinary Pharmacology and Therapeutics* **27**, 265–281

Mathur S, Syme H, Brown CA *et al.* (2002) Effects of the calcium channel antagonist amlodipine in cats with surgically induced hypertensive renal insufficiency. *American Journal of Veterinary Research* **63**, 833–839

Peterson JC, Adler S, Burkart JM *et al.* (1995) Blood pressure control, proteinuria, and the progression of renal disease. The Modification of Diet in Renal Disease Study. *Annals of Internal Medicine* **123(10)**, 754–762

Sent U, Gössl R, Elliott J *et al.* (2015) Comparison of efficacy of long-term oral treatment with telmisartan and benazepril in cats with chronic kidney disease. *Journal of Veterinary Internal Medicine* **29**, 1479–1487

Syme H (2011) Hypertension in small animal kidney disease. *Veterinary Clinics of North America: Small Animal Practice* **41**, 63–89

Yue W, Kimura S, Fujisawa Y *et al.* (2001) Benidipine dilates both pre-and post-glomerular arteriole in the canine kidney. *Hypertension Research* **24**, 429–436

Chapter 19

Effects of other endocrine diseases on kidney function

David J. Polzin

Hyperadrenocorticism and the kidneys

Canine Cushing's syndrome (hyperadrenocorticism, HAC) is commonly characterized by increased glomerular filtration rate (GFR), proteinuria, hypertension and decreased urine concentrating ability. These effects occur with both spontaneous and iatrogenic HAC. Differentiating the effects of glucocorticoids from concurrent or consequent kidney disease can be challenging. In addition, the long-term effects of HAC on the kidneys remain poorly understood. Observations in both dogs and humans suggest the possibility of long-term adverse effects of HAC on the kidneys.

Glomerular filtration rate

Untreated HAC is commonly characterized by an increase in GFR detectable by measuring iohexol or creatinine clearance. Conversely, owing to relative insensitivity, changes in GFR as measured by serum creatinine concentration typically remain within the laboratory reference range in most dogs with HAC. As a consequence, these changes in GFR are usually inapparent, although small reductions in serum creatinine concentration may occur.

Several mechanisms have been suggested to explain the cortisol-associated increase in GFR observed in HAC, including increased renal blood flow, decreased renal vascular resistance, nitric oxide-mediated vasodilatation, alterations in prostaglandins and glucocorticoid catabolic-induced increased plasma concentrations of vasodilatory amino acids (Smets et al., 2012). In contrast to glucocorticoids elevating systemic blood pressure, they promote vasodilatation of the renal cortical vasculature, which in turn reduces filtration fraction. It has been suggested that these changes in the intra-renal vasculature may result, at least in part, from reduced renal cortical angiotensin II activity. Presumably, glucocorticoids elevate GFR by causing increased renal blood flow despite the decline in fractional filtration (Kobuta et al., 2001).

Urine concentrating ability

Polyuria and polydipsia are among the most common clinical signs of canine HAC and have been documented to occur in up to 80–85% of affected dogs. Pet owners may report water intake from 2 to 10 times normal (Behrend, 2015). Urine specific gravities are typically below 1.020 and sometimes hyposthenuric. Water deprivation and/or administration of antidiuretic hormone analogues results in limited or no increase in urine concentration in dogs with HAC (see Chapter 2).

Several mechanisms have been proposed to explain the impairment in urine concentration in canine HAC. Excess cortisol may alter osmoregulation of arginine vasopressin (AVP) at the level of the hypothalamus and/or neurohypophysis, resulting in an increased osmotic threshold for AVP. Cortisol may also promote renal resistance to AVP. In addition, cortisol may downregulate renal urea transporters important in generating the renal medullary osmolality (Smets et al., 2010).

Treatment of canine HAC with trilostane has been reported to restore renal concentrating ability in at least some dogs after 6–12 months of therapy (Smets et al., 2012). However, some dogs continue to have impaired renal concentrating ability 12 months post-treatment. In contrast, treatment of canine HAC by hypophysectomy fails to restore renal concentrating ability, at least in part because hypophysectomy ablates AVP production. Renal concentrating ability may be improved by administration of antidiuretic hormone analogues in some dogs.

In contrast to dogs, it is uncommon for cats with HAC to have polyuria and polydipsia as a consequence of cortisol-associated urine concentration impairment (Feldman, 2015). Cats with HAC and polyuria are more likely to have diabetes mellitus or chronic kidney disease (CKD) as the cause for their polyuria. Of the owners of 72 cats with naturally occurring HAC, 57 (79%) reported that their cat had polyuria/polydipsia (Feldman, 2015). However, of 58 cats diagnosed with HAC and polyuria and polydipsia, 32 cats had concurrent diabetes mellitus while only 8 cats with polyuria/polydipsia did not have diabetes mellitus (Feldman, 2015).

Proteinuria

Proteinuria reportedly occurs in 44–75% of dogs with HAC (Smets et al., 2010; 2012). The magnitude of proteinuria measured as the urine protein to creatinine (UPC) ratio is typically mildly to moderately increased, with values in the lower to mid-single digits; however, occasionally dogs may have markedly higher values, even into the mid-teen range (Smets et al., 2012; Behrend, 2015). In one study, the mean UPC ratio for 19 dogs with HAC was 1.66, with a range of 0.01–16.32 (Smets et al., 2012). Proteinuria in dogs with HAC has been shown to include elevated urine levels of

BSAVA Manual of Canine and Feline Nephrology and Urology, third edition. Edited by Jonathan Elliott, Gregory F. Grauer and Jodi L. Westropp. ©BSAVA 2017

albumin, immunoglobulin (Ig)G and retinal binding protein, thus indicating the presence of a non-selective glomerular permselectivity defect (albumin and IgG) and impaired renal tubular reabsorption of small molecular weight proteins (retinal binding protein) (Smets *et al.*, 2012). The impairment of renal tubular reabsorption may be due, at least in part, to renal tubular protein overload. Proteinuria may occur in association with both adrenal tumours and pituitary-dependent HAC. The magnitude of the UPC ratio does not appear to allow reliable differentiation between these two forms of HAC (Behrend, 2015).

Exogenous administration of glucocorticoids is also associated with proteinuria. Seven of nine dogs receiving prednisone at a dosage of 2.2 mg/kg q24h developed proteinuria, with a peak mean UPC ratio of 1.27 ± 1.02 after 28 days of treatment, with seven of nine dogs having a UPC ratio >0.5 (Waters *et al.*, 1996). Urine protein electrophoresis revealed that the proteinuria was primarily albuminuria in this study. Similarly, administration of 8 mg/kg q24h of hydrocortisone for 12 weeks was associated with an increase in mean UPC ratio from 0.17 (0.15–0.28) to 0.38 (0.18–1.78) (Schellenberg *et al.*, 2008). Proteinuria resolved within 1 month after withdrawal of hydrocortisone.

Renal lesions observed in dogs receiving hydrocortisone include generalized hypercellular glomerular tufts, suggesting mesangial proliferation. Immunoglobulin deposition in the glomeruli was not found by direct immunofluorescence (Schellenberg *et al.*, 2008).

Hypoalbuminaemia

Hypoalbuminaemia does not typically develop in dogs with HAC and proteinuria. As a consequence, development of hypoalbuminaemia in dogs with HAC and proteinuria should prompt consideration of the possibility that concurrent primary glomerular disease may be present. In such instances, other possible causes for hypoalbuminaemia should be investigated and excluded. Once alternative explanations for hypoalbuminaemia have been excluded, renal biopsy including light, electron and immunofluorescent microscopy should be considered to define the cause of glomerular proteinuria.

The magnitude of proteinuria often declines with treatment and it may resolve; however, proteinuria appears to persist in 20–40% of treated dogs (Behrend, 2015). In a study of 19 dogs, UPC ratio values were significantly reduced by 1 month post-treatment (mean UPC ratio 0.41; 0.06–4.96) and the UPC ratio remained low for at least 12 months post-treatment (mean UPC ratio 0.28; 0.08–7.47) (Smets *et al.*, 2012). It is uncertain whether the persistence of proteinuria in some treated dogs reflects inadequate treatment, irreversible HAC-associated renal lesions or proteinuria of non-HAC origin.

The mechanisms underlying proteinuria in HAC are not well understood. Possible causes for proteinuria include glomerular hypertension and hyperfiltration, structural/functional alterations of the glomerular barrier (primarily glomerulosclerosis and podocytopathy), and decreased protein reabsorption by the renal tubules.

Hypertension

Hypertension affects 31–86% of dogs with HAC, and systolic blood pressures typically range from approximately 160 mmHg to 200 mmHg, with most showing mild to moderate hypertension (Behrend, 2015). While blood pressure often improves with therapy for HAC, hypertension may persist despite therapy in some dogs. Anti-hypertensive therapy (see Chapter 15) should be considered when systolic blood pressure remains >180 mmHg despite adequate treatment for HAC. While hypertension in general has the potential to promote renal injury and proteinuria, its role in kidney injury in HAC is unclear. The pathogenesis of hypertension in HAC is incompletely understood, but increased cardiac output, total peripheral resistance and renal vascular resistance appear to contribute.

HAC and CKD

A causal relationship between HAC and CKD has not been confirmed in dogs or humans. Nonetheless, the effects of glucocorticoids on various renal functions and observations from humans with HAC have prompted consideration of a possible link between HAC and subsequent development of CKD. Concurrent HAC and CKD have been recognized in dogs and humans; however, this is uncommon in both species (Smets *et al.*, 2010). Proteinuria and hypertension, common effects of glucocorticoids, may promote renal injury and are risk factors for progression of CKD. In humans who have been treated for Cushing's disease, their creatinine clearance has been reported to be lower than that of healthy controls, although the differences were not statistically significant (Faggiano *et al.*, 2002; 2003). In addition, increased endogenous glucocorticoid production has been reported in humans to be significantly correlated with the rate of progression of CKD (Walser and Ward, 1988).

There is limited evidence that HAC may be a risk factor for development of CKD in dogs. The GFR has been shown to decline following treatment of HAC (Smets *et al.*, 2010). This apparent decline in GFR may or may not reflect development of renal injury due to an extended period of corticosteroid-induced elevated GFR (glomerular hyperfiltration), systemic hypertension and/or proteinuria. In a study of 19 dogs with pituitary-dependent HAC where 12 dogs were treated with trilostane and seven dogs by trans-sphenoidal hypophysectomy, post-treatment GFR declined (Smets *et al.*, 2010). Serum creatinine and urea nitrogen concentrations increased, but remained within the laboratory reference range. In another study, kidney function, measured as plasma clearance of exo-iohexol, did not differ between a group of 25 dogs with active HAC and age- and bodyweight-matched healthy controls (Smets *et al.*, 2010). However, two of the dogs with HAC had concurrent CKD. In addition, the dogs with HAC had significantly higher glomerular (proteinuria) and tubular (urinary retinol-binding protein and urinary *N*-acetyl-beta-D-glucoseaminidase) biomarkers than the control dogs, suggesting active kidney injury. Taken together, the observations that dogs may have reduced post-treatment GFR, persistent proteinuria and hypertension, and renal lesions including glomerulosclerosis suggest that long-standing, untreated canine HAC may cause renal injury and ultimately development of CKD that may not become apparent until the effects of HAC are revealed by treatment. Based on these associations, long-term monitoring of kidney function, proteinuria and blood pressure should be considered for dogs following treatment for HAC (Smets *et al.*, 2012).

Establishing the presence of HAC in patients with CKD may be complicated by overestimation of cortisol resulting from impaired renal excretion of cortisol and decreased cortisol binding to albumin promoting increased free cortisol levels. In addition, cortisol metabolites may accumulate due to decreased clearance and then interfere with cortisol measurement. Typically, >90% of circulating cortisol is bound to cortisol-binding globulin (CBG or transcortin); however, free cortisol is the physiologically active form. Free cortisol levels change independently, and accurately reflect the clinical status of the patient. Thus, free cortisol is deemed to be the most reliable test for glucocorticoid status.

Glomerular disease

The principal concern for dogs with persistent HAC-associated proteinuria, regardless of whether they have been treated for HAC or not, is whether the continuing proteinuria and hypertension are indeed solely the result of HAC or are due to the development of additional glomerular disease attributable to HAC and/or causes of glomerular disease. Possible associations between HAC and glomerular disease have been described in humans, including nephrotic syndrome, focal segmental glomerulosclerosis, membranoproliferative glomerulonephritis and minimal change disease (Smets et al., 2010). Glomerulonephritis, glomerulosclerosis and renal amyloidosis have been reported in dogs with spontaneous or hydrocortisone-induced and prednisone-induced HAC (Smets et al., 2010).

Nephrolithiasis and urolithiasis

Humans cured of Cushing's disease remain at increased risk for the development of calcium-containing nephroliths. While nephroliths are uncommon in dogs when compared with humans, dogs with HAC have been reported to be at a 10-fold increased risk of developing calcium-containing uroliths (primarily of the lower urinary tract) compared with control dogs (Hess et al., 1998). Nonetheless, while the incidence of urolithiasis in dogs with HAC is not known, it suggested to be quite low (Behrend, 2015).

Hypoadrenocorticism and the kidneys

Hypoadrenocorticism (Addison's syndrome) is characterized by serious derangements in body water and electrolytes, in particular sodium, potassium and chloride. It typically involves deficiencies of glucocorticoid and mineralocorticoid hormones produced by the adrenal glands. However, an uncommon atypical form of hypoadrenocorticism is pure glucocorticoid deficiency disease. While glucocorticoid and mineralocorticoid hormones have wide and diverse effects in the body, both may influence fluid and electrolyte balance. Glucocorticoid deficiency can lead to hyponatraemia secondary to stimulation of vasopressin secretion. Glucocorticoid deficiency promotes vasopressin secretion by causing hypotension and lack of negative feedback of cortisol on the paraventricular nucleus in the hypothalamus (Scott-Moncrieff, 2015). Inappropriately elevated vasopressin levels result in impaired free water excretion by the kidneys, free water retention and hyponatraemia. Hyponatraemia and loss of the renal medullary concentration gradient can lead to polyuria in isolated glucocorticoid deficiency.

Mineralocorticoids increase reabsorption of sodium and secretion of potassium in the renal tubules, therefore aldosterone is critical in conserving body salt and preventing hyperkalaemia. The main site of action of aldosterone is the principal cells of the connecting segment and collecting tubules of the distal nephron. Aldosterone increases the number of sodium and potassium channels in the luminal membrane and increases activity of the Na^+-K^+-ATPase pump in the basolateral membrane. At the basolateral membrane, sodium is pumped out of the cell in exchange for potassium entering the cell to maintain low intracellular sodium levels and high intracellular potassium levels. The concentration gradient across the luminal membrane then favours absorption of sodium into the cell and excretion of potassium into the tubular lumen. Sodium is also reabsorbed in exchange for hydrogen ions in the intercalated cells of the cortical collecting tubules.

Deficiency of aldosterone leads to hyponatraemia, hypochloraemia, hyperkalaemia and metabolic acidosis. Polyuria results from the aldosterone deficiency-induced natriuresis and associated loss of the renal medullary concentration gradient. The resultant inappropriate polyuria leads to dehydration, hypovolaemia, hypotension, impaired cardiac output and decreased GFR. The decreased GFR results in pre-renal azotaemia. Because the urine concentrating ability is impaired in hypoadrenocorticism, it may be difficult to differentiate pre-renal azotaemia from renal azotaemia. Confirmation of pre-renal azotaemia can be established on the basis of a fluid-volume challenge (intravenous administration of fluids sufficient to restore adequate renal perfusion). Resolution of azotaemia subsequent to the fluid challenge, typically within 24 hours, confirms that the azotaemia is of pre-renal origin, thereby discriminating from acute kidney injury (AKI). Gastrointestinal complications of hypoadrenocorticism such as vomiting, anorexia and diarrhoea further deplete body salt and water. The volume-induced reduction in GFR promotes further potassium retention.

Hypoadrenocorticism and kidney disease (particularly AKI) present with many similar clinical and biochemical findings which may cause these two diseases to be confused diagnostically. Common clinical findings in hypoadrenocorticism and kidney disease include polyuria, polydipsia, anorexia, vomiting, dehydration, lethargy depression, weight loss, weakness and abdominal pain. Biochemical abnormalities that may be observed in both conditions include azotaemia hyperphosphataemia, hyperkalaemia, hyponatraemia, hypochloraemia, metabolic acidosis and dilute urine despite azotaemia and/or dehydration. In addition, the onset of clinical signs in both kidney disease and hypoadrenocorticism may be acute or gradual, or the condition may wane and wax, although waxing and waning is more suggestive of hypoadrenocorticism. The clinical and laboratory response to acute fluid administration is similar in that clinical signs, azotaemia and electrolyte abnormalities may improve or resolve quickly, and improvement may be transient with either condition. Given that many of the clinical manifestations of hypoadrenocorticism can be directly linked to salt and water deficiency, compensation for these losses, either in the form of fluid therapy or oral intake, can mitigate the clinical effects.

While blood urea nitrogen, serum creatinine, serum phosphorus, serum electrolytes and acid–base abnormalities appear similar in patients with hypoadrenocorticism and those with AKI, their response to appropriate fluid therapy is usually quite different. The typically relatively rapid and complete clinical and biochemical responses to fluid therapy differentiate patients with hypoadrenocorticism from those with AKI, where azotaemia persists despite aggressive fluid therapy. Azotaemia that fails to respond to fluid resuscitation supports the diagnosis of renal azotaemia. In patients with renal azotaemia, it is important to establish that the patient produces urine at an adequate rate, to avoid overhydration.

The principal laboratory findings prompting consideration of hypoadrenocorticism are hyponatraemia, hyperkalaemia, eosinophilia, and lack of a stress response on the complete blood count, although non-regenerative anaemia, hypercalcaemia, hypoalbuminaemia, hypercholesterolaemia, hypoglycaemia, metabolic acidosis and elevated liver enzymes may also support the diagnosis. It is important to remember that some dogs with oliguric AKI may have hyperkalaemia and hyponatraemia similar to that observed in hypoadrenocorticism. When hypoadrenocorticism is suspected, measuring a basal cortisol concentration is a rapid means of excluding a diagnosis of hypoadrenocorticism. A basal cortisol concentration of <2.0 µg/dl has been reported to be 100% sensitive for diagnosis of hypoadrenocorticism, but some dogs with clinically similar non-adrenal disease may also have values below 2.0 µg/dl (63.3% specificity) (Bovens *et al.*, 2014). Thus, it is necessary to confirm the diagnosis by performing an adrenocorticotrophic hormone (ACTH) response test.

Stage	Duration of diabetes mellitus	Functional/structural lesions
1	0–5 years	Renal hypertrophy, increased GFR (hyperfiltration)
2	3–7 years	Hyperfiltration continues; some patients with type 2 diabetes develop elevated blood pressure; early renal lesions develop including basement membrane thickening and mesangial expansion
3	7–15 years	Persistent microalbuminaemia, hyperfiltration continues, elevated blood pressure
4	15–20 years	Proteinuria (overt), arterial hypertension, decreased GFR
5	After 15–25 years	End-stage renal disease (ESRD – chronic, irreversible kidney disease requiring renal replacement therapy)

19.1 The five stages of diabetic nephropathy recognized in humans with diabetes. GFR = glomerular filtration rate.
(Caramori, 2009; Bloom, 2013)

Diabetes mellitus and the kidneys

Diabetic nephropathy, a form of CKD that may develop as a consequence of diabetes mellitus, is the leading cause of kidney disease in humans in the United States and Europe. It is generally a progressive condition that manifests many years (usually a decade or more) after the initial diagnosis of diabetes mellitus. Typical findings in humans with diabetic nephropathy may include microalbuminuria, overt proteinuria, glomerular lesions, arterial hypertension, azotaemia and, ultimately, azotaemic CKD. It is an important cause of death in humans with diabetes mellitus.

While there is evidence that renal lesions and some of the biochemical manifestations characteristic of diabetic nephropathy in humans may be observed in dogs and cats with diabetes mellitus, the clinical significance of these findings in dogs and cats remains uncertain. Because development of diabetic nephropathy in humans occurs after a decade or more of the diabetic state, it may be that most dogs and cats do not survive long enough with diabetes to develop clinically significant kidney disease. However, dogs and cats with concurrent diabetes and CKD and/or glomerulopathy are recognized and the cause of these renal diseases is often poorly understood. As a consequence, it may be that at least some dogs and cats do develop some form of diabetic nephropathy.

Human diabetic nephropathy

Diabetic nephropathy is defined as structural and/or functional kidney lesions that develop as a consequence of diabetes mellitus. It reportedly occurs in approximately 25–35% of humans patients with diabetes, with a peak incidence after 20 years of the condition (Caramori and Mauer, 2009). It is categorized into five sequential stages reflecting progressively more advanced kidney disease (Figure 19.1). The stages typically develop serially over many years, although not all patients develop the most advanced forms. Stages 1, 2 and 3 are characterized largely by subclinical abnormalities including increased GFR (hyperfiltration), glomerular lesions and microalbuminuria. Stage 4 diabetic nephropathy is CKD characterized by reduced GFR, proteinuria and arterial hypertension, and Stage 5 diabetic nephropathy is advanced, irreversible CKD typically requiring renal replacement therapy (e.g. dialysis).

Renal lesions typical of diabetic nephropathy appear to be predominantly related to extracellular matrix (ECM) accumulation (Caramori and Mauer, 2009). Accumulation of ECM occurs predominantly in the glomerular and tubular basement membranes and is the principal cause of mesangial expansion. It also contributes to interstitial expansion in late CKD due to diabetic nephropathy. Accumulation of ECM appears to be secondary to an imbalance between ECM synthesis and degradation, and is thought to be causally linked to high ambient glucose concentrations.

While typical ultrastructural lesions of diabetic nephropathy, including thickening of the glomerular and tubular basement membranes, expansion of mesangial matrix and loss of podocytes, are recognized in patients with both type 1 and type 2 diabetes, ultrastructural lesions in patients with type 2 diabetes may be more heterogeneous (Bloom and Rand, 2013). Some type 2 diabetic patients with normal kidney function may have reasonably normal glomeruli or atypical renal injury including global glomerulosclerosis, advanced glomerular arteriolar hyalinosis and tubulointerstitial lesions. Type 2 diabetic patients with reduced kidney function may develop atypical diabetic nephropathy characterized by interstitial and vascular changes, and renal ultrastructural lesions more characteristic of non-diabetic renal disease.

A combination of initiators and promotors is thought to facilitate development of diabetic nephropathy in humans (Bloom and Rand, 2013). Initiators include hyperglycaemia and genetic factors, while promotors include hyperglycaemia and insulin resistance, hypertension, dyslipidaemia, extended duration of diabetes, anaemia, a procoagulant state, ethnicity and smoking. Hyperglycaemia and poor glycaemic control are widely recognized as major risk factors in both type 1 and type 2 diabetic nephropathy. Hyperglycaemia promotes microvascular changes including vasoconstriction and increased vascular permeability. Growth factors, cytokines and inflammatory factors appear to mediate these microvascular injuries. Most organ systems are at risk of injury from these changes, but the kidneys (glomeruli), retina and peripheral nerves are particularly susceptible to these effects. Systemic hypertension is recognized more often in the earlier stages of diabetic nephropathy because the conditions promoting type 2 diabetes commonly also promote hypertension (e.g. obesity, metabolic syndrome). When present, arterial hypertension may promote glomerular hypertension, hyperperfusion and hyperfiltration as well as glomerular injury. An association between dyslipidaemia and micro-albuminuria or macroalbuminuria has also been recognized in humans with diabetes. Presumably, the dyslipidaemia contributes to microvascular dysfunction including development of renal vascular atherosclerosis. Dyslipidaemia is more common in patients with type 2 diabetes because of the metabolic derangements that promote hyperglycaemia.

Diabetic nephropathy in dogs

Some characteristics of diabetic nephropathy have been described in dogs including arterial hypertension, proteinuria and glomerular lesions. Evidence that diabetes leads to CKD, AKI or nephrotic syndrome is lacking. As described above, the advanced stages of diabetic nephropathy are late complications of diabetes and their development in dogs may be limited by canine lifespan and the duration of therapy for diabetes mellitus.

Spontaneous diabetes mellitus has been reported to be associated with an increased prevalence of systemic hypertension. In a longitudinal study of 17 dogs with spontaneous diabetes mellitus, 6/17 (35.3%) had systolic hypertension (defined as >150 mmHg) and 10/17 (59%) had diastolic hypertension (defined as >95 mmHg) (Herring et al., 2014). The highest systolic pressure was 165 mmHg and the highest diastolic pressure was 124 mmHg. Concurrent systolic and diastolic hypertension was present in 4/17 (23.5%) dogs. In another study of 20 diabetic dogs, systolic blood pressure ranged from 88 to 203 mmHg, and 7/20 (35%) dogs were found to be hypertensive (hypertension was defined as systolic pressure >160 mmHg) (Mazzi et al., 2008). The highest recorded prevalence of systolic and diastolic hypertension in 11 dogs followed for 2 years was 55 and 64%, respectively (Herring et al., 2014).

Proteinuria is commonly recognized in dogs with diabetes mellitus. Elevated levels of urine albumin:creatinine and both urine albumin:creatinine and protein:creatinine were detected in 5/20 (25%) and 6/20 (30%) dogs with diabetes mellitus, respectively (Mazzi et al., 2008). In another study, the prevalence of microalbuminuria and overt proteinuria in dogs with diabetes was 7/11 (64%) and 7/16 (44%), respectively, at initial evaluation (Herring et al., 2014). Using a UPC ratio >0.5 as abnormal, the prevalence of abnormal UPC ratio ranged from 48.3% to 60% over 2 years of investigation. Three microalbuminuric dogs in this study did not have a concurrent elevation of UPC ratio. Two of these three dogs with only micro-albuminuria at diagnosis subsequently developed overt proteinuria, but their UPC ratio remained below 1.0 (Herring et al., 2014). This observation is consistent with the observation in humans that microalbuminuria commonly precedes the onset of overt glomerular disease and proteinuria. However, the overall range of UPC ratio values in this study remained stable, suggesting that progression of glomerular injury may not have occurred over the 2 years of follow-up (Herring et al., 2014).

There is limited evidence that morphological lesions of early stage diabetic nephropathy may develop in dogs with diabetes mellitus. Similar to findings in humans with diabetic nephropathy, linear staining for IgG and albumin was observed in glomerular and tubular basement membranes in 12 dogs with spontaneous diabetes mellitus but not in 16 clinically normal control dogs (Jeraj et al., 1984). Uninephrectomized dogs with alloxan-induced diabetes developed structural lesions consistent with early diabetic nephropathy, including increases in mesangial thickening, fractional volumes of mesangium (cellular and matrix) and

width of the glomerular basement membrane, after 1 year of diabetes (Steffes et al., 1982). However, in a 5-year study of dogs with alloxan-induced diabetes, morphological lesions consistent with Stage 2 human diabetic nephropathy were observed (Kern and Engermann, 1987).

It is difficult to determine whether advanced diabetic nephropathy (Stages 4 and 5) occurs in dogs with naturally occurring diabetes mellitus. In 16 diabetic dogs monitored over 2 years, serum urea and creatinine concentrations remained stable and within the reference range (Herring et al., 2014). In a study of concurrent diseases in 221 dogs with diabetes mellitus, there were no dogs identified as having azotaemic CKD (Hess et al., 2000). In this study, 56/208 (27%) diabetic dogs had elevated creatinine values and 45/208 (22%) had elevated blood urea nitrogen values; however, it does not appear that any of these azotaemic dogs was confirmed as having primary kidney disease. Abdominal ultrasonography was performed in 127/221 (57%) dogs and identified 14 dogs with pyelectasia, five with decreased renal corticomedullary junction distinction, three with renal cysts and three with renal calculi. Post-mortem examinations were performed on 20/221 (9%) dogs: two had severe lymphoplasmacytic interstitial nephritis and one dog had severe chronic pyelonephritis. Seemingly none of these findings is consistent with typical diabetic nephropathy as it is recognized in humans. Thus, it appears that Stage 4 and 5 diabetic nephropathy may be very rarely, if ever, recognized in dogs.

Taken together, available studies in dogs with diabetes mellitus suggest that the early stages of diabetic nephropathy, including hyperfiltration, hypertension, microalbuminuria, proteinuria and microscopic and ultrastructural lesions, do occur in dogs. However, evidence of advanced diabetic nephropathy (Stages 4 and 5) is lacking to date. It is reasonable to speculate that dogs with spontaneous diabetes mellitus may not develop the advanced forms of diabetic nephropathy because they do not survive long enough with diabetes mellitus to develop clinically significant loss of kidney function. With improved quality of diabetic management, and particularly with development of diabetes in younger dogs, it may be prudent to consider providing appropriate monitoring and management protocols to delay or prevent more advanced stages of diabetic nephropathy in dogs. Monitoring diabetic dogs for hypertension, microalbuminuria and proteinuria would appear appropriate. Standard therapies for managing proteinuria and hypertension are well established and can be found in Chapters 18, 23 and 24.

Diabetic nephropathy in cats

Chronic kidney disease is common in cats; however, the cause of CKD in cats is rarely determined. Because CKD and diabetes mellitus may be found concurrently in some cats, it has been speculated that diabetic nephropathy could be one of the underlying diseases responsible for development of CKD in cats (Bloom and Rand, 2013). In addition, diabetic cats may have some risk factors for diabetic nephropathy including microalbuminuria, proteinuria and hypercholesterolaemia (Crenshaw and Peterson, 1996; Al-Ghazlat et al., 2011; Bloom and Rand, 2013). In a study of 66 diabetic cats, 46/66 (70%) had microalbuminuria and 50/66 (75%) had proteinuria, as defined by the International Renal Interest Society (IRIS) as UPC ratio >0.4 (Al-Ghazlat et al., 2011). In contrast, unlike human and canine diabetes, systemic hypertension appears to be an uncommon characteristic of diabetes in cats, although blood pressure in diabetic cats has been reported to be higher than in normal cats (Maggio *et al.*, 2000; Sennello *et al.*, 2003; Al-Ghazlat *et al.*, 2011). It is also controversial whether cats with CKD may have pathological characteristics of diabetic nephropathy. In a study of six diabetic cats, three were described as having glomerular lesions consistent with diabetic nephropathy (Bloom and Rand, 2013). However, a more recent study of 32 cats with diabetes mellitus failed to confirm lesions consistent with diabetic nephropathy (Zini *et al.*, 2014). Taken together, the evidence currently available in cats fails to make a convincing case for diabetic nephropathy as a cause for some cases of feline CKD. Nonetheless, proteinuria does appear to be plausible evidence for renal injury developing in some diabetic cats, and the lack of evidence that early diabetic proteinuria leads to overt advanced diabetic nephropathy and CKD may, as with dogs, reflect inadequate time for renal lesions to develop in cats on treatment for diabetes.

Discovery of a causal relationship between diabetes mellitus and CKD is difficult in cats because both conditions develop predominantly in the same demographic: middle-aged and old cats. CKD is common in geriatric cats. In one study, 30.5% of cats over 9 years of age developed azotaemia within 12 months (Jepson *et al.*, 2009). CKD has been reported to occur concurrently in 13–31% of diabetic cats (Bloom and Rand, 2013). However, concurrent diagnosis of these two conditions may be confounded by the impact of glucosuria on urine specific gravity. Differentiating renal azotaemia from pre-renal azotaemia is usually based on urine specific gravity. Depending on the concentration of the urine, glucosuria may increase or decrease urine specific gravity, thereby potentially rendering interpretation of azotaemia difficult or impossible on a single sample. At first contact, cats concurrently hyperglycaemic and azotaemic may present a significant diagnostic challenge and careful follow-up may be required to diagnose the patient's condition(s) accurately. A recent study reported that major changes in kidney function could not be demonstrated in 36 feline diabetic patients (Paepe *et al.*, 2015). In another study, histological lesions of kidney disease were found not to occur more frequently in diabetic cats than in cats dying of other causes (Zini *et al.*, 2012).

In contrast with dogs, proteinuric kidney disease (glomerular disease) is less common in cats. Thus, finding renal azotaemia and proteinuria in a cat with diabetes mellitus raises suspicion, but does not prove that the kidney disease is causally related to diabetes. Further studies will be needed to confirm a clear relationship between diabetes and CKD in cats. However, it appears reasonable to recommend that diabetic cats should be monitored for evidence of proteinuria, systemic hypertension and azotaemia. When discovered, proteinuria and hypertension should be managed as described elsewhere in this text, and increased monitoring for evidence of developing CKD should be instituted.

Hypothyroidism and the kidneys

The principal effect of hypothyroidism on the kidneys is a reduction in renal function (van Hoek and Daminet, 2009). While an important part of this reduction in renal function is a consequence of hypothyroid-associated reduction in cardiac output, hypothyroidism also directly affects specific renal functions. Most of the studies assessing the link between hypothyroidism and renal function have been performed in humans and rodents, but some data are available from dogs. Although extensive data are available on the effect of hyperthyroidism on renal function in cats (see Chapter 17), little information is available on the effects of spontaneous hypothyroidism in cats.

The GFR may decline by <40% in hypothyroid humans (van Hoek and Daminet, 2009). Thyroid supplementation can reverse the decline in GFR. Thyroidectomy and thyroid deficiency are also associated with significant reductions in GFR in dogs. Likewise, the reduction in GFR in dogs has been shown to be reversible, at least in part, with thyroid supplementation (Gommeren *et al.*, 2008). These observations suggest that the change in GFR is functional rather than pathological in origin. Mechanisms proposed to explain the reduction in GFR include increased systemic vascular resistance and vasoconstriction of the efferent arterioles, reduced cardiac output and renal blood flow, decreased activity of the renin–angiotensin–aldosterone system, and decreased tubuloglomerular feedback due to impaired renal tubular reabsorption of chloride. Glomerular lesions have been reported in hypothyroidism in dogs and humans, and they may contribute to the reduction in GFR (Hess *et al.*, 2006; Iglesias and Díez, 2009; Mariani and Berns, 2012). Lesions observed in dogs include thickening of the glomerular membranes and increases in glomerular matrix. At least some glomerular lesions observed in humans with hypothyroidism appear to be immune-mediated (Iglesias and Díez, 2009; Mariani and Berns, 2012).

As predicted, serum creatinine concentrations may increase in hypothyroid dogs and cats. Reduction in GFR is the principal mechanism underlying this increase; however, increased creatinine generation due to myopathy and rhabdomyolysis has been proposed to contribute to the increase (van Hoek and Daminet, 2009). In humans, clinically important decreases in GFR and elevations in serum creatinine may occur. It has been recommended that screening for hypothyroidism be considered in human patients with unexplained increases in serum creatinine (Mariani and Berns, 2012).

Mild proteinuria and albuminuria have been reported with hypothyroidism in humans and rats, and albuminuria may precede the decline in GFR (van Hoek and Daminet, 2009). Isolated cases of reversible proteinuria and biopsy-proven glomerulonephritis (GN) associated with hypothyroidism and hyperthyroidism, most commonly in relation to autoimmune thyroiditis, have been reported in animals, as well as in both children and adult humans (Mariani and Berns, 2012). When available, renal histopathology in humans has revealed membranous nephropathy, minimal change membranoproliferative GN and IgA nephropathy. Although a direct pathogenic link between autoimmune thyroid disease and glomerular disease has not been confirmed, immune-mediated processes affecting both have been proposed in human patients.

Hypothyroidism also influences renal tubular function; however, the impact is related to the duration of thyroid hormone deficiency (van Hoek and Daminet, 2009). The principal effect of hypothyroidism is a general reduction in tubular reabsorption. If hypothyroidism is of recent onset, the proximal tubules appear to be primarily affected, whereas long-term hypothyroidism tends to affect all tubule segments. The principal effect is downregulation of Na^+-K^+-ATPase activity, which is central to most solute reabsorption in the renal tubules. Urine acidification and urine concentrating ability are also both impaired with hypothyroidism. Sodium reabsorption via the Na^+/H^+ exchanger is decreased. Urine concentration may be impaired as a result of the decreased osmotic driving force, the impaired vasopressin response to osmotic stimuli, and impaired renal water and electrolyte handling. These effects are reversible with restoration of adequate thyroxine levels.

Hypothyroidism in patients with kidney disease

Humans with CKD, AKI and/or nephrotic syndrome may have alterations in thyroid gland physiology that affect thyroid function and the testing of thyroid function (Mariani and Berns, 2012). It has been proposed that hypothyroidism may have beneficial effects in CKD, as amelioration of proteinuria and slowed decline in GFR have been observed in rats with hypothyroidism and CKD. Factors that may explain these potential renal protective effects include reductions in intraglomerular haemodynamic factors including hypertension, hyperperfusion and hyperfiltration, reduced proximal renal tubular reabsorption demand and decreased oxidative stress. In contrast, therapeutic correction of hypothyroidism in patients with CKD may increase GFR and reduce azotaemia and the retention of some uraemic toxins. This approach is sometimes recommended for cats with CKD that develop hypothyroidism following [131]iodine therapy for hyperthyroidism (see Chapter 17 for further details).

Directional changes in thyroid hormones reported in humans with CKD include normal or decreased total (TT4) and free (fT4) thyroxine, decreased total (TT3) and free (fT3) tri-iodothyronine, and normal reverse (r)T3 and thyroid-stimulating hormone (TSH) (Kovalik and Kovalik, 2009). Humans with CKD may have lower concentrations of TT4, fT4 and T3 due to euthyroid sick syndrome (van Hoek and Daminet, 2009). Non-thyroidal illnesses can suppress TT4 concentration below the normal range in dogs. Differentiation between hypothyroidism and non-thyroidal illness is usually established by measurement of thyrotropin (TSH) levels in dogs.

Hypercalcaemia and the kidneys

The kidneys are particularly susceptible to hypercalcaemia. Elevation in blood ionized calcium concentrations may be associated with functional and/or structural changes in the kidneys that may lead to reversible or irreversible kidney injury. The severity of the impact on the kidneys may be influenced by the rate of increase of ionized calcium concentration, the magnitude and duration of hypercalcaemia and the nature of the underlying disease (Kruger and Osborne, 2011).

The earliest clinical signs of hypercalcaemia are polyuria and polydipsia. Urine specific gravity in dogs is typically <1.020. Polyuria and polydipsia are less commonly recognized in cats than in dogs, but 66% of cats with hypercalcaemia have urine specific gravities <1.020. Initially, polyuria is largely the result of an inability to respond to antidiuretic hormone (arginine vasopressin; AVP). Lack of response to AVP is further compounded by reduced medullary tonicity and disruption of medullary osmotic gradients, probably related to decreased sodium reabsorption resulting from calcium-sensor receptor-mediated downregulation of renal sodium transporters in the thick ascending loop of Henle. Increases in renal medullary blood flow and subsequent medullary washout further contribute to disruption of medullary osmotic gradients and the ability to respond to AVP. Early in the onset of hypercalcaemia the loss of urine concentrating ability is largely functional and potentially reversible. However, when hypercalcaemia persists for longer periods, structural injuries due to hypercalcaemia-induced calcification of tubular epithelium, interstitium and blood vessels may become irreversible.

Hypercalcaemia may also promote a reduction in GFR and result in azotaemia. The azotaemia may be pre-renal, primary renal or a combination of both. Hypercalcaemia may directly alter renal haemodynamics and glomerular filtration; moderate to severe hypercalcaemia consistently leads to reduced renal blood flow and GFR due to renal vasoconstriction and a decrease in the glomerular ultra-filtration coefficient (Kruger and Osborne, 2011). As with urinary concentration, reductions in renal blood flow and GFR are potentially reversible early in the disease process and reduction in blood ionized calcium to normal can result in rapid correction of GFR. However, persistent and severe hypercalcaemia promotes sustained renal vasoconstriction, nephrocalcinosis and progression to intrinsic renal tubular injury and irreversible loss of renal function. Hypercalcaemia may also lead to dysfunction of specific renal tubular functions such as tubular reabsorption and secretion.

Confirmation of hypercalcaemic nephropathy requires a demonstration that the total serum hypercalcaemia reflects an elevated ionized calcium concentration. The total serum calcium concentration does not reliably predict blood ionized calcium concentration. Because total serum calcium concentrations and ionized calcium concentrations are commonly discordant in dogs and cats with CKD, measurement of ionized calcium concentration is necessary to establish the diagnosis (Schenck and Chew, 2003).

In non-azotaemic animals, ionized hypercalcaemia is likely to be the result of a non-renal disorder. However, when an animal is azotaemic, it becomes necessary to establish whether the azotaemia is caused by hypercalcaemia or whether the hypercalcaemia is a consequence of kidney disease. When it is possible to establish that the hypercalcaemia preceded the azotaemia, it can usually be assumed that the hypercalcaemia is the cause of the azotaemia. When it is not possible to determine whether azotaemia or hypercalcaemia developed first, establishing the origin of the elevated ionized calcium concentration may be more challenging, and it may be necessary to rule out other causes of hypercalcaemia.

The diagnosis and treatment of hypercalcaemia are beyond the scope of this chapter; however, identifying the cause of the elevated ionized calcium concentration is essential for management of the hypercalcaemia and associated renal injury. The medical history, physical examination findings, routine haematology, serum chemistry, urinalysis and measurement of blood ionized calcium concentration are paramount in pursuing the diagnosis of hypercalcaemia. Figure 19.2 provides an outline of the diagnostic approach to common causes of ionized hypercalcaemia.

Given that the magnitude and duration of hypercalcaemia determine the extent and reversibility of hypercalcaemic nephropathy, early diagnosis and therapeutic intervention are essential, particularly when azotaemia and polyuria are present. The initial goal is to bring the blood ionized calcium concentration into the reference range or as close to normal as possible. The approach to acute management of hypercalcaemia has been reviewed elsewhere (Groman, 2012).

Cause of ionized hypercalcaemia	PO₄	PTH	PTHrP	25-OH Vit D	1,25 (OH)₂ Vit D
Hypercalcaemia of malignancy	N, ↑	↓	↑, N	N	↓, N, ↑
Primary hyperparathyroidism	N, ↓	N, ↑	N	N	N, ↑
Chronic kidney disease (azotaemic)	↑	↑	N	N, ↓	N, ↓
Vitamin D intoxication	N, ↑	↓	N	↑	N, ↑
Feline idiopathic hypercalcaemia	N, ↑	N, ↓	N	↓, N, ↑	↓, N, ↑

19.2 Diagnostic findings for common causes of ionized hypercalcaemia in dogs and cats. 1,25 (OH)₂ Vit D = 1,25 dihydroxyvitamin D; 25-OH Vit D = 25-hydroxyvitamin D; N = normal; PO₄ = serum inorganic phosphorus; PTH = parathyroid hormone assay; PTHrP = immunoreactive parathyroid hormone-related peptide.

References and further reading

Al-Ghazlat SA, Langston CE, Greco DS et al. (2011) The prevalence of microalbuminuria and proteinuria in cats with diabetes mellitus. Topics in Companion Animal Medicine 26, 154–157

Behrend EN (2015) Canine hyperadrenocorticism. In: Canine and Feline Endocrinology, 4th edn, ed. EC Feldman, RW Nelson, C Reusch, et al., pp. 377–451. Elsevier, St. Louis

Bloom CA and Rand JS (2013) Diabetes and the kidney in human and veterinary medicine. Veterinary Clinics of North America: Small Animal Practice 43, 351–365

Bovens C, Tennant K, Reeve J et al. (2014) Basal serum cortisol concentration as a screening test for hypoadrenocorticism in dogs. Journal of Veterinary Internal Medicine 28(8), 1541–1545

Caramori ML and Mauer M (2009) Pathogenesis and pathophysiology of diabetic nephropathy. In: Primer on Kidney Diseases, 5th edn, ed. A Greenberg, pp. 214–223. Saunders, Philadelphia

Crenshaw KL and Peterson ME (1996) Pretreatment clinical and laboratory evaluation of cats with diabetes mellitus: 104 cases (1992–1994). Journal of the American Veterinary Medical Association 209, 943–949

Faggiano A, Pivonello R, Melis D et al. (2002) Evaluation of circulating levels and renal clearance of natural amino acids in patients with Cushing's disease. Journal of Endocrinological Investigation 25(2), 142–151

Faggiano A, Pivonello R, Melis D et al. (2003) Nephrolithiasis in Cushing's disease: prevalence, etiopathogenesis, and modification after disease cure. Journal of Clinical Endocrinology and Metabolism 88(5), 2076–2080

Feldman EC (2015) Hyperadrenocorticism in cats. In: Canine and Feline Endocrinology, 4th edn, ed. EC Feldman, RW Nelson, C Reusch, et al., pp. 452–484. Elsevier, St. Louis

Gommeren K, Lefebvre HP, Benchekroun G et al. (2008) Effect of thyroxine supplementation on glomerular filtration in hypothyroid dogs. Journal of Veterinary Internal Medicine 22, 734

Groman RP (2012) Acute management of calcium disorders. Topics in Companion Animal Medicine 27, 167–171

Herring IP, Panciera DL and Were SR (2014) Longitudinal prevalence of hypertension, proteinuria, and retinopathy in dogs with spontaneous diabetes mellitus. Journal of Veterinary Internal Medicine 28, 488–495

Hess RS, Kass PH and Van Winkle TJ (2006) Association between atherosclerosis and glomerulopathy in dogs. International Journal of Applied Research in Veterinary Medicine 4, 224–230

Hess RS, Kass PH and Ward CR (1998) Association between hyperadrenocorticism and development of calcium-containing uroliths in dogs with urolithiasis. Journal of the American Veterinary Medical Association 15, 1889–1891

Hess RS, Saunders HM, Van Winkle TJ and Ward CR (2000) Concurrent disorders in dogs with diabetes mellitus: 221 cases (1993–1998). Journal of the American Veterinary Medical Association 217, 1166–1173

Iglesias P and Díez JJ (2009) Thyroid dysfunction and kidney disease. European Journal of Endocrinology 160, 503–515

Jepson RE, Brodbelt D, Vallance C et al. (2009) Evaluation of predictors of the development of azotemia in cats. Journal of Veterinary Internal Medicine 23, 806–813

Jeraj K, Basgen J, Hardy RM et al. (1984) Immunofluorescence studies of renal basement membranes in dogs with spontaneous diabetes. American Journal of Veterinary Research 45, 1162–1165

Kern TS and Engermann RL (1987) Kidney morphology in experimental hyperglycemia. Diabetes 36(2), 244–249

Kovalik J and Kovalik EC (2009) Endocrine and neurologic manifestations of chronic Disease. In: Primer on Kidney Diseases, 5th edn, A Greenberg, pp. 514–524. Saunders, Philadelphia

Kruger JM and Osborne CA (2011) Calcium disorders. In: Nephrology and Urology of Small Animals, 1st edn, ed. J Bartges and DJ Polzin, pp. 642–656. Wiley-Blackwell, Ames

Kubota E, Hayashi K, Matsuda H et al. (2001) Role of intrarenal angiotensin II in glucocorticoid-induced renal vasodilation. Clinical and Experimental Nephrology 5, 186–192

Maggio F, DeFrancesco TC, Atkins CE et al. (2000) Ocular lesions associated with systemic hypertension in cats: 69 cases (1985–1998). Journal of the American Veterinary Medical Association 217, 695–702

Mariani LH and Berns JS (2012) The renal manifestations of thyroid disease. Journal of the American Society of Nephrology 23, 22–26

Mazzi A, Fracassi F, Dondi F et al. (2008) Ratio of urinary protein to creatinine and albumin to creatinine in dogs with diabetes mellitus and hyperadrenocorticism. Veterinary Research Communications 32, S299–S301

Paepe D, Ghys LFE, Smets P et al. (2015) Routine kidney variables, glomerular filtration rate and urinary cystatin C in cats with diabetes mellitus, cats with chronic kidney disease and healthy cats. Journal of Feline Medicine and Surgery 17(10), 880–888

Schellenberg S, Mettler M, Gentilini F et al. (2008) The effects of hydrocortisone on systemic arterial blood pressure and urinary protein excretion in dogs. Journal of Veterinary Internal Medicine 22, 273–281

Schenck PA and Chew DJ (2003) Determination of calcium fractionation in dogs with chronic renal failure. American Journal of Veterinary Research 64, 1181–1184

Scott-Moncrieff JC (2015) Hypoadrenocorticism. In: Canine and Feline Endocrinology, 4th edn, ed. EC Feldman, RW Nelson, C Reusch et al., pp. 485–520. Elsevier, St. Louis

Sennello KA, Schulman RL, Prosek R and Siegel AM (2003) Systolic blood pressure in cats with diabetes mellitus. Journal of the American Veterinary Medical Association 223, 198–201

Smets P, Lefebvre HP, Meij BP et al. (2012) Long-term follow-up of renal function in dogs after treatment for ACTH-dependent hyperadrenocorticism. Journal of Veterinary Internal Medicine 26, 565–573

Smets P, Meyer E, Maddens B and Daminet S (2010) Cushing's syndrome, glucocorticoids and the kidney. General and Comparative Endocrinology 169, 1–10

Steffes MW, Buchwald H, Groppoli TJ et al. (1982) Diabetic nephropathy in the uninephrectomized dog: microscopic lesions after one year. Kidney International 21, 721–724

van Hoek I and Daminet S (2009) Interactions between thyroid and kidney function in pathological conditions of these organ systems: A review. General and Comparative Endocrinology 160, 205–215

Walser M and Ward L (1988) Progression of chronic renal failure is related to glucocorticoid production. Kidney International 34, 859–866

Waters CB, Adams LG, Scott-Montcrieff JC et al. (1996) Effects of glucocorticoid therapy on urine protein-to-creatinine ratios and renal morphology in dogs. Journal of Veterinary Internal Medicine 11, 172–177

Zini E, Benali S, Coppola L et al. (2012) Renal morphology and function in cats with diabetes mellitus (abstract). Journal of Veterinary Internal Medicine 26, 1537

Chapter 20

Effects of non-steroidal anti-inflammatory drug treatment on the kidney

Ludovic Pelligand and Jonathan Elliott

The population of animals that develop kidney disease are often elderly with multiple problems. It is not uncommon to have a clinical need to provide pain relief, often on a chronic basis, for dogs and cats with chronic kidney disease (CKD). Usually this pain relief is provided by using non-steroidal anti-inflammatory drugs (NSAIDs), which have a number of effects on the kidney. This group of drugs has the potential to cause acute kidney injury (AKI) when applied in a particular situation. This chapter will review:

- The pharmacology of NSAIDs, defining the important properties of the main drugs used clinically
- The role of the main target of NSAIDs (cyclo-oxygenase) in normal renal physiology
- The mechanisms whereby NSAID renal toxicity is most likely to occur
- The evidence for the harm/benefit assessment for the use of NSAIDs in canine and feline patients with CKD and the recommendations for the use of these drugs in patients with kidney disease.

Pharmacology of NSAIDs

The NSAIDs are a diverse class of chemical compounds widely used in veterinary medicine for their antipyretic, analgesic and anti-inflammatory actions. This section describes the discovery of their pharmacological effects as well as their main pharmacodynamic and pharmacokinetic properties, with a view to understanding their effects on the kidney.

Mechanism of action of NSAIDs

The acetyl ester of salicylic acid (aspirin) was the first NSAID, industrially produced from the end of the 19th century. The main known mechanism of action of NSAIDs is through inhibition of a cell membrane-bound enzyme: cyclooxygenase (COX). The principal role of COX is to transform its main substrate, arachidonic acid, which is released from membrane phospholipids by phospholipase A_2. The product of the reaction is an intermediate product, prostaglandin $(PG)H_2$, which is the common parent to physiologically active eicosanoids subsequently generated by prostaglandin synthases further down the cascade (Figure 20.1). Secondary mechanisms of action of some NSAIDs include inhibition of lipoxygenase (5-LO) (dual inhibitors) and inhibition of the nuclear factor (NF)-κB pathway.

Eicosanoids are a family of fatty acid derivatives composed of 20 carbon units. These mediators act locally as autacoid agents in transmembrane signalling cascades. The main eicosanoids of interest in renal physiology are PGE_2, PGI_2 (also named prostacyclin) and thromboxane $(Tx)A_2$. Specific G protein-coupled receptors have been described for each eicosanoid: four types of receptors for PGE_2 (EP_1 to EP_4), IP receptor for PGI_2 and TP receptor for TxA_2 (Figure 20.1). The EP_2, EP_4 and IP receptors (coupled with G_s alpha-subunit) stimulate cyclic adenosine monophosphate (cAMP) to cause vasodilation. The EP_3 receptor (coupled to G_i alpha-subunit) modulates the generation of cyclic AMP from previous receptors and subsequent vasodilation. The TP and EP_1 receptors (coupled with G_q alpha-subunit) increase cell calcium through phospholipase C activation, resulting in vasoconstriction.

Two isoforms of cyclooxygenase, COX-1 and COX-2, encoded by two different genes, were identified in 1991. The understanding, at the time, was that COX-1 was expressed constitutively in a variety of tissues and was involved in the maintenance of physiological 'house-keeping' functions. It would ensure: protection of the gastric mucosa against acid pH and increase epithelial perfusion; maintenance of glomerular filtration rate; and generation of TxA_2 from platelets for initiation of aggregation and blood clotting. The COX-2 isoform was considered to be an inducible isoform that played a leading role, through generation of PGE_2, in the clinical manifestation of inflammation following an injury. The pharmaceutical industry postulated during the 1990s that preferentially or selectively inhibiting COX-2 rather than COX-1 would result in a lower incidence of gastrointestinal (GI) adverse effects. Current knowledge is that COX-2 is actually expressed constitutively in several mammalian tissues, including the kidney (see below) and the digestive tract (where it plays a protective and healing role) in the absence of inflammation (Warner et al., 1999). Older NSAIDs and COX-2 inhibitors (COXIBs) authorized for use in the UK are summarized in Figure 20.2 for the dog and Figure 20.3 for the cat. The tables summarize the isoenzyme selectivities, indications, dose and route of administration, and duration of treatment.

In the sections that follow, the role of COX-1 and COX-2 in the normal physiological functions of the kidney are reviewed. This knowledge underpins the understanding of the adverse effects seen when these drugs are used clinically.

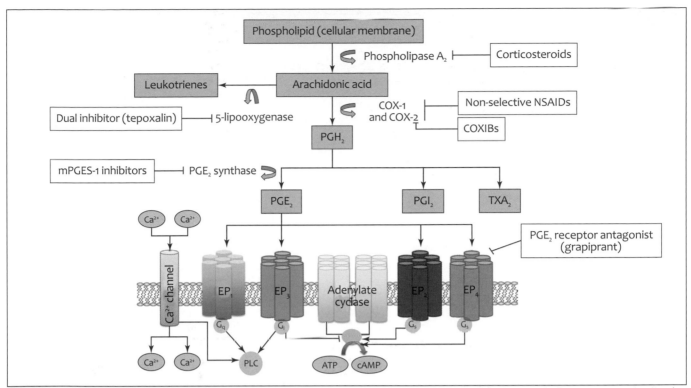

20.1 Arachidonic acid cascade from membrane phospholipids to intracellular effects of its metabolites (with particular focus on prostaglandin E_2). Enzyme actions are represented by a curved green arrow. The actions of enzyme inhibitors or receptor blockers are represented along the cascade by red arrows with flat ends. COX = cyclooxygenase; COXIB = COX-2 inhibitor; EP = G protein-coupled eicosanoid receptor; G_s, G_i, G_q = alpha-subunits of the G protein-coupled receptor; NSAIDs = non-steroidal anti-inflammatory drugs; PG = prostaglandin; PLC = phospholipase C; TX = thromboxane.
(Reproduced from Nasrallah et al. 2014 with permission from the *American Journal of Physiology*)

Drug	COX-1:COX-2 selectivity	Formulation	Dose/route	Indication	Duration of treatment
Non-steroidal anti-inflammatory drugs (NSAIDs)					
Carprofen	COX-2 preferential IC_{50} ratios: S+ carprofen = 17.6 :1[b] R- carprofen = 5.8:1[b] Rac-carprofen = 6.5:1[c] Rac-carprofen = 17.2:1[e]	Injectable: 50 mg/ml	4 mg/kg i.v. or s.c.	Perioperative pain and inflammation (orthopaedic and soft tissue)	One injection; another injection (2 mg/kg) may be given after 24 hours if necessary or oral treatment up to 5 days
		Tablets: 20 and 50 mg; palatable tablets: 20, 50 and 100 mg	2–4 mg/kg per day orally (in one or two administrations)	Chronic inflammation and postoperative pain	Unlimited duration Up to 7 days at this dose, then 2 mg/kg per day In one administration
Ketoprofen	Non-selective IC_{50} ratio = 0.88:1[b] IC_{50} ratio = 0.6:1[c]	Injectable: 10 mg/ml	2 mg/kg i.v., i.m. or s.c.	Pain and inflammation (musculoskeletal)	Injectable: can be repeated for up to 3 days
		Tablets: 5 and 20 mg	1 mg/kg per day	Acute pain and inflammation	Acute: up to 5 days (or 4 days if after injection)
			0.25 mg/kg per day	Chronic osteoarthritis	Chronic: up to 30 days
Meloxicam	COX-2 preferential IC_{50} ratio = 7.3:1[b] IC_{50} ratio = 10:1[c]	Injectable: 5 mg/ml	0.2 mg/kg i.v. or s.c.	Perioperative pain (orthopaedic/soft tissue)	May be followed by oral administration 24 hours after injection
		Oral suspension: 1.5 mg/ml	0.2 mg/kg loading dose then 0.1 mg/kg per day	Acute and chronic musculoskeletal disorders	Dose may be tapered down to lowest effective individual dose after 4 days Re-evaluate at 10 days Unlimited duration
Tepoxalin[a]	Not published	Oral lyophilisates 50, 100 and 250 mg	10 mg/kg per day	Acute and chronic musculoskeletal disorders	Up to 10 days
Tolfenamic acid	COX-2 preferential IC_{50} ratio = 13.3:1[d]	Injectable: 40 mg/ml	4 mg/kg i.m. or s.c.	Perioperative pain	May be repeated once after 24 hours
		Tablets: 6, 20 and 60 mg	4 mg/kg	Acute episodes of inflammation and pain in chronic locomotor disease	Treatment up to 3 days, course may be repeated after 7 days

20.2 Summary of isoform selectivity, formulations, route and doses, indications and duration of treatment for the older non-steroidal anti-inflammatory drugs (NSAIDs) authorized for use in dogs in the UK (generics omitted for clarity) and for the cyclooxygenase (COX)-2 inhibitors (COXIBs) authorized for use in dogs in the UK. IC_{50} = 50% inhibitory concentration. [a]At the time of publication tepoxalin is no longer available in the UK. It is included because of its unique combination of dual COX and lipoxygenase inhibition and in case the drug is re-introduced at any point in the future. (continues) ▶

([b]King *et al.*, 2009; [c]Brideau *et al.*, 2001; [d]Wilson *et al.*, 2004; [e]Lees *et al.*, 2014)

Drug	COX-1:COX-2 selectivity	Formulation	Dose/route	Indication	Duration of treatment
Cyclooxygenase (COX)-2 inhibitors (COXIBs)					
Mavacoxib	COX-2 preferential IC_{50} ratio = 22.1:1[e]	Chewable tablets: 6, 20, 30, 75 or 95 mg	2 mg/kg	Pain and inflammation associated with degenerative joint disease	Repeated after 14 days, and thereafter once a month Maximum duration 6.5 months
Firocoxib	COX-2 selective IC_{50} ratio = 380:1 (manufacturer data)	Chewable tablets: 57 and 227 mg	5 mg/kg	Perioperative pain	If preoperative: 2 hours before surgery, up to 3 days after surgery
				Osteoarthritis	Depending on response, evaluated for up to 90 days for osteoarthritis treatment
Robenacoxib	COX-2 selective IC_{50} ratio = 129:1[b]	Injectable: 20 mg/ml	2 mg/kg s.c.	Perioperative pain (soft tissue and orthopaedic surgeries)	One injection only
		Flavoured tablets: 5, 10, 20, 40 mg	1–2 mg/kg	Pain and inflammation associated with chronic osteoarthritis in dogs	Dose may be tapered down to lowest effective per individual Re-evaluate at 10 days Unlimited duration
Cimicoxib	Not published	Chewable tablets: 8, 30 or 80 mg	2 mg/kg once daily	Perioperative pain due to orthopaedic or soft tissue surgeries	One dose 2 hours prior to surgery, followed by 3–7 days of treatment
				Pain and inflammation associated with osteoarthritis	6 months

20.2 (continued) Summary of isoform selectivity, formulations, route and doses, indications and duration of treatment for the older non-steroidal anti-inflammatory drugs (NSAIDs) authorized for use in dogs in the UK (generics omitted for clarity) and for the cyclooxygenase (COX)-2 inhibitors (COXIBs) authorized for use in dogs in the UK. IC_{50} = 50% inhibitory concentration.
([b] King et al., 2009; [c] Brideau et al., 2001; [d] Wilson et al., 2004; [e] Lees et al., 2014)

Drug	COX-1:COX-2 selectivity	Formulation	Dose/route	Indication	Duration of treatment
Carprofen	COX-2 preferential IC_{50} ratio = 25.6:1[a] IC_{50} ratio = 5.5:1[d]	Injectable: 50 mg/ml	4 mg/kg s.c. or i.v.	Perioperative pain	One injection only
		No oral forms available registered for use in the cat			
Ketoprofen	COX-1 preferential IC_{50} ratio = 1:0.05[c]	Injectable: 10 mg/ml	2 mg/kg s.c.	Pain and inflammation (musculoskeletal)	Can be repeated for up to 3 days
		Tablets: 5 and 20 mg	1 mg/kg per day	Acute pain and inflammation	Up to 5 days (or 4 days if injection started treatment course)
Meloxicam	Non-selective (particularly at 0.3 mg/kg; see text)	Injectable: 5 mg/ml	0.3 mg/kg s.c.	Perioperative pain	One injection only (e.g. feral cat)
		Injectable: 2 mg/ml (new)	0.2 mg/kg s.c.	Perioperative pain (soft tissue and orthopaedic surgery) and postoperative period	One injection followed followed by oral maintenance dose (0.05 mg/kg for up to 5 days)
		Oral suspension: 0.5 mg/ml	0.1 mg/kg loading dose then 0.05 mg/ kg per day	Acute and chronic inflammation and pain in musculoskeletal disorders	Re-evaluate effect between between 7 and 14 days Unlimited duration
Tolfenamic acid	Not determined	Injectable: 40 mg/ml	4 mg/kg s.c.	Upper respiratory disease in association with antimicrobial therapy	May be repeated once after 24 hours
		Tablets: 6, 20 mg	4 mg/kg per day	Adjuvant for treatment of febrile syndromes	Up to 3 days (or 2 days if after injection)
Robenacoxib	COX-2 selective: IC_{50} ratio = 502:1[b] IC_{50} ratio = 32.2:1[c]	Injectable: 20 mg/ml	2 mg/kg s.c.	Perioperative pain (soft tissue and orthopaedic surgery)	One injection only, followed by once-daily treatment at the same dose for up to 2 days
		Flavoured tablets: 6 mg	1–2.4 mg/kg	Acute pain and inflammation associated with musculoskeletal disorders in cats	Up to 6 days in EU (11 days in Switzerland) Oral tablets can be given prior to orthopaedic surgery

20.3 Summary of isoform selectivity, formulations, route and doses, indications and duration of treatment for the older non-steroidal anti-inflammatory drugs (NSAIDs) and cyclooxygenase (COX)-2 inhibitors (COXIBs) authorized for use in cats in the UK (generics omitted for clarity). IC_{50} = 50% inhibitory concentration.
([a] Giraudel et al., 2005; [b] Giraudel et al., 2009; [c] Schmid et al., 2010; [d] Brideau et al., 2001)

Pharmacodynamic classification of NSAIDs

The inhibition of COX by NSAIDs is usually via competitive inhibition of COX. The compounds occupy the hydrophobic pocket of COX, preventing the access of arachidonic acid to the active site. The duration of this reversible inhibition is therefore related to the persistence of NSAIDs in the body. Aspirin is an exception because it chemically reacts with the enzyme covalently adding its acetyl group to the serine$_{530}$ residue of COX, leading to irreversible inhibition. Paracetamol is related to NSAIDs, being a weak inhibitor of COX-1 and COX-2, although its action at the molecular level is still unclear. It should never be used in cats. The dual inhibitor tepoxalin prevents the conversion of arachidonic acid to leukotrienes, which are mainly involved in chemotaxis and bronchoconstriction. The 'piprants' are a new class of compounds (grapiprant, now FDA approved for canine use) with an alternative mechanism of action as they act as selective EP$_4$ prostaglandin receptors.

The selectivity of NSAIDs for COX-1 and COX-2 relies on a conformational difference between these two iso-enzymes. Owing to the substitution of a couple of amino acids, the catalytic cavity of COX-2 is larger than that of COX-1. The traditional NSAIDs (ketoprofen, carprofen, meloxicam, tolfenamic acid) are small compounds able to inhibit both forms of the enzyme (Figure 20.4a). Synthetic selective COX-2 inhibitors (COXIBs) authorized for use in veterinary medicine belong to different chemical families: methylsulphone (firocoxib), sulphonamide (mavacoxib, cimicoxib) or carboxylic acid (robenacoxib). Their relatively bulky structure limits COX-1 inhibition by steric hindrance, thus conferring COX-2 selectivity (Figure 20.4b).

20.4 Chemical formulae of non-steroidal anti-inflammatory drugs (NSAIDs) authorized for use in the UK. (a) Chemical formulae for arachidonic acid and traditional NSAIDs: aspirin (salicylate), ketoprofen/carprofen (aryl propionic acid family; (*) denotes the presence of an asymmetrical carbon), tolfenamic acid (fenamate family) and meloxicam (oxicam family). (b) Chemical formulae for COX-2 inhibitors (COXIBs) authorized for use in companion animals: firocoxib (methylsulphone family), mavacoxib/cimicoxib (sulphonamide family) and robenacoxib (carboxylic acid family).

Pharmacodynamic (PD) ranking of NSAIDs by selectivity against each isoform is clinically useful because the more COX-1 sparing (i.e. COX-2 preferential or selective) the drug, the lower the risk of GI adverse events (Warner *et al.*, 1999). This can be determined with *in vitro* whole blood assays reproducing conditions relevant to the tissues of the whole animal. These assays became the gold standard for determining potency for COX-1 and COX-2. Potency curves are obtained from spiking a COX-1 and COX-2 stimulation assay with increasing concentrations of an NSAID (Giraudel *et al.*, 2005). The results are displayed as a characteristic sigmoidal inhibition curve (Figure 20.5a). The curve inflection point corresponds to the concentration which inhibits 50% of the response (IC_{50} COX-1 and IC_{50} COX-2). This allows ranking of NSAIDs by increasing IC_{50} COX-1:COX-2 potency ratios. For a guideline, see the text box and Figure 20.5b below.

Classification	IC_{50} COX-1:COX-2
Highly COX-2 selective	superior to 100:1
Moderately COX-2 selective	between 50:1 and 100:1
COX-2 preferential	between 5:1 and 50:1
Non-selective	between 0.2:1 and 5:1
COX-1 preferential	inferior to 0.2:1

The potency and selectivity of NSAIDs (in terms of COX-1:COX-2 ratios) are species-specific and there are important differences between dogs and cats. Owing to the presence of a chiral centre, NSAIDs of the aryl propionic family (ketoprofen and carprofen) coexist as (R)-(–) and (S)-(+) enantiomers characterized by different potencies as COX inhibitors. The absolute values of the ratio may vary for the same compound owing to slight methodological differences between laboratories. Consequently, NSAIDs can only rigorously be ranked if evaluated within the same assay. For more information, the reader is referred to the reviews by Lees (2004, 2009).

The IC_{50} COX-1:COX-2 potency ratios have to be considered alongside the drug pharmacokinetics (PK/PD integration, i.e. simultaneous consideration of PD in relation to PK data). The ideal NSAID would sustain concentrations in plasma or inflamed tissue above IC_{80} COX-2 for as long as possible during the inter-dosing interval to guarantee a good clinical effect. On the safety side, concentrations should exceed IC_{20} COX-1 for as short a duration as possible (>20% inhibition is correlated with GI adverse effects). The relative slopes of COX-1 and COX-2 inhibition curves are also considered, because they determine the overlap between the two effects within the range of concentrations clinically observable. For example, the subcutaneous dose

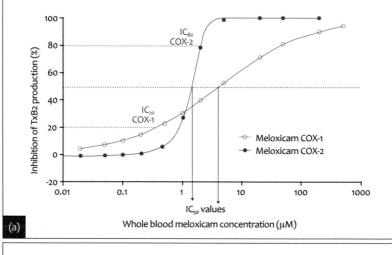

(a)

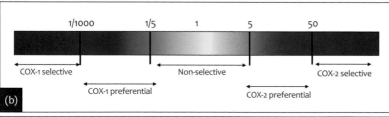

(b)

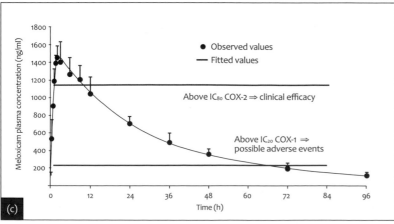

(c)

20.5 Integration of pharmacokinetic (PK) and pharmacodynamic (PD) data applied to the administration of an original dose of 0.3 mg/kg of meloxicam subcutaneously in the cat. (a) *In vitro* feline whole blood assays for meloxicam (Giraudel *et al.*, 2005). Cyclooxygenase inhibition potencies were 4.1 µM for IC_{50} COX-1 (1440 ng/ml) and 1.35 µM for IC_{50} COX-2 (474 ng/ml). From the graph, one can extrapolate to the IC_{20} COX-1 and IC_{80} COX-2. (b) Spectrum of NSAID selectivity based on the IC_{50} COX-1:COX-2 potency ratio. COX-1 selective compounds are on the left and COX-2 selective COXIBs are on the right. (c) Plasma concentration–time curve of meloxicam (0.3 mg/kg s.c.) in the cat (Giraudel *et al.*, 2005). The time during which plasma meloxicam remains above IC_{20} COX-1 and IC_{80} COX-2 can be visualized directly on the figure. IC_{50} = 50% inhibitory concentration; Tx = thromboxane.

of 0.3 mg/kg of meloxicam is associated with plasma concentrations inhibiting 80% of COX-2 for 8.8 hours but results in 20% COX-1 inhibition for 64 hours (Figure 20.5c). This is due to the long plasma half-life of meloxicam (37 hours), the low selectivity (IC_{50} COX-1:COX-2 = 3.05:1) and the shallow slope of the COX-1 inhibition curve, overlapping that of COX-2 (Giraudel et al., 2005). These findings contributed to the rationale for lowering the routine injectable dose to 0.2 mg/kg for meloxicam in the cat.

Pharmacokinetic properties of NSAIDs

All NSAIDs have similar physicochemical characteristics. They are weak acids (pK_a in the order of 3.5 to 6), moderately water soluble and have similar dose-dependent pharmacological action and toxicity.

Oral absorption

The oral availability of NSAIDs is generally good owing to an efficient ion trapping mechanism from the stomach to the plasma. As weak acids, NSAIDs are predominantly non-ionized at the acidic stomach pH, thus readily absorbable into the gastric mucosa, and transported away as the ionized form in pH-neutral blood. Oral NSAIDs are usually administered concomitantly with food but there are exceptions. The bioavailability of mavacoxib is higher in fed dogs than in fasted dogs, while food has the opposite effect on robenacoxib bioavailability in dogs and cats.

Tissue distribution and plasma protein binding

All NSAIDs are highly bound (in the order of 95–99%) to plasma proteins, mainly to albumin. This limits the distribution of traditional NSAIDs (weak carboxylic acids) and robenacoxib (carboxylic acid carrier COXIB), which all have small apparent volumes of distribution approximating plasma volume. In contrast, the methylsulphone and sulphonamide COXIBs are non-ionized at physiological pH, less restricted by their protein binding and have a much wider volume of distribution. Protein binding explains, to some extent, the long half-lives of robenacoxib and ketoprofen in feline inflammatory exudates, thus accounting for the longer clinical duration of action than their short half-lives in plasma would have predicted (Pelligand et al., 2014). This tissue selectivity is advantageous in minimizing side effects when long-lasting COX inhibition in richly vascularized organs such as the kidney is not desired.

Hypoproteinaemia and increased NSAID toxicity have often been associated, and this is relevant to dogs with nephrotic syndrome. A putative increase in NSAID free fraction resulting from the combination of hypoalbuminaemia and displacement by other highly protein-bound drugs is frequently advocated as a factor aggravating NSAID toxicity. Displacement studies have often been performed in vitro; however, these conditions may differ from those in vivo. The impact of hypoproteinaemia has long been overstated because, in vivo, the free concentration of the drug rapidly falls to normal levels owing to faster distribution to larger tissue protein pools, metabolism or excretion (Toutain and Bousquet-Melou, 2002). In the case of liver disease, the association between hypoproteinaemia and increased NSAID toxicity is explained by loss of blood proteins into the ulcerated GI tract (more common in animals with hepatic disease) or by the liver insufficiency accounting for slower hepatic clearance.

Drug clearance mechanisms

The high degree of protein binding limits renal excretion of NSAIDs because only the small free fraction can be filtered through the glomerulus. NSAIDs are not actively secreted but may be reabsorbed if present in the non-ionized form in urine. Alkalinizing the urine increases NSAID ionization, and therefore reduces their reabsorption.

The elimination of NSAIDs is predominantly hepatic. They are either excreted unchanged in the bile or transformed into metabolites. The purpose of these transformations is to increase the polarity of the NSAID for easier excretion in bile or urine. Polar metabolites are usually inactive as they lose their ability to competitively inhibit COX. These transformations occur in the liver and consist of phase I (oxidation, reduction, hydrolysis) and phase II (conjugation reactions, glucuronidation for most NSAIDs) reactions. Cats are deficient in some of the conjugation pathways. This results in slower excretion of carprofen and salicylic acid than in dogs, possibly due to deficits in glucuronidation and glycination, respectively (Court, 2013). Conversely, cats have the ability to oxidize the -oxicams such as piroxicam and meloxicam, whose clearance is not dependent on glucuronidation. Both robenacoxib and mavacoxib are authorized for use in the dog and represent the two extremes in terms of elimination half-lives and clearances. Robenacoxib is cleared extremely quickly (clearance 13.5 ml/kg/min, terminal half-life 0.63 hours). At the other end of the spectrum, mavacoxib is eliminated very slowly, owing to: very efficient enterohepatic recycling; the virtual absence of transformation by the liver; and a large volume of distribution. This results in terminal half-lives of ≥17 days in laboratory dogs, which can extend up to 44 days in older dogs with clinical osteoarthritis. Mavacoxib should not be used in cats.

Effect of kidney disease on the PK properties of NSAIDs

In human patients, clearance of NSAIDs is not dependent on glomerular filtration rate (GFR). Decreased renal function is expected to have no detrimental effect on the clearance of NSAIDs in dogs. However, this has only been demonstrated for tolfenamic acid in dogs, where there was no effect of experimentally-induced renal failure on clearance of the drug. Azotaemia can decrease albumin binding of weak acids and may increase liver and renal clearance driven by the free fraction, but this was not the case for tolfenamic acid in the experimental study. Decreased renal function can also alter tissue binding of drugs, thus changing the volume of distribution. Clearance of polar metabolites may rely more on renal filtration, leading to saturation of the metabolic pathway, with a decrease in kidney function.

Clinically relevant PK and PD drug interactions

Interactions are classified as: drugs that affect NSAID toxicity; and drugs affected by NSAIDs (subdivided into dynamic and kinetic interactions), and are summarized in Figure 20.6.

Summary

A good understanding of NSAID pharmacodynamics and pharmacokinetics provides the pharmacological basis for understanding the effects of COX-1 and COX-2 inhibition by NSAIDs on renal physiology and toxicity in the clinical setting.

Drugs that affect NSAID toxicity	Effect	Management options/considerations
Histamine H₂-receptor blockers (cimetidine and famotidine) Proton pump inhibitors (omeprazole) Aluminium hydroxide	Increased gastric pH and possibly decreased oral absorption and bioavailability	Possible loss of efficacy of NSAIDs
Some specific CYP2D inhibitors: • Quinidine • Possibly fluoxetine	Possibly decrease clearance of NSAIDs (experimental evidence with celecoxib)	Monitor for adverse NSAID reactions because of prolonged duration Reduce NSAID dose
Synthetic PGE₁ (misoprostol), sucralfate and antacid drugs	Local gastroprotective action and counteract the effects of COX inhibition in the GI tract	Prescribe to reduce incidence of gastroduodenal irritation by NSAIDs
Corticosteroids	Overlapping mechanisms of action (inhibition of phospholipase A₂) Well characterized increase in GI toxicity	Withhold NSAIDs until decision to give corticosteroids or not is taken
Drugs affected by NSAIDs	**Effect**	**Management options/considerations**
Pharmacokinetic interaction		
Renal OAT substrates Penicillins, cephalosporins Methotrexate	NSAIDs possibly inhibit OAT in proximal tubule Reduced renal clearance of these drugs	Avoid methotrexate and NSAID combinations
Aminoglycosides (gentamicin, amikacin)	NSAIDs possibly inhibit aminoglycoside renal clearance and cause additive nephrotoxicity	Use in association contraindicated
Pharmacodynamic interaction		
Loop diuretics (furosemide)	Lack of GFR compensation in the face of dehydration Possible limitation of diuretic effect	Follow-up patient on a regular basis Avoid dehydration and monitor renal function closely
Spironolactone	Possible hyperkalaemia	Monitor potassium
Angiotensin-converting enzyme inhibitors or angiotensin receptor blockers	Vasodilation of renal efferent arteriole, drop in GFR and pre-renal azotaemia	Follow-up patient on a regular basis Monitor renal function closely
Beta-blockers (atenolol, propranolol)	Reduced ability to contract afferent renal arteriole Impairment of tubuloglomerular feedback	Monitor blood pressure and dehydration

20.6 Clinically relevant drug interactions with non-steroidal anti-inflammatory drugs (NSAIDs). COX = cyclooxygenase; CYP2D = cytochrome P450 2D6; GFR = glomerular filtration rate; GI = gastrointestinal; OAT = organic anion transporter; PG = prostaglandin.

Role of COX enzyme products in normal kidney physiology

Understanding of the lipid metabolites produced by COX enzymes in renal physiology has developed significantly since the recognition that both COX-1 and COX-2 are involved in important physiological functions of a number of tissues. There are three main areas in which COX products are thought to play an important role in regulating homeostatic mechanisms in the kidney. These are in the:

- Process of tubuloglomerular feedback which ensures that the GFR, and therefore the filtered load that the tubules have to deal with, remains stable over a range of perfusion pressures (intrinsic autoregulation)
- Response of the kidney to reduced water intake, ensuring that the concentrating mechanisms of the kidney function effectively without leading to kidney damage
- Response of the kidney to increased sodium intake, ensuring that sodium excretion increases to match sodium intake (natriuresis).

In a well hydrated normotensive dog or cat taking in a standard amount of sodium in its diet, inhibition of COX enzymes is unlikely to lead to any untoward physiological effects, however renal production of prostanoids helps the kidney to achieve its homeostatic functions under stressful situations. This makes it hard to predict and reproduce the harmful effects of NSAIDs at therapeutic dose rates in the experimental setting.

COX expression in the kidney

The realization that COX-2 is constitutively expressed in the kidney, and that its expression can be altered by changing dietary sodium intake or restricting water intake, suggests that selective COX-2 inhibitors may interfere with normal physiological functions of the kidney. An understanding of the role of the different isoforms of COX-1 and COX-2 has come from work performed in experimental animals. However, the distribution of these enzymes across the different components of the nephron and associated tissues varies with species.

In general, use of the dog as an experimental model overestimates the renal effects of COX-2 inhibition for human medicine. For veterinary interest, this probably means that renal function in the dog will be significantly affected by COX-2 inhibitors. Figure 20.7 shows the relative expression of COX-1 and COX-2 in four different species (including humans). This is overly simplified because relative COX-1 and COX-2 expression is affected by age, and COX-2 is required for normal renal development. In general, COX-2 is expressed most abundantly in the macula densa, the thick ascending limb of the loop of Henle, and the medullary interstitium, whereas COX-1 is most highly expressed in glomerular mesangial cells, the renal vasculature and the collecting ducts. Preliminary data from the cat (Pelligand *et al.*, 2015) suggest that the situation is somewhat intermediate between those in dogs and humans. For example, both COX-1 and COX-2 appear to be expressed in the feline macula densa, suggesting that both may play a role in regulating renin secretion.

Site	Dog	Rat	Monkey	Human
COX-1 site				
Renal vasculature	+	+	+	+
Collecting ducts	+++	+++	++	++
Interstitial cells	–	+	+	+
COX-2 site				
Glomerulus	–	–	+	+
Thick ascending limb of the loop of Henle	+ (+++)	+ (+++)	– (–)	–
Macula densa	+ (+++)	+ (+++)	– (–)	–
Interstitium	+	+	-	–
Renal vasculature	+/–	–	+	+

20.7 Relative expression of cyclooxygenase (COX)-1 and COX-2 in four different species, according to Kahn *et al.* (1998). Data in parentheses indicate a change in intensity of immunohistochemical staining following volume depletion.

Tubuloglomerular feedback

A stable filtrate load is ideal for tubular physiology; fluctuations in the tubular load of filtrate make it difficult for the kidney to fulfil its regulatory functions. Feedback from the tubule to the glomerulus allows the glomerulus to adjust GFR depending on the amount of solute reaching the macula densa (Figure 20.8). In response to sensing high amounts of chloride flowing into the distal tubule, the macula densa secretes a signal (most probably adenosine) that constricts the afferent arteriole, lowering the glomerular capillary pressure and reducing GFR. If the macula densa senses low amounts of chloride, then prostaglandins (PGE_2 and PGI_2; via COX-2 in the dog and possibly COX-1 and -2 in the cat) and nitric oxide are released which signal to the juxtaglomerular apparatus to secrete renin. Prostanoids and nitric oxide dilate the afferent arteriole and relax the mesangial cells, whereas renin release results in production of angiotensin II, which constricts the efferent arteriole. Constriction of the efferent arteriole in combination with afferent arteriolar dilatation and mesangial cell relaxation leads to an increase in GFR.

The above mechanism maintains GFR in the face of reduced renal perfusion (e.g. haemorrhage, or hypotension which occurs during anaesthesia). The chloride sensor is thought to be the sodium–potassium–chloride cotransporter that is present also in the thick ascending limb of the loop of Henle and is the target site for the loop diuretic furosemide. Treatment with furosemide leads to rapid activation of the renin–angiotensin–aldosterone system (RAAS) as a result of inhibition of the chloride sensing mechanism. Loop diuretic treatment, administration of angiotensin-converting enzyme inhibitors (ACEi) or angiotensin receptor blockers (ARBs) and restriction of dietary sodium chloride intake all result in upregulation of COX-2 in the macula densa of the kidney. Experimental treatment of dogs with furosemide results in a small decrease in GFR;

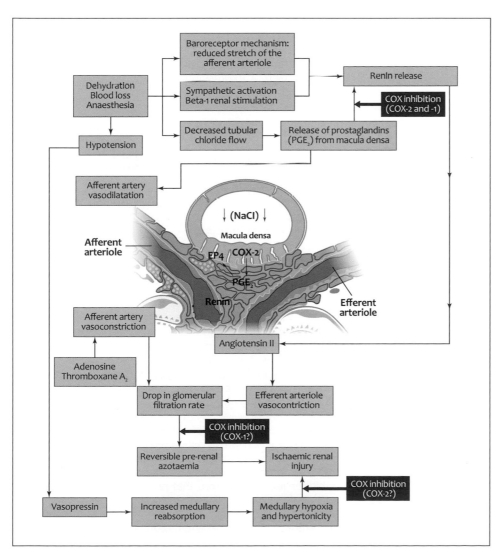

20.8 Flowchart summarizing the relationship between hypotension, renin–angiotensin–aldosterone system (RAAS) activation, cyclooxygenase (COX) dependency and renal injury mechanisms. GFR = glomerular filtration rate; MD = macula densa.

co-administration of furosemide and COX inhibitors (non-selective and COX-2 selective) results in a greater decrease in GFR than furosemide alone, suggesting that furosemide-induced volume contraction leads to a greater reduction in GFR in the absence of this protective mechanism (Surdyk et al., 2012). Preliminary data in the cat, adopting a similar experimental approach, showed that renin secretion in response to furosemide treatment is probably mediated by prostanoids produced by both COX-1 and COX-2, a finding compatible with the immunohistochemistry results suggesting that both enzymes are expressed in the macula densa of the cat (Pelligand et al., 2015).

COX enzymes and water balance

The kidneys of dogs and cats are well adapted to produce concentrated urine in response to water deprivation. The cat in particular is able to concentrate its urine to >2800 mOsm/l, which is 10-fold higher than plasma osmolality and far in excess of that which a human kidney can achieve. The loop of Henle, medullary interstitium and collecting ducts are involved in the renal counter-current mechanism, which generates the solute gradients necessary for conservation of water under the control of anti-diuretic hormone. These are all sites at which COX are expressed, with COX-2 expression in the thick ascending limb of the loop of Henle, interstitial medullary cells and the vasa recta, and COX-1 being expressed in the collecting duct epithelium.

Experimental data from mice and rats show that water deprivation leads to an upregulation of COX-2 in the medulla of the kidney. It appears that COX-2 is required to allow the interstitial cells to survive the hypertonic stress that results from the increased osmolality generated in the interstitium in response to water deprivation. Activity of COX-2 is linked to the ability of these cells to generate increased intracellular osmolality by way of organic osmolytes, and therefore avoid osmotic stress. PGE_2 has been shown to prevent caspase-3 activation in the short term while the cells adapt to the hypertonicity, which requires time. If COX-2 is inhibited pharmacologically at the same time as water deprivation occurs, the interstitial cells undergo apoptosis (programmed cell death, mediated by caspase-3). This information results from experiments in rodents; the situation in dogs and cats has not been investigated but the distribution of COX enzymes within the kidneys of dogs and cats suggests that it may be pertinent. It seems likely that papillary necrosis, a pathological lesion associated with NSAID renal toxicity observed in the dog (and rat), is related to removal of this protective mechanism (Figure 20.9).

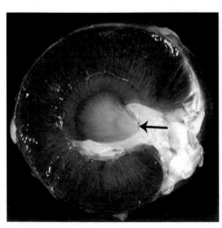

20.9

Gross pathology of naproxen-mediated renal papillary necrosis in a dog.
(Reproduced from Radi et al., 2009 with permission from Toxicologic Pathology)

COX and natriuresis

The thick ascending limb of the loop of Henle transports 25% of the filtered load of sodium, and small changes in sodium transport in this region could make a large difference to sodium homeostasis, extracellular fluid volume and blood pressure. The cells of this segment of the nephron strongly express COX-2. Lowering sodium intake in the diet leads to upregulation of COX-2 in the macula densa and the thick ascending limb of the loop of Henle in the cortex of the kidney (see above). By contrast, feeding excessively high amounts of sodium upregulates COX-2 in the medullary portions of the thick ascending limb of the loop of Henle. Moreover, inhibition of COX-2 in the face of increased dietary sodium intake blunts the normal natriuretic response that is thought to be COX-2 generated in the medullary thick ascending limb of the loop of Henle. This physiology may help to explain why some humans have increased blood pressure when taking NSAIDs and an increased tendency to develop oedema if receiving treatment for heart failure. The relevance of this basic understanding of physiological regulation of renal handling of sodium for canine and feline medicine remains to be determined.

Summary

It is clear that the kidney expresses COX-2 constitutively and that the prostanoids it generates play key roles in helping the kidney adapt to a number of stressful stimuli. The PGs generated locally in the kidney are renoprotective, especially in the inner medullary and papillary areas, when animals become dehydrated. The renoprotective COX is not just COX-1, as might be the case in other tissues; COX-2 expression is influenced by a number of physiological stimuli and the prostanoids it generates in the kidney assist in maintaining homeostasis.

Renal toxicity of NSAIDs

The above discussion of the importance of arachidonic acid metabolites in renal physiology explains the following observations.

Toxic effects of NSAIDs:

- Are dependent on the physiological state of the animal, with dehydration and hypovolaemia being important risk factors
- Vary with species and with drug according to species because of the relative importance of the different isoforms (COX-1 and COX-2) for kidney function (e.g. in the dog COX-2 is important in the kidney whereas in humans it is less important)
- Are difficult to reproduce in safety studies in target animal species conducted in well hydrated laboratory dogs or cats fed a normal diet.

Acute renal toxicity of NSAIDs was first recognized in the 1990s when pre-emptive analgesia became common practice and AKI following anaesthesia and surgery was most commonly associated with the non-selective COX inhibitor flunixin. Factors that predisposed to this adverse effect of flunixin are likely to include:

- Withholding of food and therefore reduced fluid intake prior to surgery

- Hypotensive effects of anaesthesia during surgery
- Haemorrhage and blood loss resulting from the surgical procedure
- Further stress on fluid balance in the postoperative recovery period if water intake is delayed.

Toxicity related to acute use

The combination of hypotension due to anaesthesia and blood loss plus dehydration results in renal production of prostaglandins to counterbalance the decreased renal blood flow, as follows (summarized in Figure 20.8):

- Hypotension activates the RAAS through reduced stretch of the afferent arteriole and renal sympathetic nerves, triggering renin release as a general systemic response
- The macula densa would normally release vasodilatory prostanoids (PGE_2 and PGI_2) as the third mechanism stimulating renin release; these are important locally to dilate the afferent arteriole. The vasoconstrictor effect of angiotensin II here and elsewhere in the kidney is less well counterbalanced if prostanoid production is inhibited
- The GFR is less well maintained in the absence of afferent arteriolar dilatation by prostanoids, and nitrogenous waste products accumulate and may add to the reduced water intake in the recovery period. The reduced blood flow to the kidney causes azotaemia at this stage and would be reversible with adequate fluid therapy; if it persists, however, ischaemic damage may result
- In response to dehydration and hypotension, vasopressin is released by the posterior pituitary; this acts to upregulate the counter-current mechanism and urea recycling to increase medullary hypertonicity
- The blood flow to the medulla is normally sluggish and in the absence of PG production the medulla becomes even more hypoxic
- Cells in the interstitial area of the medulla are not protected against the hypertonicity which increases with sluggish blood flow and stimulation of the counter-current multiplier system.

The end result of this sequence of events is ischaemic and hypertonic damage to the kidney, leading to papillary necrosis in particular and tubular damage in general (see Figure 20.9). This occurs at therapeutic dose rates, which are effective in blocking renal PG production at a time when it is needed. In normotensive, well hydrated dogs, such kidney lesions are not observed in toxicity trials even at multiples of the recommended therapeutic dose rates because the kidneys are not stressed. However, in toxicity trials, at dose rates where gastric ulceration occurs, blood loss and reduced food and fluid intake can stress the kidneys, similar to the scenario described above, and papillary necrosis and tubular damage can occur at multiples of the therapeutic dose rate.

AKI can occur with NSAID use in clinical patients in the absence of anaesthesia, if other reasons for dehydration and hypovolaemia occur. In addition, clinically evident AKI may be the tip of the iceberg. Clinical studies have shown that GFR is reduced when measured 24 hours after anaesthesia and surgery (routine castration). Both carprofen (COX-2 selective in the dog) and ketoprofen (non-selective) used at clinical dose rates led to a 26–34% lower GFR 24–48 hours after surgery in healthy male dogs undergoing routine castration when compared with the placebo-treated group (Forsyth et al., 2000). These dogs were not reported to show signs of adverse effects at the time, but

the reversibility of this effect was not determined. Thus NSAID-induced AKI in the dog can arise with COX-2 selective inhibitors and non-selective COX inhibitors for the very reason that COX-2 is a constitutively expressed enzyme in the canine kidney.

The situation in the cat in terms of NSAIDs and AKI is less well characterized than in the dog, primarily because the cat is not used as a laboratory animal species in human drug development and toxicity testing. The veterinary profession has also tended to be more cautious in using NSAIDs in cats because of their perceived sensitivity to these drugs (e.g. aspirin). From our rudimentary understanding of the role of COX enzymes in renal physiology, cats may be less sensitive to selective COX-2 inhibition and it is possible that both COX-1 and COX-2 have to be inhibited before many of the stress protective mechanisms in the feline kidney are blocked. There may be more redundancy built in to the feline kidney compared with the canine kidney.

Toxicity related to chronic use

Having discussed the acute effects of NSAIDs on the kidney and the way in which AKI develops, a more difficult issue to understand is whether low-grade, long-term damage occurs with chronic use of NSAIDs. Chronic kidney damage occurs in humans secondary to lifetime abuse of NSAIDs; NSAID use is most common in elderly humans (and dogs and cats), where the prevalence of CKD is also at its highest. However, human epidemiological data from Scotland show reduced prescribing of NSAIDs when estimated GFR (eGFR) reporting was implemented, which resulted in significant improvements in renal function in those patients that stopped taking NSAIDs (Wei et al., 2013). eGFR reporting was introduced because of the insensitivity of plasma creatinine in determining renal function in elderly patients with low muscle mass, in particular. These data suggest that chronic NSAID use reduces GFR and that this effect is reversible when the drugs are stopped. Other human epidemiological data, however, showed that a decline in eGFR of ≥15 ml/min/1.73 m^2 was linearly associated with the cumulative dose of NSAID, regardless of whether the drug was COX-2 selective or non-selective (Gooch et al., 2007).

Such large-scale epidemiological studies are lacking in veterinary medicine. There is a trend in veterinary medicine to use NSAIDs continuously over several months to achieve better control of pain than with intermittent treatment. The authorization of the long-acting COX-2 selective drug mavacoxib facilitates continuous COX inhibition owing to its long half-life and once-monthly dosing. Relatively large clinical trials in older dogs with osteoarthritis have not revealed significant renal related adverse events (Lees et al., 2015). The number of dogs involved in registration and post-registration pharmacovigilance studies is an order of magnitude larger than most veterinary clinical trials; more than 800 dogs were treated continuously for 6 months and the renal related adverse events reported were very low (Six et al., 2012; Payne-Johnson et al., 2015). It has to be acknowledged that these studies compared mavacoxib with carprofen rather than with a placebo, because a placebo-controlled study in old dogs with osteoarthritis is likely to be considered unethical. Furthermore, the onset of clinical signs of kidney disease does not occur until significant renal pathological damage has occurred and therefore pharmacovigilance studies may not have detected NSAID-induced renal damage.

Contrary to the above discussion, it has been suggested that in some forms of kidney disease upregulation of COX enzymes may drive intrinsic progression via their involvement in altering renal haemodynamics and creating the conditions for hyperfiltration to occur. There is some evidence that COX-2 may be involved in this process in experimental renal reduction models in the rat, particularly when used in combination with inhibitors of angiotensin II (Gonçalves et al., 2004). This may be due in part to upregulation of COX-2 expression in the macula densa contributing to hyperfiltration in rat remnant kidney studies. In the same experimental renal reduction models, COX-2 is also upregulated in the glomeruli, arterioles and the cortical interstitium, mostly at inflamed or sclerosing areas, and celecoxib inhibited the inflammation and renal injury occurring in this model (Fujihara et al., 2003).

Summary

In conclusion, NSAIDs (non-selective COX inhibitors and COX-2 selective inhibitors) are associated with AKI under certain circumstances. The risk factors for this are well defined. Evidence for chronic, cumulative damage to the kidney resulting from long-term treatment of dogs and cats with NSAIDs is currently lacking. Nevertheless, experience from human medicine suggests that NSAIDs should be used with caution in ageing patients with deteriorating kidney function, owing to the reliance on PGs generated by COX enzymes (both isoforms) in protecting the kidney in the face of dehydration and hypotension. Some species (e.g. the laboratory rat) are protected from progressive renal injury by the administration of a COX-2 selective inhibitor. Our lack of knowledge as to whether this is the case in cats and dogs represents an important gap that should be filled in the future.

Benefit/harm assessment of the use of NSAIDs in patients with kidney disease

This section describes the indications for NSAID therapy in dogs and cats. The dilemma of whether to use NSAIDs or not occurs mainly with cats, which are more prone to spontaneous CKD. This section will focus on two clinical situations where the interaction between NSAIDs and the kidney is particularity relevant and the risk:benefit ratio has to be evaluated on a case-by-case basis: when NSAIDs are administered to an animal with normal renal function but whose kidneys are exposed to risk factors (intraoperative period, drug interaction, long treatment duration); and when NSAIDs are administered to patients with some evidence of CKD.

Management of acute musculoskeletal and chronic pain of osteoarthritis or other causes

NSAIDs are the cornerstone of the pharmaceutical treatment of osteoarthritis (OA) in veterinary patients. The recognition that animals can develop OA-related pain and the approval of NSAIDs with species-specific dosage regimens have greatly improved the quality of life of companion animals. At the site of injury, NSAIDs inhibit the facilitatory effect of PGE_2 on other mediators, such as bradykinin and histamine, to produce peripheral hyperalgesia and oedema. In addition, NSAIDs have a central antihyperalgesic effect, where PGE_2 participates in neuroplasticity within the spinal cord.

In dogs, caprofen, ketoprofen, meloxicam and tolfenamic acid are older NSAIDs authorized for the treatment of inflammation and musculoskeletal pain (see Figure 20.2). Firocoxib, robenacoxib, mavacoxib and cimicoxib are the more recent COXIBs approved for management of pain and inflammation related to canine OA (see Figure 20.2). There is no limit on oral treatment duration for carprofen (2 mg/kg per day), meloxicam (0.1 mg/kg per day) or firocoxib and robenacoxib. Owing to its long half-life, mavacoxib treatment is initiated with two oral doses (2 mg/kg) administered at a 14-day interval, then administered once a month for a maximum of 6 months.

In cats, the only NSAIDs authorized for treatment of inflammation and musculoskeletal pain are ketoprofen (up to 5 days), robenacoxib (up to 6 days) and meloxicam (unlimited duration). Restricted indications exist for tolfenamic acid (febrile syndrome) and carprofen (perioperative pain) in the cat. There are three authorized doses for meloxicam. The single 0.3 mg/kg subcutaneous dose is associated with long-term COX-1 inhibition and should not be followed by a maintenance dose. The 0.2 mg/kg subcutaneous dose is used perioperatively and can be continued with oral treatment. Finally, oral treatment may be initiated with a loading dose of 0.1 mg/kg and maintained with a daily dose of 0.05 mg/kg.

Specific use in patients with kidney disease and proteinuric glomerulonephritis

The use of low-dose aspirin in dogs with proteinuric glomerulonephritis has been recommended for the prevention of thromboembolic complications in nephrotic syndrome (see Chapter 24). Aspirin should be considered for hypoalbuminaemic dogs (plasma albumin <10 g/l), as well as for dogs with low serum levels of antithrombin III (<30% of normal). In dogs with marked proteinuria and serum albumin <20 g/l, low-dose aspirin therapy (2.5–5 mg/kg/q24h orally) is appropriate alongside other therapies, unless melaena is present or gastric ulceration is suspected (Brown, 2013). In human patients, aspirin has an antiproteniuric effect mediated by local blockade of TxA_2-induced vasoconstriction, whereas the renoprotective effects of non-selective NSAIDs (mentioned above) are mediated by vasomodulatory effects of PGE_2 inhibition (Vogt et al., 2010).

Perioperative use for prevention of soft tissue and orthopaedic surgical pain

The concept of pre-emptive analgesia supposes that preincisional administration reduces pain or the analgesic dose required to a greater extent than does post-incisional administration. This approach, in theory, should provide better patient comfort and earlier hospital discharge. In the dog, carprofen, meloxicam, tolfenamic acid and robenacoxib can be injected at the time of surgical preparation. Firocoxib and cimicoxib are also authorized for use preoperatively but are only available as oral forms. In the cat, only carprofen, meloxicam and robenacoxib are approved for intraoperative pain.

During drug development, rigorous target animal safety studies evaluated NSAIDs safety at supra-therapeutic levels in healthy conscious laboratory dogs and cats. Little is known about the margin of safety of their use under general anaesthesia in real patients susceptible to hypotension or the adverse effects of drug interactions. Acute alteration of renal function is only rarely documented in elective surgical procedures when NSAIDs have been administered preoperatively, but this may be the tip of the iceberg. By suppressing the PG link between decreased tubular flow rate and renin release, non-selective and COX-2 selective inhibitors may cause transient loss of autoregulation. Postoperative renal dysfunction in a surgical patient may result from hypoxic damage to medullary nephrons secondary to hypotension or hypovolaemia, which may be exacerbated by the use of NSAIDs. A higher incidence of lower grade acute renal dysfunction or injuries (see Chapters 13 and 21, RIFLE classification) may occur subclinically but could be diagnosed by sensitive tests (transient GFR changes and urinary AKI biomarkers such as neutrophil gelatinase-associated lipocalin (NGAL)). Renal function recovers after the initial insult (normalization of GFR and plasma creatinine) but the loss of a significant number of nephrons may predispose the animal to renal disease later in life.

It should be emphasized at this point that the association of anaesthesia and surgery does not constitute a contraindication for preoperative NSAID administration in routine procedures. The risk of developing renal injury is greatly reduced by keeping renal perfusion above the lower limit of autoregulation (mean arterial pressure (MAP) >65–70 mmHg). This is achieved by attentive monitoring of blood pressure and tissue perfusion, good surgical principles and provision of supportive care (optimization of circulating volume, use of balanced anaesthesia and inotropes). In patients with sepsis, dehydration or expected significant blood loss, NSAIDs should be withheld until recovery from anaesthesia. Use of iodinated contrast media or hydroxyethyl starches does not seem to be a risk factor for AKI in veterinary medicine.

The concept of pre-emptive analgesia was derived from unequivocal evidence in experimental rodents. However, the benefit of pre-emptive administration of NSAIDs in clinical patients is less clear than with other analgesic classes. The demonstration of the benefit of preoperative administration certainly requires well thought out experimental designs and choice of the right timing of administration. The only published study supporting the concept of pre-emptive analgesia conferred by NSAIDs in companion animals is from Lascelles et al. (1998). In bitches undergoing ovariohysterectomy, nociception scores on recovery were lower with preoperative carprofen compared to postoperative administration. In the same study, however, the area under the plasma concentration–time curve of carprofen was significantly smaller when carprofen was administered preoperatively in comparison to postoperatively. Alteration of liver perfusion and volume of distribution during anaesthesia and surgery may therefore alter NSAID pharmacokinetics.

The dilemma of animals with CKD and degenerative joint disease

The common co-occurrence of CKD and degenerative joint disease in the cat (Marino et al., 2014) means that the question regarding the safety of chronic NSAID administration to cats with CKD is important yet difficult to answer. The question is also of clinical importance in the dog, even though CKD is less common in the ageing dog.

Lomas et al. (2013) monitored the medium- (28 days) to long-term (6 months) effect of the dual inhibitor tepoxalin on the renal function of 16 client-owned dogs with stable CKD (IRIS CKD Stages 2 and 3) confirmed by two successive GFR measurements. Renal function was maintained in all dogs except in one that progressed from Stage 2 to Stage 3 before stopping tepoxalin. This dog had been receiving enalapril and amlodipine concomitantly with tepoxalin. It has been suggested, based on uncontrolled longitudinal retrospective studies, that meloxicam (at a median maintenance dose of 0.02 mg/kg) treatment of cats with CKD (IRIS Stages 1–3) may slow progression (Gowan et al., 2011) and improve long-term survival (Gowan et al., 2012). The median survival duration of cats with CKD treated with meloxicam for more than 6 months was 1608 days, which compares favourably with other published survival data for cats with CKD. There are many biases in the selection of cases for these studies that could explain these observations without there being a direct causative effect of meloxicam on longevity or progression of CKD. Direct evidence to support the hypothesis based on this observation is inconclusive.

Surdyk et al. (2013) treated cats with experimentally reduced renal mass leading to hyperfiltration with meloxicam or acetylsalicylic acid for 7 days and found no effect on GFR or urine protein to creatinine ratio, suggesting that COX-derived products were not major factors involved in driving the hyperfiltration occurring in this model. Preliminary data from the authors' own group have identified upregulation of COX enzymes in renal tissue from cats with CKD in all areas of the kidney examined (Suemanothan et al., 2009), but no association between proteinuria or progressive kidney disease and the level of COX-enzyme expression was found, suggesting that COX enzyme upregulation does not appear to be linked to progressive kidney disease in the cat. As mentioned above, selective COX-2 inhibition can reduce proteinuria without reduction of blood pressure in rat models (renal reduction, diabetic nephropathy and polycystic kidney disease). In human patients, NSAIDs were used for renoprotection in proteinuric CKD before the introduction of drugs blocking the RAAS. Treatment with NSAIDs induced preglomerular vasoconstriction that limited intraglomerular pressures and protein leakage but also caused proportional reductions in GFR, especially during sodium restriction. Recent reappraisal of the renal risk:benefit ratio and small proof of concept studies suggested an overall benefit of NSAID inclusion when a combination of two drugs acting on the RAAS fails to reduce proteinuria (Vogt et al. 2010).

Current guidelines on long-term NSAID use

When it comes to tailoring NSAID therapy in companion animals, a full benefit/harm assessment has to be carried out for the individual patient (Sparkes et al., 2010). All important factors to be considered in the risk assessment of NSAID use are summarized in Figure 20.10.

Individual patient factors

A thorough clinical examination and full history should be taken for each new patient. Each animal will be different, based on age, genetics, illnesses and other drugs administered. There should be particular focus on hydration status, signs of renal or liver functional compromise or the presence of cardiac disease compromising cardiac output. Hydration should be improved by feeding wet food.

Evaluate NSAIDs benefit/harm ratio taking into account the following considerations. If in doubt, consider pharmaceutical or non-pharmaceutical alternatives.

Patient factors:
- Animal health status and hydration
- Renal, hepatic or cardiac functional compromise
- Genetic predisposition

Prudent therapy:
- Document baseline (blood pressure, renal and liver panel, serum protein)
- Identify lowest efficacious dose
- Go low, go slow (use lean weight, no loading dose)
- Pulse dosing

Favourable formulation:
- Clear instructions
- Precise dosing
- Palatable formulation
- Ease of administration

Drug interactions:
- ACEi
- Furosemide
- Anti-hypertensive (calcium channel and beta-blockers ?)
- NSAIDs washout time

Clinical monitoring:
- Efficacy for clinical improvement (QoL, orthopaedic disability)
- Known signs of toxicity
- Validation of new biomarkers for monitoring renal toxicity (GFR measurement, enzymuria)

Pharmacological knowledge of NSAIDs:
- Pharmacokinetic/pharmacodynamic
- Tissue distribution
- Sources of variability in clinical population

Owner participation:
- Motivation/dedication
- Good compliance
- Education (signs of toxicity)
- Monitoring clinical efficacy daily in home environment

20.10 Factors to be considered in the risk assessment for long-term non-steroidal anti-inflammatory drug (NSAID) use. ACEi = angiotensin-converting enzyme inhibitor; BP = blood pressure; GFR = glomerular filtration rate; PD = pharmacodynamics; PK = pharmacokinetics; QoL = quality of life.

Recognize and rationalize drug interactions

Clinically relevant drug interactions are summarized in Figure 20.6. Caution is warranted with ACEi or ARBs owing to their vasodilatory effects on the efferent renal arteriole. Only one study reports the absence of deleterious effect of co-administration of tepoxalin and enalapril for 28 days on GFR in laboratory dogs (Fusellier *et al.*, 2005), but little is known about the tolerability of the combination of NSAIDs and ACEi in clinical patients. The addition of non-selective or COX-2 selective NSAIDs to furosemide administration for 8 days caused a significant but reversible decrease in GFR in volume-depleted experimental dogs (Surdyk *et al.*, 2012). There are no published data on the combined administration of calcium channel inhibitors and beta-blockers with NSAIDs in companion animals. It should be recognized, however, that patients with later stage CKD (IRIS CKD Stages 3 and 4) can easily become unstable, and maintenance of GFR may be dependent on RAAS activation. NSAIDs inhibit tubuloglomerular feedback, and beta-blockers inhibit sympathetic nervous system stimulation of renin secretion. Both of these therapeutic regimens will be additive or synergistic with drugs directly inhibiting the RAAS (ACEi and ARBs), which means that these patients will be more susceptible to suffering an azotaemic crisis in response to dehydration or hypotension (see Figure 20.8). Experts advise waiting at least five drug half-lives before switching from one NSAID to another.

Prudent therapy

As a basis for prudent therapy, the authors advise documentation of baseline laboratory results (urine specific gravity, urine protein to creatinine ratio, renal and liver parameters, serum protein). The lowest clinically efficacious dose should be identified by trial and error, while keeping in mind that dose may be adjusted back up during a flare in pain. When in doubt, the adage 'go low, go slow' is a good general rule; indeed, starting with a lower dose initially is acceptable. Good pharmacological knowledge of the PK and PD of NSAIDs can help inform clinical decisions.

Efficacy and safety monitoring

Frequent monitoring is paramount to ensure clinical efficacy and early detection of signs of toxicity. Owner assessment focused on daily activity, mobility, social interaction and grooming (for cats) helps to provide accurate assessment of the clinical improvement of the animal in its natural environment. Initial reassessment should be performed 1 week after the start of treatment and follow-up visits should occur after 1 month and every 2–6 months, depending on perceived risk.

In the future, evaluation of GFR (see Chapters 10 and 12) and enzymuria (see Chapter 21) may be part of a sensitive panel to detect adverse effects of NSAIDs on renal function.

Owner participation

Once educated, owners will be able to evaluate clinical improvement and identify signs of renal toxicity as soon as they occur, contact the practice for advice and withhold the medication. Administering NSAIDs with food will help to improve treatment compliance and stop dosing if inappetence or vomiting (which can be early indicators of GI complication) occurs. Occasional NSAID withdrawal allows confirmation that the dose identified is efficacious and the pain/disability assessment tool is sensitive enough. Some animals may only need pulse dosing to manage the intermittent signs of the underlying disease.

Favourable formulation

Innovative formulations such as a palatable liquid suspension or oromucosal sprays can increase treatment compliance in animals with poor appetite. However, care should be taken not to treat an anorexic animal. Instructions to the owner regarding dosing should be clear. Liquid formulations allow greater precision in dose reduction.

Alternatives to NSAIDs

Alternatives to NSAIDs should be considered if the risk:benefit ratio is judged to be too adverse. Pharmaceutical and non-pharmaceutical options presented below can be used, based on available evidence or clinical judgement (KuKanich, 2013).

Pharmaceutical options:
- Other analgesics (tramadol, gabapentin, amantadine).
- Nutraceuticals (glucosamine and chondroitin).
- Prescription diets containing omega-3 fatty acids or green-lipped mussels.

Non-pharmaceutical options:
- Invasive management: surgical intervention, intra-articular treatment.

- Holistic approach: maintenance of muscle strength and joint mobility with physiotherapy, hydrotherapy, acupuncture.
- Other options: weight reduction, mild to moderate routine exercise, adjustment of the environment to cope with the disability.

Conclusions

Judicious use of NSAIDs in dogs and cats with chronic pain and inflammation and concomitant CKD may be considered. If the therapeutic response to the NSAID is good, the improvement in the quality of life of the animal may outweigh the potential harm these drugs might cause to the kidney. If the CKD is stable and the patient continues to eat well, maintains good hydration status and is free from GI side effects, continuous therapy may be possible, although the dose should be titrated to the lowest possible. Care should be taken to ensure owners are aware that dogs and cats on NSAIDs are susceptible to sudden deterioration in renal function should they go off their food or develop GI side effects and urgent attention should be sought should this happen. Care should be taken to be aware of all drugs the patient is receiving, and the clinician should be aware that certain combinations heighten the risk of a uraemic crisis.

References and further reading

Brideau C, Van Staden C and Chan CC (2001) *In vitro* effects of cyclooxygenase inhibitors in whole blood of horses, dogs and cats. *American Journal of Veterinary Research* 62, 1755–1760

Brown SA (2013) Glomerular disease in small animals. Available at: www.merckmanuals.com/vet/urinary_system/noninfectious_diseases_of_the_urinary_system_in_small_animals/glomerular_disease_in_small_animals.html

Court MH (2013) Feline drug metabolism and disposition: pharmacokinetic evidence for species differences and molecular mechanisms. *Veterinary Clinics of North America: Small Animal Practice* 43, 1039–1054

Forsyth SF, Guilford WG and Pfeiffer DU (2000) Effect of NSAID administration on creatinine clearance in healthy dogs undergoing anaesthesia and surgery. *Journal of Small Animal Practice* 41, 547–550

Fujihara CK, Antunes GR, Mattar AL *et al.* (2003) Cyclooxygenase-2 (COX-2) inhibition limits abnormal COX-2 expression and progressive injury in the remnant kidney. *Kidney International* 64, 2172–2181

Fusellier M, Desfontis JC, Madec S *et al.* (2005) Effect of tepoxalin on renal function in healthy dogs receiving an angiotensin-converting enzyme inhibitor. *Journal of Veterinary Pharmacology and Therapeutics* 28, 581–586

Giraudel JM, Toutain PL, King JN and Lees P (2009) Differential inhibition of cyclooxygenase isoenzymes in the cat by the NSAID robenacoxib. *Journal of Veterinary Pharmacology and Therapeutics* 32, 31–40

Giraudel JM, Toutain PL and Lees P (2005) Development of *in vitro* assays for the evaluation of cyclooxygenase inhibitors and predicting selectivity of nonsteroidal anti-inflammatory drugs in cats. *American Journal of Veterinary Research* 66, 700–709

Gonçalves AR, Fujihara CK, Mattar AL *et al.* (2004) Renal expression of COX-2, ANG II, and AT1 receptor in remnant kidney: strong renoprotection by therapy with losartan and a nonsteroidal anti-inflammatory. *American Journal of Physiology. Renal Physiology* 286, F945–F954

Gooch K, Culleton BF, Manns BJ *et al.* (2007) NSAID use and progression of chronic kidney disease. *American Journal of Medicine* 120, 280.e1–7

Gowan RA, Baral RM, Lingard AE *et al.* (2012) A retrospective analysis of the effects of meloxicam on the longevity of aged cats with and without overt chronic kidney disease. *Journal of Feline Medicine and Surgery* 14, 876–881

Gowan RA, Lingard AE, Johnston L *et al.* (2011) Retrospective case–control study of the effects of long-term dosing with meloxicam on renal function in aged cats with degenerative joint disease. *Journal of Feline Medicine and Surgery* 13, 752–761

Khan KN, Venturini CM, Bunch RT *et al.*, (1998) Interspecies differences in renal localization of cyclooxygenase isoforms: implications in nonsteroidal antiinflammatory drug-related nephrotoxicity. *Toxicologic Pathology* 26(5), 612–20

King JN, Rudaz C, Borer L *et al.* (2009) *In vitro* and *ex vivo* inhibition of canine cyclooxygenase isoforms by robenacoxib: A comparative study. *Research in Veterinary Science* 88, 497–506

KuKanich B (2013) Outpatient oral analgesics in dogs and cats beyond nonsteroidal antiinflammatory drugs: an evidence-based approach. *Veterinary Clinics of North America: Small Animal Practice* 43, 1109–1125

Lascelles BD, Cripps PJ, Jones A *et al.* (1998) Efficacy and kinetics of carprofen, administered preoperatively or postoperatively, for the prevention of pain in dogs undergoing ovariohysterectomy. *Veterinary Surgery* 27, 568–582

Lees P (2009) Analgesic, antiinflammatory, antipyretic drugs. In: *Veterinary Pharmacology and Therapeutics, 9th edn,* ed. JE Riviere and MG Papich, pp.461–486. Wiley Blackwell Publishers, Ames

Lees P, Giraudel J, Landoni MF and Toutain PL (2004) PK–PD integration and PK–PD modelling of nonsteroidal anti-inflammatory drugs: principles and applications in veterinary pharmacology. *Journal of Veterinary Pharmacology and Therapeutics* 27, 491–502

Lees P, Pelligand L, Elliott J *et al.* (2015) Pharmacokinetics, pharmacodynamics, toxicology and therapeutics of mavacoxib in the dog: a review. *Journal of Veterinary Pharmacology and Therapeutics* 38, 1–14

Lomas AL, Lyon SD, Sanderson MW *et al.* (2013) Acute and chronic effects of tepoxalin on kidney function in dogs with chronic kidney disease and osteoarthritis. *American Journal of Veterinary Research* 74, 939–944

Marino CL, Lascelles BD, Vaden SL *et al.* (2014) Prevalence and classification of chronic kidney disease in cats randomly selected from four age groups and in cats recruited for degenerative joint disease studies. *Journal of Feline Medicine and Surgery* 16, 465–472

Payne-Johnson M, Becskei C, Chaudhry Y *et al.* (2015) Comparative efficacy and safety of mavacoxib and carprofen in the treatment of canine osteoarthritis. *Veterinary Record* 176, 284

Pelligand L, King JN, Hormazabal V *et al.* (2014) Differential pharmacokinetics and pharmacokinetic/pharmacodynamic modelling of robenacoxib and ketoprofen in a feline model of inflammation. *Journal of Veterinary Pharmacology and Therapeutics* 37, 354–366

Pelligand L, Suemanothan N, King JN *et al.* (2015) Effect of cyclooxygenase (COX)-1 and COX-2 inhibition on furosemide-induced renal responses and immunolocalization in the healthy cat kidney. *BMC Veterinary Research* 11, 296

Radi ZA (2009) Pathophysiology of cyclooxygenase inhibition in animal models. *Toxicologic Pathology* 37, 34–46

Schmid VB, Seewald W, Lees P and King JN (2010) *In vitro* and *ex vivo* inhibition of COX isoforms by robenacoxib in the cat: a comparative study. *Journal of Veterinary Pharmacology and Therapeutics* 33, 444–452

Six H, Mitchell J, Anton C *et al.* (2012) Efficacy and safety of mavacoxib in comparison with carprofen in the treatment of pain and inflammation associated with degenerative joint disease in dogs presented as veterinary patients. *Journal of Veterinary Pharmacology and Therapeutics* 35, 56

Sparkes AH, Heiene R, Lascelles BD *et al.* (2010) ISFM and AAFP consensus guidelines: long-term use of NSAIDs in cats. *Journal of Feline Medicine and Surgery* 12, 521–538

Suemanothan N, Borhane Y, Syme H *et al.* (2009) Urinary prostanoids in feline chronic kidney disease. *Proceedings of the 19th ECVIM-CA Congress, Porto,* pp.213–214

Surdyk KK, Brown CA and Brown SA (2013) Evaluation of glomerular filtration rate in cats with reduced renal mass and administered meloxicam and acetylsalicylic acid. *American Journal of Veterinary Research* 74, 648–651

Surdyk KK, Sloan DL and Brown SA (2012) Renal effects of carprofen and etodolac in euvolemic and volume-depleted dogs. *American Journal of Veterinary Research* 73, 1485–1490

Toutain PL and Bousquet-Melou A (2002) Free drug fraction *versus* free drug concentration: a matter of frequent confusion. *Journal of Veterinary Pharmacology and Therapeutics* 25, 460–463

Vogt L, Laverman GD and Navis G (2010) Time for a comeback of NSAIDs in proteinuric chronic kidney disease? *Netherlands Journal of Medicine* 68, 400–407

Warner TD, Giuliano F, Vojnovic I *et al.* (1999) Nonsteroid drug selectivities for cyclo-oxygenase-1 rather than cyclo-oxygenase-2 are associated with human gastrointestinal toxicity: a full *in vitro* analysis. *Proceedings of the National Academy of Sciences of the United States of America* 96, 7563–7568

Wei L, MacDonald TM, Jennings C *et al.* (2013) Estimated GFR reporting is associated with decreased nonsteroidal anti-inflammatory drug prescribing and increased renal function. *Kidney International* 84, 174–178

Wilson JE, Chandrasekharan NV, Westover KD, Eager KB and Simmons DL (2004) Determination of expression of cyclooxygenase-1 and -2 isozymes in canine tissues and their differential sensitivity to non-steroidal anti-inflammatory drugs. *American Journal of Veterinary Research* 65, 810–818

Chapter 21

Acute kidney injury

Sarah Crilly Guess and Gregory F. Grauer

Acute kidney injury (AKI) is most often caused by an ischaemic, toxic or infectious insult and may result in acute renal failure (ARF), which is usually defined as an acute onset of azotaemia superimposed on an inability to concentrate urine (see Chapter 12 for a discussion of AKI grading). Renal tubular epithelial cells are most commonly affected because of their high metabolic rates and dependence on oxygen and substrate delivery. AKI is often reversible but, in some cases, tubular damage may be severe enough to be irreversible.

Physiologically, the kidneys are responsible for regulation of body fluid homeostasis. The kidneys also regulate acid–base and electrolyte balance in the body, produce and metabolize hormones, and excrete metabolic waste products and foreign substances (xenobiotics). When AKI occurs, these functions are compromised to varying degrees, resulting in clinical signs and biochemical changes.

Pathophysiology

The kidneys are uniquely susceptible to acute injury, because they receive approximately 20% of cardiac output, the highest of any organ in the body in relation to organ weight (Epstein, 1995). The cortical and outer medullary structures receive the majority of renal blood flow, and therefore these regions have greater risk of toxic or ischaemic insults (Vetterlein et al., 1986). Within the renal cortex, the epithelial cells of the proximal tubule and thick ascending limb of the loop of Henle are most frequently affected by ischaemia and toxicant-induced injury because of their transport functions and high metabolic rates.

The pathophysiology of AKI is considered to have four main phases (Figure 21.1). The **initiation** phase (phase 1) starts with the insult itself and usually occurs over the first minutes to hours of AKI. The **extension** phase (phase 2), which is the continuation of the initial injury by ongoing hypoxia, lasts hours to days. This second phase blends into the maintenance phase, when cellular repair may start but damage often continues. The **maintenance** phase (phase 3) usually starts around day 3 and lasts days to weeks. The **recovery** phase (phase 4) occurs over weeks to months, when repair continues and normal function begins to return. While much overlap exists among these four phases of AKI, a basic understanding of each phase helps facilitate early diagnosis as well as management of the injury.

The initiation phase (phase 1) of AKI begins with the insult itself, which may be ischaemic, infectious or nephrotoxic. In ischaemic AKI, renal blood flow is compromised, leading to severe depletion of adenosine triphosphate (ATP) and causing cell damage and dysfunction. The insult could also be directly nephrotoxic, interfering with normal cell processes, such as cellular metabolism and energy production, and causing tubular and glomerular cell death. Identification and initiation of therapy in this phase can attenuate the severity of damage and improve clinical outcome. The type of insult (toxic, ischaemic, infectious) determines the length of time to the onset of clinical signs (if any) and the severity of clinical disease if and when it occurs (Stromski et al., 1986). Although evaluation of new biomarkers to increase the sensitivity and specificity of diagnosis in the initiation phase is ongoing, this first phase of AKI often goes undetected and the opportunity for early intervention is missed, unless patients who are at risk are recognized and screened.

The second phase, the extension phase, is often associated with most cellular damage and the efficacy of therapeutic intervention becomes debatable. This phase is marked by continued hypoxia and a developing inflammatory response (Sutton et al., 2002; Figure 21.2). Cellular injury during the extension phase stems from lack of production of ATP, which causes diminished activity of the Na^+-K^+-ATPase pump, leading to cytosolic accumulation of sodium and cell swelling. Furthermore, the intracellular calcium concentration increases because of impaired calcium transporters, leading to activation of proteases and phospholipases, which disrupt the cytoskeleton and impair mitochondrial energy metabolism. These processes either directly cause or lead to initiation of pathways resulting in cellular swelling, apoptosis and necrosis (Padanilam, 2003). Inflammation is propagated by the release of inflammatory mediators, chemokines and cytokines from the damaged cells, which recruit leucocytes to the affected area (Ysebaert et al., 2000). These leucocytes enhance injury as they cause mechanical obstruction to small vessels, release more cytokines, vasoactive eicosanoids and reactive oxygen species (ROS) and exacerbate the inflammatory response (Segerer et al., 2000; Bonventre, 2003). Associated with tubular cell damage, the basement membrane may become exposed by the desquamation of viable and non-viable cells. Finally, endothelial cell damage in peritubular vessels probably plays a role in the ongoing renal ischaemia.

The maintenance phase (phase 3) is characterized by both ongoing cellular damage and, in many cases,

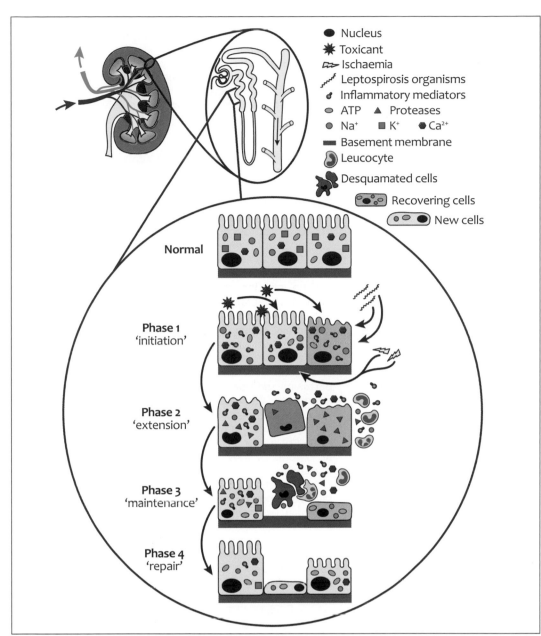

21.1 In this schematic representation of the four phases of acute kidney injury (AKI), normal proximal tubular epithelial cells are represented in the first row. In phase 1, the infectious/ischaemic/toxic insult causes increased presence of inflammatory mediators, and decreased intracellular adenosine triphosphate (ATP), leading to phase 2, when increased intracellular sodium (Na⁺) and calcium (Ca²⁺) concentrations and further destruction of the brush border occur. The basement membrane may also become exposed as cells are desquamated. Leucocytes migrate to the site of damage in phase 2. Phase 3 shows ongoing damage (apoptosis) and early repair. Phase 4 is when epithelial cells are further repaired and proliferate to cover the exposed basement membrane. This figure demonstrates the continuum of AKI that occurs over these four phases. K⁺ = potassium.
(Courtesy of Mal Rooks Hoover, CMI, Kansas State University)

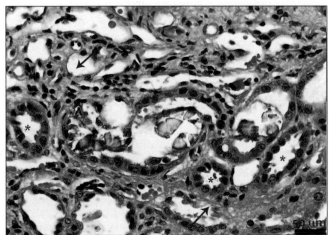

21.2 Photomicrograph of the renal cortex of a cat with ethylene glycol toxicosis. The proximal renal tubules frequently contain semi-transparent, refractile calcium oxalate crystals associated with renal tubular epithelial attenuation and loss (arrowed) with regeneration (*) and infiltrates of lymphocytes and plasma cells in the interstitial spaces.
(Courtesy of Chanran K. Ganta BVSc PhD DACVP, Kansas State University Veterinary Diagnostic Laboratory)

simultaneous cellular repair. Damage to the kidney peaks in this phase and it may or may not be reversible. During this phase, cells may undergo repair, migration, apoptosis and proliferation, with cellular integrity and function being re-established (Sutton *et al.*, 2002). Large areas of focal necrosis may no longer be present, but some cell injury may continue. Most studies suggest that the glomerular filtration rate (GFR), which declines during the extension phase, is maintained at its nadir during the maintenance phase and later improves during recovery (Devarajan, 2006). The extent of damage sustained by the time the maintenance phase begins is dependent on both the initial insult and the timeliness of early intervention.

Finally, recovery predominates in the fourth and final phase of AKI. This phase is characterized by ongoing cellular repair and reorganization, which results in progressively improving cellular function and, eventually, overall kidney function. The exposure of the basement membrane that occurred during the extension phase as a result of cellular desquamation may be repaired. The process relies on epithelial cell spread and proliferation to cover exposed areas (Pawar *et al.*, 1995). In some cases, the damage and inflammation is so severe that fibrosis and scarring occur, causing total and permanent loss of function of the nephrons in that area (Furuichi et al., 2009) and leading to chronic kidney disease (CKD). Compensation by the remaining nephrons, leading to nephron hypertrophy, can also contribute to improved kidney function in the recovery phase.

These four phases should not be thought of as mutually exclusive steps in the injury process, but rather as an overlapping continuum of complex biological events and interactions, the mechanisms of which have yet to be fully elucidated. Furthermore, AKI is not necessarily a single process in itself, but rather a spectrum of damage and clinical illness. Intervention should be tailored to the individual patient, keeping in mind the phases of injury to the kidney, treatment of the underlying disease and prevention of further damage. Early recognition and intervention, including correction of the underlying cause, may improve the prognosis.

Aetiology

For simplification, acute azotaemia is classically divided into pre-renal, renal and post-renal categories. These should be thought of as aids for diagnosis and treatment, knowing that there is the potential for overlap of the categories.

Pre-renal azotaemia involves decreased renal perfusion and renal haemodynamic compromise. A functional decline in glomerular filtration results from deficient renal blood flow or perfusion pressure, or excessive renal vasoconstriction. This form of azotaemia is usually associated with a hypersthenuric urine (urine specific gravity (USG) >1.030 for dogs and >1.035 for cats). Pre-renal azotaemia may, in some cases, be superimposed on an inability to concentrate urine (e.g. with diuretic therapy, hypercalcaemia, pyometra, hypoadrenocorticism (Addison's disease), diabetic ketoacidosis). The cornerstone of the treatment of pre-renal azotemia is correction of hypovolaemia or hypotension as well as the underlying disease. Pre-renal azotaemia is rapidly reversed with appropriate therapy, but could lead to cellular damage/ARF in severe or prolonged cases and therefore is still classified as AKI by the International Renal Interest Society (IRIS) AKI grading system (see Chapter 12).

Renal azotaemia implies intrinsic renal damage/ disease associated with a direct insult to the kidney, such as acute tubular necrosis, interstitial nephritis, embolic disease, glomerulonephritis or vasculitis. Renal azotaemia is superimposed on the inability to concentrate urine (i.e. urine is minimally concentrated or isosthenuric). Causes include nephrotoxic agents, infectious or immune-mediated diseases and ischaemic events. Pre-renal azotaemia may contribute to the severity of renal damage and there is usually some degree of overlap between pre-renal and renal azotaemia. Fluid therapy for renal azotaemia is similar to that for pre-renal azotaemia and is designed to improve renal perfusion and increase urine production. In addition, specific treatment may be indicated in cases where the cause of AKI is known (e.g. alcohol dehydrogenase inhibitors for ethylene glycol toxicity or antibiotics for leptospirosis). Renal azotaemia carries the least favourable prognosis compared with pre- and post-renal azotaemia.

Post-renal azotaemia is most often caused by obstruction or rupture of the excretory pathway. The USG is typically not helpful in making the diagnosis, because it varies with hydration status. Long-term obstruction can lead to intrinsic renal azotaemia and permanent renal damage (more common with more proximal obstructions), hence post-renal azotaemia is also included in the IRIS AKI grading system (see Chapter 12). Treatment involves relieving the obstruction and/or repairing the leakage, treating any dehydration, electrolyte abnormalities or hypotension, and addressing the underlying cause of the urinary obstruction/leakage.

Risk factors

Specific risk factors for AKI include dehydration, preexisting kidney disease, advanced age, electrolyte imbalances, nephrotoxic drug administration, decreased cardiac output, anaesthesia and multiple organ dysfunction. Of these risk factors, dehydration is one of the most common and most important. Studies in humans indicate that volume depletion increases the risk of development of AKI by a factor of 10 (Brezis et al., 1991). Hypovolaemia not only decreases renal perfusion, which can enhance ischaemic damage, but also decreases the volume of distribution of nephrotoxic drugs, resulting in decreased tubular flow rates and enhanced tubular reabsorption of toxicants. In addition to hypovolaemia, renal hypoperfusion may be caused by decreased cardiac output, decreased plasma oncotic pressure, increased blood viscosity, systemic hypotension, decreased vasodilatory renal prostaglandin synthesis (e.g. secondary to administration of a non-steroidal anti-inflammatory drug (NSAID) or chronic kidney disease) or renal arterial thrombus formation.

Pre-existing CKD can increase the risk of AKI. Careful attention should be given to avoiding or minimizing other potential risk factors in patients with known CKD. In a study of nearly 20,000 humans, those with AKI were significantly older and had lower baseline creatinine clearances than non-AKI patients admitted to a hospital within the same time period (Chertow et al., 2005). These findings emphasize pre-existing renal disease and advancing age as risk factors for development of AKI. Mechanistically, advancing age and pre-existing renal disease can increase the risk of AKI by altering the pharmacokinetics of potentially nephrotoxic drugs, decreasing the ability to compensate for pre-renal influences and compromising local production of prostaglandins that help maintain renal blood flow.

Multiple organ dysfunction syndrome (MODS) is defined as 'the presence of altered organ function in an acutely ill patient such that homeostasis cannot be maintained without intervention' (ACCP/SCCM Consensus Conference, 1992). This syndrome has been recently recognized in veterinary medicine, and should be considered in critically ill patients that suddenly develop azotaemia. MODS, by definition, affects multiple target organs, usually as a result of severe trauma, sepsis, neoplasia or systemic inflammation. Specifically in the case of AKI, MODS can lead to renal tubular cell apoptosis caused by production of inflammatory cytokines and endotoxins, even in cases without renal hypoperfusion (Osterbur et al., 2014). The development of AKI in humans with MODS markedly increases mortality (Wang et al., 2012).

Another potential risk factor for AKI is the dietary protein level. The quantity of protein fed to dogs prior to a nephrotoxic insult can affect the subsequent renal damage and dysfunction. Feeding high dietary protein prior to and during gentamicin administration in dogs with initially normal renal function reduces nephrotoxicity, enhances gentamicin clearance and results in a larger volume of distribution compared with feeding medium or low protein (Grauer *et al.*, 1994). The beneficial effects of high dietary protein are probably associated with increased glomerular filtration and, therefore, improved toxicant excretion. High dietary protein also results in increased urinary excretion of protein, which may compete for nephrotoxicant reabsorption by tubular epithelial cells. Although dietary protein conditioning prior to use of a potentially nephrotoxic drug is unlikely to be a viable clinical option, reduced protein intake (i.e. in anorexic or vomiting dogs or cats) should be recognized as potentially increasing the risk of developing nephrotoxic AKI.

Early detection of AKI

Urinary and serum biomarkers

Detection of enzymes in the urine, such as gamma-glutamyl transferase (GGT) and *N*-acetyl-beta-D-glucosaminidase (NAG), has been proven to be a sensitive indicator of early renal tubular damage (Greco *et al.*, 1985). The acute onset of low-level proteinuria/albuminuria and/or normoglycaemic glucosuria may be observed in dogs and cats early in the course of AKI as a consequence of tubular cell damage and decreased resorptive function. Newer serum and urine biomarkers, such as neutrophil gelatinase associated lipocalin (NGAL), urine or plasma symmetric dimethylarginine (SDMA), urine clusterin and urinary kidney injury molecule (KIM-1), may improve the sensitivity and specificity for early detection of AKI (De Loor *et al.*, 2013). Urine clusterin is very useful for detecting early changes in acute kidney injury and is more sensitive and specific for AKI than blood urea nitrogen (BUN) and serum creatinine. Furthermore, urinary and serum biomarkers for detection of AKI can be anatomically specific (i.e. they can differentiate between glomerular and tubular injury) (Dieterle *et al.*, 2010). While novel urine and serum biomarkers have important potential diagnostic utility, additional research in veterinary patients is necessary before routine clinical use of these biomarkers can be recommended.

Evaluation of patients with suspected AKI

Signalment

A patient's signalment can provide clues to a possible cause for acute azotaemia. For example, geriatric patients should be considered at increased risk for pre-existing CKD, while younger animals may be at increased risk for nephrotoxicant ingestion.

History

Owners should be questioned specifically about exposure to specific nephrotoxicants. If possible, a list of medications in the home, as well as any common nephrotoxicants such as lilies, antifreeze, chicken jerky treats (which can cause acquired Fanconi syndrome) and raisins/grapes, should be obtained. Furthermore, an understanding of the patient's surrounding environment is key in evaluating the acutely azotaemic patient. An outdoor cat would be considered at higher risk for antifreeze toxicity than an indoor-only cat, and *vice versa* for lily ingestion. Any recent anaesthesia and current medications are paramount in establishing a prioritized list of exclusions for acute azotaemia.

Physical examination

In a patient with suspected AKI, specific aspects of the physical examination should be emphasized. Hydration status and pulse quality should be evaluated, as well as body condition. An accurate weight must be obtained prior to initiation of fluid therapy, because bodyweight is an important parameter for evaluation of the response to fluid therapy during treatment. The heart, lungs and pulse should be evaluated for evidence of murmurs, arrhythmias, crackles or pulse deficits. If the heart rate is inappropriately low, serum potassium concentration and a lead II electrocardiogram (ECG) rhythm strip (see Figure 21.5) should be evaluated as quickly as possible. The kidneys should be palpated for size, shape and pain (see Chapter 4). The abdomen should also be palpated and, if the presence of fluid is suspected, uroabdomen must be ruled out. The character of the faeces should be noted during a rectal examination and the presence or absence of melaena recorded.

Early general monitoring

A baseline complete blood count (CBC), serum biochemistry profile and urinalysis should be obtained for all patients with known or suspected AKI. Monitoring packed cell volume (PCV), plasma total protein and bodyweight in comparison with baseline values will often suggest changes in hydration status. Blood pressure measurement will identify hypotensive and hypertensive patients, both of whom may be at increased risk for renal injury. Leptospirosis should be ruled out (via serology and urine polymerase chain reaction) in all dogs with AKI of unknown aetiology.

Urinalysis and urine production

Numerous urine parameters can herald the development of AKI in at-risk patients. Changes in urine volume may signal AKI because both oliguria (0.5–1 ml urine/kg/hour) and polyuria (>2–3 ml urine/kg/hour) can be observed in AKI. Increased urine turbidity or changes in urine sediment (increasing numbers of renal epithelial cells, cellular or granular casts or cellular debris) are often indications of acute ongoing tubular damage. The acute onset of tubular glucosuria (normoglycaemic glucosuria) or tubular proteinuria (urine protein to creatinine ratio (UPC) >0.5 but <2) may also be indicative of tubular cell damage, as previously described. The interpretation of all of the above parameters is enhanced by comparison with the baseline values.

Therapy

Pre-renal *versus* renal azotaemia

Clinical signs associated with pre-renal azotemia are often non-specific and may be similar to those associated with AKI. Although the initial fluid therapy may be the same for all azotaemic patients, the subsequent treatment and prognosis differ greatly between pre-renal azotaemia and established kidney injury. Any condition that decreases renal blood flow may result in pre-renal azotaemia, including hypovolaemia (e.g. dehydration, hypoadrenocorticism, haemorrhage), hypotension (e.g. anaesthesia, shock) and aortic or renal arterial thrombus formation. In most patients with pre-renal azotaemia the azotaemia is rapidly reversed with fluid therapy, and no lasting functional damage to the kidney occurs unless the decreased renal perfusion is prolonged or severe. Pre-renal azotaemia is usually associated with the production of hypersthenuric urine, but can be associated with any urine concentration (see above and Chapter 2).

Differentiating pre-renal from renal azotaemia may be more difficult if urine concentrating ability is impaired in patients with pre-renal azotaemia. Examples of this pre-renal syndrome include hypoadrenocorticism, pyometra and paraneoplastic hypercalcaemia, all of which can compromise urine concentrating ability and result in dehydration secondary to vomiting. The response to fluid therapy is key in these cases. Azotaemia caused by decreased renal perfusion should resolve quickly with replacement of volume deficits and restoration of renal perfusion, whereas renal azotaemia will not resolve completely with fluid therapy alone.

Fluid therapy for patients with suspected pre-renal azotaemia should be administered intravenously, with the fluid volume calculated on the basis of percentage dehydration, maintenance fluid requirements and continuing fluid losses (see Figure 21.3). Many patients with suspected pre-renal azotaemia have fluid losses associated with vomiting and diarrhoea, and therefore polyionic isotonic fluid solutions for replacement, such as lactated Ringer's solution, are good initial fluid choices. The magnitude of azotaemia as well as any electrolyte abnormalities (e.g. hypokalaemia, hyperkalaemia or hypercalcaemia) should be confirmed in serum obtained prior to initiation of fluid therapy. Rechecking a biochemistry profile to assess the patient's responses to fluid therapy is typically accomplished after 24–48 hours of fluid administration.

Supportive treatment for established AKI

Most dogs and cats with AKI are dehydrated because of gastrointestinal fluid loss as well as their urine concentrating deficits. Replacement of volume deficits will correct the pre-renal component of the disease and help protect against any additional ischaemic renal tubular damage. Once the patient is rehydrated, establishing or augmenting diuresis can facilitate excretion of solutes that are reabsorbed and secreted by renal tubular cells (e.g. urea nitrogen and potassium) and decrease the risk of overhydration or pulmonary oedema.

Fluid therapy

The goal of fluid therapy for established AKI is the correction of renal haemodynamic disorders and alleviation of water and solute imbalances in order to buy time for nephron repair and eventual compensation. A positive response to therapy is indicated by an increase in glomerular filtration (reduction in serum creatinine concentration) and an increase in urine production (if the patient was oliguric). However, the GFR is frequently unchanged in the early stages of fluid therapy, and any increased urine production observed with diuresis is usually the result of a relative decrease in the tubular reabsorption of filtrate. Increased urine production alone does not indicate an improvement in glomerular filtration.

Typically, the large volume of fluid and rapid administration rate necessary in AKI requires that fluids be given intravenously. Deficit fluid requirements should be replaced over the first 4–6 hours of treatment, unless the patient has a cardiopulmonary disorder that requires a slower administration rate. The purpose of replacing volume deficits over the first 4–6 hours rather than over the normal 12–24 hours is to attempt to improve renal perfusion rapidly and decrease the likelihood of continued ischaemic damage. Normal 0.9% physiological saline or lactated Ringer's solution are good first choices for rehydration. If the patient is hypernatraemic, a solution containing 0.45% saline and 2.5% dextrose can be used. Once the patient is rehydrated, a maintenance fluid (instead of a replacement fluid) such as Normosol-M™ can be used to decrease the likelihood of inducing hypernatraemia (this type of solution is not on the veterinary market in the UK; however, 0.18% sodium chloride (NaCl) plus 4% dextrose is available, and potassium chloride (KCl) can be added to this to approximate Normosol-M). The volume of fluid required to restore extracellular fluid deficits can be calculated by multiplying the estimated percentage of dehydration by the patient's bodyweight in kilograms (Figure 21.3).

Requirement	Volume of fluid
Deficit replacement for a 20 kg dog 7% dehydration = 0.07 x 20 kg = 1.4 kg (1400 ml)	1400 ml
Daily maintenance requirements 60 ml/kg x 20 kg	1200 ml
Continuing needs (administer as they occur) Dog vomits five times over 24-hour period with an estimated loss of 125 ml fluid per episode	625 ml
Total 24-hour[a] fluid replacement	3225 ml

21.3 Example of daily fluid requirements for a vomiting dog (20 kg) with suspected pre-renal azotaemia. [a] Deficit replacement can be administered more rapidly (e.g. over 4–6 hours).

During the rapid rehydration phase, the patient should be closely monitored for signs of overhydration, which is a common complication of fluid therapy in patients with AKI, especially those with oliguria. Once overhydration has occurred, the risk of pulmonary oedema increases. Overhydration is very difficult to correct (without dialysis) in an oliguric patient. Frequent assessment of bodyweight, PCV, central venous pressure (CVP) and plasma protein will help to detect overhydration at an early stage. An increase in the CVP of >5–7 cm of water (H_2O) over baseline values suggests the likelihood of overhydration. Physical manifestations of overhydration include:

- Increased bronchovesicular sounds
- Tachycardia
- Restlessness
- Chemosis
- Serous nasal discharge.

These signs, as well as auscultation of overt crackles and wheezes, may not occur prior to established pulmonary oedema.

Urine production should be measured and electrolyte and acid–base status assessed during the period of rehydration. Urine production (ml/kg/hr) should be measured so that maintenance fluid needs can be accurately determined. Approximately two-thirds of normal maintenance fluid needs are due to fluid loss in urine, therefore oliguric and non-oliguric patients can have large variations in their maintenance fluid needs (Figure 21.4). Urinary catheters

Parameter	Normal	Oliguric AKI	Non-oliguric AKI
Insensible fluid loss (ml/kg/day)	20	20	20
Urine production (ml/kg/day)	40	10	160
Total maintenance fluid needs (ml/kg/day)	60	30	180

21.4 Hypothetical daily fluid requirements for oliguric and non-oliguric patients with acute kidney injury (AKI), compared with those of a normal animal.

and manual collection of voided urine are methods used to collect and measure urine volume. With indwelling urinary catheters, strict aseptic technique and closed collection systems must be used. In cats, weighing the litter tray before and after voiding is a useful, although less accurate, method for assessing urine production. Observation of urine voiding and urinary bladder palpation are the least reliable methods for determining the volume of urine produced.

Correction of sodium and chloride imbalances

Initially, most patients with AKI have normal serum sodium and chloride concentrations because of isonatraemic fluid loss. Hypernatraemia can develop, however, after several days of therapy with fluids containing large amounts of sodium (0.9% NaCl, lactated Ringer's solution) and/or in association with sodium bicarbonate treatment of metabolic acidosis. If hypernatraemia occurs, the use of fluids containing 0.45% NaCl with 2.5% dextrose or conversion to a maintenance solution (which has a lower sodium content of about 40 mmol/l) will usually correct the problem.

Correction of calcium imbalances

Disorders of calcium balance can also occasionally manifest in patients with AKI. If moderate to severe hypercalcaemia is observed with elevated ionized calcium, a primary hypercalcaemic disorder (e.g. neoplasia or vitamin D3 intoxication) should be considered as the cause of the AKI. Immediate treatment for hypercalcaemia includes rehydration with 0.9% NaCl followed by diuresis with furosemide. Calcium-containing fluids should be avoided (e.g. lactated Ringer's). Glucocorticoids may also help to lower calcium concentrations by decreasing intestinal absorption and facilitating renal tubular excretion, but their use may interfere with diagnosis of the underlying disorder (e.g. lymphosarcoma).

Hypercalcaemia can have deleterious side effects, such as nausea, vomiting, polyuria/polydipsia and soft tissue mineralization. As a general rule, if a patient has a calcium–phosphorus product (Ca x PO$_4$) >70 mg^2/dl^2, they are at risk for soft tissue mineralization and can have a comparatively low survival rate (Langston, 2010; Lippi et al., 2014; to convert total calcium and phosphate concentrations from mmol/l to mg/dl, multiply by 4 and 3.1, respectively). In these cases, fluid therapy to induce diuresis is recommended. Hypocalcaemia can be observed in dogs and cats with AKI associated with ethylene glycol intoxication. However, clinical evidence of hypocalcaemia is rare in these cases, because the metabolic acidosis tends to maintain ionized calcium concentrations by displacing calcium ions from albumin.

Correction of potassium imbalances

Oliguric patients with AKI are at risk of hyperkalaemia. Serum potassium concentrations >6.5–7 mmol/l can cause cardiac conduction disturbances (bradycardia, atrial standstill, idioventricular rhythms, ventricular tachycardia, fibrillation and asystole) and ECG changes (peaked T waves, prolonged PR intervals, widened QRS complexes or the loss of P waves) (Figure 21.5). Mild to moderate hyperkalaemia is largely resolved with the administration of potassium-free fluids (dilution) and improved urine flow (increased excretion). More severe hyperkalaemia (>7–8 mmol/l) or hyperkalaemia resulting in ECG abnormalities should be treated using agents that decrease serum potassium concentrations or counteract the effects of hyperkalaemia on cardiac conduction. Sodium bicarbonate will help counteract metabolic acidosis and lower serum potassium concentration by cation exchange (intracellular hydrogen ions exchange with serum potassium). Glucose and insulin can also be used to encourage intracellular shifting of potassium. Regular insulin is administered at a dosage of 0.1–0.25 IU/kg i.v. followed by a dextrose bolus of 1–2 g per unit of insulin given. Blood glucose monitoring for hypoglycaemia should be maintained for several hours following administration of insulin.

Alternatively, if the hyperkalaemia is not very severe, a dextrose bolus at a dose of 1 ml/kg 50% dextrose diluted 1:2 can be given intravenously to stimulate insulin release and decrease extracellular potassium. Calcium gluconate (10% w/v; 0.5–1 ml/kg i.v. over 10–15 minutes) will counteract the cardiotoxic effects of hyperkalaemia without lowering the serum potassium level, and can be used in emergency situations. The effects of the above regimens are relatively short-lived, and fluid and acid–base therapy to initiate and maintain diuresis, and to maintain blood pH and bicarbonate within the physiological range (see below), are important to maintain potassium excretion and normokalaemia.

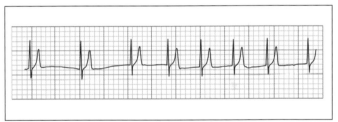

21.5 Electrocardiogram (ECG) showing absent P waves, bradycardia and tall T waves, suggestive of hyperkalaemia. (Paper speed: 25 mm/s; heart rate: 40 beats/min; 1 cm = 1 mV). (Courtesy of Dr Justin Thomason, Kansas State University)

Correction of acidosis

Mild to moderate metabolic acidosis also commonly resolves with fluid therapy, and specific treatment is not usually necessary unless the blood pH is <7.2 or total CO$_2$ (TCO$_2$) is <12 mmol/l. Bicarbonate requirements can be calculated by utilizing the base deficit as determined from arterial blood gas analysis, or an estimated base deficit:

Bodyweight (kg) x 0.3 x base deficit, or (20 − TCO$_2$) = mmol bicarbonate required

Optimally, one-quarter to one-half of the calculated bicarbonate dosage should be administered slowly intravenously over 15–30 minutes and then acid–base parameters reassessed. Overzealous bicarbonate administration may result in ionized calcium deficits, paradoxical cerebral spinal fluid acidosis and/or cerebral oedema (DiBartola, 2006).

Volume expansion

If signs of overhydration are not present and oliguria persists after apparent rehydration, mild volume expansion (3–5% of the patient's bodyweight in fluid) may be initiated, because dehydration of this magnitude is difficult to detect clinically. If volume expansion is attempted, the possibility of inducing overhydration increases and close patient monitoring is necessary. Unfortunately, most patients that present with oliguria will remain oliguric despite rehydration and volume expansion.

Diuretic/vasodilator therapy

In the past, diuretic therapy has been recommended for patients that are persistently oliguric or anuric in the face of appropriate fluid therapy. In comparison with patients with diminished urine production, polyuric AKI patients are thought to have less severe tubular injury, improved excretion of solutes that are reabsorbed or secreted (e.g. urea nitrogen or potassium) and a lower risk of developing overhydration and pulmonary oedema. Unfortunately, there are no prospective or randomized studies in veterinary medicine addressing the benefit and/or efficacy of loop or osmotic diuretics in AKI. Because of the potential for adverse effects and the lack of supportive evidence, the use of diuretics in patients with AKI has become controversial. However, it remains common practice to use either furosemide or mannitol in an attempt to induce a diuresis. Furosemide, in the case of oliguric or anuric renal failure, is given at a dose of 2–6 mg/kg i.v. q8h in cats, or as a constant-rate infusion (CRI) at 0.66 mg/kg/hr in dogs after a 0.66 mg/kg i.v. loading dose. Mannitol can be used at a dose of 0.5–1 g/kg i.v. over 15–20 minutes. Urine output should increase within 1 hour if either treatment is effective. Dopamine is not recommended owing to its unpredictable effects on renal blood flow, GFR and the cardiovascular system.

Whether or not diuresis can be established, fluid therapy should be tailored to match urine volume and other losses, including insensible losses (e.g. water loss due to respiration) and continuing losses (e.g. fluid loss due to vomiting or diarrhoea). Insensible losses are estimated at 20 ml/kg/day. Urine output can be quantified at intervals of 6–8 hours, and that amount plus insensible and continuing losses should be replaced over an equivalent subsequent time period. If hypernatraemia and hyperkalaemia are not present and diuresis has been established, polyionic maintenance fluids should be utilized. In the recovery phase of AKI, urine volume and electrolyte losses can be great. Potassium supplementation may be necessary, especially if the patient is vomiting or anorexic.

Dialysis

Peritoneal dialysis (see Chapter 22) may be considered for patients with severe, persistent uraemia, acidosis and hyperkalaemia. Peritoneal dialysis may also be used to treat overhydration and hasten elimination of a dialysable toxicant. Recently, haemodialysis has become more commonly used in veterinary medicine and is associated with a decreased mortality rate in AKI and improved outcome in patients who survive. This treatment modality is especially beneficial for patients that are refractory to standard fluid therapy. In a study of the long-term outcome of cats and dogs with AKI that were treated with intermittent haemodialysis, although the mortality rate prior to hospital discharge was still high for patients with AKI, those patients receiving haemodialysis and surviving to discharge had a higher probability of long-term survival (Eatroff et al., 2012). Haemodialysis protocols vary widely; this treatment method requires special training and equipment, and is available only at a few academic or specialty centres. Haemodialysis should be considered for patients that do not respond optimally to conventional fluid therapy.

Control of nausea and vomiting

Control of nausea and vomiting in dogs and cats with AKI is important in order to facilitate caloric intake and decrease ongoing fluid losses that can contribute to morbidity and mortality. Furthermore, vomiting increases the risk of aspiration pneumonia, which can significantly complicate the management of AKI. Management of nausea and vomiting in patients with AKI is similar to that for patients with advanced-stage CKD (see Chapter 23).

Longer term care

When fluid therapy is successful in inducing or maintaining diuresis, the daily volume of fluid administered to the patient will eventually need to be decreased. Indications for tapering intravenous fluid volume include: reductions in BUN and phosphorus concentrations with stable creatinine concentrations, control of vomiting and diarrhoea, and the patient beginning to eat and drink. These benchmarks rarely occur prior to 5–6 days of intense fluid therapy/diuresis and may require 10 or more days of treatment. Gradually reducing maintenance fluid requirements by 25% each day or every other day is usually recommended for fluid tapering. If the patient loses weight or increases are observed in PCV, total protein, BUN and/or creatinine concentrations, tapering should be discontinued and the previous rate of fluid administration reinstated. If the patient does not respond to appropriate fluid therapy or if the diagnosis is in question, renal biopsy should be considered to help determine the potential for nephron repair and reversibility of lesions.

Prognosis

The long-term prognosis for dogs or cats with AKI is usually fair to good if the patient survives the initial phases of AKI. One study showed that negative prognostic indicators specifically in cats include anaemia, hypoalbuminaemia, hypoglycaemia, advancing age and lower body temperature (Lee et al., 2012). Other studies have demonstrated an inverse correlation between urine output and initial serum potassium concentrations with survival (Worwag and Langston, 2008). The literature shows conflicting results regarding the severity of initial azotaemia and overall prognosis. Survival rates in veterinary studies are approximately 50% (Behrend et al., 1996; Vaden et al., 1997; Worwag and Langston, 2008; Lee et al., 2012). AKI grading systems have been developed (see Chapter 12) and these can help to establish the initial prognosis. The patient's response to treatment (e.g. reduction in serum creatinine and increased urine output associated with fluid therapy) is usually thought to be a better prognostic indicator than is the magnitude of initial dysfunction. Animals with AKI may require weeks of hospitalization, diligent monitoring and follow-up. Overall amelioration of the effects of AKI is dependent on the type and severity of damage, the timeliness of proper diagnosis and an appropriate therapeutic plan.

References and further reading

American College of Chest Physicians/Society of Critical Care Medicine Consensus Conference (1992) Definitions for sepsis and organ failure and guidelines for the use of innovative therapies in sepsis. *Critical Care Medicine* **20**, 864–874

Behrend E, Grauer GF, Mani I *et al.* (1996) Hospital-acquired acute renal failure in dogs: 29 cases (1983–1992). *Journal of the American Veterinary Medical Association* **208(4)**, 537–541

Bonventre JV (2003) Dedifferentiation and proliferation of surviving epithelial cells in acute renal failure. *Journal of the American Society of Nephrology* **14**, S55–S61

Bonventre JV and Weinberg JM (2003) Recent advances in the pathophysiology of ischemic acute renal failure. *Journal of the American Society of Nephrology* **14**, 2199–2210

Bonventre JV and Zuk A (2004) Ischemic acute renal failure: An inflammatory disease? *Kidney International* **66**, 480–485

Brezis M, Rosen S and Epstein FH (1991) Acute renal failure. In: *The Kidney*, ed. BM Brenner and FC Rector, pp.993–1061. WB Saunders, Philadelphia

Chertow GM, Burdick E, Honour M *et al.* (2005) Acute kidney injury, mortality, length of stay, and costs in hospitalized patients. *Journal of the American Society of Nephrology* **16**, 3365–3370

De Loor J, Daminet S, Smets P *et al.* (2013) Urinary biomarkers for acute kidney injury in dogs. *Journal of Veterinary Internal Medicine* **27**, 998–1010

Devarajan P (2006) Update on mechanisms of ischemic acute kidney injury. *Journal of the American Society of Nephrology* **17**, 1503–1520

DiBartola SP (2006) Metabolic acid–base disorders. In: *Fluid, Electrolyte, and Acid–Base Disorders in Small Animal Practice*, ed. SP DiBartola, pp.251–282. Saunders Elsevier, St Louis

Dieterle F, Perentes E, Cordier A *et al.* (2010) Urinary clusterin, cystatin C, β2-microglobulin and total protein as markers to detect drug-induced kidney injury. *Nature Biotechnology* **28**, 463–469

Eatroff AE, Langston CE, Chalhoub S *et al.* (2012) Long-term outcome of cats and dogs with acute kidney injury treated with intermittent hemodialysis: 135 cases (1997–2010). *Journal of the American Veterinary Medical Association* **241**, 1471–1478

Epstein FH (1995) Hypoxia of the renal medulla – Its implications for disease. *New England Journal of Medicine* **332(10)**, 647–655

Furuichi K, Kaneko S and Wada T (2009) Chemokine/chemokine receptor-mediated inflammation regulates pathologic changes from acute kidney injury to chronic kidney disease. *Clinical and Experimental Nephrology* **13**, 9–14

Grauer GF, Greco DS, Behrend EN *et al.* (1994) The effects of dietary protein conditioning on gentamicin-induced nephrotoxicosis in healthy male dogs. *American Journal of Veterinary Research* **55**, 90–97

Greco DS, Turnwald GH, Adams R *et al.* (1985) Urinary gamma-glutamyl transpeptidase activity in dogs with gentamycin-induced nephrotoxicty. *American Journal of Veterinary Research* **46**, 2332–2335

Langston C (2010) Acute uremia. In: *Textbook of Veterinary Internal Medicine*, ed. SJ Ettinger and EC Feldman, pp.1969–1985. Saunders Elsevier, St Louis

Lee YJ, Chan JPW, Hsu WL *et al.* (2012) Prognostic factors and a prognostic index for cats with acute kidney injury. *Journal of Veterinary Internal Medicine* **26**, 500–505

Lippi I, Guidi G, Marchetti V *et al.* (2014) Prognostic role of the product of serum calcium and phosphorus concentrations in dogs with chronic kidney disease: 31 cases (2008–2010). *Journal of the American Veterinary Medical Association* **245**, 1135–1140

Osterbur K, Mann FA, Kuroki K and DeClue A (2014) Multiple organ dysfunction syndrome in humans and animals. *Journal of Veterinary Internal Medicine* **28**, 1141–1151

Padanilam BJ (2003) Cell death induced by acute renal injury: a perspective on the contributions of apoptosis and necrosis. *American Journal of Physiology: Renal Physiology* **284**, F608–F627

Pawar S, Kartha S and Toback FG (1995) Differential gene expression in migrating renal epithelial cells after wounding. *Journal of Cellular Physiology* **165**, 556–565

Segerer S, Nelson PJ and Schlondorff D (2000) Chemokines, chemokine receptors, and renal disease: From basic science to pathophysiologic and therapeutic studies. *Journal of the American Society of Nephrology* **11**, 152–176

Stromski ME, Cooper K, Thulin G *et al.* (1986) Chemical and functional correlates of postischemic renal ATP levels. *Proceedings of the National Academy of Sciences USA* **83**, 6142–6145

Sutton TA, Fisher CJ and Molitoris BA (2002) Microvascular endothelial injury and dysfunction during ischemic acute renal failure. *Kidney International* **62**, 1539–1549

Vaden SL, Levine J, Breitschwerdt EB *et al.* (1997) A retrospective case–control of acute renal failure in 99 dogs. *Journal of Veterinary Internal Medicine* **19**, 794–801

Vetterlein F, Petho A and Schmidt G (1986) Distribution of capillary blood flow in rat kidney during postischemic renal failure. *American Journal of Physiology* **20**, H510–H519

Wang HE, Muntner P, Chertow GM *et al.* (2012) Acute kidney injury and mortality in hospitalized patients. *American Journal of Nephrology* **35**, 349–355

Worwag S and Langston CE (2008) Acute intrinsic renal failure in cats: 32 cases (1997–2004). *Journal of the American Veterinary Medical Association* **232**, 728–732

Ysebaert DK, De Greef KE, Vercauteren SR *et al.* (2000). Identification and kinetics of leukocytes after severe ischaemia/reperfusion renal injury. *Nephrology Dialysis Transplantation* **10**, 1562–1574

Chapter 22

Haemodialysis and peritoneal dialysis

Sheri Ross and Cathy Langston

Principles of dialysis

Dialysis is a method of treating kidney failure and certain types of toxicities, and includes haemodialysis (HD) and peritoneal dialysis (PD). The principles are similar for HD and PD. However, during HD, the exchange of solutes and water between the patient's blood and the prepared dialysate solution occurs extracorporeally, across a manufactured membrane, whereas during PD this exchange occurs within the abdominal cavity using the peritoneum as the membrane.

Methods of clearance

Solute and fluid removal during dialysis occurs via four different mechanisms: diffusion, ultrafiltration, convection and adsorption (Figure 22.1). The relative contribution of each of these mechanisms to the removal of solutes will depend upon the properties of the semipermeable membrane, the solute of interest and the relative pressures acting across the membrane.

Diffusive transfer of solute relies on the random movement of particles through the pores of the dialyser membrane (or the peritoneum) from a solution of higher concentration to a solution of lower concentration. Once concentration equilibrium has been achieved between the two solutions, an equal bidirectional exchange continues, with no net change in the solute concentration on either side of the membrane. During HD, constant replenishment of fresh dialysate within the dialyser prevents equilibrium from being established, thus maintaining active diffusion. The efficiency of diffusion is further increased by using a countercurrent direction of flow between blood and dialysate that maximizes the concentration gradient. Molecular weight strongly influences the kinetic motion of a solute and this is inversely related to the rate of diffusion. For this reason, small solutes such as urea (60 Da) diffuse more readily than larger molecules such as creatinine (113 Da). Movement of larger solutes, plasma proteins and cellular components of blood across the dialyser membrane is limited by the size of the membrane pores.

Ultrafiltration is the removal of excess plasma water from the patient. In the context of HD, ultrafiltration is accomplished by means of a transmembrane pressure gradient that moves water from the blood to the dialysate. The amount of water removed depends on the permeability and surface area of the membrane and the hydrostatic pressure gradient across the membrane. Most HD platforms allow the rate and total amount of ultrafiltration to be set for each treatment. During PD, the removal of

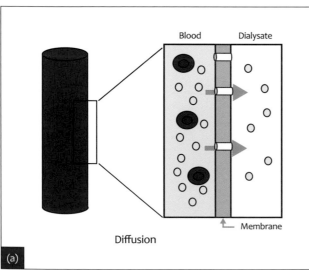
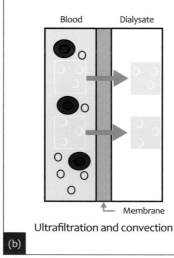
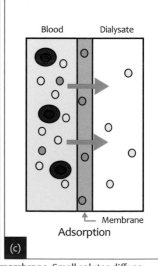

22.1 Solute and fluid removal during dialysis. (a) Blood flows through hollow fibres made of a semipermeable membrane. Small solutes diffuse through pores in the membrane in response to the concentration gradient. (b) Water that is removed from the blood compartment through hydrostatic forces (ultrafiltration) also removes any solutes that are dissolved in that water (convection or solute drag). (c) Substances may adhere to the membrane (adsorption) and thus be removed from the bloodstream.

BSAVA Manual of Canine and Feline Nephrology and Urology, third edition. Edited by Jonathan Elliott, Gregory F. Grauer and Jodi L. Westropp. ©BSAVA 2017

excess plasma water is accomplished through osmosis. The addition of varying concentrations of dextrose (or occasionally other solutes) to the dialysate produces a hyperosmolar solution. The resulting osmotic gradient aids in the removal of excess plasma water. The rate of fluid removal may be controlled by adjusting the concentration of dextrose in the dialysate.

Convection is the simultaneous transport of solutes along with water across a semipermeable membrane during ultrafiltration. Solutes are carried with the water by a process known as solvent drag. The efficiency of convective clearance of solutes is determined by the size of the solute and the pore size and surface area of the membrane. Convective clearance contributes little to the overall solute removal during standard intermittent HD and PD treatments. However, some renal replacement modalities rely on convection as the major mechanism of clearance, using high ultrafiltration rates with simultaneous replacement of intravenous fluids to maintain vascular volume (haemofiltration). When this technique is combined with diffusive clearance during standard HD, the process is referred to as haemodiafiltration. As the molecular size of the solutes to be removed increases, convective clearance becomes more efficient than diffusive clearance. Convective transport does not require a concentration gradient across the membrane and does not generate diffusive gradients or alter serum concentrations.

Adsorptive solute removal depends on the physical and chemical properties of the dialyser membrane and of the solute being absorbed. In general, with standard dialysers, adsorption of solutes is typically limited to proteins, with very little adsorption of solutes with low molecular weights. More extensive adsorption is used in a technique called charcoal haemoperfusion (see below).

Indications and patient selection

In veterinary medicine, dialysis is used most commonly for acute kidney injury (AKI). Dialysis is indicated for patients with anuria or oliguria, life-threatening fluid overload (e.g. pulmonary oedema) or refractory hyperkalaemia, if attempts to induce urine production are unsuccessful. Uraemic signs, progressive azotaemia, or azotaemia that does not improve with standard medical therapy are indications for dialysis, even if urine output is adequate or increased. Whether initiating dialysis early in the course of AKI improves outcome compared with later initiation is unresolved. Some studies have shown an advantage to early initiation, although others have not (Gettings *et al.*, 1999; Bouman *et al.*, 2002; Liu *et al.*, 2006). In many situations, AKI is reversible, and because there are no studies that clearly predict which patients will need dialysis, it is possible that results of studies on early *versus* late initiation will be biased towards early initiation because of the inclusion of patients in the early group that did not need dialysis. Despite the lack of an adequate study to answer this question, waiting until uraemic signs are severe and the condition of the patient has deteriorated may be disadvantageous. The risk of early initiation in a patient that may not need dialysis must be weighed against the potential risks and cost of renal replacement therapy.

Dialysis is reserved until standard medical management has been attempted (see Chapter 21). Standard medical management includes adequate volume expansion, but overhydration worsens renal function and outcome. Because dehydration of <5% cannot be clinically detected, patients that appear normally hydrated but not over-hydrated should receive a dose of intravenous fluid equal to 5% of bodyweight. The systemic blood pressure should be adequate to perfuse the kidneys (>80–100 mmHg systolic or >60–80 mmHg mean arterial pressure). The use of diuretics is widespread in both human and veterinary medicine despite lack of conclusive evidence of a positive impact on outcome (Bagshaw *et al.*, 2008). If ensuring adequate renal perfusion (i.e. correcting dehydration and/or hypotension) fails to induce adequate urine production within hours, early referral for dialysis is appropriate.

In humans, haemodialysis is used primarily to treat end-stage renal disease. Human patients may be maintained on chronic HD for years while waiting for a renal transplant, or for decades if transplantation is not possible. Transplantation is generally preferred over chronic HD, because it replaces renal function more completely, but transplantation is not readily available for dogs. Chronic HD is an alternative in these cases, and in cats where there are clear contraindications to transplantation (e.g. nephrolithiasis). The goal of chronic HD is to maintain a satisfactory quality of life, which should take precedence over longevity. Chronic HD should be recommended when the signs of uraemia are no longer controlled by medical management. In these cases the serum creatinine concentration is generally >5 mg/dl and, in some patients, the main sign of uraemia may be anorexia. If few other uraemic signs are present or they can be controlled, placement of a feeding tube prior to initiating dialysis may be prudent. Although patients may decompensate acutely and unpredictably, the decision to initiate chronic dialysis ideally should be planned in advance, allowing scheduling of surgical placement of a permanent HD catheter in conjunction with feeding tube placement. Although return of a normal appetite is expected with adequate dialysis, anorexia can be seen during prolonged interdialysis intervals, when catheter function is temporarily inadequate, or when concurrent illness is present. Enteral feeding via oesophageal feeding tubes during these times allows better overall patient care.

Patients weighing <2.5 kg are difficult to treat with HD because of the relatively large volume of blood required to fill the blood circuit. Given the prolonged and intimate operator contact with the patient, aggressive patients are inappropriate candidates. The choice among the modalities (intermittent haemodialysis (IHD), continuous renal replacement therapy (CRRT), hybrid extracorporeal therapies and PD) depends on a variety of factors. There is no outcome benefit between the extracorporeal therapies, and the choice is usually made on the basis of availability. PD requires no specialized equipment, and thus can be performed in any practice with 24-hour care, but experience appears to decrease complications and improve outcomes, making referral to regional experts warranted. Small patients or patients with hypotension who are poor candidates for extracorporeal therapy may be more suited for PD. In addition, if a peritoneal catheter is already in place (e.g. because of uroabdomen), PD may be a suitable choice.

Other indications for extracorporeal therapy

Very large molecules or those that are protein-bound cannot be removed by standard HD, but may be removed using haemoperfusion. During haemoperfusion, anticoagulated blood is passed through a column containing adsorbent particles. Most perfusion devices contain activated charcoal, which allows the non-selective removal of large, or protein-bound, toxins from the blood (Figure 22.2). Haemoperfusion devices may also contain resins that improve the clearance of lipid-soluble compounds. Antibody- or antigen-coated resins have also been used for selective removal of specific substances such as endotoxin, cytokines or antibodies (Cruz, 2009). In many cases, one or two treatments can remove substantial amounts of toxins, and this may be more cost-effective than prolonged supportive care.

Therapeutic apheresis is an extracorporeal blood purification technique, which is designed for the removal of either plasma (plasmapheresis) or cellular blood components (cytopheresis). Plasmapheresis can be performed through a centrifugal or a membrane filtration technique. The most frequently used centrifugal method of plasmapheresis is represented by therapeutic plasma exchange (TPE or PEX), in which the plasma removed is replaced by frozen plasma or albumin solution. Plasma exchange represents a non-selective procedure to remove the offending agent. The membrane filtration technique allows the separation of plasma from the blood cells by a plasma filter. The cascade filtration technique is a semi-selective procedure in which the separated plasma is further processed through a plasma fractionator to remove different macromolecules, such as immunoglobulin (Ig)G, IgA, IgM, immune complexes and low-density lipoprotein (LDL) cholesterol. Therapeutic plasma exchange has also been used to treat immunologically mediated diseases such as myasthenia gravis and immune-mediated haemolytic anaemia.

Isolated ultrafiltration is a technique in which fluid is removed from the patient to control volume overload, most notably from congestive heart failure.

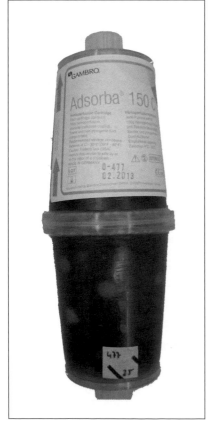

22.2 Charcoal haemoperfusion device. Blood is percolated through the cartridge. Toxins bind to the charcoal and thus are removed from the blood.

Outcome

The overall survival rate of dogs and cats treated with haemodialysis for AKI is 41–52%, but survival is dependent on aetiology, with infectious and ischaemic causes faring better than toxic causes, in general (Figure 22.3; Langston, 2011). Of the non-surviving patients, about half die or are euthanased as a result of extra-renal conditions (e.g. pancreatitis, respiratory complications). About one-third of non-survivors are euthanased because of a failure to recover renal function. Ongoing uraemic signs, dialysis complications and unknown causes account for the remaining deaths. Of the surviving patients, approximately half regain normal renal function (defined by normal serum creatinine concentration) and half have persistent chronic kidney disease (CKD), which tends to be mild and non-progressive.

Category	Survival rate
Obstructive (cats)	70–75%
Infectious	58–86%
Metabolic/haemodynamic	56–72%
Toxic	18–35%
Other	29–56%

22.3 Survival rates with intermittent haemodialysis for acute kidney injury of various aetiologies.

The outcome with CRRT has not been reported as extensively. In one study, 44% of 16 cats survived; among them, 70% had normal blood urea nitrogen (BUN) and creatinine. For dogs, 41% of 17 dogs survived, and 43% of the survivors had BUN and serum creatinine concentrations that returned to the reference ranges (Diehl and Seshadri, 2008).

With PD, 22% of 27 dogs and cats survived to discharge in an older report (Crisp et al., 1989). In a more recent report, 46% of 22 cats survived to discharge (Cooper and Labato, 2011), although five of six cats survived to discharge in another recent study (Dorval and Boysen, 2009), and four of five dogs with leptospirosis survived in a third report (Beckel et al., 2005).

Haemodialysis

Vascular access

For all extracorporeal modalities, vascular access is essential for the delivery of a large and continuous flow of blood through the extracorporeal circuit. In veterinary medicine, dual-lumen catheters placed in the jugular vein are the most frequently used vascular access ports for extracorporeal therapies.

As a general rule, it is advisable to use the largest catheter that may be safely placed in the jugular vein to maximize blood flow. Blood flow is proportional to the catheter diameter and inversely proportional to its length. A 7–8 Fr catheter is generally suitable for a cat or a small dog, while a 12–14 Fr catheter is appropriate for a medium to large dog.

Temporary catheters are designed for placement using the percutaneous 'over-a-wire' or Seldinger technique. With strict adherence to asepsis and very careful maintenance, these catheters may remain functional for several weeks (Figure 22.4). If the patient is likely to require chronic therapy, a permanent catheter is placed surgically and

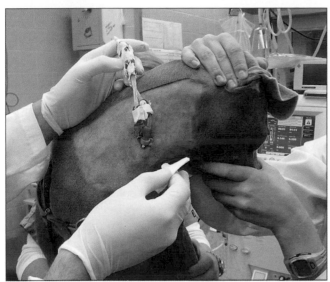

22.4 A dog with a non-cuffed, non-tunnelled percutaneously placed temporary dialysis catheter in the jugular vein.

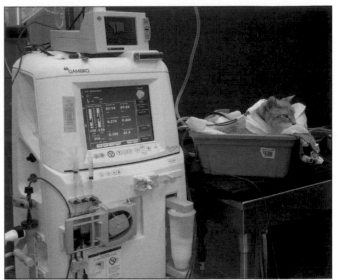

22.5 A cat being treated with intermittent haemodialysis using a Gambro Phoenix® machine.

tunnelled subcutaneously from the cutaneous exit site to the site of entrance to the jugular vein. Although typically more expensive and difficult to place, long-term catheters can be used for months to years with appropriate care.

Catheters should be dedicated to HD treatments only and be handled aseptically. Dialysis catheters should not be used for intravenous fluids, medications, blood sampling, parenteral nutrition or anything else, to minimize the risk of contamination. Each time the catheter is accessed, and at the beginning and end of each dialysis treatment, the catheter should be isolated with a sterile drape and a surgical scrub of the ports performed.

Between dialysis treatments, both lumens are filled with an anticoagulant solution, generally unfractionated heparin or citrate. As a preventive measure, antimicrobials may be added to the heparin locking solutions. One common addition is cefazolin. Sodium citrate may be used as a catheter locking solution. It has both anticoagulant and antibacterial properties, but can cause hypocalcaemia if inadvertently flushed into the patient instead of being removed and discarded when the catheter is used. In addition to anticoagulant locking solutions, most patients undergoing haemodialysis also receive oral aspirin or clopidogrel to minimize catheter-associated thrombosis.

Machines

Several different types of machine are available to provide extracorporeal therapy. There is only one machine (available in Japan) that is made specifically for small animals; all others are made for treating adult humans. In the past, machines were intended either for intermittent treatments or for continuous treatment, but newer machines have a greater range of capabilities and the line between the machine types has become blurred. Some machines (typically used for IHD) generate dialysate by mixing purified water with a concentrated electrolyte solution (Figure 22.5). Large quantities (20–50 l/h) of dialysate can be produced with these machines, allowing rapid and extensive diffusive clearance of uraemic solutes in a short period of time. A water purification system is necessary to provide the water for dialysate production. Some machines can generate replacement fluid (fluid administered into the bloodstream to replace the fluid removed for convective clearance) when providing haemodiafiltration. Other

machines (typically used for CRRT) use prepackaged sterile dialysate fluid. These machines provide much slower clearance and are designed to be able to use a combination of diffusive and convective clearance (Figure 22.6). A prototype machine has been developed that provides solely convective clearance (i.e. no dialysate is needed) and is intended for use in human neonates and infants.

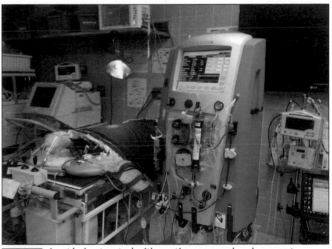

22.6 A cat being treated with continuous renal replacement therapy using a Gambro Prismaflex® machine.

Schedules and prescriptions

The goals of individual HD treatments may vary significantly between and within patients. One of the primary considerations when planning the dialysis prescription is the total **volume of the extracorporeal circuit**. Selection of the dialyser should focus on the priming volume, surface area of the dialyser, characteristics of the filtration membrane and biocompatibility. Smaller and low-flux dialysers are more appropriate for smaller patients, or when a low-efficiency treatment is required, such as in severe azotaemia (Figure 22.7). Conversely, high-flux dialysers are generally preferred if more intense treatments or high convective clearance is required. **Treatment intensity** is another key point of the prescription. It is a function of the total volume of blood processed through the

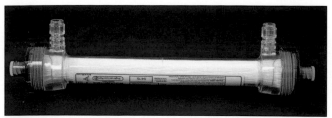

22.7 The dialyser houses the semipermeable membrane. Blood travels through the fibres while dialysate fills the space surrounding the fibres.

dialyser during the dialysis session in machines with high dialysate flow rates (i.e. IHD), and a function of the total volume of dialysate and replacement fluid in machines with limited fluid flow rates (i.e. CRRT).

The two main measures of the adequacy of dialysis are the urea reduction ratio (URR) and *Kt/V*, where *K* is a measurement of urea clearance, *t* is the time on dialysis, and *V* is the volume of distribution. Short, highly efficient dialysis treatments can induce dramatic changes in BUN in small patients with severe azotaemia, which predisposes the patient to life-threatening conditions, such as dialysis disequilibrium syndrome. Several methods of slowing the efficiency of treatment are advisable in this setting. With IHD-type machines, limiting the blood flow rate will decrease the amount of clearance, but it may not be possible to maintain a blood flow slow enough to reduce BUN safely because of the risk of clotting in the extracorporeal circuit with slow flow rates. Alternating dialysis treatment periods with bypass periods can slow clearance. During bypass, the blood continues to move throughout the circuit, but the dialysate flow is stopped, preventing further diffusion once equilibrium has been established. Alternatively, diverting part of the dialysate flow in an IHD-type machine, such that the blood is exposed to only a limited volume of dialysate, can provide safe rates of clearance for high-risk patients. Such devices are not commercially available. CRRT-type machines can provide controlled amounts of clearance and are ideal for these patients. Initially, treatments are provided for several hours (6–12 hours) daily, or continuously, for several days until the patient is more stable.

Once the severe uraemia has been reduced over the first few days of treatment, more intensive treatment prescriptions can provide rapid solute clearance over several hours of treatment. IHD-type machines excel at this type of prescription, although CRRT-type machines can provide moderately intense treatments for small to medium-sized patients when needed. During this phase, 4–6-hour treatments every other day may control the uraemia adequately.

Other important factors to consider when formulating the dialysis prescription include **dialysate composition** and **temperature**. Conventional dialysate formulations for IHD-type machines contain a mix of different electrolytes, such as sodium (about 145 mmol/l in dogs and 150 mmol/l in cats), potassium (0–3 mmol/l), bicarbonate (25–40 mmol/l), chloride (about 113 mmol/l in dogs and 117 mmol/l in cats), calcium (1.5 mmol/l), magnesium (1 mmol/l) and glucose (200 mg/dl). The sodium concentration of the dialysate may be increased or decreased during dialysis according to the patient's needs. A low bicarbonate concentration (25 mmol/l) is generally preferred in patients with severe metabolic acidosis, to prevent rapid correction of the acidosis, which could cause paradoxical cerebral acidosis. With CRRT-type machines, changing the dialysate (or replacement fluid) composition involves simply changing the bag of dialysate to one with a different formulation.

Occasionally, certain additions to the dialysate may be required. For example, in patients with acute ethylene glycol intoxication (prior to the development of renal failure), ethanol may be added to the dialysate in order to raise and maintain the patient's blood alcohol level. Patients with a normal to low serum phosphate concentration being treated for non-renal toxicities may require the addition of phosphate to the dialysate in order to avoid hypophosphataemia.

The temperature of the dialysate is regulated by the IHD machine and may have a significant effect on the haemodynamic stability of the patient. Warm dialysate temperatures may promote vasodilation and hypotension, while cooler temperatures result in vasoconstriction and increasing blood pressure. With CRRT-type machines, external devices to warm the blood are necessary to prevent hypothermia.

The blood in the extracorporeal circuit is prone to clotting. Anticoagulation sufficient to prevent thrombosis of the extracorporeal circuit without causing excessive bleeding in the patient is usually required. Unfractionated heparin is the mainstay of anticoagulant therapy in intermittent HD, and typically consists of the systemic administration of a standard dose of heparin (10–50 IU/kg) given as a bolus 5 minutes before starting the dialysis treatment, followed by a continuous infusion of heparin (10–50 IU/kg/h) into the access limb of the circuit, to maintain an activated clotting time of 1.6–2 times normal. The heparin infusion may be discontinued up to 30 minutes prior to the end of the treatment.

Citrate may be used as an alternative to heparin. Citrate exerts its effect by chelating calcium, which prevents coagulation. Although the majority of calcium–citrate complexes are lost into the effluent dialysate, some citrate returns to the patient to be metabolized by the liver into bicarbonate. In order to prevent systemic hypocalcaemia, the patient's physiological levels of serum calcium are maintained with a constant rate infusion of calcium.

In patients with active bleeding or with a recent history of surgery or haemorrhagic episodes, HD procedures may be performed without any anticoagulation. During a no-heparin treatment, frequent saline boluses are needed to flush fibrin strands from the circuit and minimize clotting.

Complications

Complications encountered during dialytic management may be a result of the dialysis procedure or of the underlying renal failure. Dialysis disequilibrium syndrome is a condition characterized by a rapid decline in blood osmolality caused by rapid removal of osmoles (especially urea) by dialysis. The relatively high intracellular osmolality in the brain promotes central nervous system (CNS) oedema, causing CNS signs (i.e. seizures, mentation changes, coma, death). In small animals, removal of the blood volume necessary to fill the dialysis circuit frequently results in hypotension, although hypertension related to the kidney injury and fluid overload is commonly encountered in the dialysis patient population. Haemorrhage related to heparin anticoagulation is most likely during the first few dialysis treatments, while the individual response to heparin is being determined, and with prolonged sessions (>6 hours). With inadequate anticoagulation, clotting in the extracorporeal circuit is likely, which prevents return of the full amount of blood at the end of treatment, in addition to decreasing the efficiency of treatment. Thrombosis at the tip of the dialysis catheter in the right atrium is common with catheters kept in place for over 3 weeks, and impairs adequate blood flow. Although the blood in the extracorporeal circuit is returned to the patient at the end of treatment, a small amount usually remains in the dialyser. Because erythropoietin production is typically diminished, dialysis patients are unable to correct the ensuing anaemia.

Peritoneal dialysis

Catheters

PD catheters can be placed percutaneously or surgically (Figure 22.8). The general design of PD catheters includes multiple fenestrations at the tip of the catheter to allow fluid ingress and egress. A variety of catheters are available that are made specifically for this purpose, or a fenestrated chest tube or Jackson Pratt suction drain may be used. For percutaneous placement, local anaesthesia in conscious animals or a short-acting injectable anaesthetic may be used. The urinary bladder should be emptied to avoid perforation. With the patient in dorsal recumbency, a stab incision through the skin lateral to the midline at the level of the umbilicus allows introduction of a trocar threaded through the dialysis catheter. The trocar is tunnelled under the skin for 1–2 cm before puncturing the abdominal musculature. The trocar should be directed toward the opposite hip. Having the abdomen slightly distended with fluid facilitates percutaneous placement. After the trocar has been introduced, the catheter is advanced off the trocar. The tip of the catheter should rest near the urinary bladder to facilitate fluid drainage. If the catheter is placed during surgery, a partial omentectomy can be performed to diminish catheter occlusion. Ideally, the catheter would not be used for 24 hours after placement to allow formation of a fibrin seal, but the animal's condition rarely allows this. When the catheter must be used immediately, a small volume of dialysate (half the standard volume) should be used for each exchange for the first 24 hours.

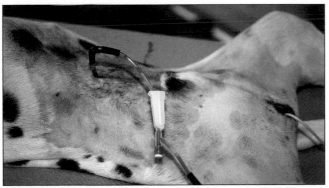

22.8 Peritoneal dialysis catheter placed percutaneously. A urinary catheter has been placed in a prescrotal urethrostomy.

Peritoneal dialysate solutions

Peritoneal dialysate solutions are provided as prepackaged sterile fluids made specifically for PD. The dialysate must contain physiological concentrations of readily diffusible substances such as sodium, chloride, calcium and magnesium. Dextrose or other osmotically active agents can be added to create a mildly to moderately hyperosmolar solution, which creates an osmotic gradient to promote fluid removal from an overhydrated patient. If no fluid removal is desired, a dextrose concentration of

1.5% is typically used. Dextrose concentrations of 2.5% or 4.25% are used to promote ultrafiltration. The typical 2 litre volume of 1.5% glucose dialysate instilled in a human will cause ultrafiltration of 50–100 ml after 1 hour and 150–200 ml after 2 hours. A 4.25% glucose dialysate will create 300–400 ml of ultrafiltrate in the first hour and 400–600 ml in 2 hours. However, after 3 hours, glucose has been absorbed and metabolized, and the peritoneum will reabsorb the ultrafiltrate. Long-term exposure to dextrose can decrease the ability of the peritoneum to filter, and therefore a glucose polymer, icodextrin, has been developed to replace dextrose. Because icodextrin is not metabolized, ultrafiltration continues during the entire dwell period. Heparin (250–1000 IU/l) should be added to the dialysate for the first few days after catheter placement to minimize fibrin clot formation. Magnesium should be added after several days of dialysis to achieve a concentration of 1.5 mmol/l. Although dialysate can be improvised from saline by adding the necessary substances, each additive to the dialysate increases the risk of contamination and formulation error.

Exchange procedure

Frequent dialysate exchanges are necessary in dogs or cats with acute oliguric or anuric renal failure, with hyperkalaemia, or those that are overhydrated. Initially, exchanges may be as frequent as every 45–60 minutes. As the uraemia improves (typically after 24–48 hours), the frequency of exchanges can be gradually decreased to 4 times a day, with the goal of maintaining the BUN concentration between 60 and 100 mg/dl. The volume of dialysate to instill is 40 ml/kg per exchange. The dialysate should be warmed to 38°C to maintain body temperature and to improve peritoneal permeability. Dogs and cats need to be closely observed for signs of abdominal discomfort or respiratory compromise.

Peritonitis is a frequent complication of PD, so the catheter and all connections should be handled as aseptically as possible. The connection ports should be covered with antiseptic-soaked gauze and should be scrubbed prior to any connection or disconnection. A mask and sterile gloves should be worn when handling the equipment, and the frequency of connection and disconnection should be kept to a minimum. Most contamination occurs when connecting the catheter to the dialysate bags. A Y-connector (or stopcock) can be placed on the catheter and connected to a multidose bag of fresh dialysate and to an empty bag to collect spent dialysate. At the start of each exchange, a small amount of fresh dialysate is flushed directly into the drain bag with the catheter closed to the animal. This will help to flush any contaminants that may have been introduced during the connection process into the drain bag and not into the abdomen. After flushing 10–20 ml into the drain bag, the drain bag is clamped and the catheter unclamped. The dose of dialysate should then be instilled into the abdomen by gravity, usually taking <10 minutes. The fresh dialysate bag should then be clamped and the catheter closed to the dog or cat during the dwell time. After the appropriate dwell time, the catheter is opened to allow drainage of the abdominal fluid into the drain bag. The drain bag must be positioned lower than the catheter to allow gravity drainage. Gentle ballottement of the abdomen and repositioning the animal can facilitate more complete drainage. After draining ceases (approximately 15–30 minutes), fresh dialysate is again instilled into the abdomen. If the entire volume of the fresh dialysate bag is infused per exchange, the empty bag should be clamped after the infusion and left attached. After the dwell time, the clamp should be opened and the bag used as the drain bag (Figure 22.9).

The volume of dialysate instilled and the volume recovered should be monitored carefully, as should urine output and the volume of administered fluids, medications and feed. When hypertonic dialysate is used (e.g. 4.25% dextrose), a larger volume of dialysate should be recovered than instilled, indicating net fluid removal from the animal. The dog or cat should be monitored for evidence of dehydration. If less dialysate is being recovered than is being instilled, the catheter tubing should be checked for kinks or occlusion and the animal repositioned. The catheter can be flushed forcefully with heparinized saline, or tissue plasminogen activator can be instilled in the catheter for 2–3 hours to dislodge fibrin clots or omentum. If these measures do not restore flow, the catheter may need to be repositioned or replaced.

In addition to meticulous attention to fluid balance, several other parameters should be monitored routinely. Blood glucose concentration should be monitored once or twice daily. If hyperglycaemia is documented, low doses of insulin may need to be administered. Packed cell volume (PCV), total solids and electrolytes should be monitored twice daily. Initially, BUN, creatinine and albumin should be monitored once or twice daily. Fluid analysis with cytology should be performed on the spent dialysate on a daily basis, and the dialysate should be cultured weekly or if it becomes cloudy.

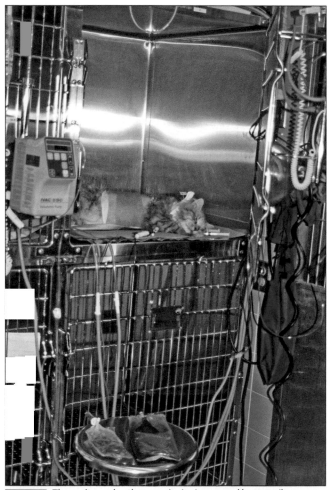

22.9 The peritoneal catheter exit site is covered by a sterile bandage. The spent dialysate is being collected in the bag on the right. Blood may be present in the first few exchanges after catheter placement. Urine volume is also being monitored (bag on left).

Complications

Peritonitis is a major complication of PD. Meticulous attention to aseptic technique is necessary to decrease this risk. Diagnosis is made by the presence of clinical signs (e.g. abdominal pain, fever), cloudy dialysate, or >100 inflammatory cells per ml of dialysate. Because *Staphylococcus* is the most common organism isolated, systemic cephalosporins are recommended pending culture results. Intraperitoneal administration of antibiotics may be helpful (e.g. 125 mg cefalothin per litre of dialysate). Although peritonitis may be successfully managed while continuing dialysis, removal of the PD catheter may be required to allow resolution of unresponsive peritonitis.

Catheter occlusion is a common problem with PD. The omentum has tremendous migratory capability and can rapidly encompass the catheter. Acute PD catheters may occlude within 24–72 hours of placement. A partially occluded catheter drains more slowly and incompletely. Incomplete emptying of the dialysate decreases the efficiency of toxin removal and risks overdistension of the abdomen, with concomitant problems (abdominal or respiratory distress). Other catheter-related complications include dialysate leakage or infections of the exit site and subcutaneous tunnel.

Hypoalbuminaemia is one of the most common complications of PD and can be partially addressed by providing adequate nutrition either enterally or parenterally. Enteral feeding is frequently difficult, because of anorexia or vomiting. Gastrostomy or jejunostomy tubes are contraindicated in PD owing to exit site leaks and increased risk of infection. Dialysate containing amino acids may provide partial nutrition but should not be used unless adequate non-protein calories are being provided.

Discontinuing dialysis

Intermittent rest periods, in which no dialysate dwells in the abdomen, with close evaluation of the animal's clinical and biochemical status can be used to determine when dialysis can be discontinued. When the dog or cat can maintain homeostasis without dialysis for several days, the catheter should be removed.

Cost and availability

As with most intensive and highly specialized therapies, the cost of dialysis can be high. Although many types of dialysis machine are not excessively expensive, the disposable supplies can range from modest to high cost. Sometimes the cost can be decreased by partnership with an affiliated human hospital with a large caseload eligible for bulk discounts. The biggest expense with these therapies (IHD, CRRT and PD) is expert care. While operation of the dialysis machine can be learned relatively quickly, the investment in learning to manage dialysis patients is high for the veterinary surgeon (veterinarian) and nurse (technician). Each treatment requires a nurse to be present for the duration of therapy. A proficient veterinary nurse may be able to treat two to three patients simultaneously, but in most settings only a single patient requires treatment at a time (or only one machine may be available). The training time and the intensive time required to administer each treatment make the labour costs of dialysis high. Dialysis is available in a limited number of veterinary hospitals (Figure 22.10), although the number of dialysis units is increasing worldwide.

Europe/Middle East	
Clinic of Small Animal Medicine, Ludwig Maximilians University of Munich, Munich, Germany	Hospital Veterinario das Laranjeiras, Lisbon, Portugal
Tierärztliche Klinik für Kleintiere, Norderstedt, Germany	Hospital Veterinario Montenegro, Porto, Portugal
Koret School of Veterinary Medicine, The Hebrew University of Jerusalem Rehovot, Israel	Hospital Veterinario do Porto, Porto, Portugal
Anubi Companion Animal Hospital, Moncalieri, Italy	Romanian Society for Veterinary Minimally Invasive Surgery, Bucharest, Romania
Universita Di Pisa, Pisa, Italy	University of Cordoba Veterinary Teaching Hospital, Cordoba, Spain
Clinica Veterinaria Roma Sud Rome, Italy	Vetsuisse Faculty University of Berne Small Animal Clinic, Berne, Switzerland
Elwet-Warsaw Veterinary and Animal Hospital, Warsaw, Poland	Queen Mother Hospital for Animals, Royal Veterinary College, London, UK
Hospital Veterinario do Restelo, Lisbon, Portugal	
North America	
Auburn University College of Veterinary Medicine, Auburn, Alabama, USA	Tufts University Foster Hospital for Small Animals, School of Veterinary Medicine, North Grafton, Massachusetts, USA
City of Angels Veterinary Specialty Center, Culver City, California, USA	Weare Animal Hospital, Weare, New Hampshire, USA
University of California Veterinary Medical Center, San Diego, California, USA	Veterinary Referral & Emergency Center of Westbury, Westbury, New York, USA
William R. Pritchard Veterinary Medical Teaching Hospital – University of California Davis, Davis, California, USA	North Carolina State University College of Veterinary Medicine, Raleigh, North Carolina, USA
Animal Hospital Specialty Center, Highlands Ranch, Colorado, USA	Ohio State University, Columbus, Ohio, USA
Colorado State University – James L. Voss Veterinary Teaching Hospital, Fort Collins, Colorado, USA	University of Pennsylvania – Matthew J. Ryan Veterinary Hospital, Philadelphia, Pennsylvania, USA
University of Florida Small Animal Hospital, Gainesville, Florida, USA	Center for Veterinary Specialty Care, Carrollton, Texas, USA
University of Georgia College of Veterinary Medicine, Athens, Georgia, USA	Advanced Veterinary Care, Salt Lake City, Utah, USA
Chicago Veterinary Kidney Center, Buffalo Grove, Illinois, USA	Animal Critical Care and Emergency Services, Renton, Washington, USA
Louisiana State University, Baton Rouge, Louisiana, USA	University of Wisconsin – Madison, Madison, Wisconsin, USA
VCA Boston Road Animal Hospital, Springfield, Massachusetts, USA	Ontario Veterinary College, University of Guelph, Guelph, Ontario, Canada
South America	
Renal Vet- Bauru, Bauru, São Paulo, Brazil	Renal Vet – Santos, Santos, Brazil
Renal Vet Ribeirao Preto, Ribeirao Preto, Brazil	Renal Vet – Sorocaba, Sorocaba, Brazil
Canne & Gatto Small Animal Hospital, Rio de Janeiro, Brazil	Renal Vet – Uberlandia, Uberlandia, Brazil
Renal Vet São Paulo, São Paulo, Brazil	Renal Vet Medellin – Colombia, Medellin, Colombia
Asia/Australia	
Greencross Vets Ku-Ring-Gai, Sydney, Australia	Manhattan Veterinary Hospital, Taipei, Taiwan
Greencross Vets South Tamworth Animal Hospital, South Tamworth, Australia	National Taiwan University Veterinary Hospital, Taipei, Taiwan
Chungnam National University Veterinary Medicine Teaching Hospital, Daejeon, Korea	Kasetsart University Faculty of Veterinary Medicine, Bangkok, Thailand
Matsubara Animal Hospital, Osaka, Japan	

22.10 Veterinary dialysis units.

Summary

With modern technology and techniques, dialysis is technically feasible, safe, efficacious and indispensable for the management of both dogs and cats with life-threatening uraemia. Haemodialysis is an outstanding bridging mechanism that often permits life-saving repair of renal injury in patients when no other therapeutic options exist, but clients must understand that dialysis does not 'fix' damaged kidneys. The prognosis and duration of therapy vary tremendously from patient to patient and depend on the aetiology and degree of renal insult, as well as patient condition and comorbidities.

References and further reading

Bagshaw SM, Bellomo R and Kellum JA (2008) Oliguria, volume overload, and loop diuretics. *Critical Care Medicine* **36**, S172–S178

Beckel NF, O'Toole TE, Rozanski EA and Labato MA (2005) Peritoneal dialysis in the management of acute renal failure in 5 dogs with leptospirosis. *Journal of Veterinary Emergency and Critical Care* **15**, 201–205

Bouman C, Oudemans-Van Straaten HM *et al.* (2002) Effects of early high-volume continuous venovenous hemofiltration on survival and recovery of renal functions in intensive care patients with acute renal failure: a prospective, randomized trial. *Critical Care Medicine* **30**, 2205–2211

Cooper RL and Labato MA (2011) Peritoneal dialysis in cats with acute kidney injury: 22 cases (2001–2006). *Journal of Veterinary Internal Medicine* **25**, 14–19

Crisp MS, Chew DJ, DiBartola SP and Birchard SJ (1989) Peritoneal dialysis in dogs and cats: 27 cases (1976–1987). *Journal of the American Veterinary Medical Association* **195**, 1262–1266

Cruz D, Bobek I, Lentini P *et al.* (2009) Machines for continuous renal replacement therapy. *Seminars in Dialysis* **22**, 123–132

Diehl SH and Seshadri R (2008) Use of continuous renal replacement therapy for treatment of dogs and cats with acute or acute-on-chronic renal failure: 33 cases (2002–2006). *Journal of Veterinary Emergency and Critical Care* **18**, 370–383

Dorval P and Boysen SR (2009) Management of acute renal failure in cats using peritoneal dialysis: a retrospective study of six cases (2003–2007). *Journal of Feline Medicine and Surgery* **11**, 107–115

Gettings L, Reynolds HN and Scalea T (1999) Outcome in post-traumatic acute renal failure when continuous renal replacement therapy is applied early *versus* late. *Intensive Care Medicine* **25**, 805–813

Langston CE (2011) Hemodialysis. In: *Nephrology and Urology of Small Animals*, ed. JW Bartges and DJ Polzin, pp. 255–285. Wiley-Blackwell Publishing, Ames

Liu KD, Himmelfarb J, Paganini EP *et al.* (2006) Timing of initiation of dialysis in critically ill patients with acute kidney injury. *Clinical Journal of the American Society of Nephrology* **1**, 915–919

Chapter 23

Management of chronic kidney disease

Rosanne Jepson and Harriet Syme

For patients that develop chronic kidney disease (CKD), the underlying aetiology may never be identified. Irrespective of the inciting injury, the histopathological response to injury in the kidney is the same, and tubulo-interstitial nephritis and fibrosis with variable degrees of secondary glomerulosclerosis and mineralization are usually identified. Having made a diagnosis (see Chapter 10) and staged a patient with CKD (see Chapter 12), the goals of managing CKD are to slow or halt progression to end-stage disease, to reduce the frequency of episodes of uraemic crisis, and to manage any secondary complications associated with CKD, whilst ensuring quality of life for both the patient and the owner. With any intervention, careful monitoring is required to ensure that the benefits of treatment outweigh adverse effects and enable the veterinary surgeon (veterinarian) to respond and modify treatment as necessary based on the individual patient.

Factors associated with progression of CKD

A number of different factors have been implicated in the progression of CKD. An appreciation of these factors is important in order to understand the rationale for therapeutic interventions that are recommended for the management of patients with CKD where the goal is to slow progression.

Mineral and bone disorder

Mineral and bone disorder (MBD) is the term which is now used in place of renal secondary hyperparathyroidism and this is discussed in greater detail in Chapter 11. This change in terminology reflects the advances in our understanding of the regulatory hormones, which become activated as renal function declines prior to the development of azotaemia.

In CKD, as nephrons are lost and renal function declines, the ability of the kidney to excrete phosphorus decreases. Alteration in calcium and phosphorus homeostasis drives a series of pathophysiological events that stimulate the production of fibroblast growth factor 23 (FGF-23) and subsequently parathyroid hormone (PTH), and result in a relative deficiency in 1,25-dihydroxycholecalciferol (calcitriol). Increased production of PTH and FGF-23, at least in the early stages of CKD (International

Renal Interest Society (IRIS) Stage 1 and 2), maintain normophosphataemia by increasing the capacity of remaining nephrons to excrete phosphate. However, in the later stages of CKD (azotaemic IRIS CKD Stage 2, IRIS CKD Stages 3 and 4), when there is a further reduction in the capacity of the kidney to excrete phosphate, hyperphosphataemia develops.

If a high calcium × phosphate product exists (>6 $mmol^2/l^2$ or 70 mg^2/dl^2), the patient is at risk of metastatic mineralization of soft tissues, including the kidneys, which may lead to progression of CKD. In addition, the chronic action of PTH on bone can result in the development of renal osteodystrophy, and PTH itself is considered to be a uraemic toxin. Methods to reduce the incidence and severity of MBD are therefore advantageous in slowing the progression of CKD. Control of PTH, FGF-23 and phosphate concentrations can be achieved in most CKD patients by introducing a phosphate-restricted prescription renal diet, either alone or in combination with oral phosphate binders. In certain situations calcitriol therapy may be considered.

Systemic hypertension

The kidney is one of the main target organs for hypertensive damage, and the association between systemic hypertension and the kidney is discussed in Chapter 18. Renal autoregulation is the capacity of the kidney to regulate renal blood flow independently of systolic blood pressure and occurs as a result of the myogenic properties of the vessel walls and tubuloglomerular feedback. Autoregulation of pressure within the afferent arteriole supplying each glomerulus ensures stable glomerular capillary pressure, glomerular filtration and hence glomerular filtration rate (GFR). However, autoregulation only occurs within a certain range of mean systemic arterial pressures (70–150 mmHg). Outside this systemic pressure range, autoregulation is no longer able to maintain stable glomerular capillary pressures. In patients with systemic hypertension, high pressures entering the afferent arteriole will be transferred to the glomerular capillary network, resulting in glomerular hypertension, damage to the glomerulus (glomerulosclerosis) and secondary proteinuria. Systemic hypertension can therefore contribute to the progression of kidney disease, not only through direct damage to the glomerular architecture but also through proteinuria (see below). The diagnosis (see Chapter 15) and control of systemic hypertension (see Chapter 18) are fundamental to management of CKD.

Proteinuria

Patients with tubulointerstitial nephritis typically only have a low level of proteinuria, which occurs predominantly as a consequence of reduced tubular absorption of filtered proteins (see Chapter 5), although in those patients with glomerular injury, increased filtration of proteins may also play a role. *In vitro* studies suggest that protein processing by proximal tubular cells can result in increased production of pro-inflammatory mediators (e.g. interleukin (IL)-6, transforming growth factor (TGF)-beta, IL-8, monocyte chemoattractant protein), which may promote tubulointerstitial inflammation. Large-scale studies in human patients with CKD indicate that control of proteinuria is beneficial in terms of improving survival and reducing progression of kidney disease. It is hypothesized that similar benefits may be appreciated in cats and dogs, although direct experimental evidence, or evidence from randomized controlled clinical trials assessing the progression of CKD, is not available to support this hypothesis. Treatment of proteinuria includes provision of a reduced protein diet, polyunsaturated fatty acid (PUFA) supplementation and pharmacological reduction in glomerular capillary pressure.

Hypoxia, hypoperfusion and ischaemia

Hypoxia, hypoperfusion and ischaemia may contribute to the progression of CKD. The kidney generally and the tubular cells in particular have a high level of metabolic activity. Hypoxia can occur as a result of:

- Reduced perfusion of the renal parenchyma secondary to hypovolaemia/dehydration
- Alteration in renal haemodynamics
- Reduced oxygen delivery due to chronic anaemia.

The architecture of the blood supply to the kidney means that, in health, the renal medulla operates at a low oxygen tension and is particularly susceptible to hypoxia. With loss of nephrons, a haemodynamic response occurs in order to maintain and increase GFR in the remaining nephrons. This haemodynamic response includes vasoconstriction of the efferent arteriole in order to preserve glomerular capillary pressures and hence GFR. However, glomerular injury and vasoconstriction of the efferent arteriole can lead to decreased post-glomerular peritubular capillary blood flow. This may exacerbate hypoxia in the renal medulla, where tubular cells are dependent on oxygen delivery by diffusion. Angiotensin II is the main mediator of this efferent arteriolar vasoconstriction and is also a direct stimulus for oxidative stress. Increase in inflammatory cell numbers and fibrosis between the peritubular capillaries and tubular cells may also impair oxygen diffusion, contributing to hypoxia.

Oxidative stress is the imbalance that occurs between the production of reactive oxygen species (ROS) (e.g. the hydroxyl radical, superoxide anions) and antioxidant mechanisms which can be either enzymatic (e.g. superoxide dismutase, catalase, nitric oxide synthase) or non-enzymatic (e.g. glutathione, vitamins E and C). ROS are highly reactive, causing damage to cellular structures such as lipids, proteins, DNA and carbohydrates. This can lead to structural and functional changes that ultimately result in cellular apoptosis, necrosis and inflammation. In CKD, a number of stimuli including angiotensin II, ageing, tubular hypermetabolism, proteinuria and hypoxia can all stimulate the production of ROS, with oxidative stress being compounded by a relative deficiency in antioxidants (Brown, 2008).

Few published studies have evaluated oxidative stress and hypoxia in either canine or feline CKD but there is preliminary evidence that oxidative stress does occur in feline CKD (Keegan and Webb, 2010). Chronic non-regenerative anaemia is identified in approximately 20% of dogs and cats with CKD and is more evident as kidney disease progresses. This chronic anaemia is typically considered to be due to reduced erythropoietin production, although other factors such as subclinical gastrointestinal bleeding, reduced red blood cell lifespan, red cell fragility and iron deficiency may also contribute. Population studies in cats have identified that a low haematocrit is associated with survival and the progression of CKD. Anaemia not only contributes to renal hypoxia but is also likely to have a substantial impact on activity levels and quality of life in patients in the later stages of CKD. In both canine and feline patients with CKD, chronic dehydration and hypovolaemia can contribute to reduced renal perfusion and hence hypoxia. In addition, the presence of chronic dehydration can have an important impact on quality of life, in particular on activity levels and development of constipation. Methods for managing hypoxia and oxidative stress include ensuring adequate hydration to prevent periods of dehydration and hypovolaemia, antioxidant and PUFA supplementation and administration of erythrocyte-stimulating agents when required.

Treatment and management strategies for patients with CKD

Nutritional management and control of MBD

Nutritional management goals

The clinical goals associated with nutrition in patients with CKD are to maintain bodyweight, to maintain muscle and body condition, and to ensure continued calorie intake while providing all required nutrients. Substantial morbidity in patients with CKD relates to malnutrition and inadequate attention to nutritional intake. Reduced appetite can be a particular problem in both cats and dogs in IRIS CKD Stages 3 and 4, as a consequence of the nausea and vomiting associated with uraemia, although other factors, for example dental disease and uraemic stomatitis, may play a role. Inadequate caloric intake can result in catabolism, with loss of body condition and weight. Nutrition in all patients with CKD therefore requires careful consideration. Recording of bodyweight, body condition score and muscle condition score is recommended at every visit so that any decline can be documented and, where possible, rectified through alteration in management.

Prescription renal diets are widely advocated for both dogs and cats diagnosed with CKD. The rationale for introduction of a renal diet and the appropriate IRIS stage for introduction of these diets are discussed later (see 'Suggested management protocols'). Any dietary change in cats and dogs with CKD should be made gradually to allow acceptance of the diet, typically over a period of 1–2 weeks. Acceptance of dietary change is often easier in the early stages of CKD while the appetite remains good. In those patients with later stage CKD, the transition to a renal diet may need to be made more gradually (e.g. over 3–6 weeks). While the goal in transitioning to a prescription renal diet should be that the patient eats the renal diet exclusively, in some instances this cannot be achieved. In this scenario, the patient may accept the prescription renal diet when it is mixed with a small volume of their regular diet, or a senior diet. Particularly in cats, selection and alternation of a variety of different commercial renal diets, in terms of both flavour and composition (i.e. dry *versus* wet diets), can be beneficial to encourage adequate intake.

Many renal diets are calorie dense, which can be advantageous for the CKD patient with a reduced appetite in order to maintain caloric intake. However, supportive measures such as gastroprotectant therapy, anti-emetics, appetite stimulants and nutritional support (via an oesophageal or percutaneous endoscopic gastrostomy (PEG) tube) may need to be considered (see 'Additional therapies') in patients whose appetite remains poor or where there is concern about either a gradual decline in body condition or malnutrition (see Figure 23.7). Both dry and wet prescription renal diet formulations are available and there is no evidence that one is superior to the other.

Prescription renal diets

Protein reduction: Catabolism of protein from the diet contributes to the production of nitrogenous waste products, which have been implicated as uraemic toxins contributing to the clinical signs of uraemia. The ideal amount of protein that should be fed to patients with CKD is unknown. However, protein reduction is advocated in order to ameliorate the clinical signs associated with uraemia, which are usually seen in patients in the later stages of CKD (IRIS CKD Stages 3 and 4). The benefit of protein reduction in patients with early CKD (IRIS CKD Stage 1 and 2) prior to the onset of clinical signs of uraemia is less clear, and to date it has not been confirmed that protein reduction itself slows progression of CKD in the early stages of disease. However, protein reduction does play a role in modulating proteinuria, which may be beneficial in patients with IRIS CKD Stages 1 and 2 that are suspected to have primary glomerular disease and where persistent proteinuria has been demonstrated.

Phosphate restriction: Control of MBD (previously referred to as renal secondary hyperparathyroidism) can be achieved through introduction of a prescription renal diet. Such diets are markedly phosphate restricted in comparison with commercially available adult diets, with phosphate restriction being achieved in these diets by protein reduction.

In cats with IRIS CKD Stages 2 and 3, studies have demonstrated that introduction of a prescription renal diet is associated with improved survival, and in dogs with IRIS CKD Stages 3 and 4, feeding a prescription renal diet has been associated with both reduced occurrence of episodes of uraemic crisis and reduced renal-related mortality. However, it is important to appreciate that the compositional changes in a prescription renal diet not only reflect reduced phosphate intake, but also reduced protein intake, mild sodium restriction and supplementation of PUFA. Renal diets for cats are also often potassium supplemented. While it is considered likely that the significant differences identified in survival are the consequence of phosphate restriction, these additional dietary modifications must be taken into consideration when interpreting these studies.

In patients with IRIS CKD Stages 2, 3 and 4 that demonstrate hyperphosphataemia, it is anticipated that introduction of a phosphate-restricted diet will significantly reduce phosphate, PTH and FGF-23 concentrations, although the latter two parameters are rarely monitored in clinical practice. No change in creatinine concentration should be expected with introduction of a renal diet.

A recent study has evaluated the effect of introduction of a prescription phosphate-restricted renal diet to cats in IRIS CKD Stage 2 that are normophosphataemic. This study demonstrated that, while phosphate and PTH concentrations remain unchanged, FGF-23 concentrations (which were elevated at baseline) significantly decreased with the introduction of a renal diet. This indicates that the early increase in FGF-23 is likely to be a determinant of maintaining normal phosphate concentrations in these cats and that introduction of a phosphate-restricted renal diet has an impact on phosphate homeostasis even if changes in serum phosphorus concentration cannot be appreciated on a routine biochemical profile (Geddes *et al.*, 2013). The clinical impact of an early introduction of a renal diet in cats (i.e. before the onset of azotaemia) in terms of improvement in survival requires further study.

Commercially available senior diets tend to have a phosphate content that falls between that of an adult maintenance and a prescription renal diet, and therefore may be a second choice of diet for those patients who refuse to eat a prescription renal diet. However, this approach is unlikely to maintain normophosphataemia adequately for patients that initially present with hyperphosphataemia or with more advanced CKD (IRIS CKD Stages 3 and 4).

Introduction of a prescription renal diet should be carefully monitored both in terms of the patient's nutritional status and also in relation to the IRIS targets for phosphate control (Figures 23.1 and 23.2). Based on the available evidence, the target for phosphate control is not only to achieve a plasma phosphate concentration within the reference interval but also, in those patients with IRIS CKD Stage 2 and 3, for the phosphate concentration to be at the lower end of the reference interval. Patients should have a repeat plasma phosphate assessed approximately 4–6 weeks after introduction of a renal diet. For patients with IRIS CKD Stage 2, transition to a phosphate-restricted renal diet may be sufficient to return plasma phosphate concentrations to within the IRIS target. However, for those patients in IRIS CKD Stages 3 and 4, it is common that dietary management alone will be insufficient and addition of oral phosphate binders will be required (see below).

Polyunsaturated fatty acids: Many of the prescription renal diets are supplemented with omega-3 PUFA with the goal of altering the balance towards reduced production of inflammatory prostaglandins (e.g. PGE_2) and increased production of prostaglandins with less inflammatory properties (e.g. PGE_3) and reducing oxidative stress. Experimental studies performed in dogs showed that there was a reduction in renal histopathology changes (e.g. glomerulosclerosis, tubulointerstitial fibrosis and inflammation) associated with very high level supplementation of omega-n3 PUFA. However, the benefit of more moderate omega-n3 PUFA supplementation and the optimal ratio of omega-6:omega-3 PUFA has not been established, nor is there evidence that supplementation beyond that already available in prescription renal diets will provide additional benefit to patients with CKD.

IRIS CKD Stage	Phosphate target
2	<1.45 mmol/l (<4.5 mg/dl)
3	<1.6 mmol/l (<5 mg/dl)
4	<1.9 mmol/l (<6 mg/dl)

23.1 International Renal Interest Society (IRIS) targets for phosphate regulation.

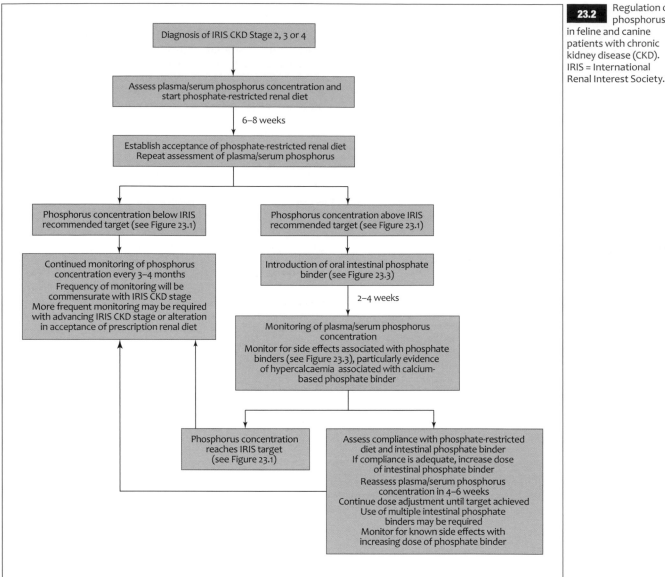

23.2 Regulation of phosphorus in feline and canine patients with chronic kidney disease (CKD). IRIS = International Renal Interest Society.

Potassium supplementation: Both dogs and cats with CKD can develop hypokalaemia although clinical manifestations of hypokalaemia are more commonly appreciated in cats. Hypokalaemia develops owing to increased urinary excretion, reduced dietary intake and activation of the renin–angiotensin–aldosterone system (RAAS). In cats in particular, hypokalaemia can have a marked impact on quality of life because of the associated muscle weakness, but hypokalaemia has also been reported to have a negative impact on renal function and to be associated with progression of tubulointerstitial nephritis in experimental rodent studies.

Prescription renal diets are supplemented with potassium in order to try and prevent the development of clinically significant hypokalaemia. However, in some patients, additional parenteral potassium supplementation may be required (potassium gluconate or potassium citrate 1–2 mmol/kg orally q24h). When potassium supplementation is started, serum potassium concentrations should be reassessed in approximately 2–4 weeks to ensure normalization of potassium concentrations.

The presence of severe persistent hypokalaemia and an inadequate response to potassium supplementation should prompt clinical assessment for concurrent conditions that could be contributing to hypokalaemia (e.g.

hyperaldosteronism). Rarely, patients with IRIS CKD Stage 4 receiving prescription renal diets may develop hyperkalaemia. This is more likely to occur in patients receiving enteral nutrition via a feeding tube that ensures caloric requirements are met, and/or those receiving additional potassium-sparing medications (e.g. aldosterone inhibitors, angiotensin receptor blockers or angiotensin converting enzyme inhibitors) and clinically is appreciated more often in the dog than the cat.

Metabolic acidosis: Metabolic acidosis has been associated with protein catabolism, uraemia and skeletal and cardiovascular effects in CKD. It is uncommon in the early stages of CKD but has been reported in up to 50% of cats with clinical signs of uraemia. Prescription renal diets are alkalinizing and it is rare for additional alkalinizing therapy to be warranted. Indeed, evidence that alkalinizing therapy will have a significant clinical impact in either cats or dogs is lacking.

Current IRIS treatment guidelines recommend that, in the patient with persistent marked acidosis after stabilization on a renal diet (dog: bicarbonate (HCO_3^-) <18 mmol/l; cat: HCO_3^- <16 mmol/l), additional oral alkalinizing therapy can be used (sodium bicarbonate 8–12 mg/kg orally q8h, potassium citrate 2 mmol/kg orally q12h) to maintain HCO_3^-

between 18 and 24 mmol/l. In cats, the use of potassium citrate may offer the combined benefit of treating acidosis and hypokalaemia concurrently. Venous blood gases should be reassessed 10–14 days after initiating supplementation.

Sodium restriction: There is limited evidence regarding the role of sodium restriction and its effect on renal function. Diets that are excessively sodium restricted may result in stimulation of the RAAS. Most commercially available renal diets are mildly sodium restricted, and further modification of sodium intake is therefore not required. High-sodium diets should be avoided.

Antioxidants and vitamin supplementation: Oxidative stress is a key mechanism that may contribute to the development and progression of CKD, although evidence to document this specifically in veterinary medicine is lacking. Prescription renal diets are frequently supplemented with antioxidants and are formulated to provide vitamin requirements. There is no current evidence that supplementation beyond that provided by a prescription renal diet is beneficial.

Additional measures for control of mineral and bone disorder

Oral phosphate binders: For those patients in IRIS CKD Stages 2, 3 and 4 where introduction of a phosphate-restricted renal diet does not allow IRIS targets for serum phosphate to be reached (see Figures 23.1 and 23.2), addition of an oral phosphate binder is recommended. Oral phosphate binders complex with dietary phosphate, preventing absorption of phosphate from the intestinal tract. It is therefore imperative that phosphate binders are administered with food and at every meal. Commonly used phosphate binders are listed in Figure 23.3. Several of the available phosphate binders contain calcium. Care should be taken when these phosphate binders are prescribed that the patient does not have evidence of hypercalcaemia. This is particularly important in cats, where both idiopathic hypercalcaemia and hypercalcaemia associated with CKD may be present. Plasma phosphate concentrations should be monitored 2–4 weeks after starting an oral phosphate binder and the dose of binder gradually titrated

upwards until the required IRIS target is achieved. The palatability of oral phosphate binders is universally poor in patients with advanced CKD and adequate administration to reach the target may require feeding tube placement.

In patients that will not tolerate a prescription renal diet it has been anecdotally advocated that use of a phosphate binder alone (i.e. used with the maintenance diet) may be beneficial. However, the high phosphate content of maintenance canine and feline diets means that prohibitively large quantities of phosphate binder would be required in order to achieve phosphate targets for azotaemic CKD patients. A single study has evaluated the use of a maintenance diet with or without chitosan/calcium carbonate in cats with IRIS CKD Stage 1 and 2 (Brown et al., 2008). This study demonstrated that mean serum phosphorus and PTH concentrations were significantly lower in cats that received the phosphate binder. However, it should be recognized that the cats included in this study represented cats with only very mild CKD. While recognizing that renal diets have other potential beneficial effects in addition to phosphate restriction, for cats with IRIS CKD Stages 1 and 2 that have borderline phosphate concentrations, the use of an intestinal phosphate binder may be of some benefit. However, it is unlikely that management of cats with more severe CKD (IRIS CKD Stage 3 or 4) and evidence of hyperphosphataemia with intestinal phosphate binders alone will be successful. In this scenario every attempt should be made to encourage consumption of a renal diet to which phosphate binders can be added.

Calcitriol therapy: As part of the mineral and bone disorder complex (previously referred to as renal secondary hyperparathyroidism), a decrease in 1,25-dihydroxycholecalciferol (calcitriol) may be present. The enzyme 1-alpha-hydroxylase, which is found in the kidney, is required for the conversion of 25-hydroxycholecalciferol to active calcitriol. Increased concentrations of phosphate and FGF-23 have a direct inhibitory action on the activity of 1-alpha-hydroxylase, again reducing the production of calcitriol. A decrease in calcitriol therefore occurs as a consequence of both reduced functional renal mass, which leads to a decrease in the availability of 1-alpha-hydroxylase, and the decreased activity of 1-alpha-hydroxylase itself.

Drug	Dosage	Comment
Aluminium hydroxide	30–90 mg/kg orally q24h in divided doses with each meal	• Can cause constipation • High dose: neurological aluminium toxicity
Chitosan and calcium carbonate	1 g/5 kg orally q12h with each meal	• Can cause constipation • Monitor for hypercalcaemia
Calcium carbonate	30–90 mg/kg orally q24h in divided doses with each meal	• Can cause constipation • Monitor for hypercalcaemia • Efficacy influenced by pH
Calcium acetate	60–90 mg/kg orally q24h in divided doses with each meal	• Can cause constipation • Efficacy less influenced by pH • Monitor for hypercalcaemia
Lanthanum carbonate octahydrate	400–800 mg/cat orally q24h in divided doses with each meal	• Also contains kaolin and vitamin E • Gastrointestinal side effects above recommended dose range
Lanthanum carbonate	12.5–25 mg/kg orally q24h in divided doses with each meal	• Gastrointestinal side effects above recommended dose range
Sevelamer hydrochloride	90–160 mg/kg orally q24h in divided doses with each meal	• Pills are hygroscopic • Can cause constipation • Expensive • Reported efficacy is poor

23.3 Commonly used intestinal phosphate binders. Note that these products are marketed as food supplements rather than drugs and as such are not covered by the prescribing cascade. Ideally, phosphate binders should be mixed with the food rather than administered directly to the animal.

This cascade of events can be partially ameliorated by feeding a phosphate-restricted diet, but additional benefit may be gained from calcitriol administration. Calcitriol acts to increase calcium and phosphate absorption from the intestinal tract and to inhibit PTH production. Based on current evidence, calcitriol therapy may be of benefit to dogs in IRIS CKD Stage 3 or 4 and may improve demeanor and increase appetite, activity and survival (Nagode et al., 1996; de Brito Galvao et al., 2013). Currently, data supporting a beneficial effect of calcitriol therapy in cats are not available and therefore calcitriol therapy, although anecdotally used by some clinicians, is not currently recommended by IRIS.

Calcitriol therapy in dogs requires careful and frequent monitoring of plasma or serum phosphate, ionized calcium and PTH concentrations, and it should never be considered in patients where phosphate targets have not been met or cannot be maintained, or in patients with documented ionized hypercalcaemia. Development of hypercalcaemia associated with the administration of calcitriol can result in renal mineralization and progression of renal injury. Figure 23.4 outlines a protocol for initiating and monitoring calcitriol therapy. Calcitriol must be administered life-long for clinical benefits to be appreciated. Calcitriol therapy has been challenging owing to a lack of appropriately sized formulations. Compounding pharmacies are routinely used in some countries to facilitate calcitriol administration.

Control of systemic hypertension

Systemic hypertension is a common complication of CKD and may itself promote glomerulosclerosis and proteinuria. Anti-hypertensive agents should always be provided for patients that are diagnosed with systemic hypertension, and this is a life-long therapy. The measurement of blood pressure is discussed in Chapter 15 and the association between hypertension and the kidney and treatment of systemic hypertension are presented in Chapter 18. In the cat, the first-line anti-hypertensive agent is the L-type calcium channel blocker amlodipine besylate, to which most cats demonstrate an excellent response. Second-line anti-hypertensive agents, when required, include angiotensin-converting enzyme inhibitors (ACEi) and angiotensin receptor blockers (ARBs). Management of systemic hypertension in the dog is more challenging because the response to either ACEi or amlodipine besylate is typically poor. Multimodal anti-hypertensive therapy is therefore frequently required in the dog.

Irrespective of the anti-hypertensive agent used, all patients require careful monitoring of blood pressure, typically 7–14 days after starting anti-hypertensive therapy or after any dose adjustment. Anti-hypertensive agents should be gradually titrated upwards to reach target blood pressure with the goal of achieving a gradual but persistent decline in blood pressure such that there is reduced risk for ongoing target-organ damage and the risk of hypotension is avoided. The currently recommended target according to the American College of Veterinary Internal Medicine (ACVIM) hypertension guidelines is to reduce systolic blood pressure (SBP) into the normotension (<150 mmHg) or borderline hypertension (151–159 mmHg) categories, which carry a minimal or mild risk of target-organ damage, respectively. There is currently no evidence that lowering dietary sodium concentration will reduce blood pressure in either canine or feline patients. Indeed, sodium restriction may stimulate the RAAS. However, high-sodium diets should be avoided.

Control of proteinuria

In patients that are diagnosed with CKD, proteinuria should be assessed by measuring the urine protein to creatinine ratio (UPC). Samples for UPC assessment may be obtained either by free catch or by cystocentesis although it is imperative to exclude the presence of urinary tract infection, which may sometimes falsely increase UPC values. Intervention for proteinuria is recommended for all IRIS CKD stages if the UPC is persistently >0.4 in cats or >0.5 in dogs on at least two occasions 2–4 weeks apart. Antiproteinuric therapy has three main components: introduction of a reduced protein diet; inhibition of the RAAS; and supplementation with omega-n3 PUFA.

Dietary therapy

There is evidence in patients with primary glomerular disease that protein reduction may alter renal glomerular haemodynamics and therefore reduce proteinuria, although the significance of protein reduction specifically in patients with CKD and primarily tubular disease is less clearly defined. Most azotaemic patients will already be receiving

23.4 The use of daily calcitriol therapy in dogs with IRIS CKD Stages 3 and 4 . CKD = chronic kidney disease; IRIS = International Renal Interest Society; PTH = parathyroid hormone.

a prescription renal diet, which has a reduced protein content. Protein reduction beyond this is not advocated. Non-azotaemic patients with persistent proteinuria should be started on a low-protein prescription renal diet (Figure 23.5).

PUFA supplementation

Omega-n3 PUFA supplementation may aid in the reduction of proteinuria. Most prescription renal diets are supplemented with PUFA. The optimal ratio of omega-n6 to omega-n3 PUFA is unknown, although a ratio of 5:1 is advocated. Patients with non-azotaemic or azotaemic CKD and persistent proteinuria should be started on a prescription renal diet. There is currently no evidence that omega-n3 PUFA supplementation above that provided by commercial renal diets is superior to the use of dietary therapy alone.

RAAS inhibition

The mainstay of anti-proteinuric therapy is inhibition of angiotensin II production or activity. This can either be achieved with ACEi, which reduce conversion of angiotensin I to angiotensin II, or with ARBs, which inhibit the action of angiotensin II at the angiotensin type 1 (AT_1) receptor. Despite hypothetical benefits of the use of ARBs in providing more complete blockade of angiotensin II-mediated effects, clinical data to support this are lacking. In dogs, first-line therapy is usually with an ACEi, given the greater experience with the use of this type of medication (Figure 23.6). However, for the cat, both the ACEi benazepril and the ARB telmisartan are available and authorized in Europe for the management of proteinuria associated with CKD (Figure 23.6).

Careful monitoring is required after introduction of either an ACEi or ARB, which both cause preferential dilation of the efferent arteriole, reduction in glomerular capillary pressure and a decline in glomerular filtration rate. It is anticipated that plasma creatinine concentration will increase after introduction of either medication but this increase is typically <25% of baseline creatinine.

Monitoring of renal function, electrolytes (potassium) and blood pressure is recommended 7–14 days after starting either ACEi or ARB therapy (see Figure 23.5). If an increase in plasma creatinine >25% is noted, the patient develops hyperkalaemia (K^+ >6 mmol/l) or a deterioration in clinical signs is observed, the ACEi or ARB medication

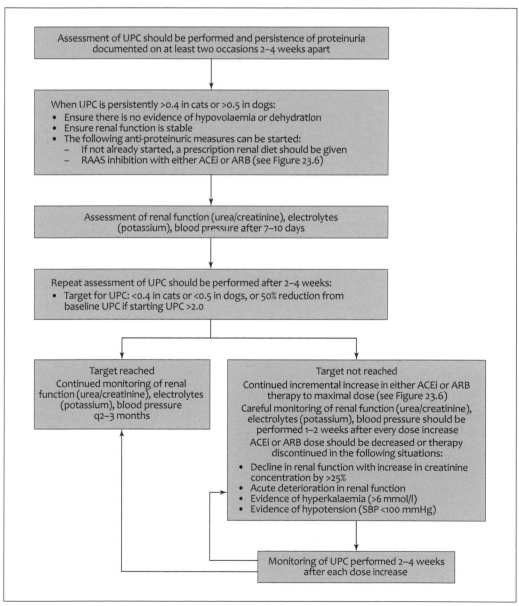

23.5 Management of proteinuria in dogs and cats with confirmed IRIS CKD Stages 1 to 3. ACEi = angiotensin-converting enzyme inhibitor; ARB = angiotensin receptor blocker; RAAS = renin–angiotensin–aldosterone system; SBP = systolic blood pressure; UPC = urine protein to creatinine ratio.

Assessment of UPC should be performed and persistence of proteinuria documented on at least two occasions 2–4 weeks apart

When UPC is persistently >0.4 in cats or >0.5 in dogs:
- Ensure there is no evidence of hypovolaemia or dehydration
- Ensure renal function is stable
- The following anti-proteinuric measures can be started:
  - If not already started, a prescription renal diet should be given
  - RAAS inhibition with either ACEi or ARB (see Figure 23.6)

Assessment of renal function (urea/creatinine), electrolytes (potassium), blood pressure after 7–10 days

Repeat assessment of UPC should be performed after 2–4 weeks:
- Target for UPC: <0.4 in cats or <0.5 in dogs, or 50% reduction from baseline UPC if starting UPC >2.0

Target reached
Continued monitoring of renal function (urea/creatinine), electrolytes (potassium), blood pressure q2–3 months

Target not reached
Continued incremental increase in either ACEi or ARB therapy to maximal dose (see Figure 23.6)
Careful monitoring of renal function (urea/creatinine), electrolytes (potassium), blood pressure should be performed 1–2 weeks after every dose increase
ACEi or ARB dose should be decreased or therapy discontinued in the following situations:
- Decline in renal function with increase in creatinine concentration by >25%
- Acute deterioration in renal function
- Evidence of hyperkalaemia (>6 mmol/l)
- Evidence of hypotension (SBP <100 mmHg)

Monitoring of UPC performed 2–4 weeks after each dose increase

Drug	Drug class	Starting dose	Escalating dose
Benazepril	ACEi (hepatic metabolism) Authorized for the reduction of proteinuria in cats with CKD and for treatment of congestive heart failure in dogs in the UK	0.5 mg/kg orally q24h	Increase daily dose by 0.5 mg/kg to a maximum dose of 2 mg/kg May consider divided dosage
Enalapril	ACEi (renal excretion) Authorized for treatment of dogs with congestive heart failure in dogs in the UK No product authorization for cats	0.5 mg/kg orally q24h	Increase daily dose by 0.5 mg/kg to a maximum dose of 2 mg/kg
Telmisartan	ARB Authorized for the treatment of proteinuria in cats with CKD in the UK No product authorization in dogs	1 mg/kg orally q24h	Increase daily dose by 0.5 mg/kg up to maximum dose of 2 mg/kg
Spironolactone	Aldosterone inhibitor Authorized for use in combination with standard therapy for the treatment of congestive heart failure in dogs in the UK No product authorization for cats Facial excoriations may be seen as a side effect in cats	1–2 mg/kg orally q12h	–

23.6 Agents used in the management of proteinuria. ACEi = angiotensin-converting enzyme inhibitor; ARB = angiotensin-receptor blocker; CKD = chronic kidney disease.

should be discontinued or the dose reduced, depending on the patient's clinical status and the severity of the abnormality detected. ACEi and ARB therapy should be used with extreme caution in patients with IRIS CKD Stage 3 or greater. Their use in IRIS CKD Stage 3 should be reserved for those patients where stable renal function has been documented. ACEi and ARB should be used with extreme caution in patients with IRIS CKD Stage 4 and their use should be avoided in patients with acute kidney injury (AKI), dehydration and/or hypovolaemia where preservation of renal function may be RAAS-dependent. Proteinuria should be monitored 3–4 weeks after starting an ACEi or ARB by repeat assessment of UPC. Dose increments in either ACEi or ARB can be made providing renal function remains stable and hyperkalaemia and/or hypotension are not observed.

The target for control of proteinuria is dependent on the severity of proteinuria at diagnosis. In those patients with mild proteinuria (UPC <2.0), the goal of therapy should be a UPC <0.4 (cat) or <0.5 (dog). However, for patients with severe proteinuria (UPC >2.0), a minimum of 50% reduction in baseline UPC should be the goal (see Figure 23.5). In both cats and dogs with mild to moderate proteinuria (UPC <2.0), monotherapy with either an ACEi or an ARB is usually sufficient to control proteinuria. It has been hypothesized that the combined use of an ACEi and an ARB can afford a greater degree of RAAS blockade as a consequence of the different modes of action of these drugs. For individual patients with marked proteinuria attributable to primary glomerular disease, when gradual up-titration of monotherapy has failed to provide adequate control of proteinuria, the combined use of an ACEi and an ARB has been reported (Bugbee et al., 2014) and may be beneficial in terms of controlling proteinuria. However, in human medicine, large-scale studies comparing monotherapy with the use of dual ACEi and ARB RAAS blockade in patients with CKD and diabetic nephropathy have demonstrated an increased risk of adverse effects (e.g. AKI and hyperkalaemia) without significant benefit in terms of cardiovascular or renal morbidity (Gentile et al., 2015). Without an appropriate evidence base of superiority, the routine use of combined ACEi and ARB is currently not recommended for cats and dogs with CKD.

Additional therapies

Gastroprotectants

Gastrin is one of the determinants of gastric acid secretion and undergoes renal excretion. Cats and dogs with reduced renal function develop hypergastrinaemia which, for a long time, has been considered to contribute to the development of a uraemic gastropathy and secondary nausea, vomiting, reduced appetite and weight loss. Recently, a study comparing gastric pathology among cats with CKD and non-azotaemic cats has revealed that the most common histopathological abnormalities detected were gastric fibrosis (43%) and gastric mineralization (38%) (McLeland et al., 2014). The cats did not exhibit ulceration, oedema, vascular fibrinoid change or haemorrhage, which have been reported in other species including the dog (McLeland et al., 2014).

Nevertheless, both dogs and cats may benefit from gastroprotectant therapy, including histamine receptor agonists (H_2 blockers) or proton pump inhibitors (PPI; Figure 23.7). Given the lack of histopathological evidence of uraemic gastropathy in cats, it has been suggested that, where medication is challenging and nausea/reduced appetite are believed to be affecting quality of life, prioritization should be given to the use of anti-nausea or appetite-stimulating medications.

Anti-nausea and anti-emetic medication

The combination of uraemic gastropathy and an increase in the circulation of uraemic toxins can lead to nausea and vomiting which may have secondary effects on appetite, weight loss, body condition and quality of life. A number of anti-emetic medications, including metoclopramide, maropitant and ondansetron, are available and can be used on a short- or longer-term basis in patients with CKD (see Figure 23.7). Mirtazapine, a $5\text{-}HT_3$ antagonist, is traditionally considered to be an appetite stimulant but may also have anti-nausea properties (Quimby and Lunn, 2013). A recent study has evaluated the pharmacokinetics of ondansetron, another $5\text{-}HT_3$ antagonist, in healthy cats (Quimby et al., 2014). This study demonstrated that subcutaneous administration results in greater bioavailability and a longer half-life than either intravenous or oral administration. Further studies are required to assess the use of ondansetron in patients with CKD.

Appetite stimulants

In a patient with advancing CKD and the onset of clinical signs of uraemia, the appetite may wax and wane. This may have a substantial impact on acceptance and tolerance of renal or other diets. In such patients, appetite stimulants may be considered (see Figure 23.7).

Mirtazapine is a tricyclic antidepressant with central (presynaptic) alpha-2 adrenoceptor antagonist properties that lead to increased concentrations of noradrenaline (norepinephrine) and 5-hydroxytryptamine (5-HT) within the brain. It is believed to have both anti-emetic and appetite-stimulating effects via inhibition of the 5-HT$_3$ receptor and the histamine H$_1$ receptor. A placebo-controlled cross-over study in young cats has demonstrated the appetite-stimulating properties of this drug at a dose of 1.88 mg/cat. At higher doses (3.75 mg/cat) side effects were appreciated including increased vocalization and activity, hyperexcitability and muscle tremors. The half-life

of mirtazapine in healthy cats is reported to be approximately 10 hours (Quimby et al., 2011b). However, the pharmacokinetics of mirtazapine may be influenced by a number of factors including sex, age and hepatic and renal impairment, the latter two as a consequence of both hepatic and renal excretion of the drug. In a study comparing cats with CKD with age-matched control cats with normal renal function, the half-life of mirtazapine was 15 hours and 12 hours, respectively. Although no concern regarding accumulation was documented in young healthy cats, in cats with CKD drug accumulation is a concern and therefore the current recommendation for cats with CKD is 1.88 mg/cat q48–72h (Quimby et al., 2011a). A placebo-controlled cross-over study showed that cats with CKD receiving mirtazapine demonstrated significantly improved appetite, increased activity levels, had a decreased frequency of vomiting and gained a significant amount of weight compared with when they were receiving placebo (Quimby and Lunn, 2013).

To date, there have been no studies specifically evaluating mirtazapine in dogs with CKD, although it may have the same effect on appetite (at 1.1–1.3 mg/kg orally q24h). Pharmacokinetic studies performed in Beagles suggest

Drug	Mechanism of action	Dose range
Gastroprotectant therapy		
Ranitidine	Histamine (H$_2$) antagonist No veterinary product authorization in dogs and cats in the UK	Dogs: 2 mg/kg slow i.v., s.c., orally q8–12h Cats: 2 mg/kg q24h i.v. constant rate infusion, 2.5 mg/kg slow i.v. q12h, 3.5 mg/kg orally q12h
Cimetidine	Histamine (H$_2$) antagonist Authorized for use in dogs in the UK; not authorized for use in cats	Dogs: 5–10 mg/kg i.v., i.m., orally q8h Cats: 2.5–5 mg/kg i.v., i.m., orally q12h
Famotidine	Histamine (H$_2$) antagonist No veterinary product authorization in dogs and cats in the UK	Dogs and cats: 0.5–1 mg/kg orally q12–24h
Omeprazole	Proton pump inhibitor No product authorization in dogs and cats in the UK (authorized for use in horses)	Dogs: 0.5–1.5 mg/kg i.v., orally q8h for maximum 8 weeks Cats: 0.75–1.0 mg/kg q24h for maximum 8 weeks
Anti-emetic agents		
Maropitant	Neurokinin (NK1) receptor antagonist Authorized for use in dogs and cats in UK for prevention of vomiting and reduction of nausea	Dogs and cats: 1 mg/kg s.c. q24h or 2 mg/kg orally q24h [a]
Metoclopramide	Central dopamine (D$_2$) receptor antagonist and high-dose 5-HT$_3$ antagonist at chemoreceptor trigger zone Authorized for use in dogs and cats for the symptomatic treatment of vomiting in chronic nephritis	Dogs and cats: 0.25–0.5 mg/kg i.v., i.m., s.c., orally q12h or 0.17–0.33 mg/kg i.v., i.m., s.c., orally q8h, or 1–2 mg/kg i.v. over 24 hours as a constant rate infusion
Ondansetron	5-HT$_3$ antagonist with central and peripheral effects No veterinary product authorization for dogs and cats in the UK	Dogs and cats: 0.5 mg/kg i.v. loading dose followed by 0.5 mg/kg/h infusion for 6 hours, or 0.5–1 mg/kg orally q12–24h
Appetite stimulants		
Mirtazapine	Tricyclic antidepressant acting on central alpha-2 receptors. Inhibition of serotonin receptors and histamine (H$_1$) receptors No veterinary product authorization in dogs and cats in the UK	Dogs: 1.1–1.3 mg/kg orally q24h Cats: 1.88–3.75 mg/kg q48–72h Note that mirtazapine and cyproheptadine must not be co-administered Side effects including hyperactivity and increased vocalization have been reported in cats. Dose reduction should be considered if such effects are reported Do not use in patients with pre-existing haematological disease
Cyproheptadine	Histamine (H$_1$) and serotonin antagonist No veterinary product authorization in dogs and cats in the UK	Dogs and cats: 0.1–0.5 mg/kg orally q8–12h Note that mirtazapine and cyproheptadine must not be co-administered Side effects include sedation, polyphagia, weight gain; may reduce seizure threshold

23.7 Commonly used gastroprotectant, anti-emetic agents and appetite stimulants for dogs and cats with chronic kidney disease. [a] The use of oral maropitant in the cat is off-label.

that the metabolism of mirtazapine may be different in dogs from that in cats and humans (Giorgi and Yun, 2012). Use of diazepam is not advocated as an appetite stimulant, particularly in cats, where idiosyncratic reactions can result in irreversible hepatotoxicity.

Assisted feeding

In many patients with advancing CKD, maintaining nutritional support and administering the required medications can become challenging. In such patients, placement of either an oesophageal feeding tube or a PEG tube may provide the means to ensure adequate and appropriate nutrition, maintenance of fluid balance and easy administration of medications. Oesophageal feeding tubes are easily placed and well tolerated long term by many feline patients. Guidance on the placement of both oesophageal and PEG tubes can be found in the *BSAVA Guide to Procedures in Small Animal Practice*.

Erythrocyte-stimulating analogues

Non-regenerative anaemia is reported in approximately 20–30% of feline patients with CKD. Whilst it is uncommon to identify anaemia in cats with IRIS Stage 2 CKD, the prevalence of anaemia increases with IRIS stage and approximately 50% of cats in IRIS Stage 4 CKD will be anaemic. In patients with packed cell volumes (PCV) ≤20% or where anaemia is believed to be having a clinical consequence on quality of life, consideration should be given to the use of erythrocyte-stimulating agents. Dogs may manifest clinical signs attributable to anaemia associated with CKD at a higher PCV (e.g. 25–30%) than cats, which may appear to cope well with mild anaemia. Traditionally, human erythropoietin and synthetic human erythropoietin analogues have been administered. However, approximately 20% of dogs and cats receiving these agents will develop anti-erythropoietin antibodies with the subsequent development of aplastic anaemia, which renders the patients dependent on transfusions.

More recently, a long-acting synthetic human erythropoietin compound, darbepoetin, has been manufactured. Darbepoetin has been modified by the addition of two *N*-linked oligosaccharides. The goal of this modification in human medicine was to reduce the required frequency of administration. The same effect has been reported in cats and dogs but with the additional benefit that the prevalence of anti-erythropoietin antibody production is anecdotally reduced. Despite this, some caution and careful discussion are still required when initiating darbepoetin because long-term blood transfusion therapy in the event of aplastic anaemia is unlikely to be feasible either financially or clinically for most individuals. Other potential side effects of the administration of erythrocyte-stimulating agents include the development of systemic hypertension and polycythaemia. It is important that blood pressure monitoring is considered routine during administration of erythrocyte-stimulating agents.

Studies report that the response to darbepoietin therapy in cats is variable and may be dose-dependent. Although initial reports suggested a darbepoetin dose of 0.5 μg/kg q7 days, it is now widely accepted that a higher starting dose of 1 μg/kg q7 days is more effective. Similar dosing can be used in dogs (1 μg/kg q7 days). Iron supplementation with parenteral iron dextran administration (50 mg/cat i.m. or 10 mg/kg i.m. in dogs) is recommended concurrently with the first administration of darbepoetin. The subsequent requirement for iron supplementation should be based on monitoring of a complete blood count for evidence of iron deficiency (e.g. microcytic hypochromic anaemia), the reticulocyte count and failure to respond to darbepoetin therapy. Evaluation of an iron panel may also be considered. Approximately 60% of cats are reported to show improved regenerative response with darbepoetin therapy. The underlying reason for cats failing to respond is often not identified although some will subsequently respond to an increased dose of darbepoetin (up to 2 μg/kg q7 days). Similar dose increments may be considered for dogs that fail to respond.

Careful monitoring is required with darbepoetin therapy. It is recommended that, as a minimum, the PCV/total protein is monitored on a weekly basis prior to administration. A suggested monitoring protocol for darbepoetin therapy is provided in Figure 23.8.

Maintenance of hydration

Patients with CKD without adequate water intake are predisposed to dehydration due to polyuria. It can be beneficial to increase the patient's water intake through a number of methods. Water intake may be increased by switching to a wet rather than a dry diet, and it has been shown that both cats and dogs will increase water intake following an increase in the frequency of feeding. Other adjustments, for example the use of water fountains, can be helpful although evidence that such interventions increase water consumption or prevent dehydration is limited.

For patients presenting with uraemia or severe dehydration/hypovolaemia, hospitalization for intravenous fluid therapy may be required. In the longer-term, patients who are demonstrating chronic dehydration or an inability to maintain fluid balance may benefit from subcutaneous fluid administration. Either sodium chloride 0.9% or lactated Ringer's solution may be administered using a butterfly needle, needle and syringe, or a via a needle and giving set. The volume of fluid required and frequency of administration is patient-dependent and the response to administration of subcutaneous fluids should be carefully monitored. However, typically patients will require between 10 and 20 ml/kg, with the frequency ranging between three times per week and daily administration. Particular care should be taken in cats with cardiac disease because volume overload and congestive heart failure can be induced with subcutaneous fluid therapy. Subcutaneous ports have been advocated for repeated administration of subcutaneous fluids. However, failure of ports and localized infection anecdotally limit their utility. If a more permanent method for fluid administration is required, placement of an oesophageal feeding tube or PEG tube should be considered, given the additional benefits of providing sodium-free water, and being able to provide nutritional support and medication without the requirement for frequent tableting.

Urinary tract infections

Urinary tract infection (UTI) is a common complication in both cats and dogs with CKD because of reduced host defense mechanisms. Patients with CKD should have a full urinalysis and ideally urine culture performed at regular intervals (i.e. every 3–4 months) in order to identify occult UTI. It is important to note that, particularly in cats with CKD, clinical signs of bacterial cystitis may not be apparent. Treatment of UTI is discussed in greater detail in Chapter 29 but in all instances appropriate antimicrobial

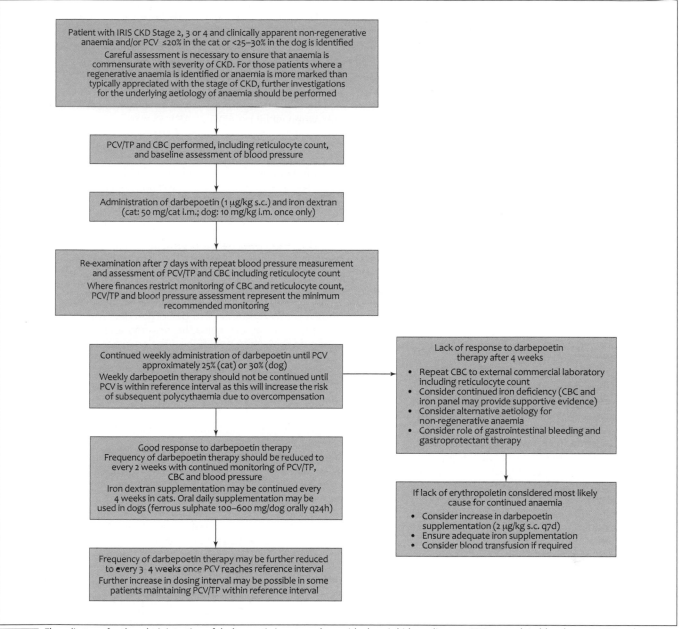

23.8 Flow diagram for the administration of darbepoetin in cats or dogs with chronic kidney disease. CBC = complete blood count; CKD = chronic kidney disease; PCV = packed cell volume; TP= total protein.

therapy should be based on culture and sensitivity results. The duration of antibiotic therapy will vary, depending on the individual patient and whether any complicating factors are present (e.g. the presence/suspicion of pyelonephritis or recurrent infections). Monitoring for successful resolution of the UTI and any improvement in azotaemia is strongly recommended and, particularly in patients with recurrent UTI, repeat culture both during therapy and 1–2 weeks after completion of antibiotic therapy is recommended.

Management according to IRIS CKD stage

The IRIS has published guidelines for the management of both cats and dogs according to their stage of CKD based on plasma creatinine concentrations. These guidelines are evaluated and updated on an annual basis. For the most up-to-date version of the IRIS guidelines please visit www.iris-kidney.com. For all canine and feline patients, certain key recommendations can be made:

- Potentially nephrotoxic drugs should be identified and where possible discontinued
- Pre-renal and/or post-renal abnormalities should be identified and treated:
  - Dehydration and/or hypovolaemia should be corrected with isotonic polyionic replacement fluid therapy (e.g. compound sodium lactate, 0.9% sodium chloride). The route of fluid administration, subcutaneous *versus* intravenous, will be dependent on the patient's presentation and severity of dehydration and/or hypovolaemia as well as client-related factors e.g. finance
- Complicating conditions such as UTIs, pyelonephritis and/or urolithiasis should be identified and treated.

Further recommendations for management and treatment are made on the basis of the severity of CKD and hence IRIS stage. The requirements for supportive management escalate with increasing severity of disease.

Suggested management protocols

Managing patients with IRIS CKD Stage 1

- There is currently no evidence supporting the introduction of a renal diet for cats or dogs with IRIS CKD Stage 1.
- Patients should be carefully assessed for the presence of persistent proteinuria:
  - Dogs and cats with proteinuria should be started on anti-proteinuric therapy including a renal diet and RAAS inhibition with either an ACEi or an ARB. Note that the use of either agent for RAAS inhibition is contraindicated in the presence of dehydration or hypovolaemia, which, when initiating ACEi or ARB therapy, may result in a precipitous decline in GFR and decompensation
  - Low-dose aspirin therapy (1–5 mg/kg orally q24h) should be considered for patients demonstrating protein-losing nephropathy and hypoalbuminaemia (albumin concentration <20 g/l)
  - Careful monitoring with assessment of blood pressure, renal function and electrolytes (potassium) is recommended 1–2 weeks after starting either ACEi or ARB therapy. If decline in renal function (increase in creatinine concentration by >25%), hyperkalaemia or hypotension is identified the dose of ACEi or ARB should be reduced or therapy discontinued
  - The target for anti-proteinuric therapy should be UPC <0.5 (dogs) or <0.4 (cats). For patients with more marked proteinuria at diagnosis a reduction in UPC by 50% from baseline may be a more realistic goal. Gradual dose increase may be required in order to achieve these targets (see Figure 23.5) but should be performed only with careful monitoring of renal function, electrolytes (potassium) and blood pressure.
- Systolic blood pressure (SBP) should be assessed in all dogs and cats with IRIS CKD Stage 1:
  - For those patients with SBP persistently in the IRIS hypertension (AP2; SBP 160–179 mmHg) or severe hypertension (AP3; SBP ≥180 mmHg) category or patients with hypertensive target-organ damage (hypertensive encephalopathy or hypertensive retinopathy/choroidopathy), anti-hypertensive therapy should be initiated. For patients in IRIS CKD Stage 1 care should be taken to ensure that white coat hypertension is not contributing to elevated blood pressure readings
  - Anti-hypertensive therapy and monitoring are discussed in greater detail in Chapter 18.
- Most dogs and cats with IRIS CKD Stage 1 will be clinically asymptomatic. For patients where clinical signs such as decreased appetite, nausea, vomiting, which might be related to uraemia in a more severely azotaemic patient, are identified, an alternative aetiology should be investigated.
- It is rare for patients with IRIS CKD Stage 1 to demonstrate evidence of anaemia. If anaemia is identified, an alternative aetiology other than CKD should be investigated.
- Although polyuria and polydipsia may be identified in patients with IRIS CKD Stage 1 it is uncommon for such patients to demonstrate persistent hypokalaemia. The presence of such a biochemical finding should prompt further investigation for other underlying causes of hypokalaemia.
- Frequency of monitoring of patients with IRIS CKD Stage 1 will depend on the underlying nature of their presentation. For non-proteinuric or borderline proteinuric patients without evidence of systemic hypertension, re-examination on a 6-monthly to annual basis may be adequate, with re-examination prompted sooner should there be a change in the clinical status of the patient. However, for those patients demonstrating either proteinuria or systemic hypertension, re-examination should be commensurate with the severity of their disease process. Once stable, for such patients monitoring every 3–4 months is recommended. Routine monitoring should include physical examination with assessment of bodyweight, body condition, muscle condition, serum biochemistry, packed cell volume with total solids, urinalysis (specific gravity, dipstick, sediment examination, urine culture), UPC ratio and non-invasive blood pressure measurement. Again, more frequent monitoring may be indicated should the patient demonstrate a change in clinical presentation or with any alteration in medical therapy.

Managing patients with IRIS CKD Stage 2

- Dietary management should be recommended for all patients with azotaemic IRIS CKD Stage 2. There is no evidence to support the introduction of a renal diet for non-proteinuric, non-azotaemic patients in IRIS CKD Stage 2. Transition to a renal diet may be more easily accomplished in the earlier stages of disease:
  - With advancing disease and loss of excretory function, the prevalence of hyperphosphataemia increases. Evidence supports phosphate restriction in order to maintain plasma phosphorus <1.45 mmol/l but not < 0.9 mmol/l. Phosphorus restriction should be achieved in patients with azotaemic IRIS CKD Stage 2 through introduction of a renal diet with subsequent monitoring of response to the diet after 6–8 weeks (see Figure 23.2)
  - For most patients in IRIS CKD Stage 2, dietary management alone will be sufficient to control phosphorus concentrations. However, with continued decline in renal function additional intestinal serum phosphate binders may be required, with further monitoring performed after 4–6 weeks. The dose of intestinal phosphate binder required will depend on the severity of renal disease and the phosphate content of the diet. A gradual increase in the dose of intestinal phosphate binders may be required until the target is achieved, with careful monitoring for known adverse effects (see Figures 23.2 and 23.3).
- Patients should be carefully assessed for the presence of persistent proteinuria:
  - Dogs with UPC persistently >0.5 and cats with UPC persistently >0.4 should be started on anti-proteinuric therapy including a renal diet and RAAS inhibition with either an ACEi or an ARB. Note that the use of either

▶

Managing patients with IRIS CKD Stage 2 *continued*

- agent for RAAS inhibition is contraindicated in the presence of dehydration or hypovolaemia, which, when initiating ACEi or ARB therapy, may result in a precipitous decline in GFR and decompensation
- Careful monitoring with assessment of blood pressure, renal function and electrolytes (potassium) is recommended 1–2 weeks after starting either ACEi or ARB therapy. If decline in renal function (increase in creatinine by >25%), hyperkalaemia or hypotension is identified the dose of ACEi or ARB should be reduced or therapy discontinued
- Low-dose aspirin therapy (1–5 mg/kg orally q24h) should be considered for patients demonstrating protein-losing nephropathy and hypoalbuminaemia (albumin <20 g/l)
- The target for anti-proteinuric therapy should be UPC <0.5 (dogs) or <0.4 (cats). For patients with more marked proteinuria at diagnosis a reduction in UPC by 50% from baseline may be a more realistic goal. A gradual dose increase may be required in order to achieve these targets but should be performed only with careful monitoring of renal function, electrolytes (potassium) and blood pressure (see Figure 23.5).
- Systolic blood pressure should be assessed in all dogs and cats with IRIS CKD Stage 2. The approach to the diagnosis, management and monitoring of systemic hypertension is reviewed under IRIS CKD Stage 1 and in Chapter 18.
- Some dogs and cats with early non-azotaemic IRIS CKD Stage 2 will be clinically asymptomatic. However, as azotaemia progresses clinical signs relating to uraemia such as decreased appetite, nausea and vomiting may become apparent. For such patients the use of anti-emetics, gastroprotectants and appetite stimulants may be indicated (see Figure 23.7).
- It is uncommon for patients with IRIS CKD Stage 2 to demonstrate evidence of anaemia. If moderate to severe anaemia is identified, an aetiology other than CKD should be investigated.
- Patients demonstrating hypokalaemia may require supplementation. Supplementation may be achieved through introduction of a renal diet; however, as CKD progresses some patients will require additional oral potassium supplementation. For patients where management of hypokalaemia is challenging despite introduction of a renal diet and oral supplementation, alternative aetiologies for the hypokalaemia (e.g. hyperaldosteronism) should be investigated.
- Patients diagnosed with azotaemic IRIS CKD Stage 2 should be monitored in terms of physical examination, bodyweight, body condition, muscle condition, serum biochemistry, packed cell volume with total protein, urinalysis (specific gravity, dipstick, sediment examination, urine culture), UPC and blood pressure every 3–4 months. More frequent monitoring may be indicated should the patient demonstrate a change in clinical presentation or with any alteration in medical therapy.

Managing patients with IRIS CKD Stage 3

- Dietary management should be recommended for all patients with IRIS CKD Stage 3:
  - Phosphate restriction should be achieved with the introduction of a renal diet with subsequent monitoring of response after 6–8 weeks. For dogs and cats in IRIS CKD Stage 3, a target for phosphate control of 1.6 mmol/l is recommended. In IRIS CKD Stage 3, intestinal phosphate binders are frequently required in order to reach this target, with further monitoring performed 4–6 weeks after introduction. The dose of intestinal phosphate binder required will depend on the severity of renal disease and the phosphate content of the diet. A gradual increase in the dose of intestinal phosphate binders and combined use of intestinal phosphate binders may be required to achieve this target. Careful monitoring for known adverse effects is required (see Figures 23.2 and Figure 23.3)
  - For dogs in IRIS CKD Stage 3, there is evidence that calcitriol therapy prolongs survival. Calcitriol therapy should only be considered in dogs where tight regulation of serum phosphorus has been achieved and when careful monitoring of plasma ionized calcium, phosphorus and PTH concentrations will be feasible. Details regarding calcitriol therapy are provided above and in Figure 23.4. Currently there is no published evidence to support calcitriol therapy in cats.
- Diagnosis and management of systemic hypertension should be performed as for IRIS Stage 1 and described in Chapter 18.
- Diagnosis and management of proteinuria should be performed as for IRIS CKD Stage 2:
  - With advancing CKD, greater caution is required to ensure there is no evidence of dehydration or hypovolaemia at the time that either ACEi or ARB therapy is started. Careful monitoring with assessment of blood pressure, renal function and electrolytes (potassium) is recommended 1–2 weeks after starting either ACEi or ARB therapy. If decline in renal function (increase in plasma creatinine by >25%), hyperkalaemia or hypotension is identified the dose of ACEi or ARB should be reduced or therapy discontinued.
- With advancing CKD, clinical signs relating to uraemia may become more evident. In such patients, supportive therapy including gastroprotectants, anti-emetics and appetite stimulants may be considered (see Figure 23.7).
- For patients demonstrating recurrent episodes of dehydration, introduction of subcutaneous fluid therapy may be beneficial, particularly to prevent uraemic episodes. Additional use of laxative agents may be required for patients with recurrent constipation. The use of feeding tubes for nutritional support, administration of medications and provision of fluid may be considered.
- For patients with persistent hypokalaemia, oral potassium supplementation may be required.
- With continued loss of renal mass and progression of CKD, a non-regenerative anaemia may be identified. In those patients with PCV <20% or clinically affected by anaemia, which may be earlier in dogs (i.e. PCV <25–30%), erythrocyte-stimulating agents may be started. Potential side effects should be carefully discussed (see Figure 23.8).

Managing patients with IRIS CKD Stage 4

- Dietary management should be recommended for all patients with IRIS CKD Stage 4 although acceptance of a renal diet may be variable and challenging:
  - For IRIS Stage 4 CKD patients, a target for phosphate control of 1.9 mmol/l is recommended. With declining renal function, a renal diet alone will less commonly achieve this phosphate target and intestinal phosphate binders will often be required. Serum phosphate concentrations should be reassessed 4–8 weeks after introduction of a phosphate-restricted renal diet and 4–6 weeks after introduction of a phosphate binder. A gradual increase in intestinal phosphate binder dose and combined use of intestinal phosphate binders may be required in order to achieve the recommended target. However, palatability and the development of constipation are frequent limitations in IRIS CKD Stage 4 patients. Patients should be carefully monitored for recognized side effects of intestinal phosphate binders as doses are increased (see Figures 23.2 and 23.3).
- Diagnosis and management of systemic hypertension should be performed as for IRIS CKD Stage 1 and described in Chapter 18. Amlodipine besylate may be preferred as a first-line anti-hypertensive agent in dogs with IRIS CKD Stage 4 in order to avoid use of an ACEi or ARB, which may contribute to decline in GFR.
- Proteinuria should be carefully evaluated in patients and can be managed with the introduction of a low protein renal diet. However, use of ACEi or ARBs is contraindicated in most patients with IRIS CKD Stage 4 due to the potential for decline in GFR and decompensation and the limited evidence that such patients will benefit from the long-term effects of these medications.
- As for IRIS CKD Stage 3, with advancing CKD supportive therapy with gastroprotectants, anti-emetics, appetite stimulants, potassium supplementation and erythrocyte-stimulating agents may be required (see Figures 23.7 and 23.8).
- For patients demonstrating recurrent episodes of dehydration, introduction of subcutaneous fluid therapy may be beneficial, particularly to prevent uraemic episodes. Severe dehydration may more effectively be managed by hospitalization for intravenous fluid therapy. Provided adequate consideration has been given to preventing dehydration, laxative therapy may also be required in those patients demonstrating constipation. The use of feeding tubes for nutritional support, administration of medications and provision of fluid may be considered.

Advanced renal therapies

Renal replacement therapy

Renal replacement therapy can be provided by either continuous renal replacement therapy or intermittent haemodialysis (see Chapter 22). Renal replacement therapy is frequently utilized in human medicine for patients with CKD and end-stage renal disease while awaiting renal transplantation. However, the current availability of chronic dialysis is limited and the associated costs are typically prohibitive for most veterinary patients. For those patients where renal transplantation is considered, short-term haemodialysis may be used to ensure stability of the patient prior to transplantation.

Renal transplantation

Renal transplantation is not currently available in Europe but is performed at certain centres in the USA for cats with CKD. Renal transplantation is typically only considered for cats in late IRIS CKD Stage 3 and IRIS CKD Stage 4, and cats must be free from other systemic and infectious diseases. Post-transplantation acute rejection is prevented by the use of immunosuppression, typically with ciclosporin and prednisolone. Life-long immunosuppression with ciclosporin is required and, despite this, chronic graft rejection is possible. Currently centres in the USA report that 90–95% of cats undergoing renal transplantation are discharged and that 60–70% of the cats remain alive and continue to do well 1 year post-transplantation. A requirement to rehome the donor cat is typically made at American institutions offering renal transplantation in cats. See also the Royal College of Veterinary Surgeons (RCVS) website and RCVS Council (2016) for information about feline renal transplantation in the UK.

Renal transplantation has been performed in dogs but survival in canine patients has been poor. A recent study evaluating 26 dogs undergoing renal transplantation reported a median survival time of 24 days and a 100-day survival probability of 36%. Thromboembolic disease was a frequent cause of mortality (Hopper *et al.*, 2012).

Stem cell therapy

There has been much interest recently in the potential role of stem cell therapy to advance the treatment of patients with CKD but evidence in veterinary medicine is currently sparse. In experimental rodent models of CKD, mesenchymal stem cell therapy has resulted in improvement in renal function with reduced renal fibrosis and glomerulosclerosis. The mechanism by which stem cell therapy causes this beneficial effect is incompletely understood; however, it is likely that paracrine effects (e.g. a reduction in inflammation) are more important than direct incorporation of cells into the nephron.

To date only a limited number of studies have evaluated autologous mesenchymal stem cell therapy in cats (Quimby and Dow, 2016). In the first study, six cats (four healthy and two with CKD) received a single intra-renal injection of autologous bone marrow- or adipose tissue-derived mesenchymal stem cells using ultrasound guidance. No immediate or long-term benefits in terms of renal function were identified with 30 days of follow-up (Quimby *et al.*, 2011c). A subsequent study has evaluated intravenous administration of adipose-derived allogeneic mesenchymal stem cells in a randomized placebo-controlled study (n = 8 cats) (Quimby *et al.*, 2015). However, again no significant alteration in renal function was identified, although the study only extended to 8 weeks and was therefore unable to ascertain whether there would be longer-term benefits of stem cell administration. Further studies are required to understand fully the potential benefits of stem cell therapy for patients with renal disease in veterinary medicine.

Conclusions

The overall goal of managing a patient with CKD is to provide therapies and treatment that will slow the progression of disease while at the same time improving and maintaining the quality of life. An early diagnosis of CKD (see Chapter 10) is fundamental to the management of CKD because damage that occurs to the kidney should be considered irreversible and therefore there is the greatest potential to impact on disease progression if therapies are introduced early in the disease course. In the later stages of disease, quality of life and abrogating the secondary effects of kidney disease become much more important but should always be tailored to the individual requirements of both patient and client.

References and further reading

Bexfield N and Lee K (2014) *BSAVA Guide to Procedures in Small Animal Practice, 2nd edn.* BSAVA Publications, Gloucester

Brown SA (2008) Oxidative stress and chronic kidney disease. *Veterinary Clinics of North America: Small Animal Practice* **38**, 157–166

Brown SA, Rickertsen M and Sheldon S (2008) Effects of an intestinal phosphorus binder on serum phosphorus and parathyroid hormone concentration in cats with reduced renal function. *International Journal of Applied Research in Veterinary Medicine* **6**, 155–160

Bugbee AC, Coleman AE, Wang A, Woolcock AD and Brown SA (2014) Telmisartan treatment of refractory proteinuria in a dog. *Journal of Veterinary Internal Medicine* **28**, 1871–1874

de Brito Galvao JF, Nagode LA, Schenck PA and Chew DJ (2013) Calcitriol, calcidiol, parathyroid hormone, and fibroblast growth factor-23 interactions in chronic kidney disease. *Journal of Veterinary Emergency and Critical Care* **23**, 134–162

Geddes RF, Elliott J and Syme HM (2013) The effect of feeding a renal diet on plasma fibroblast growth factor 23 concentrations in cats with stable azotomic chronic kidney disease. *Journal of Veterinary Internal Medicine* **27(6)**, 1354–1361

Gentile G, Remuzzi G and Ruggenenti P (2015) Dual renin–angiotensin system blockade for nephroprotection: still under scrutiny. *Nephron* **129**, 39–41

Giorgi M and Yun H (2012) Pharmacokinetics of mirtazapine and its main metabolites in Beagle dogs: a pilot study. *The Veterinary Journal* **192**, 239–241

Hopper K, Mehl ML, Kass PH, Kyles AE and Gregory C (2012) Outcome after renal transplantation in 26 dogs. *Veterinary Surgery* **41**, 316–327

Keegan RF and Webb CB (2010) Oxidative stress and neutrophil function in cats with chronic renal failure. *Journal of Veterinary Internal Medicine* **24**, 514–519

McLeland SM, Lunn KF, Duncan CG, Refsal KR and Quimby JM (2014) Relationship among serum creatinine, serum gastrin, calcium-phosphorus product, and uremic gastropathy in cats with chronic kidney disease. *Journal of Veterinary Internal Medicine* **28**, 827–837

Nagode LA, Chew DJ and Podell M (1996) Benefits of calcitriol therapy and serum phosphorus control in dogs and cats with chronic renal failure. Both are essential to prevent or suppress toxic hyperparathyroidism. *Veterinary Clinics of North America: Small Animal Practice* **26**, 1293–1330

RCVS Council (2016) Kidney transplants in cats: RCVS considers its guidance. *Veterinary Record* **178**, 332–334

Quimby JM and Dow SW (2015) Novel treatment strategies for feline chronic kidney disease: A critical look at the potential of mesenchymal stem cell therapy. *The Veterinary Journal* **204(3)**, 241–246

Quimby JM, Gustafson DL and Lunn KF (2011a) The pharmacokinetics of mirtazapine in cats with chronic kidney disease and in age-matched control cats. *Journal of Veterinary Internal Medicine* **25**, 985–989

Quimby JM, Gustafson DL, Samber BJ and Lunn KF (2011b) Studies on the pharmacokinetics and pharmacodynamics of mirtazapine in healthy young cats. *Journal of Veterinary Pharmacology and Therapeutics* **34**, 388–396

Quimby JM, Lake RC, Hansen RJ, Lunghofer PJ and Gustafson DL (2014) Oral, subcutaneous, and intravenous pharmacokinetics of ondansetron in healthy cats. *Journal of Veterinary Pharmacology and Therapeutics* **37**, 348–353

Quimby JM and Lunn KF (2013) Mirtazapine as an appetite stimulant and anti-emetic in cats with chronic kidney disease: a masked placebo-controlled crossover clinical trial. *The Veterinary Journal* **197**, 651–655

Quimby JM, Webb TL, Gibbons DS and Dow SW (2011c) Evaluation of intrarenal mesenchymal stem cell injection for treatment of chronic kidney disease in cats: a pilot study. *Journal of Feline Medicine and Surgery* **13**, 418–426

Quimby JM, Webb TL, Randall E *et al.* (2016) Assessment of intravenous adipose-derived allogeneic mesenchymal stem cells for the treatment of feline chronic kidney disease: a randomized, placebo-controlled clinical trial in eight cats. *Journal of Feline Medicine and Surgery* **18(2)**,165–71

Chapter 24

Management of glomerulopathies

David J. Polzin and Larry D. Cowgill

Glomerular disease is a common and often severe form of kidney disease in dogs. In contrast, it appears to be a relatively uncommon cause of kidney disease in cats. It is often a challenging condition to manage, in part because of limited understanding of the causes of glomerular disease and limited clinical studies on which to develop an evidence-based approach to management. In the absence of adequate evidence-based studies, guidelines for the management of glomerulopathies have been developed on the basis of review of pertinent literature in animals, expert opinion and subsequent validation by a formal consensus methodology (Polzin and Cowgill, 2013; Segev *et al.*, 2013). Here the authors have summarized those recommendations with editorial comment on gaps or modifications in the recommendations since their adoption. The text depicted in this chapter in inverted commas is abstracted directly from the consensus guidelines; the other text and comments are provided in the context of the consensus guidelines but represent the opinions of the authors and may not represent explicitly those of the consensus panels. The recommendations herein are generally intended for application in dogs and are not specifically designed for cats.

Diagnostic approach to glomerular disease

The clinical presentation of glomerular disease occurs as several different pathogenic phenotypes and clinical presentations with the common characteristic of proteinuria. The International Renal Interest Society (IRIS) Consensus Clinical Practice Guidelines for Glomerular Disease in Dogs proposed that 'Tiers be recommended for grouping dogs with glomerular diseases into categories based on major clinical manifestations of the disease to appropriately match diagnostic recommendations to each dog's clinicopathologic circumstances' (Figure 24.1) (Littman *et al.*, 2013). These three tiers are subcategorized further according to the presence or absence of hypertension, clinical complications of hypoalbuminaemia, or concurrent hypoalbuminaemia with azotaemia. The clinical utility of categorizing dogs with glomerular disease into these tiers is that recommendations for therapy can be linked to the patient's specific tier.

Glomerular lesions and proteinuria may develop in many ways. Primary glomerulopathies are diseases in which

Tier I – Persistent renal proteinuria without hypoalbuminaemia or azotaemia

- **Tier I-A** – Persistent subclinical renal proteinuria that is not accompanied by any discernible renal-related signs or sequelae
- **Tier I-B** – Persistent renal proteinuria with hypertension as the only discernable renal-related sign or sequelae, with or without evidence of target-organ damage

Tier II – Renal proteinuria associated with hypoalbuminaemia, but not azotaemia

- **Tier II-A** – Persistent renal proteinuria with hypoalbuminaemia, with or without any of its associated complications or sequelae (mainly oedema and thromboembolic events), but without hypertension or azotaemia
- **Tier II-B** – Persistent renal proteinuria with hypoalbuminaemia, with or without any of its associated complications or sequelae (mainly oedema and thromboembolic events), plus hypertension (with or without evidence of target-organ damage), but without azotaemia

Tier III – Renal proteinuria associated with renal azotaemia

- **Tier III-A** – Renal proteinuria with renal azotaemia but not hypertension or hypoalbuminaemia
- **Tier III-B** – Renal proteinuria with renal azotaemia and hypertension (with or without evidence of target-organ damage), but not hypoalbuminaemia
- **Tier III-C** – Renal proteinuria with renal azotaemia and hypoalbuminaemia, with or without any of its associated complications or sequelae (mainly oedema and thromboembolic events), which often (but not always) are accompanied by hypertension (with or without evidence of target-organ damage)

24.1 Tiers recommended for grouping dogs with glomerular diseases. Apply tier classification criteria after initial patient stabilization, including correction of dehydration, if present.

intrinsic glomerular injury initiates the renal damage. In contrast, secondary glomerulopathies develop consequent to renal tubular, interstitial or whole nephron injury and involve the glomerulus secondarily. Dogs with chronic kidney disease (CKD) arising from renal tubular or whole nephron injury commonly manifest proteinuria in association with glomerular hypertension, hyperfiltration and secondary segmental glomerulosclerosis (Polzin *et al.*, 1988). This last group of dogs, with CKD and secondary glomerular disease, should be managed primarily for CKD (see Chapter 23). Indeed, Tiers III-A and III-B overlap with dogs with CKD and, in fact, dogs with chronic primary glomerular disease may present as having CKD. It may be possible to differentiate primary and secondary glomerular diseases by renal biopsy. However, renal biopsy (see Chapter 13) is usually not recommended for dogs with IRIS CKD Stage 4 or dogs with small kidneys owing to the increased risk of complications and the lower probability of finding reversible lesions.

Discovery of proteinuria is usually the prompt that leads to the diagnostic consideration of glomerular disease. Localization, persistence and magnitude of proteinuria are essential considerations in ascertaining its significance. While proteinuria is the hallmark of glomerular disease, proteinuria *per se* is not always of glomerular origin. It is essential to confirm that proteinuria is primarily of glomerular origin before considering therapy for glomerular disease. Details on confirming the glomerular origin of proteinuria are beyond this discussion and are described elsewhere (Littman *et al.*, 2013) (see Chapter 5).

For the purpose of staging dogs with glomerular disease into the appropriate tier and seeking possible clues as to the origin (causation) and type of glomerular disease, the IRIS Consensus Clinical Practice Guidelines for Glomerular Disease state that all dogs with suspected glomerular disease should receive a problem-specific panel of diagnostics. These diagnostics are intended to detect and assess the severity of various sequelae of glomerular disease (i.e. tier characteristics: azotaemia, hypoalbuminaemia, hypertension, hypercoagulopathy and fluid balance), identify underlying infections or conditions likely to be causing the glomerular injury, and characterize the pathological changes in the kidneys (Littman *et al.*, 2013). Recommended diagnostics included in the initial minimum database are summarized in Figure 24.2. If any abnormalities are found in this initial minimum database, appropriate problem-specific investigation of the detected abnormalities should be pursued further. Depending on the patient's location and travel history, testing for regional specific infectious diseases known to be associated with glomerulonephritis should be considered as well. 'Additional diagnostics are recommended for dogs with suspected glomerular disease associated with high magnitude (urine protein to creatinine ratio (UPC) ≥3.5) or progressive proteinuria, hypertension, hypoalbuminaemia, and/or azotaemia' in order to document infectious diseases and concurrent extra-renal abnormalities and disease. It is further recommended that 'diagnostic priorities be based on the patient's glomerular disease tier'.

In dogs with glomerular disease, UPC can be quite variable (Nabity *et al.*, 2007). Therefore, regardless of the initial magnitude of proteinuria, multiple UPC measurements should be obtained before initiating therapy to provide a reliable estimate of the magnitude of pretreatment proteinuria and to use as a comparison for post-treatment measurements to assess the response to therapy. In addition, serial monitoring of the magnitude of proteinuria is essential for establishing the progression of proteinuria and glomerular disease.

Renal biopsy is useful for identifying the type and severity of renal lesions when samples are properly obtained, processed and interpreted. Renal biopsy findings provide guidance in planning treatment and establishing prognosis.

- Comprehensive medical history
- Physical examination (including body condition score, retinal examination, rectal examination, and blood pressure measured on at least two occasions)
- Complete blood count
- Comprehensive biochemical profile (including at least BUN, creatinine, phosphorus, calcium, sodium, potassium, chloride, albumin, globulin, glucose, alanine aminotransferase, alkaline phosphatase, bilirubin, cholesterol and, if possible, total CO_2)
- Urinalysis
- Urine protein to creatinine ratio (repeated on at least two visits)
- Urine culture (if indicated).

24.2 Recommended diagnostics for dogs and cats with suspected glomerular disease. BUN = blood urea nitrogen.

A key purpose for renal biopsy is to determine whether the glomerular lesions are immune-mediated because this influences therapeutic recommendations. However, in order for renal biopsy to provide guidance in planning therapy, it is usually essential to obtain ultrastructural (i.e. transmission electron microscopy), immunostaining (i.e. immunofluorescence microscopy), as well as light microscopic observations obtained with specialized techniques including 3 μm sections and appropriate special stains (Cianciolo *et al.*, 2013; Littman *et al.*, 2013). In addition, collection of suitable biopsy samples containing sufficient glomeruli for analysis and submitted in suitable fixatives is required for proper interpretation of the renal lesions. Equally important, the evaluation and interpretation of the biopsy specimen should be performed by an experienced veterinary nephropathologist. In most cases, light microscopic examination alone is inadequate for determining whether immune-mediated glomerular disease is present.

Renal biopsy is most likely to have the greatest interpretive and therapeutic impact early in the course of glomerular disease when the condition is most likely to be reversible and/or amenable to treatment. Renal biopsy samples obtained from dogs with advanced disease (IRIS CKD Stage 4) are less likely to facilitate clinical decisions because renal lesions are more difficult to recognize and the renal damage, such as fibrosis, is less likely to respond to therapy.

Standard therapy of glomerular disease

'Standard therapy' of glomerular disease is indicated for dogs (and cats) with glomerular proteinuria, regardless of the inciting cause of the glomerular disease, morphology of the glomerular lesions and whether the renal lesions are primary or secondary. It consists of suppression of the renin–angiotensin–aldosterone system (RAAS), dietary therapy and antithrombotic therapy. In addition, when indicated, it also may include treatment of systemic hypertension (including any associated target-organ damage) and fluid management including hydration and management of oedema. Recommendations for 'standard therapy' presented here are from the IRIS Consensus Clinical Practice Guidelines for Glomerular Disease in Dogs (Brown *et al.*, 2013).

The magnitude of proteinuria, as measured by serial UPC values, should be used to guide therapeutic recommendations. Dogs with spontaneous glomerular disease have been shown to exhibit more adverse outcomes when UPC values exceed 1.0 (Jacob *et al.*, 2005). In dogs with induced kidney disease, lesions associated with secondary glomerular disease improved when therapy reduced UPC values below 0.5 (Brown *et al.*, 2013). Based on these observations, 'standard therapy' should be considered whenever renal proteinuria persistently exceeds a UPC value of 0.5 (Brown *et al.*, 2013). Reduction of the UPC to below 0.5, or alternatively a 50% reduction in the nadir UPC from the baseline values, should be considered as evidence of therapeutic success (Brown *et al.*, 2013). Although evidence that reducing proteinuria improves clinical outcomes in dogs (and cats) with spontaneous glomerular disease is limited, drug-induced reduction in albuminuria in humans has been reported to alter renal outcomes favourably in a wide range of studies (Heerspink *et al.*, 2014).

Inhibition of the RAAS

Inhibition of the RAAS has been shown to reduce the magnitude of proteinuria, using a variety of drug strategies (Figure 24.3). The magnitude of proteinuria reduction achieved appears to be greater than could be explained solely by the anti-hypertensive benefit of these drugs (Brown *et al.*, 2013). Rather, the anti-proteinuric benefit of inhibiting the RAAS is thought to derive from modifying renal haemodynamics. Principal drug classes used to target the RAAS include angiotensin-converting enzyme inhibitors (ACEi), angiotensin receptor blockers (ARBs) and aldosterone receptor blockers. Although not commonly used in dogs, renin inhibitors have also been used successfully to suppress the RAAS in human patients.

While there is evidence that inhibition of the RAAS reduces proteinuria and may be renoprotective, ACEi and ARBs can also be associated with adverse effects. Suppression of the RAAS may reduce renal function and promote hypotension and hyperkalaemia. Reduced renal function and hypotension are the result, at least in part, of vasodilatory consequences of reducing angiotensin II concentrations systemically and locally within the kidneys, while hyperkalaemia results from reduced aldosterone concentrations. As a consequence, serum creatinine and potassium concentrations as well as blood pressure should be monitored regularly. Small increases in creatinine and potassium concentrations and decreases in blood pressure are expected and not of concern. However, large changes beyond the reference ranges should prompt careful reconsideration of drug and dose choices and investigation of other factors that may predispose to these adverse events.

ACEi therapy

Administration of ACEi is considered 'standard therapy' for dogs with glomerular disease because these agents reduce proteinuria and may preserve renal function and structure by decreasing efferent glomerular arteriolar resistance, thus promoting a decline (or normalization) in glomerular hydraulic pressure. Other proposed mechanisms by which suppression of the RAAS may reduce the magnitude of proteinuria include preservation of glomerular heparin sulphate, decreased size of glomerular capillary endothelial pores, improved lipoprotein metabolism, slowed glomerular mesangial growth and proliferation, and inhibition of bradykinin degradation (Lefebvre *et al.*, 2007).

ACEi used for management of glomerular disease in dogs include enalapril, benazepril, ramipril and imidapril (Figure 24.4). While the renal actions of these drugs are similar, their pharmacokinetics vary. Benazepril and its active metabolite, benazeprilat, are excreted largely via the biliary route with a lesser portion excreted in urine, whereas enalapril and its active metabolite, enalaprilat, are excreted largely by the kidneys. Changes in the patient's renal function may have divergent effects on blood concentrations of these two drugs. However, the pharmacokinetics of both drugs are complex and unpredictable, and there currently are no published studies justifying a preferred recommendation for any one ACEi over others in the class.

It is recommended that ACEi therapy begin at the lowest recommended (or starting) dose, given once daily. Serum creatinine should be measured immediately before and shortly after beginning ACEi treatment to assess the impact of therapy on renal function. Creatinine levels should be measured 3–5 days after beginning ACEi therapy in dogs with serum creatinine values >177 μmol/l (>2.0 mg/dl) and after about 7–14 days in dogs with serum creatinine values ≤177 μmol/l (≤2.0 mg/dl).

The ACEi can induce a small reduction in glomerular filtration rate which is recognized as an increase in serum creatinine concentration secondary to its effects on reducing glomerular hydraulic pressure. A small increase in creatinine concentration indicates effective reduction of glomerular hydraulic pressure, and in most dogs this increase is not clinically important. However, the degree to which worsening of renal function can be tolerated varies according to the IRIS CKD stage. Dogs with IRIS CKD Stages 1 and 2 can usually tolerate an increase in serum creatinine concentration of ≤30% above baseline. However, the occasional dog will respond with a greater

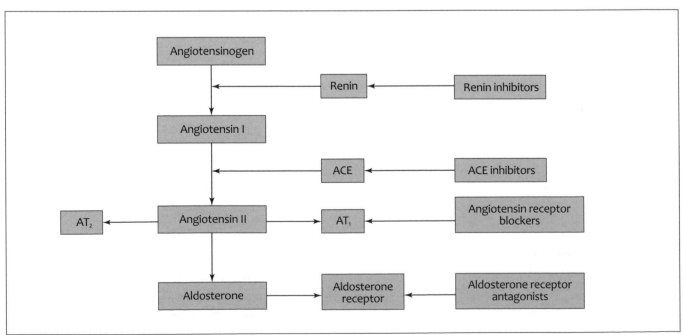

24.3 Diagram of the renin–angiotensin–aldosterone system and the various pharmacological strategies for suppressing the effects of the system. ACE = angiotensin-converting enzyme; AT_1 = angiotensin type 1 receptor; AT_2 = angiotensin type 2 receptor.

Drug	Mechanism	Initial dose	Escalating dose scheme
Benazepril	ACEi	0.5 mg/kg orally q24h	Increase by 0.5 mg/kg q24h to a maximum of 2 mg/kg q24h
Enalapril	ACEi	0.5 mg/kg orally q24h	Increase by 0.5 mg/kg q24h to a maximum of 2 mg/kg q24h
Ramipril	ACEi	0.125 mg/kg orally q24h	Increase by 0.125 mg/kg q24h to a maximum of 0.5 mg/kg q24h
Imidapril	ACEi	0.25 mg/kg orally q24h	Increase by 0.25 mg/kg q24h to a maximum of 5 mg/kg orally q24h. Usually given q24h
Telmisartan	ARB	1.0 mg/kg orally q24h	Increase by 0.5 mg/kg q24h to a maximum of 2 mg/kg q24h
Losartan	ARB	0.125 mg/kg orally q24h 0.5 mg/kg orally q24h	0.25 mg/kg q24h in azotaemic dogs 1 mg/kg q24h in non-azotaemic dogs
Spironolactone	Aldosterone receptor blocker	1–2 mg/kg orally q12h	Not applicable

24.4 Commonly used angiotensin-converting enzyme inhibitors (ACEi), angiotensin receptor blocking (ARB) and aldosterone receptor blocking drugs used in the management of proteinuria in dogs with glomerular disease.

increase in serum creatinine concentration (i.e. an increase >30% above the measured baseline value) that may be accompanied by clinical consequences. Most commonly this occurs in dogs with volume contraction due to dehydration. In contrast to dogs with IRIS CKD Stages 1 and 2, stable renal function should be the goal in dogs with IRIS CKD Stages 3 and 4. In these patients, reduction in renal function should prompt therapeutic intervention, with fluid therapy and possibly dosage reduction. Dogs with IRIS CKD Stage 4 are particularly susceptible to developing a uraemic crisis should renal function decline after initiating ACEi therapy. As a consequence, ACEi should be initiated conservatively and monitored closely in dogs with more advanced renal dysfunction, and supportive therapeutic intervention should be provided as needed.

The goal of ACEi therapy is to reduce the UPC to <0.5 or, if values <0.5 cannot be achieved, to reduce the UPC by at least 50% of the pretreatment baseline. Since the starting dose of ACEi rarely reduces UPC values to the stated goal, the dose should be increased progressively either until the treatment goal is achieved or to a maximum dose of 2.0 mg/kg q24h. Although the renoprotective benefits of ACEi appear to be independent of baseline renal function in humans, and they are therefore appropriate at all levels of renal dysfunction, caution is warranted in dogs with serum creatinine values >440 µmol/l (>5 mg/dl) (Brown et al., 2013). At a minimum, increased monitoring of renal function is indicated in these patients, and an abrupt decline in renal function should prompt reconsideration of the dose and/or use of an ACEi. Serum potassium and blood pressure should also be monitored as dosage increases are instituted to optimize control of proteinuria (Brown et al., 2013).

ARBs therapy

The ARBs suppress the RAAS by blocking the angiotensin II type 1 receptor. Losartan and telmisartan have been used in dogs with glomerular proteinuria (see Figure 24.4), and telmisartan is approved in Europe for the treatment of proteinuria in cats with CKD (Brown et al., 2013; Bugbee et al., 2014). While these drugs have been used extensively in humans with glomerular disease and found to reduce proteinuria, similar to ACEi, experience with ARBs in dogs is limited. Until recently, losartan has been used most commonly in dogs. There is evidence confirming that it has predictable pharmacodynamic effects in dogs, despite the apparent inability of dogs to produce one of the major active metabolites of losartan (Christ et al., 1994). Preliminary evidence also suggests that telmisartan may be effective in reducing proteinuria and blood pressure in dogs (Brown et al., 2013; Bugbee et al., 2014). Telmisartan has a longer half-life, and has a higher affinity for the angiotensin II type 1 receptor, than losartan and may prove to be superior in dogs (Brown et al., 2013). Telmisartan has shown more efficacy than losartan and enalapril in attenuating the blood pressure response to angiotensin I administration (Bugbee et al., 2014).

Combined therapy with ACEi and ARB (dual drug therapy)

When treatment with a single class of drug fails to achieve the recommended UPC treatment goal or adverse effects are seen with a single agent (see below), combining ACEi and ARBs is a reasonable next strategy. An ACEi may incompletely block formation of angiotensin II, particularly within the kidneys, and blockage of the angiotensin II receptor with an ARB can promote a compensatory increase in renin activity and incomplete block of the RAAS (Brown et al., 2013; Laverman, 2002). Thus, blocking both ACE and the angiotensin II type 1 receptor is likely to be more effective than monotherapy with either drug class in suppressing angiotensin II activity and reducing proteinuria. An additional potential benefit of combining these drugs is that it may be possible to reduce the doses of both drugs, thus reducing the risk of adverse side effects of either.

The safety and effectiveness of dual drug therapy in dogs with glomerular disease has not been documented. The results of studies on the safety and effectiveness of dual drug therapy in humans have been inconsistent (Mallat, 2013). A meta-analysis/meta-regression of trials in human patients with primary glomerulonephritis showed that the anti-proteinuric response to ACEi plus ARB therapy versus either monotherapy was consistently greater, and was strictly related to baseline proteinuria, with only a moderate increase in serum potassium levels (Catapano et al., 2008). A more recent systematic review and meta-analysis of all randomized controlled trials reported between January 1990 and August 2012 comparing dual blockers of the RAAS with monotherapy showed that, while dual drug therapy had seemingly beneficial effects on surrogate endpoints (e.g. proteinuria), it failed to reduce mortality and was associated with an excessive risk of adverse events such as hyperkalaemia, hypotension and renal failure, when compared with monotherapy (Makani et al., 2013). The authors of this comprehensive meta-analysis indicated that the risk:benefit ratio argues against using dual drug therapy in humans. While these results are specifically intended for humans with glomerular disease, it appears prudent to be particularly cautious and vigilant when using dual drug therapy for dogs with glomerular disease.

Aldosterone receptor blockers

In humans receiving ACEi and/or ARB drugs, it is common for serum aldosterone levels to increase progressively ('aldosterone break through'). Prolonged hyperaldosteronism may have adverse effects on the heart and systemic blood vessels as well as the kidneys, where it manifests as proteinuria. Aldosterone receptor blockers have been shown to reduce proteinuria and stabilize renal function in humans treated with ACEi and ARBs. The reduction in proteinuria would be expected to be most prominent when aldosterone concentrations are high. Spironolactone and eplerenone are aldosterone receptor blockers that can be used when ACEi and/or ARB therapy is associated with persistent proteinuria and hyperaldosteronism. However, evidence that any aldosterone receptor blocking drug is effective in lowering the magnitude of proteinuria in dogs is lacking.

The IRIS Canine GN Study Group Consensus Recommendation for Managing Proteinuria with RAAS Inhibition states that 'An ACEi should be the initial treatment for most dogs with proteinuria. The initial choice of drug and starting dose may vary, but can be gradually increased to achieve a therapeutic target. The ideal therapeutic target is a reduction in the UPC to <0.5 without inappropriate worsening of renal function. However, as this ideal target is not achieved in most dogs, a reduction in UPC of 50% or greater is the recommended alternate target.'

Dietary therapy in dogs with glomerular disease

Dietary therapy is generally accepted to be important in management of CKD because it has been shown to influence renal function favourably and mitigate the magnitude of proteinuria, renal lesions and the rate of progression of kidney disease in dogs (Polzin et al., 1984; 1988; Jacob et al., 2002; Brown et al., 2013). Studies on this subject are based primarily in dogs with spontaneous or induced CKD and secondary glomerular disease. Dietary therapy has been shown to reduce proteinuria, but it has yet to be established whether diet alters the course of primary glomerular disease in dogs. Dietary components that may have a salutary impact on proteinuria and glomerular disease include polyunsaturated fatty acids (PUFA), protein and salt (Brown et al., 2013). Because diets formulated for dogs with CKD include all of these modifications, putatively they are appropriate for dogs with glomerular disease.

Dietary polyunsaturated fatty acids

The IRIS Consensus Clinical Practice Guidelines for Glomerular Disease in Dogs recommend that 'dogs with glomerular disease should be fed a diet with a reduced n-6/n-3 PUFA ratio, approximating 5:1. Where diet supplementation with n-3 PUFA by the owner is used to alter this ratio, a dosage of 0.25–0.50 g of n-3 PUFA/kg bodyweight containing eicosapentaenoic acid and docosehexaenoic acid is appropriate for a typical canine diet' (Brown et al., 2013). Although the source and type of PUFA vary by product, commercially available diets formulated for management of canine CKD are supplemented with eicosapentaenoic acid and docosehexaenoic acid with an n-6/n-3 ratio approximating 5:1. Supplementing the diet with additional PUFA increases antioxidant requirements; as a consequence, antioxidant supplementation is recommended (e.g. 1.1 IU of supplemental vitamin E per gram of added fish oil) whenever additional PUFA are added to the diet. In addition, antioxidants have been shown to increase survival in canine models of CKD, thus they may have a direct benefit in addition to limiting oxidation of n-3 PUFA supplementation (Brown et al., 2013).

Limiting dietary protein

The IRIS Consensus Clinical Practice Guidelines for Glomerular Disease in Dogs recommend that modified protein diets should be fed to dogs with glomerular disease (Brown et al., 2013). Studies in dogs with induced and spontaneous CKD have shown that reducing protein intake is associated with reduced proteinuria (Polzin et al., 1984; Jacob et al., 2002; Burkholder et al., 2004; Brown et al., 2013).

Limiting dietary salt

The IRIS Consensus Clinical Practice Guidelines for Glomerular Disease in Dogs state: 'based on evidence from laboratory studies, the study group recommends feeding diets formulated to contain reduced sodium chloride content to dogs with glomerular disease' (Brown et al., 2013). Salt restriction has been shown to enhance the anti-hypertensive efficacy and renal haemodynamic effects of some anti-hypertensive agents in dogs, particularly those that interfere with the RAAS (Navar et al., 1982).

Antithrombotic therapy in dogs with glomerular disease

Thromboembolism is a recognized complication of proteinuria in dogs, and frequently is the cause of death in dogs with the nephrotic syndrome (Pressler, 2013). The prevalence of thromboembolism in dogs with proteinuric kidney disease (glomerular diseases) has been reported to be as high as 25% (Cook and Cowgill, 1996). While the relationship between the magnitude of proteinuria and the development of thromboembolism has not been well established in dogs, it is generally accepted that the risk of thromboembolism increases as the serum albumin concentration declines as a result of proteinuria. The mechanisms underlying the thrombotic diathesis associated with proteinuria are poorly understood, but loss of antithrombotic substances into the urine is a likely contributor.

The IRIS Consensus Clinical Practice Guidelines recommend: 'daily administration of low-dose aspirin (1–5 mg/kg q24h) for thromboprophylaxis in dogs with proteinuric glomerular disease. Clopidogrel may be similarly effective to aspirin and may be used instead of aspirin; however, there is no compelling evidence that it is superior to low-dose aspirin in dogs with glomerular disease.' While evidence supporting the efficacy of aspirin as prophylaxis for thromboembolism in dogs is lacking, it has been used widely in proteinuric dogs and appears to be safe provided the dogs are well hydrated and normotensive. Most thromboembolic complications in dogs with nephrotic syndrome appear to be venous. Although anti-platelet therapy is generally not the primary approach to venous thromboembolism, limited evidence suggests that anti-platelet agents may provide some protection against venous thromboembolism in hospitalized human patients (Geerts, 2008). Direct evidence that aspirin therapy influences renal function or pathology in dogs with spontaneous glomerular disease is lacking.

Management of hypertension in glomerular disease

Blood pressure (BP) should always be measured in dogs with proteinuria because they have an increased risk of systemic hypertension. Sustained elevations in BP promote injury to the vasculature, the kidneys, heart, eyes and brain, and this is referred to as 'target-organ damage' (TOD). To address the consequences of TOD, the IRIS Consensus Clinical Practice Guidelines for Glomerular Disease in Dogs recommend that 'initial assessment of a dog with glomerular disease suspected of having systemic hypertension should include recognizing conditions that may be contributing to an elevation of BP, identifying and characterizing TOD, and determining if there are any seemingly unrelated concurrent conditions that may complicate anti-hypertensive therapy. Dogs with glomerular disease are presumed to have TOD and the general consensus is to institute therapy in a patient wherein reliable measurement of BP indicates that systolic BP exceeds 160 and/or diastolic BP exceeds 100 mmHg (hypertension). In dogs with glomerular disease and either severe hypertension or a hypertensive emergency (e.g. systolic blood pressure above 200 mmHg or evidence of ocular or neurologic target-organ damage), co-administration of two agents with different mechanisms of action (generally an ACEi or ARB plus amlodipine) is recommended. A dog with glomerular disease in IRIS CKD Stages 1 or 2 should be evaluated 3–14 days following any change in anti-hypertensive therapy. In unstable patients and those with IRIS Stage 3 or 4 CKD, this recheck should be conducted in a shorter timeframe, typically 3–5 days. Patients deemed to be hypertensive emergencies and hospitalized patients, particularly those receiving fluid therapy or pharmacological agents with cardiovascular effects, should be assessed daily. The purpose of these short-term assessments is to determine if there are any findings that are unexpected (e.g. new or worsening TOD) or adverse (e.g. marked worsening of azotemia or systemic hypotension).' Diagnosis and treatment of systemic hypertension can be found in Chapters 15 and 18.

Management of fluid balance in dogs with glomerular disease

Abnormalities in fluid balance are common in dogs with glomerular disease, and may include excesses, deficits and intercompartmental maldistribution (Brown *et al.*, 2013). Failure to diagnose accurately and properly manage the fluid status of the patient may lead to exacerbation of peripheral oedema, ascites, systemic hypertension, overhydration, dehydration, worsening azotaemia and uraemic crisis. Accurate determination of the fluid status can be challenging in these patients. Therefore, administration of fluid and diuretics therapy should be done cautiously and with careful monitoring, to avoid harming the patient.

Fluid status in nephrotic syndrome

The development of oedema and ascites has been explained traditionally by decreased intravascular colloid osmotic pressure caused by urinary loss of albumin and other proteins. In this theory (the 'underfill theory'), loss of fluid from the vascular compartment leads to hypovolaemia which, in turn, activates the RAAS, causing retention of salt and water. However, the colloid osmotic pressure of the interstitium typically declines in parallel with the reduction in plasma albumin, making it unlikely to cause translocation of fluid out of the vascular system. Indeed, most patients with the nephrotic syndrome do not have evidence of intravascular volume contraction.

More recent studies have suggested that inappropriate renal tubular sodium retention as a consequence of proteinuria promotes the oedema, ascites and hypertension (the 'overfill theory') (Palmer and Alpern, 1997; Doucet *et al.*, 2007). While this theory has not been confirmed in dogs, it is consistent with the observations of worsening of oedema following colloid administration, a high prevalence of systemic hypertension and the poor response of hypertension to RAAS blockade alone. Another possible theory, the 'vascular hyperpermeability theory', suggests that systemic vascular and glomerular capillary dysfunction leads to increased translocation of fluid outside the vascular space. In a recent review of nephrotic syndrome in dogs it was not possible conclusively to determine the cause of intercompartmental fluid redistribution (Klosterman *et al.*, 2011).

The IRIS Consensus Clinical Practice Guidelines for Glomerular Disease in Dogs state: 'since data on the prevailing mechanisms of nephrotic edema in the canine species are lacking, careful assessment of the hydration, and of the vascular volume, status of individual dogs with glomerular disease should be a priority both before and during fluid therapy. The evaluation of the fluid status of a dog with glomerular disease should be based on anamnestic data (e.g. serial bodyweight) and a complete physical examination with special emphasis on skin turgor, mucous membrane color and moisture, capillary refill time, temperature of the extremities, heart rate, pulse quality, and systemic blood pressure.'

Diuretic use in dogs with nephrotic syndrome

Fluid retention in nephrotic syndrome may range from mild subcutaneous oedema and ascites through to marked ascites that causes respiratory distress or abdominal discomfort. The clinical impact on the patient should guide the decision for the use of diuretic therapy. The IRIS Consensus Clinical Practice Guidelines for Glomerular Disease in Dogs state that: 'because there is no rationale for diuretic intervention in dogs with glomerular disease and mild peripheral edema, use of diuretics in dogs with edema should be limited to situations where organ function is critically impaired (e.g. ascites or pleural effusion that impairs respiration). When indicated in a dog with glomerular disease, diuretic therapy with furosemide or spironolactone may be instituted. Furosemide may be the first choice drug in dogs with pulmonary edema or hyperkalemia and spironolactone for dogs with pleural or abdominal effusion. Furosemide may be administered at an initial dosage of 1 mg/kg q6–12h, with incremental increases of 0.5–1 mg/kg q6–12h or conversion to continuous IV infusion at a rate of 2–15 µg/kg/min after an initial loading dose of 2 mg/kg in animals with insufficient response. Spironolactone may be started at 1 mg/kg q12–24h and titrated in increments of 1 mg/kg q12–24h to a maximum of 4 mg/kg q12–24h.'

Fluid therapy in dogs with nephrotic syndrome

Overzealous administration of fluids can be harmful or fatal to dogs with glomerular disease and the nephrotic syndrome. The IRIS Consensus Clinical Practice Guidelines for Glomerular Disease in Dogs recommend that 'fluid replacement therapy should be used with great caution in dogs with glomerular disease because they are predisposed to fluid overload. Intravenous fluid therapy is indicated for hemodynamic stabilization (e.g. a patient with dehydration, poor tissue perfusion) of the patient. Colloids or plasma/albumin should not be administered solely on the basis of decreased oncotic pressure, serum albumin concentration, or total protein concentration, or for the purpose of mobilizing edema. The endpoint of therapy should be the patient's response to therapy (i.e. correction of tissue hypoperfusion, hypotension, hypovolemia, dehydration). Judicious administration of colloids should be considered when crystalloid fluid support has failed to correct the patient's hemodynamic dysfunction.'

Therapeutic approach beyond standard therapy

There have been considerable advances in the diagnostic evaluation of glomerular diseases of dogs in the past 8 years with the establishment of the World Small Animal Veterinary Association (WSAVA) Renal Standardization Project. A fundamental lesson gleaned from this project was the extent of pathological diversity represented among dogs with glomerular disease. This diversity was revealed only with comprehensive evaluation of kidney biopsy samples using light, immunofluorescent and electron microscopy by specialized nephropathologists (Cianciolo *et al.*, 2013; Schneider *et al.*, 2013). These pathological insights predict that similar diversity might be expected for therapeutic strategies and outcomes for these diseases, and this holds the potential to improve conventional therapeutic recommendations and prognostic accuracy for dogs with glomerular disease when evidence-based observations are linked to the concurrent pathology. To date, however, therapeutic recommendations beyond 'standard therapy' for the management of glomerular diseases have not been established, on the foundations of either medical evidence in animal patients or precise categorization of the underlying disease. When there is established evidence of an immune-mediated pathogenesis in the glomerular disease, the use of immunosuppressive and anti-inflammatory therapy seems rational and indicated. However, despite this logic, compelling evidence supporting immunosuppressive strategies in dogs is lacking, and their use should balance potential benefits against predictable adverse effects (Segev *et al.*, 2013). In the interim, to provide guidance for management of glomerular diseases, consensus recommendations based on review of pertinent literature in animals, expert opinion and subsequent validation by a formal consensus methodology have been outlined in The IRIS Consensus Clinical Practice Guidelines for Glomerular Disease in Dogs (Polzin and Cowgill, 2013; Segev *et al.*, 2013).

Recently, canine glomerular diseases have been categorized into a series of statistically distinct pathological entities on the basis of comprehensive pathological imagery, including light, immunofluorescent and electron microscopy, as stated above (Cianciolo *et al.*, 2016). More broadly, these morphologically distinct categories can be divided into diseases with identifiable immunological foundations and those without. From this perspective, the IRIS Consensus Clinical Practice Guidelines for Glomerular Disease in Dogs suggest that the empirical application of immunosuppressive and anti-inflammatory therapy is rational and recommended for dogs with severe, persistent or progressive glomerular disease in which there is evidence of an active immune pathogenesis and no identified contraindication to immunosuppressive therapy (Segev *et al.*, 2013). The rationale underlying this recommendation is based on the supposition that suppression of the immune-mediated or inflammatory response will ameliorate the pathological and clinical response and positively influence the course of the injury. Despite the theoretical rationale for immunosuppressive therapy, there is limited clinical experience or evidence in animal patients to predict which agents will influence, positively or negatively, the clinical outcome, specific patterns of glomerular injury, or immunological activity. Consequently, recommendations for specific immunosuppressive therapy should be regarded as tentative and awaiting future experience and evidence.

With regard to this broader classification, approximately 50% of canine glomerular diseases have no morphological or immune foundations that would justify immunosuppressive therapy and potentially impose therapeutic risks (Schneider *et al.*, 2013; Segev *et al.*, 2013). Consequently, a documented immunopathogenesis should be established before the use of immunomodulatory therapy is recommended, and this information is only established from a properly processed and evaluated kidney biopsy specimen. 'The most compelling evidence supporting active immune-mediated mechanisms promoting the glomerular injury identified in the kidney biopsy includes identification of electron-dense deposits in subendothelial, subepithelial, intramembranous, or mesangial locations in the glomerulus or unequivocal immunofluorescent staining for IgG, IgM, IgA, light chains, and/or complement components in peripheral capillary loops and/or the mesangial compartment. Less definitive evidence supporting active immune-mediated mechanisms include identification of "red granular" staining on the capillary walls on Masson's trichrome-stained sections (probable immune deposits), identification of "spikes" along the glomerular basement membrane on Jones methenamine silver-stained sections, or identifiable "holes" within the glomerular basement membrane on Jones methenamine silver-stained sections' (Segev *et al.*, 2013). In the interpretation of these morphological features, it is important to ascertain whether they reflect active and ongoing injury or merely residual immunological material deposited in the glomerular basement membrane (GBM) during a previous immunological insult. The latter case may no longer be associated with active or ongoing immunological events susceptible to immunosuppressive therapy, or may represent non-specific immunoglobulin entrapment in lesions without an immunopathogenesis.

Therapeutic strategy for glomerular disease in dogs

The IRIS Consensus Clinical Practice Guidelines for Glomerular Disease in Dogs recommend that: 'the immunosuppressive strategy to manage dogs with documented glomerular disease of an apparent immune-mediated pathogenesis should be selected on the basis of the severity of the disease and its rate of progression. For diseases associated with UPC values >3.5, attendant hypoalbuminemia, nephrotic syndrome, or rapidly progressive azotemia, single drug, or combination therapy consisting of rapidly acting immunosuppressive drugs is recommended' (Segev *et al.*, 2013). The selection of an immunosuppression protocol should be based on the actions, adverse effects and costs of the selected agent(s) in dogs.

In most circumstances there is little evidence regarding the efficacy of any drug, and the following suggestions must be regarded as consensus recommendations until stronger evidence is available.

Glucocorticoids have an established basis in veterinary therapeutics, but they have not been advocated in the management of glomerular disease because of the characteristic adverse effects (relative to the benefits) of these agents in dogs when compared with humans and other species. The most worrisome adverse effects include increasing proteinuria, negative nitrogen metabolism, hypercatabolism and muscle wasting, increased hypercoagulable and thromboembolic potential, sodium and fluid retention, and systemic hypertension. In contrast to dogs, the management of glomerular disease in humans relies heavily on glucocorticoid therapy as a first-line treatment or in conjunction with other immunosuppressive agents for the management of many types of primary glomerular disease (Rhen and Cidlowski, 2005; Ponticelli and Passerini, 2010). These differences in therapeutic practice may reflect perceived differences in the risk:benefit ratio for glucocorticoids in humans *versus* dogs, possible differences in the immunopathogenesis of canine glomerular diseases, or the lack of documented, evidence-based efficacy for glucocorticoids in canine glomerular diseases. A proportion of human patients within most glomerular disease categories are categorized as 'steroid-resistant' owing to lack of a treatment effect, and are transitioned to other therapeutic protocols. It remains possible that specific categories of canine glomerular disease may demonstrate steroid responsiveness, but this designation will require future controlled clinical trials of carefully characterized glomerular diseases.

Until a specific treatment benefit is established for dogs, the apparent species differences in the clinical and pathophysiological responses to corticosteroids should prompt careful selection of patients if they are to be used. The IRIS Consensus Clinical Practice Guidelines for Glomerular Disease in Dogs recommends that: 'short-term administration of glucocorticoids may be appropriate in fulminant cases where immediate immunosuppression is required if their use is adjusted to minimize their adverse effects. Potential benefits of alternative treatment regimens, i.e. pulse therapy *versus* continuous therapy, should be considered. However, on the basis of current practice perceptions and anecdotal experience, the use of glucocorticoid therapy should be tapered to the minimally effective dose as quickly as possible because of predictable adverse effects. Glucocorticoids may also be appropriate in the acute management of multisystemic immune-mediated diseases where their use has proven beneficial (e.g. concurrent polyarthritis, immune-mediated hemolytic anemia)' (Segev *et al.*, 2013).

Mycophenolate is an immunosuppressive agent with a rapid onset of action that is deemed appropriate for peracute, severe or rapidly progressing glomerular diseases. Mycophenolate appears to promote less toxicity (including myelotoxicity and hepatotoxicity) than alkylating agents, which affect all tissues with a high proliferative or mitotic activity (Allison, 2005; Zwerner and Fiorentino, 2007; Whitley and Day, 2011). Gastrointestinal signs including anorexia, vomiting and diarrhoea are the main adverse effect of this drug; however, they are usually reversible upon dose reduction or drug withdrawal. Recent anecdotal experience in dogs since establishment of the IRIS consensus recommendations suggests that the prevalence of adverse gastrointestinal side effects can be minimized by starting therapy at a lower dosage (5 mg/kg q12h or q24h) without substantial loss of therapeutic efficacy in many patients. The dosage may be increased incrementally to achieve a balance between effective dosing and adverse effects. Although randomized controlled clinical trial evidence is lacking, based on preliminary, uncontrolled clinical experience and its low rate of severe complications, mycophenolate is recommended as the first choice for treatment of dogs with peracute or rapidly progressive glomerular disease with an apparent immune-mediated pathogenesis (Segev *et al.*, 2013).

The effectiveness of ciclosporin in dogs with spontaneous glomerular disease has been evaluated in a randomized controlled clinical trial, and it has been found to provide little apparent benefit (Vaden *et al.*, 1995). The lack of disease characterization and the potential for diverse categories of disease was a major limitation of this and all previous studies of specific therapeutic agents in canine glomerular diseases. Further studies on the effectiveness of ciclosporin in dogs with glomerular disease have not been reported, and its use cannot be recommended explicitly, but it warrants consideration in glomerular diseases with immune foundations that are not responsive to other therapies.

There are currently no studies in the veterinary literature to support or negate the use of cyclophosphamide in dogs with glomerular diseases. Although it has been shown to be effective in some glomerular diseases in humans, it is more likely to be associated with adverse effects than other immunosuppressant drugs. Cyclophosphamide may be administered as pulse therapy in cases of rapidly progressive disease, given its rapid onset of action. Chlorambucil generally is associated with minimal adverse effects, such as mild myelotoxicity, but its efficacy as monotherapy for the management of glomerular disease has not been demonstrated in the veterinary literature.

Azathioprine is used routinely in the management of a variety of immune-mediated disorders in veterinary medicine, including immune-mediated glomerular disease. However, in dogs with glomerular disease requiring an acute onset of drug action, azathioprine may not be an ideal selection because of its delayed onset of action: it may take 2–5 weeks or more of administration to be fully effective in dogs. There are no randomized clinical trials to support or negate the use of azathioprine for the management of glomerular diseases in dogs, but uncontrolled anecdotal clinical experience supports its efficacy, in combination with chlorambucil.

The clinical presentation of canine glomerular diseases may be peracute and rapidly progressive or active but slowly progressive. Consequently, the selection of immunosuppressive drugs for their management should be linked to their severity and rate of progression. The IRIS Consensus Clinical Practice Guidelines for Glomerular Disease in Dogs recommend that 'dogs with peracute or rapidly progressive glomerular disease should receive induction therapy with a potent immunosuppressive protocol characterized by a rapid onset of immunosuppression. Mycophenolate alone or in combination with prednisolone, or cyclophosphamide (continuous or pulse therapy) alone or in combination with prednisolone are suggested for these presentations' (Segev *et al.*, 2013).

Although the efficacy and safety of mycophenolate in dogs with glomerular disease is not well established, preliminary observations suggest it has potential in the management of fulminant canine glomerular disease, with an appropriate safety margin. Cyclophosphamide also is a reasonable option for dogs with peracute or rapidly progressive disease or as an alternative therapy when mycophenolate appears ineffective, but its use may entail greater risk of adverse effects and require more aggressive monitoring. Drugs with less rapid onset (alone or in combination) may not be less effective in dogs with more severe or progressive glomerular diseases, and they should be considered as alternatives to the rapidly acting protocols once an initial response is achieved or in response to adverse effects to rapidly acting agents. The IRIS Consensus Clinical Practice Guidelines for Glomerular Disease in Dogs state that 'there is no clear evidence to support or reject a recommendation for glucocorticoids as induction therapy in dogs with glomerular disease. To minimize the adverse effects associated with glucocorticoid therapy, its use as monotherapy is not recommended, and when used concurrently with mycophenolate or cyclophosphamide, glucocorticoids should be tapered as quickly as possible to the minimally effective dose with the goal to discontinue the corticosteroid component within as soon as possible' (Segev et al., 2013).

Dogs with active but stable or slowly progressive glomerular diseases with an immune-mediated foundation, or those with slowly progressive diseases that are only partially responsive to standard therapy, may receive induction therapy with either drugs that have a rapid onset or drugs with more protracted onset, including mycophenolate or chlorambucil alone or in combination with azathioprine on alternate days, cyclophosphamide and glucocorticoids, or ciclosporin. In the absence of overt adverse effects, at least 8 weeks of the rapid-acting immunosuppressive drug therapy (e.g. mycophenolate) and 8–12 weeks of slow-acting drug therapy (e.g. azathioprine) should be provided before altering or abandoning an immunosuppressive trial. If no response is evident or the therapeutic goals are not achieved within these time intervals, consideration should be given to an alternative drug or dosing protocol. If no therapeutic response is noted after 3–4 months, discontinuing immunosuppressive therapy may be considered. Immunosuppressive therapy should be continued for a minimum of 12–16 weeks in dogs that demonstrate a complete or partial response to initial treatment. Thereafter, consideration should be given to tapering the treatment to a dose/schedule that maintains the response without worsening of the proteinuria, azotaemia or clinical signs (Segev et al., 2013).

The kidney biopsy sample alone holds the potential to document involvement of components of the immune system in the pathogenesis of glomerular diseases. Recent evidence has confirmed that approximately 50% of canine glomerular disease contains morphological evidence of immune reactants, justifying immunosuppressive drugs in the therapeutic approach. The remaining diseases have no evident immune pathogenesis and immunosuppressive therapy has no rational indication and could predispose to adverse events. The IRIS Consensus Clinical Practice Guidelines for Glomerular Disease in Dogs emphasize the importance of identifying an underlying immune process prior to initiating immunosuppressive therapy (Segev et al., 2013). However, there are morphologically distinct glomerular diseases in human patients with no evident antibody deposition or evidence of immune reactants that demonstrate steroid or immunosuppressive responsiveness. Both minimal change disease and a specific form of focal segmental glomerulosclerosis (FSGS) are consequences of podocyte injury without detectable involvement of immune reactants. The podocyte injury is probably due to uncharacterized circulating permeability factors which can be influenced, in selected patients, by steroid and/or immunosuppressive therapies (Segarra-Medrano et al., 2013; Sethi et al., 2015). The mechanism of action of these therapies for FSGS is not known but they may influence the cellular components of the immune system independently of antibody production or complement activation.

With the advent of the WSAVA Renal Standardization Project and the use of advanced pathological imagery (Cowgill and Polzin, 2013), the recognition of FSGS in canine patients has increased (Schneider et al., 2013). By consensus criteria, adopted in the 2013 IRIS Consensus Clinical Practice Guidelines for Glomerular Disease in Dogs, this lesion would not justify immunosuppressive therapy (Segev et al., 2013). The WSAVA Renal Standardization initiative, however, has demonstrated morphological similarities between both canine and human glomerular pathology. Equally importantly, it has revealed that there are considerable differences in the glomerular diseases between these species, making it speculative to transpose classification criteria blindly, and especially therapeutic and outcomes experiences which have not been subjected to controlled clinical trial. Given this caveat, it appears prudent to expand consideration of an immune-mediated pathogenesis beyond the morphological recognition of conventional immune reactants in the kidney biopsy sample. This is not intended to provide licence for the blanket and irresponsible sanction of immunosuppressive therapy in patients without traditional evidence of an immunopathogenesis. Rather, there should be open-mindedness to clinical experiences in humans or other species where seemingly identical diseases demonstrate therapeutic benefit from these therapies.

As detailed above, a properly processed kidney biopsy sample evaluated by an experienced veterinary nephropathologist provides considerable guidance on therapeutic directions and is recommended as part of the diagnostic assessment of dogs with Tier II and Tier III glomerular disease (Littman et al., 2013). Nevertheless, there are circumstances in which a kidney biopsy cannot be performed because of medical contraindications, financial limitations or logistical constraints. The IRIS Consensus Clinical Practice Guidelines for Glomerular Disease in Dogs suggest that 'Renal biopsy should not be performed in dogs (1) with IRIS CKD Stage 4; (2) when other medical contraindications are present and cannot be mitigated (including coagulopathy, renal cystic disease, moderate-to-severe hydronephrosis, pyelonephritis, perirenal abscess, uncontrolled hypertension, severe anaemia, and pregnancy); or (3) when results of renal biopsy are deemed unlikely to alter treatment, outcome, or prognosis' (Pressler et al., 2013). Under these conditions, and without a kidney biopsy, therapeutic decisions beyond standard therapy become entirely empirical. Some patients may be denied appropriate therapy if none is provided, and some patients may be exposed to inappropriate drugs and potential adverse effects if treated non-specifically.

When the kidneys are recognized as small, end-stage or unlikely to have reversible injury, the patient has chronic azotaemia (i.e. IRIS CKD Stage 3), the pathological process is unlikely to be active, or the biopsy sample is not to be subjected to appropriate processing or pathological interpretation, the results of the kidney biopsy may not yield findings that contribute to therapeutic decisions or facilitate patient care. In these clinical circumstances, kidney biopsy is not recommended and alternative diagnostic information (e.g. serology, hereditary factors) may substitute for the pathological findings in directing therapeutic decisions. The IRIS Consensus Clinical Practice Guidelines for

Glomerular Disease in Dogs recommend, further, that 'immunosuppressive/anti-inflammatory therapy should not be administered to dogs with proteinuria before renal biopsy when (1) proteinuria is not definitively glomerular in origin; (2) immunosuppressive therapy is otherwise contra-indicated; (3) the dog breed and age of disease onset suggest that a non-immune-mediated familial nephropathy is likely; or (4) amyloidosis is the most likely histopathologic diagnosis' (Pressler *et al.*, 2013).

Alternatively, appropriate immunosuppressive/anti-inflammatory therapy may be warranted, in the absence of or before a kidney biopsy diagnosis, in patients with peracute or rapidly progressive azotaemia/proteinuria, multi-systemic immune-mediated diseases or some familial diseases (e.g. in Soft-coated Wheaten Terriers, Bernese Mountain Dogs) when sufficient clinical information is available to presume the likely diagnosis. Delay or absence of such therapy might compromise patient management or outcomes (see recommendations for when serology is positive, below). Again, the intent of these recommendations is not to diminish the value of the kidney biopsy or to circumvent its role in therapeutic decisions but rather to recognize that approximately 50% of dogs with glomerular disease are putative candidates for an immunosuppressive/anti-inflammatory therapeutic trial, and the consequences of not providing additional therapy could be notable (Klosterman *et al.*, 2011; Pressler *et al.*, 2013).

In the absence of biopsy confirmation, the conundrum confronted in providing immunosuppressive/anti-inflammatory therapy with uncertain indications and unproven benefits for such therapy is the risk imposed by the specific therapy *versus* the potential for undefined benefits. Without biopsy confirmation, there are nearly equal risks of promoting harm (including death) by withholding immunosuppressive therapy and promoting harm (including death) from the therapeutic risks and adverse effects associated with providing such therapy without indication or proven benefit. However, with judicial case selection, careful surveillance of the course of the disease, appropriate choice of therapeutic agent(s) and frequent monitoring for adverse effects of therapy, the risks of blinded therapeutic intervention can be minimized while attempting to document therapeutic benefit. This responsibility lies solely with the attending clinician, following informed consent of the client with regard to the use of these drugs in an unproven setting (Pressler *et al.*, 2013).

Another therapeutic dilemma concerns the management of glomerular disease in animals with associated infectious or serology positive aetiologies. The association of glomerular proteinuria and seropositivity for an infectious agent does not necessarily confirm that the infectious disease is active or that there is an explicit cause–effect relationship between the infectious agent and the glomerular disease. If the infectious disease is clinically active, it is compelling to conclude that the two conditions are linked, but the link is agent specific, and they may be unrelated (Goldstein *et al.*, 2013). For chronic suppurative bacterial or fungal diseases, the glomerular involvement may be either secondary immune-mediated injury or amyloidosis, which are indistinguishable on clinical criteria. For more specific infectious aetiologies, including *Borrelia burgdorferi*, *Ehrlichia* spp., *Anaplasma* spp., *Babesia* spp. or leishmaniosis, the corresponding glomerular injury is characteristically immune-mediated and predicts a therapeutic approach that includes both anti-infective therapy for the infectious component and immunosuppressive approaches beyond standard therapy for the secondary glomerular component.

The coexistence of glomerular disease and seropositivity supports the presumption of glomerular injury induced by an infectious agent and the rationale to initiate specific anti-infective treatment immediately, despite evidence for causality of the infection and the proteinuria (Goldstein *et al.*, 2013). Nephrotoxic anti-infective agents should be avoided if possible and clinical parameters including serial serology and appropriate cultures should be monitored to document resolution of the infection. For active infections characterized or documented to be associated with non-amyloid, immune-mediated glomerular injury it is necessary to decide whether or not to initiate immunosuppressive therapy. The IRIS Consensus Clinical Practice Guidelines for Glomerular Disease in Dogs recommend that: 'if the results of renal biopsy document an active immune component to the glomerular disease, appropriate immunosuppressive treatment is indicated. At this stage, the glomerular disease should be considered as having an immune-mediated component, and not infectious alone, and it is not likely to respond merely to anti-infective treatment and eradication of the infection if severe or progressive' (Goldstein *et al.*, 2013).

Initiation of immunosuppressive treatment is likely to compromise control of the presumptive predisposing infection. This is clearly a therapeutic dilemma, but the glomerular disease and the infection must be considered and managed as separate comorbid diseases. Proceeding with immunosuppressive or anti-inflammatory treatment without biopsy confirmation of their specific indications gives the potential for greater therapeutic risk in dogs with active or sequestered infection, based on positive serology, than in dogs without an infectious comorbidity. Conversely, dogs with peracute and rapidly progressive disease associated with seropositivity (e.g. Lyme-associated nephritis) often die from consequences of their glomerular disease within days of diagnosis and require immediate and aggressive immunomodulatory treatment in addition to supportive treatment for renal failure.

For peracute and rapidly progressive immune-mediated glomerular diseases such as Lyme-associated nephritis, novel immunomodulatory therapies including therapeutic plasma exchange (TPE) may be of value. The application of TPE is predicated on the foundation that the disease is caused by abnormal substances such as pathological antibodies or immune complexes in the plasma that, if removed effectively, will ameliorate or resolve the disease. To be effective, the therapy must remove a sufficient volume of pathological plasma relative to the total plasma volume of the patient to negate the causative component. In addition, the process must be provided for a sufficient duration or repeated as required to eliminate newly generated or redistributed substances (e.g. a plasma protein, IgG or IgM antibodies, immune complexes or lipoproteins) which cause re-equilibration (or recontamination) of circulating plasma from intravascular or extravascular compartments. TPE has been used for decades to manage a variety of glomerulopathies in human patients. It may alleviate clinical signs more rapidly and improve long-term outcomes when compared with historical experiences with conventional therapies in patients with comparable disease. The role of TPE in immune-mediated glomerular diseases in companion animals awaits further experience. However, for animals with acute, life-threatening presentations, it may provide immediate control of the condition until long-term therapy can be established.

Criteria for assessing effectiveness of treatment and re-evaluation of the treatment plan

Clear expectations and therapeutic goals should be established for both standard therapy and immuno-suppressive protocols. It is especially important to extend immunosuppressive therapies maximally to achieve thera-peutic goals while remaining cognizant of the predictable risks associated with these therapies. Changes in the clinical and biochemical characteristics of glomerular dis-ease provide the most time sensitive and documentable recognition of the responses to treatment. However, these parameters have not as yet been confirmed to be reliable surrogates for renal survival in dogs.

Therapeutic effectiveness for proteinuria and kidney function can be assessed most efficiently by monitoring changes in the UPC ratio and the serum albumin and serum creatinine concentrations, respectively. Responses to therapy may be categorized as a complete response, a partial response or failure to respond. With recognition of the considerable day-to-day variation in the UPC ratio in dogs, significant changes in the UPC ratio are likely to reflect beneficial (decreased UPC), or a failure or adverse responses (increased UPC), to therapy (Nabity *et al.*, 2007). Reduction of the magnitude of proteinuria has been shown to predict renal survival and the rate of progression of renal dysfunction in human patients. There is no comparable information in dogs with active glomerular disease to document whether reduction in the magnitude of proteinuria confers a favourable outcome in renal sur-vival and the patient's quality of life. Nevertheless, estab-lishing the greatest sustained nadir in the UPC should be the therapeutic goal within the constraints of therapeutic risks. The IRIS Consensus Clinical Practice Guidelines for Glomerular Disease in Dogs state: 'Response to treatment as measured by changes in UPC is defined as follows: A complete response is defined as a reduction in the UPC to less than 0.5. A partial response is defined as a reduction in the UPC by greater than 50% of the highest pretreat-ment UPC after standard therapy or with standard therapy if both were initiated simultaneously. Therapeutic failure is defined as a reduction in UPC of less than 50% of the highest pretreatment UPC after standard therapy or with standard therapy if both were initiated simultaneously' (Segev *et al.*, 2013).

It should be noted that the UPC ratio may normalize in some patients, but this magnitude of response is unlikely to be achievable in all dogs. A partial response is a favourable result of therapy, especially if the disease has produced permanent structural alterations to the glo-merular filtration barrier or the treatment incompletely controls the pathogenesis of the injury. In addition, gluco-corticoids may promote a transient or persistent increase in proteinuria. If the initial treatment fails to achieve the expected therapeutic goals, consideration should be given to maximizing therapeutic dosages, within accept-able risks of therapy, or establishing an alternative drug strategy.

In patients with an acute presentation, renal function (as assessed by serum creatinine and urea nitrogen) may return to reference ranges spontaneously or in response to standard therapy, immunosuppressive therapy or both (complete response). By contrast, in dogs with long-standing persistent proteinuria and CKD, or dogs with peracute presentation, the glomerular damage may not be repaired and may remain abnormal, progress or resolve incompletely (partial response). For azotaemic partial responders, some degree of sustained azotaemia is expected, and the maintenance of stable kidney func-tion can be regarded as a therapeutic goal. Responses to treatment also should be assessed by changes in kidney function (serum creatinine concentration) as compared with the serum creatinine concentration preceding initi-ation of therapy. The IRIS Consensus Clinical Practice Guidelines for Glomerular Disease in Dogs suggest that 'the response to treatment as measured by changes in serum creatinine concentration is defined as follows: A complete response is defined as reduction in serum creatinine concentration to less than 1.4 mg/dl (124 µmol/l) (or the patient's last known serum creatinine concentration before onset of the glomerular disease). A partial response is a sustained reduction in serum creatinine concentration by 25% or greater than baseline serum creatinine concen-tration most proximate to starting treatment. Therapeutic failure is defined as a reduction in serum creatinine con-centration less than 25% of baseline serum creatinine concentration most proximate to starting treatment' (Segev *et al.*, 2013).

Improvement in serum albumin concentration (in addition to serum globulins, total plasma protein, anti-thrombin and fibrinogen) may also represent a surrogate for improvement in glomerular permselectivity. Presump-tively, an increase in serum protein concentration reflects a decrease in urinary loss; however, it may also occur secondarily to progressive excretory failure independent of improvement in glomerular permselectivity. The IRIS Consensus Clinical Practice Guidelines for Glomerular Disease in Dogs state: 'Response to treatment as meas-ured by changes in serum albumin concentration from baseline (defined as the mean of serum albumin concen-tration values during the 30 days preceding immuno-suppressive therapy) is defined as follows: A complete response is a sustained increase in serum albumin con-centration to greater than 2.5 g/dl (25 g/l). A partial response is either (1) a sustained increase in serum albu-min concentration to 2.0–2.5 g/dl (20–25 g/l) or (2) a sus-tained increase of 50% or more in serum albumin concentration from the baseline serum albumin concen-tration. A therapeutic failure is defined as failure to increase serum albumin concentration to greater than 2.0 g/dl (20 g/l) or by less than a 50% increase from base-line serum albumin concentration' (Segev *et al.*, 2013).

Secondary therapeutic goals include (Segev *et al.*, 2013):

- An improvement in blood pressure. In conjunction with standard therapy, systolic blood pressure should be maintained at <150 mmHg
- Resolution of nephrotic signs, including peripheral and/ or pulmonary oedema, ascites and pleural effusion
- Stabilization (or improvement) of bodyweight and body condition or body composition as measures of nitrogen metabolism. Bodyweight should be compared with a historical reference or the body composition score to 'ideal'.

Summary

Glomerular disease is a complex and poorly understood syndrome. Spontaneous remission is possible in some types of glomerular disease (especially membranous nephropathy), but in general these diseases progress to CKD in many patients. Patient management and survival may be enhanced by early detection of protein-uria, determination of the morphological diagnosis of the underlying pathology and directed therapy for the primary and secondary manifestations of glomerular disease. Dogs with all forms of glomerular disease are likely to benefit from early intervention with standard therapy; however, standard therapy alone is unlikely to resolve the disease. Because of the limited benefits accruing from standard therapy, specific therapies are being proposed but need validation based on clinical evidence. A large number of dogs are euthanased after initial evaluation because of the severity of the renal fail-ure, a grave prognosis for recovery or the presence of concurrent life-threatening complications/diseases (e.g. thromboembolism, cancer, cardiovascular failure).

Aggressive immunosuppressive therapy in animals with glomerular disease with an immune-mediated aeti-ology has a reasonable potential either to control or to cure the disease, based on recent experience. A thera-peutic trial with immunosuppressive therapy is recom-mended for dogs with glomerular disease proven to have an immunological origin based on findings from a renal biopsy. In the absence of biopsy findings, there is an approximately 50% chance that the patient will have an immunological origin for their glomerular disease. In addition to these therapies, a search for possible infec-tious agents contributing to the glomerular injury should be undertaken, and therapy directed against identified infectious agents should be considered.

References and further reading

Allison AC (2005) Mechanisms of action of mycophenolate mofetil. *Lupus* **14(Suppl. 1)**, s2–s8

Brown S (2013) Renal pathophysiology: lessons learned from the canine remnant kidney model. *Journal of Veterinary Emergency and Critical Care* **23(2)**, 115 121

Brown S, Elliott J, Francey T *et al.* (2013) Consensus recommendations for standard therapy of glomerular disease in dogs. *Journal of Veterinary Internal Medicine* **27**, S27–S43

Bugbee AC, Coleman AE, Wang A *et al.* (2014) Telmisartan treatment of refractory proteinuria in a dog. *Journal of Veterinary Internal Medicine* **28**, 1871–1874

Burkholder WJ, Lees GE, LeBlanc AK *et al.* (2004) Diet modulates proteinuria in heterozygous female dogs with X-linked hereditary nephropathy. *Journal of Veterinary Internal Medicine* **18**, 165–175

Catapano F, Chiodini P, De Nicola L *et al.* (2008) Antiproteinuric response to dual blockade of the renin-angiotensin system in primary glomerulonephritis: meta-analysis and metaregression. *American Journal of Kidney Disease* **52(3)**, 475–485

Christ DD, Wong PC, Wong YN *et al.* (1994) The pharmacokinetics and pharmacodynamics of the angiotensin II receptor blocker losartan potassium (DuP 753/MK 954) in the dog. *Journal of Pharmacology and Experimental Therapeutics* **268**, 1199–1205

Cianciolo RE, Brown CA, Mohr FC *et al.* (2013) Pathologic evaluation of canine renal biopsies: methods for identifying features that differentiate immune-mediated glomerulonephritides from other categories of glomerular diseases. *Journal of Veterinary Internal Medicine* **27(Suppl. 1)**, S10–S18

Cianciolo RE, Mohr FC, Aresu L *et al.* (2016) World Small Animal Veterinary Association Renal Pathology Initiative: classification of glomerular disease in dogs. *Veterinary Pathology* **53(1)**, 113–135

Cook AK and Cowgill LD (1996) Clinical and pathological features of protein-loving glomerular disease in the dog: a review of 137 cases (1985–1992) *Journal of American Animal Hospital Association* **32**, 313–322

Cowgill LD and Polzin DJ (2013) Vision of the WSAVA Renal Standardization Project. *Journal of Veterinary Internal Medicine* **27(Suppl. 1)**, S5–S9

Doucet A, Favre G and Deschenes G (2007) Molecular mechanism of edema formation in nephrotic syndrome: therapeutic implications. *Pediatric Nephrology* **22**, 1983–1990

Geerts WH, Bergqvist D and Pineo GF (2008) Prevention of venous thromboembolism: American College of Chest Physicians Evidence-Based Clinical Practice Guidelines (8th edn). *Chest* **133**, 381S–453S

Goldstein RE, Brovida C, Fernández-Del Palacio MJ *et al.* (2013) IRIS Glomerular Disease Study Group: Consensus recommendations for treatment for dogs with serology positive glomerular disease. *Journal of Veterinary Internal Medicine* **27(Suppl. 1)**, S60–S66

Heerspink HJL, Kropelin TF, Hoekman J *et al.* (2014) Drug-induced reduction in albuminuria is associated with subsequent renoprotection: A meta-analysis. *Journal of the American Society of Nephrology* **26**, 2055–2064

Jacob F, Polzin DJ, Osborne CA *et al.* (2002) Clinical evaluation of dietary protein modification for treatment of spontaneous chronic renal failure in dogs. *Journal of the American Veterinary Medical Association* **220**, 1163–1170

Klosterman ES, Moore GE, de Brito Galvao JF *et al.* (2011) Comparison of signalment, clinicopathologic findings, histologic diagnosis, and prognosis in dogs with glomerular disease with or without nephrotic syndrome. *Journal of Veterinary Internal Medicine* **25(2)**, 206–214

Laverman GD, Navis GJ, Henning RH *et al.* (2002) Dual blockade of renin-angiotensin blockage at optimal doses for proteinuria. *Kidney International* **62**, 1020–1025

Lefebvre HP, Brown SA, Chetboul V *et al.* (2007) Angiotensin-converting enzyme inhibitors in veterinary medicine. *Current Pharmaceutical Design* **13**, 1347–1361

Littman MP, Daminet S, Grauer GF, Lees GE and van Dongen AM (2013) Consensus recommendations for the diagnostic investigation of dogs with suspected glomerular disease. *Journal of Veterinary Internal Medicine* **27**, S19–S26

Makani H, Bangalore S, Desouza KA *et al.* (2013) Efficacy and safety of dual blockade of the renin-angiotensin system: meta-analysis of randomized trials. *British Medical Journal* **346**, 360–375

Mallat SG (2013) Dual renin-angiotensin system inhibition for prevention of renal and cardiovascular events: do the latest trials challenge existing evidence? *Cardiovascular Diabetology* **12**, 108–120

Nabity MB, Boggess MM, Kashtan CE and Lees G (2007) Day-to-day variation of the urine protein: creatinine ratio in female dogs with stable glomerular proteinuria caused by X-linked hereditary nephropathy. *Journal of Veterinary Internal Medicine* **21(3)**, 425–430

Nachman PH, Jenette JC and Falk RJ (2007) Primary on glomerular diseases. In: *The Kidney, 8th edn*, ed. BM Brenner, pp.987–1066. Saunders, Philadelphia

Navar L, Jirakulsomchok D, Bell D *et al.* (1982) Influence of converting enzyme inhibition on renal hemodynamics and glomerular dynamics in sodium-restricted dogs. *Hypertension* **4(1)**, 58–68

Palmer BF and Alpern RJ (1997) Pathogenesis of edema formation in the nephrotic syndrome. *Kidney International* **Suppl. 59**, S21–S27

Polzin DJ and Cowgill LD (2013) Development of clinical guidelines for management of glomerular disease in dogs. *Journal of Veterinary Internal Medicine* **27(Suppl. 1)**, S2–S4

Polzin DJ, Leininger JR, Osborne CA and Jeraj KP (1988) Development of renal lesions in dogs after 11/12 reduction of renal mass: influence of dietary protein intake. *Laboratory Investigation* **58**, 172–183

Polzin DJ, Osborne CA, Hayden DW *et al.* (1984) Influence of reduced protein diets on morbidity, mortality and renal function in dogs with induced chronic renal failure. *American Journal of Veterinary Research* **45**, 506–517

Ponticelli C and Passerini P (2010) Management of idiopathic membranous nephropathy. *Expert Opinion in Pharmacotherapy* **11**, 2163–2175

Pressler B, Vaden S, Gerber B, Langston C and Polzin D (2013) IRIS Canine GN Study Subgroup on Immunosuppressive Therapy Absent a Pathologic Diagnosis: Consensus guidelines for immunosuppressive treatment of dogs with glomerular disease absent a pathologic diagnosis. *Journal of Veterinary Internal Medicine* **27(Suppl. 1)**, S55–S59

Rhen T and Cidlowski JA (2005) Antiinflammatory action of glucocorticoids – new mechanisms for old drugs. *New England Journal of Medicine* **353**, 1711–1723

Schneider SM, Cianciolo RE, Nabity MB *et al.* (2013) Prevalence of immune-complex glomerulonephritides in dogs biopsied for suspected glomerular disease: 501 cases (2007–2012). *Journal of Veterinary Internal Medicine* **27(Suppl. 1)**, S67–S75

Segarra-Medrano A, Jatem-Escalante E, Agraz-Pamplona I *et al.* (2013) Treatment of idiopathic focal segmental glomerulosclerosis: options in the event of resistance to corticosteroids and calcineurin inhibitors. *Nefrologia* **33(4)**, 448–461

Segev G, Cowgill LD, Heiene R, Labato MA and Polzin DJ (2013) IRIS Canine GN Study Group Established Pathology Subgroup: Consensus recommendations for immunosuppressive treatment of dogs with glomerular disease based on established pathology. *Journal of Veterinary Internal Medicine* **27(Suppl. 1)**, S44–S54

Sethi S, Glassock RJ and Fervenza FC (2015) Focal segmental glomerulosclerosis: towards a better understanding for the practicing nephrologist. *Nephrology Dialysis Transplantation* **30(3)**, 375–384

Vaden SL, Breitschwerdt EB, Armstrong PJ *et al.* (1995) The effects of cyclosporine *versus* standard care in dogs with naturally occurring glomerulonephritis. *Journal of Veterinary Internal Medicine* **9**, 259–266

Whitley NT and Day MJ (2011) Immunomodulatory drugs and their application to the management of canine immune-mediated disease. *Journal of Small Animal Practice* **52**, 70–85

Zwerner J and Fiorentino D (2007) Mycophenolate mofetil. *Dermatology and Therapy* **20**, 229–238

Manuscripts from the International Renal Interest Society Consensus Clinical Practice Guidelines for Glomerular Disease in Dogs

Brown S, Elliott J, Francey T, Polzin DJ and Vaden S (2013) Consensus recommendations for standard therapy of glomerular disease in dogs. *Journal of Veterinary Internal Medicine* **27(Suppl. 1)**, S27–S43

Goldstein RE, Brovida C, Fernández-Del Palacio MJ *et al.* (2013) IRIS Glomerular Disease Study Group: Consensus recommendations for treatment for dogs with serology positive glomerular disease. *Journal of Veterinary Internal Medicine* **27(Suppl. 1)**, S60–S66

Littman MP, Daminet S, Grauer GF, Lees GE and van Dongen AM (2013) Consensus recommendations for the diagnostic investigation of dogs with suspected glomerular disease. *Journal of Veterinary Internal Medicine* **27(Suppl. 1)**, S19–S26

Pressler B, Vaden S, Gerber B, Langston C and Polzin D (2013) IRIS Canine GN Study Subgroup on Immunosuppressive Therapy Absent a Pathologic Diagnosis: Consensus guidelines for immunosuppressive treatment of dogs with glomerular disease absent a pathologic diagnosis. *Journal of Veterinary Internal Medicine* **27(Suppl. 1)**, S55–S59

Segev G, Cowgill LD, Heiene R, Labato MA and Polzin DJ (2013) IRIS Canine GN Study Group Established Pathology Subgroup: Consensus recommendations for immunosuppressive treatment of dogs with glomerular disease based on established pathology. *Journal of Veterinary Internal Medicine* **27(Suppl. 1)**, S44–S54

Chapter 25

Management of prostatic disease

Autumn P. Davidson

Prostatic disease is common in dogs but rare in cats. In the dog, prostatic disease is the most common disorder of the male reproductive tract. Diseases of the prostate gland include benign prostatic hyperplasia (BPH), cystic benign prostatic hyperplasia (CBPH), squamous metaplasia (SM), paraprostatic cysts (PPC), infectious prostatitis/prostatic abscessation (IP) and prostatic neoplasia (PN). BPH, CBPH and IP are more common in intact dogs. PN is more common in neutered dogs than in intact dogs, and is a disease of aged dogs. SM is associated with endogenous or exogenous oestrogen exposure. PPC are more common in intact dogs and rare in cats.

Anatomy

The prostate gland is the only accessory sex gland in the dog; it surrounds the urethra just caudal to the urinary bladder and is normally easily palpated per rectum as a bilobed oval gland with a median septum. The prostate gland of the cat has four lobes and is located dorsal to the proximal urethra. The prostate gland in both species is primarily corpus (external to the urethra); the disseminate prostate (within the pelvic urethral wall) is vestigial. Additionally, the cat has bilobed bulbourethral glands found near the ischial arch on either side of the urethra (Figure 25.1).

25.1 (a) The relationship of the prostate gland to other structures in the caudal abdomen of the dog. (continues) ▶

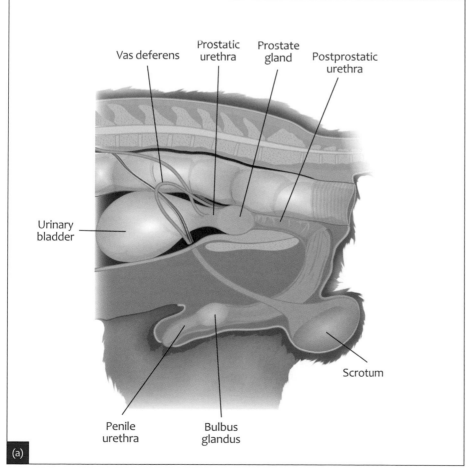

Vas deferens

Prostatic urethra

Prostate gland

Postprostatic urethra

Urinary bladder

Scrotum

Penile urethra

Bulbus glandus

(a)

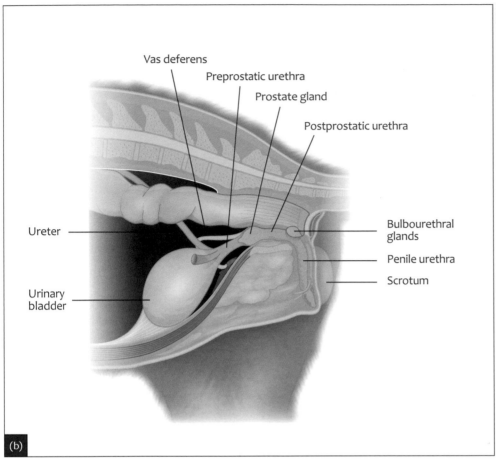

25.1 (continued) (b) The relationship of the prostate gland to other structures in the caudal abdomen of the male cat. Note that the prostate gland is more caudal to the neck of the bladder than in the dog.

Physiology

The prostate is stimulated to grow and is maintained in size and function by the presence of circulating testosterone. Several protein-type growth factors, such as urogastrone and prostatropin, may also promote prostatic growth. After testosterone from the plasma has entered the prostatic cell through diffusion it is metabolized to other steroids by a series of enzymes. Over 95% of testosterone is converted to the most important prostatic androgen, dihydrotestosterone (DHT), by the enzyme 5-alpha reductase in prostatic epithelial cells. DHT then binds to activated androgen receptors and stimulates growth of the prostate gland. In the absence of testosterone in males neutered before puberty, the prostate gland remains hypoplastic. Following neutering of the post-pubertal male, the prostate gland atrophies. Pharmacologically blocking the formation of DHT can have the same effect on the prostate gland.

The prostatic epithelial cells provide secretions that empty through ducts into the urethra to form the major component of the seminal plasma of the ejaculate. The seminal plasma has several functions: adding volume to the concentrated semen in the tail of the epididymis; providing energy for sperm cells; initiating and enhancing sperm motility; providing immunological and protective factors; and stimulating uterine contractility. In the dog, during the copulatory tie, the volume of prostatic fluid forces the sperm-rich part of the ejaculate through the cervix into the uterus, assisting conception.

Diagnostic tests

Multiple diagnostic techniques exist for evaluating the prostate gland; most are more feasible in the dog than the cat. A thorough history should be obtained, including general health, diet and supplements, and present and past medications; specific inquiry should also be made concerning urination, defecation, preputial discharge and the outcome of breeding (if any) or time of neutering. Physical examination of the prostate includes transabdominal and rectal palpation, which can require analgesia/sedation if painful (Figure 25.2). Evaluation of the size, symmetry, firmness, and the presence or absence of pain or compression of the colon and urethra should be made. Careful examination of the testes, prepuce, preputial discharge and penis should also be performed. The presence or absence of orthopaedic or abdominal pain should be noted. Most dogs under evaluation for prostatic disorders should have a complete blood count (CBC), serum biochemical panel, urinalysis with culture (cystocentesis) and *Brucella canis* screen (slide agglutination) performed.

Semen collection should be considered in intact male dogs unless it is too painful for the dog to ejaculate. Equipment for proper collection and evaluation of semen is minimal (Figures 25.3–25.5). A smooth collection of fresh semen often requires a quiet room, special footing (rubber-backed rug), an oestrous 'teaser' bitch or a toy dog treated with pheromone or oestral swab scent, and special artificial vagina equipment (Figures 25.6 and 25.7). The veterinary surgeon (veterinarians) and assistant should not wear their

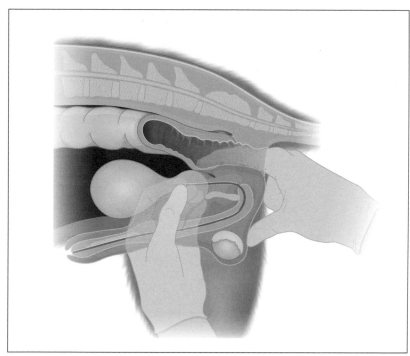

25.2 Rectal palpation of the prostate gland in a male dog. One hand should apply pressure on the caudal abdomen while the other palpates rectally. The prostate gland, when abdominal, can be palpated in the caudal abdomen as well as per rectum. The hand palpating the caudal abdomen can both evaluate the cranial aspects of the gland and push the prostate gland into or near the pelvic canal for better palpation per rectum.

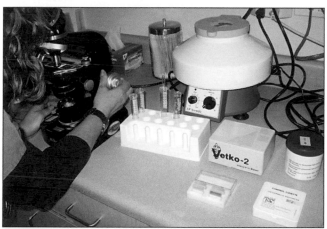

25.3 Examples of equipment for semen collection and evaluation: light microscope, slide warmer, centrifuge, automated sperm counter, frosted slides and cover slips.

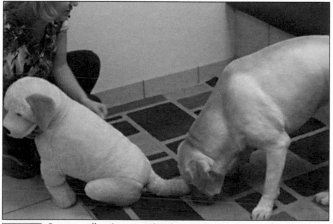

25.6 Semen collection examination room set-up: non-slip rug, 'teaser' treated with pheromone and no white coats.

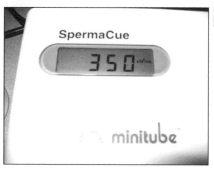

25.4 SpermaCue (Minitube®) automated sperm count machine (in this case 350 million sperm/ml are present).

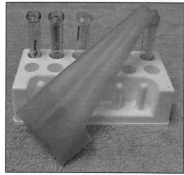

25.7 Latex artificial vagina, plastic vented and unvented semen collection tubes in rack.

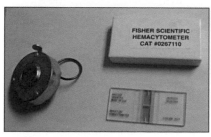

25.5 Haemocytometer.

white coats in an attempt to put the dog at ease before the collection; other diagnostics (venepuncture, cystocentesis, ultrasonography) should be performed after semen collection. When performing semen collection, try to approximate the stud dog's usual breeding environment as closely as possible. Act in a relaxed, friendly and non-threatening manner. The collection should be performed on the floor, except for toy breeds that are accustomed to being mated on a table.

Ensure that all collection equipment is at room temperature. Attach a semen collection tube with a vent hole into the small end of the latex AV (artificial vagina). The vent hole prevents a vacuum, allowing semen to flow freely into the tube. Fold the large end of the AV inside out by about 2.5 cm. The use of a lubricant is optional; use one that is not spermicidal. Have three to four additional tubes close at hand, in the test tube rack. If using a live bitch, support her in a standing position, restraining her head as necessary. Allow the stud to familiarize himself with the surroundings, the bitch and the handlers (Figure 25.8a). The examiner should be positioned next to the stud dog; right-handed people usually work best on the stud's left side (switch if left handed). Allow the stud to mount, placing the AV in front of his penis with the left hand, as he thrusts towards the bitch. If he does not mount or thrust, gently massaging the penis through the prepuce with the right hand will stimulate an erection (Figure 25.8b). When he is 50% erect or less, push the prepuce behind the bulbus glandis (Figure 25.9). If this cannot be done easily, pull the dog off the bitch, walk him away to allow his erection to subside, and bring him back to the bitch to try again, because ejaculating inside the prepuce is painful.

While the dog is thrusting, the examiner should reposition their hands to provide gentle constant pressure just behind and incorporating the bulbus glandis, keeping the AV over the penis. Rapid thrusting coincides with penetration in a natural breeding, before the copulatory tie occurs. After achieving full erection, coinciding with the tie, the stud dog will dismount and try to step over the bitch and the examiner's arm in order to turn. The dog should be helped by lifting his leg over and swinging the penis 180 degrees, so it is directed backwards between his legs (Figures 25.10 and 25.11). Keep the dogs standing near each other during the ejaculation phase, so the stud believes that mating is occurring.

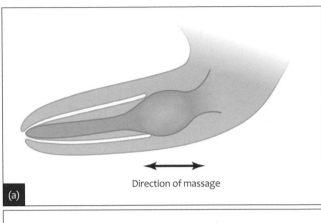

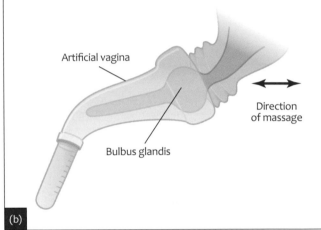

Direction of massage

Artificial vagina

Direction of massage

Bulbus glandis

25.9 (a–b) Proper extrusion of the penis into the artificial vagina. (b) The bulbus glandis is inside the artificial vagina, with the preputial skin pushed caudally.

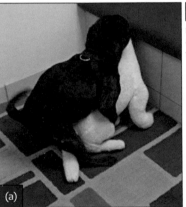

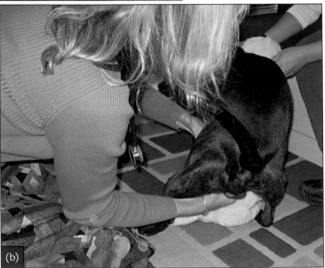

25.8 (a) Stud dog approaches and mounts the 'teaser'. (b) The collector places the artificial vagina in position.

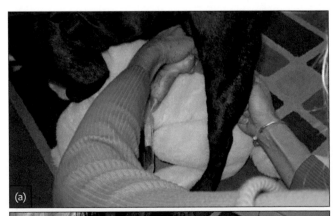

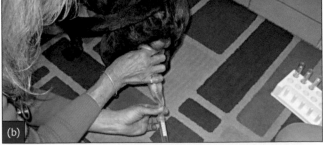

25.10 (a–b) The collector simulates the tie by bringing the penis caudally, permitting visualization of the ejaculate.

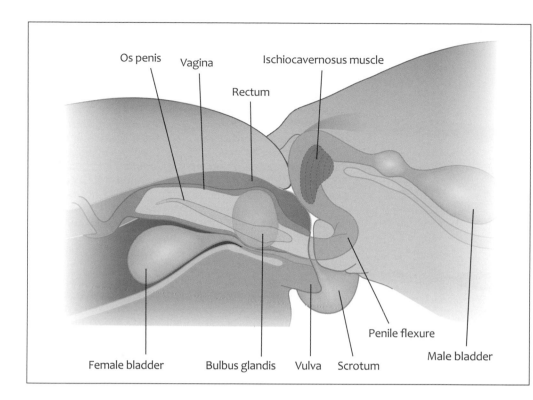

Observe the semen as it flows into the clear tubes. The three fractions are: first, normally clear and scant, from the prostate; second, white, 0.5–1.5 ml, sperm-rich fluid (SRF); third, voluminous, normally clear, prostatic. The SRF is usually released at the end of rapid thrusting, after the dog has turned. If fractionation of the ejaculate into its components is desired, an assistant should switch tubes to collect the SRF by itself. This entails rolling the end of the AV off of the first tube with a fingertip. At each switch, the collector should pinch the end of the AV above the tube, then ask the assistant to remove the tube and replace it. The assistant should put the tubes into the test tube rack to prevent spillage. When replacing subsequent tubes, the assistant should fold the end of the AV longitudinally into the tubes, rather than attaching it to the outside of the tube, because it will be slippery (Figures 25.12 and 25.13). The sample can be centrifuged with a commercially available semen separating solution if fractionation is not accomplished.

After collection is complete, the AV should be left on the stud dog until his erection has diminished. This keeps the penis more moist and comfortable (Figure 25.14). Apply some lubrication to the base of the penis, under the AV, to facilitate return of the penis within the prepuce. Always check to make sure the prepuce did not fold over the tip of the penis as it returned to the sheath, causing compression and oedema/paraphimosis. It is not necessary to walk the dog; he will lose the erection in 5–15 minutes. Care must be taken to ensure that the stud dog has undergone adequate detumescence before he is retired, because preputial skin and hair can strangulate the tip of the penis (Figure 25.15).

Semen analysis should include evaluation of morphology, motility and concentration/count. Normal canine semen has >70% progressively motile sperm with moderate speed and good quality motility. Place a drop of the SRF on a warmed slide, using a pipette. Cover with a cover slip and observe under the X10–40 microscope objective for motility. Sperm should swim across the slide

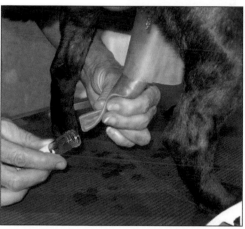

25.12 Assistant fractionating the collected ejaculate by switching tubes.

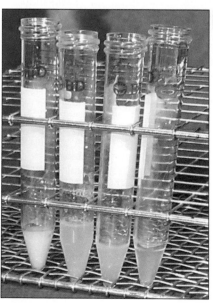

25.13 Fractions of ejaculate: sperm rich (left tube), and prostatic fluid (remaining three tubes).

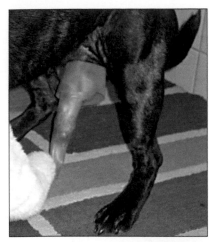

25.14 Artificial vagina left in place during detumescence.

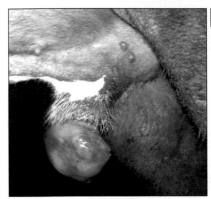

25.15 Paraphimosis of the tip of the penis following semen collection.

in a relatively straight path with minimal gyrations (good quality motility) and brisk speed (moderate to fast motility). No sperm-to-sperm agglutination should occur, but agglutination to egg yolk particles (if an extender was used) or other cells in semen may be normal. If motility is poor, prepare another drop on a new slide and double check. Observe individual live, unstained sperm cells under the X40 objective for morphology. Abnormal sperm may have coiled tails, proximal droplets, abnormally shaped heads, double tails or heads, or altered acrosomes. The acrosome is difficult to visualize without phase-contrast microscopy. Iatrogenic damage can cause detached heads and bent tails. Observing fresh sperm before staining permits evaluation for stain-induced morphological abnormalities.

Another slide should be prepared with the pipette as for a peripheral blood smear, air-dried and stained for morphological analysis. Either Wright–Giemsa or an eosin–nigrosin stain is commonly used. One to two hundred sperm should be tallied for morphology, noting normal cells and sperm cells with head abnormalities (misshapen, double), neck abnormalities (proximal droplets) and tail abnormalities (distal droplets, coiled, double). Using a differential cell counter labelled for semen morphology with the above categories is helpful. If a high number of morphological abnormalities occur post staining, a different methodology may be advisable. Note the presence of epithelial cells, white blood cells (WBCs) and erythrocytes (RBCs) (1–4+ per high-power field (hpf)).

Sperm counts can be performed by using a haemocytometer and Unopette® or an automated counter. Mix the SRF gently and draw it into the Unopette capillary tube for dispersal into the diluent chamber. Mix again gently and load the haemocytometer as for a WBC count. The haemocytometer needs to sit for 5 minutes to allow

sperm to settle at one level, permitting easier focusing. Systematically count the number of sperm cells in three representative squares of the nine primary squares in the haemocytometer grid. Multiply the number of sperm per millilitre by the volume of the SRF to obtain the number of sperm per ejaculate. Normal dogs have 200–400 million sperm or more per ejaculate; normal sperm counts correlate with the size of the dog. Culture of ejaculated semen requires special consideration for the presence of urethral and preputial normal flora; >100,000 organisms per millilitre suggests a pathogen (see 'Infectious prostatitis').

The advent of high quality ultrasound equipment and examinations in the clinical setting, usually not requiring anaesthesia, has facilitated the acquisition of urine, testicular, lymphatic and prostatic samples. Transabdominal ultrasound-guided prostatic sampling can usually be performed with mild analgesia or sedation. Prostatic massage, urethral catheterization and urethroscopy are usually reserved for sampling urethral masses when there is concern about tumour seeding (e.g. transitional cell carcinoma (TCC)). Surgical (open) biopsies are performed as indicated, usually when surgical intervention (marsupialization, excision) is planned.

Radiography remains important for evaluation of anatomical sites not amenable to ultrasonography (gas filled) and metastasis checks; computed tomography (CT) and magnetic resonance imaging (MRI) provide more precise evaluations.

Prostatic disorders

Benign prostatic hyperplasia and cystic benign prostatic hyperplasia

Pathophysiology

Dihydrotestosterone causes symmetrical progressive eccentric prostatic parenchymal enlargement (benign prostatic hyperplasia, BPH), which can become cystic (CBPH). Prostatic cell hyperplasia and hypertrophy are both contributory, but hyperplasia predominates. Benign hyperplasia occurs predictably in all intact dogs after the age of 5 years, and can be present as early as 2.5 years. An age-associated alteration in the intraprostatic oestrogen:androgen ratio potentiates the hyperplastic response to DHT.

Clinical findings

BPH and CBPH occur in the dog. Prostatic hyperplasia can occur without any clinical signs. Because prostatic enlargement in canine BPH is eccentric, urethral compression, as seen in men with concentric hyperplasia, is unlikely. Tenesmus secondary to colonic compression from marked prostatomegaly can be seen in advanced cases. The most common clinical signs of BPH and CBPH are blood (of prostatic origin) dripping from the urethra/prepuce, haemospermia and haematuria, which can be alarming to clients. Haemospermia is commonly discovered during a routine semen collection and is limited to the prostatic portion of the ejaculate (Figure 25.16). Semen quality is not affected; the sperm count, sperm cell morphology and motility are not altered. The presence of numerous RBCs in the ejaculate can make visualization of sperm difficult; centrifugation to separate the fractions of semen can help. Fertility is not impaired although attempts at cryopreservation are compromised because the presence of haemoglobin in

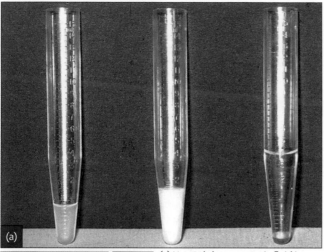

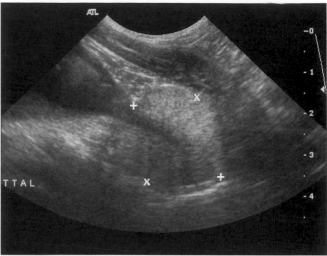

25.16 (a) Normal clear prostatic fluid in third fraction (right tube). (b) Haemospermia.

25.17 Benign prostatic hyperplasia. A sagittal ultrasound image of an intact canine prostate (between callipers) with multiple 'wagon wheel' striations radiating from the urethra to the capsule; a typical ultrasonographic finding for this disease.

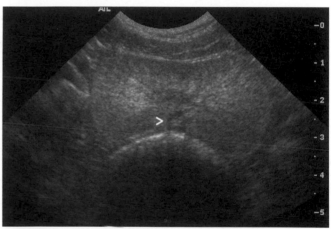

25.18 Benign prostatic hyperplasia. A transverse ultrasound image of an intact canine prostate showing hyperplastic parenchymal change. The urethra (>) is noted centrally.

semen increases sperm cell membrane fragility during the freeze/thaw process. Historically, the client commonly recalls seeing evidence of minor blood spotting in the dog's environment. Urinary outflow compromise, prostatic or lumbar pain, or deterioration of semen quality should prompt closer evaluation for more serious prostatic disorders/diseases such as prostatic carcinoma.

Diagnostic tests

The physical examination is unremarkable; the prostate is not painful upon palpation, but is usually prominent, sometimes with mild asymmetry.

When physical examination findings and semen evaluation are normal (other than haemospermia), an aggressive diagnostic evaluation is not indicated. The CBC and chemistry panel should be normal. Abdominal ultrasonography to evaluate the appearance of the prostate gland and guide the acquisition of a urine sample by cystocentesis to rule out urinary tract infection is prudent.

Benign hyperplasia and CBPH have a characteristic ultrasonographic appearance: a symmetrical parenchymal striation with increased echogenicity is apparent, with variable hypoechoic to anechoic intraparenchymal cystic structures evident. The cystic structures vary in size (Figures 25.17–25.19). No associated lymphadenomegaly is evident. Urinalysis is normal other than haematuria, and aerobic bacterial urine culture is negative.

Cytology from a prostatic parenchymal fine-needle aspirate, intraprostatic cyst aspirate or prostatic biopsy sample for histopathology can be used to confirm the diagnosis if the ultrasound examination findings are not characteristic (Figure 25.20). BPH and CBPH can accompany IP or more serious prostatic disorders in older dogs, making ultrasonographic conclusions difficult. Fluid aspirated from prostatic cysts should always be submitted for aerobic culture and sensitivity testing.

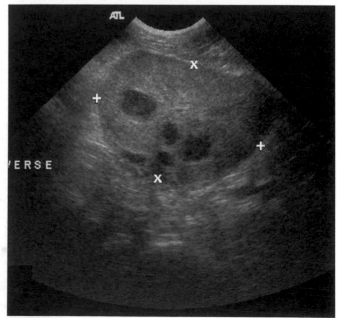

25.19 Cystic benign prostatic hyperplasia. A transverse ultrasound image of a canine prostate (between callipers) with hypoechoic parenchymal cysts.

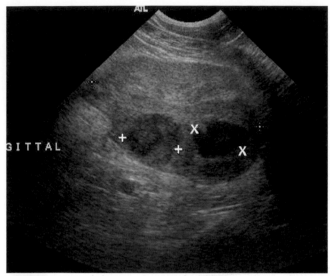

25.20 A sagittal ultrasound image of a dog suspected to have cystic benign prostatic hyperplasia (x–x); the more cranial (left) echogenic cystic structure (+–+) was an abscess.

Therapy

Castration is curative and is the most effective treatment. Atrophy of the prostate gland is noticeable in 2 weeks and this maximizes in 4 months. Failure of such atrophy following castration suggests another concurrent prostatic disease.

In valuable stud dogs, medical anti-androgen therapy is an option; it is indicated if defecation is difficult, or if the owners find the clinical signs of BPH/CBPH objectionable. Alternatively, medical anti-androgen therapy can be used until cryopreservation can be accomplished, and then castration can provide a cure. The presence of intraparenchymal cysts in CBPH may increase the potential for prostatic abscessation; anti-androgen therapy can be indicated if progression from BPH/CBPH to IP or prostatic abscessation is a clinical concern and castration is unacceptable.

Anti-androgen therapy using the 5-alpha reductase inhibitor finasteride is a potentially effective option; the conversion of testosterone to dihydrotestosterone is inhibited in the prostate gland, causing a reduction in prostatic size and cysts beginning in 1–8 weeks. The dose has been extrapolated from the human dose: 1.25–5 mg/dog orally q24h, although higher doses (0.1–0.2 mg/kg orally q24h) have been evaluated without problems other than the expense. A generic form of the drug is significantly less costly; efficacy appears to be comparable to the brand name. Libido and semen quality are not compromised, but the prostatic fluid component of the ejaculate is markedly diminished. The effect of this on fertility with natural matings, where prostatic fluid volume during the ejaculatory tie forces the SRF of the ejaculate into the uterus, is not known. Similarly, the effect of the loss of the protective effects of seminal fluid on sperm function is not known. Artificial insemination, either vaginal or transcervical, using semen extenders could be utilized if fertility seems compromised in dogs on finasteride. Finasteride is not authorized for use in dogs, but has achieved common clinical use. Finasteride is secreted in the urine, semen and faeces of dogs; repeated exposure of pregnant women to the drug during the first trimester can cause developmental abnormalities in male fetuses and should be avoided. The potential for exposure to future canine fetuses is not relevant.

Use of alternative medical therapies such as oestrogenic or progestational compounds is not advised, owing to their negative effect on circulating testosterone concentrations and spermatogenesis, and their induction of prostatic metaplasia (oestrogen), potential for myelosuppression (oestrogen), insulin and glucose dysregulation (progesterone) and mammary neoplasia (oestrogen). Over-the-counter extracts of the saw palmetto plant have no documented efficacy.

Squamous metaplasia

Pathophysiology

Squamous metaplasia (SM) occurs as a consequence of hyperoestrogenism, either of endogenous (functional Sertoli cell tumour, adrenal gland dysfunction) or exogenous (therapy for BPH, inadvertent exposure to human transdermal hormone replacement therapy) origin. Prostatic epithelial SM is accompanied by secretory stasis; intraprostatic cysts can form.

Clinical findings

The prostate gland is enlarged and is firm on palpation. Compression of the urethra and colon can cause dysuria and tenesmus. Other physical findings typical of hyperoestrogenism can be present: attractiveness to males, gynaecomastia, symmetrical alopecia, hyperpigmentation, testicular atrophy or dissymmetry (if a mass is present) and a pendulous prepuce. The presence of an abdominal (cryptorchid) testis should be ruled out when two scrotal testes are not present. Oestrogen toxicity to the bone marrow can cause pale mucous membranes (anaemia), petechiation or haemorrhage (thrombocytopenia), and/or fever (secondary to neutropenia).

Diagnostic tests

A careful history should be taken concerning possible exposure to transdermal hormone replacement therapies used by humans in contact with the dog, or past purposeful therapy with oestrogen for prostatomegaly.

A CBC, serum chemistry panel, urinalysis and aerobic bacterial urine culture should be performed to evaluate for myelotoxicity and metabolic status. Changes are variable and dependent upon oestrogen exposure, duration and dose, and the time delay between insult and testing. Generally, in the initial 2–3 weeks, both thrombocytopenia and thrombocytosis may be noted, with progressive anaemia and leucocytosis (WBC count may exceed 100,000/μl). After 3 weeks, pancytopenia with aplastic anaemia may be noted. Haematuria may occur secondary to thrombocytopenia or due to the presence of blood of prostatic origin in the urine.

In an intact dog, semen collection will show deterioration of semen quality (primarily sperm count: oligospermia or azoospermia); squamous epithelial cells can be present in the prostatic fluid, and can often be sampled from the preputial mucosa (Figure 25.21a). If a scrotal testicular mass is palpable (or discovered on ultrasonography (Figure 25.21b)), a fine-needle aspirate can reveal cytological evidence of a functional testicular neoplasm. Ultrasonography will reveal an enlarged prostate with hyperechoic parenchyma, often with cavitations; the typical striations of BPH are lacking (Figure 25.21c).

In a neutered dog with no scrotal testes, abdominal ultrasonography should be performed to screen for a cryptorchid, malignantly transformed testis (Figure 25.21de). A serum luteinizing hormone (LH) screen can support the presence of a gonad if imaging is negative. The canine

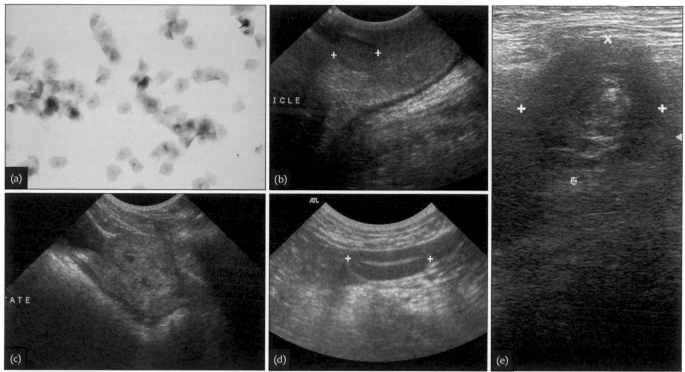

25.21 (a) Squamous cells in the prostatic fluid of a dog with squamous metaplasia of the prostate gland. (b) Sagittal ultrasonographic image of an intratesticular neoplasm (between callipers). (c) Sagittal ultrasonographic image of prostatic squamous metaplasia. Note the asymmetrical prostatic outline and hyperechoic parenchyma lacking striation, and parenchymal cysts. (d) Sagittal ultrasonographic image of an intra-abdominal testis (between callipers) in a 6-month-old Labrador Retriever. Normal intratesticular anatomy is evident. (e) Transverse ultrasonographic image of an intra-abdominal, malignantly transformed testis (between callipers) in a 9-year-old unilaterally cryptorchid Flat Coated Retriever.

anti-mullerian hormone (AMH) test (an enzyme-linked immunosorbent assay) is now most reliable for detecting cryptorchidism. Cytology can be performed on a fine-needle aspirate or biopsy specimen of the prostate to support suspicions.

Therapy

Therapy is dictated by the clinical findings: discontinuation of exogenous oestrogen exposure or therapy, or castration if functional testicular neoplasia is present. Concurrent prostatic infection or abscessation may be present and should be treated appropriately.

Paraprostatic cysts

Pathophysiology

Paraprostatic cysts (PPCs) are fluid-filled structures adjacent and attached to the prostate gland; they may or may not be patent. They can be prostatic in origin or be remnants of the uterus masculinus in both dogs and cats. They have been diagnosed in both intact and neutered dogs.

Clinical findings

The chronicity and size of PPC dictate the clinical signs, which can be minimal to marked. Large cysts can encroach on the urethra or colon, causing stranguria, incontinence or tenesmus, abdominomegaly or perineal swelling.

Diagnostic tests

Other than haematuria, the CBC, chemistry panel and urinalysis are generally unremarkable. Ultrasonography identifies a fluid-filled structure adjacent to the urinary bladder (Figure 25.22). Ultrasound-guided centesis of the PPC provides fluid for cytology and culture.

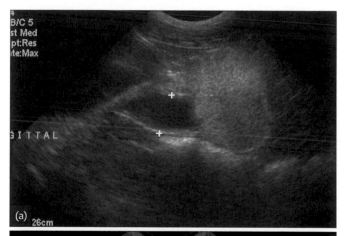

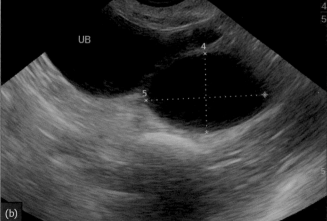

25.22 (a) Paraprostatic cysts (between callipers) seen in a sagittal ultrasound image of the prostate. (b) Uterus masculinus (between callipers) adjacent to the urinary bladder (UB) diagnosed in a neutered dog 6 months post-orchiectomy.

Therapy

Ultrasound-guided cyst drainage can relieve the clinical signs until surgical removal is performed. Castration is recommended. Antimicrobial therapy is dictated by culture and sensitivity and tailored for likely prostatic involvement.

Infectious prostatitis

Pathophysiology

Infectious prostatitis (IP) occurs most commonly with bacterial organisms; mycotic prostatitis has been rarely reported. Infection of the prostate gland can be acute and fulminant or chronic and progressive. Prostatic abscessation can occur. The most common source of infection is ascending urethral flora, but the haematogenous route of infection is also possible. The organisms most commonly isolated from the infected prostate are *Escherichia coli* and *Staphylococcus*, *Streptococcus* and *Mycoplasma* spp. Occasionally, *Proteus* spp., *Pseudomonas* spp. or anaerobic organisms are cultured. Mycotic prostatitis is uncommon and usually limited to endemic regions. Cystic benign hyperplasia predisposes dogs to IP. This alteration of the normal architecture of the prostate gland predisposes to bacterial colonization by interfering with normal defence mechanisms and by providing an environment that supports bacterial growth; infectious agents gain access to intraparenchymal cysts, flourish, and can encapsulate to form abscesses. Infectious prostatitis occurs most commonly in intact male dogs, but can occur in dogs neutered after infection is in place without appropriate antimicrobial therapy. Acute septic prostatitis can result in the later development of chronic septic prostatitis.

Clinical findings

Clinical signs of IP can be mild to fulminant. The prostate is often painful on palpation; sublumbar lymphadenopathy can be present. Dogs may exhibit stranguria, excessive preputial licking, constipation and tenesmus. Haemorrhagic and purulent urethral discharge may also be present. Dogs are commonly febrile, anorexic and lethargic, exhibiting pain on ambulation and kyphosis. Ejaculation can be painful, and affected dogs may be reluctant to breed or have semen collected. Peritonitis can cause nausea and abdominal discomfort.

Recurrent urinary tract infections imply chronic septic prostatitis. Dogs with chronic septic prostatitis may not have clinical signs, with deteriorating semen quality the only feature present. The prostate may be painful, firm and irregular on palpation. Ultrasonographic findings are nonspecific but typically the prostate will be of mixed echotexture with hyperechoic areas reflecting fibrosis. The ultrasonographic appearance can be similar to that of prostatic neoplasia. Additionally, multiple prostatic pathologies can be present in an individual patient.

Diagnostic tests

Septic prostatitis is best diagnosed on the basis of the findings from physical examination followed by ultrasonography, and cytology and culture of the prostate, with specific attention to any cystic structures within the parenchyma.

Pyuria and bacteriuria should always prompt evaluation of the prostate in any intact male dog. Because prostatic fluid normally refluxes into the urinary bladder, urinary tract infection is usually present whenever there is bacterial prostatitis and therefore aerobic bacterial urine culture is indicated. If IP is mild, semen collection can be attempted. Semen is typically abnormal, with suppurative inflammation, haemospermia, pyospermia, necrospermia and decreased prostatic fluid volume evident. Culture of semen is not ideal because normal urethral flora will be acquired. Quantitating urethral *versus* prostatic ejaculate organisms can help to differentiate the normal flora from pathogens but is expensive and laborious. Prostatic massage/wash requires sedation and also will collect urethral flora.

A CBC reflects systemic inflammation. The serum biochemical panel can be normal or reflect pre-renal azotaemia, hepatopathy, nephrogenic diabetes insipidus, sepsis or peritonitis. The urinalysis and urine culture reflect an infectious aetiology.

Ultrasonography, with appropriate analgesia/sedation, provides the best opportunity for sampling IP. IP is characterized by both hypoechoic and hyperechoic non-homogeneous parenchyma and, if abscessed, hypoechoic to isoechoic thick irregular-walled cystic structures in the parenchyma (Figure 25.23). Sublumbar lymphadenopathy can also be present.

The diagnosis of chronic septic prostatitis requires cytological and microbiological examination of urine and prostatic tissue, which may be obtained by ultrasound-guided fine-needle aspiration.

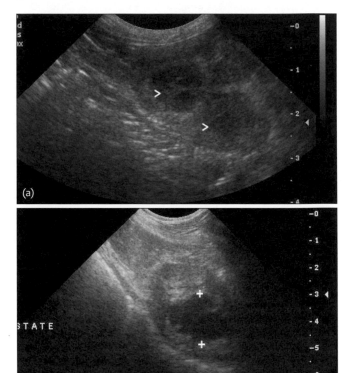

25.23 Infectious prostatitis. (a) Sagittal ultrasound image of prostatic abscessation (>). (b) Transverse ultrasound image of a cavitated intraprostatic abscess (between callipers).

Therapy

Acute IP is a serious disorder and can lead to sepsis and death. Treatment must be prompt and aggressive. Fluid therapy is necessary to correct dehydration and shock. Large prostatic abscesses are treated most effectively by surgical drainage and omentalization. Abscesses may also be drained by fine-needle aspiration under ultrasound guidance if the patient's condition is unstable. Pending the results of urine and/or prostatic fluid culture and susceptibility testing, treatment with a veterinary fluoroquinolone should be initiated. Antibiotic penetration in acute prostatitis may not be as problematic because inflammation alters the blood–prostate barrier, allowing most antimicrobials to penetrate. A negative culture of the urine or prostate should be obtained once therapy has been initiated to confirm effectiveness. Antimicrobial treatment for acute prostatitis should be continued for a minimum of 4 weeks. [Editors' note: Shorter duration therapies, which are recommended in human patients, may be appropriate in dogs.] Urine or prostatic fluid acquired using ultrasound guidance should be re-cultured 1 week after discontinuing antimicrobial therapy and again 2–4 weeks later to be certain the infection has resolved. Castration should be considered. Medical castration with finasteride is an acceptable alternative if the dog stabilizes rapidly and is valuable for breeding. Relapse is common, and can be diminished with the use of finasteride chronically.

Chronic bacterial prostatitis may be difficult to clear because the blood–prostate barrier is quite effective in preventing many drugs from penetrating into the prostatic parenchyma. In chronic prostatitis, only highly lipophilic agents cross into the prostate. Erythromycin, clindamycin, oleandomycin, trimethoprim–sulphonamide, chloramphenicol, enrofloxacin and ciprofloxacin are the agents most capable of achieving therapeutic concentrations in the prostate. Ciprofloxacin penetrates well into human prostate tissues, but in dogs its prostate:blood concentration ratios are not as high as for enrofloxacin. Antimicrobial therapy should be based on culture and susceptibility results from urine and prostatic tissue. Traditionally, treatment has been recommended for at least 4 weeks. Cultures should be repeated during and for several months after discontinuing antimicrobial therapy to ascertain whether resistance to antibiotics or persistent infection has developed. Castration, surgical or medical, improves the response to treatment of chronic bacterial prostatitis. It has been suggested that castration should be postponed until a negative urine or prostatic culture is obtained while the dog is receiving antimicrobial therapy, to avoid creating a sequestration of infectious material in an involuting gland.

Prostatic neoplasia

Pathophysiology

Transitional cell carcinoma (TCC) and prostatic adenocarcinoma (ACA) are the most common primary prostatic malignancies. TCC is more common; it is epithelial in origin, either from the transitional epithelium, extending from the bladder into the prostate, or originating from the uroepithelium of the prostatic urethra. Regional lymphatic and distant pulmonary or bone metastasis occurs in <20% of cases. Scottish Terriers (18-fold over-representation), Shetland Sheepdogs, Beagles, Wirehaired Fox Terriers, and West Highland White Terriers are the breeds most commonly affected by TCC. It occurs in middle-aged to older dogs, with a reported mean age of 11 years. Exposure to some topical insecticides, herbicides and cyclophosphamide are risk factors.

ACA is less common in dogs and rare in cats. It is of glandular origin and occurs in both intact and neutered dogs. Most ACAs do not express androgen receptors and are not influenced by androgens or anti-androgens. Prepubertal castration appears to be a risk factor for the development of ACA. ACAs are locally invasive and metastasize to regional lymph nodes, lungs and the skeleton in 24–42% of cases. There is an increased incidence in medium- to large-breed dogs >10 years of age, neutered early in life.

Squamous cell carcinoma, fibrosarcoma, leiomyosarcoma, haemangiosarcoma and lymphoma can also occur in the prostate gland.

Clinical findings

Malignant prostatomegaly commonly causes signs of tenesmus and constipation due to compression of the rectum, accompanied by sublumbar lymphadenopathy, overdistension of the urinary bladder due to urethral compression, lumbar pain from invasion into the lumbar vertebrae and nerve roots, and lower urinary tract signs of stranguria, dysuria, pollakiuria and haematuria. Concurrent urinary tract infection may be present. Pelvic limb ataxia and paresis or paralysis can occur.

Diagnostic tests

Physical examination findings commonly include prostatomegaly, sublumbar lymphadenopathy, abdominal pain and gait abnormalities. The prostate is unusually enlarged for a neutered dog (Figure 25.24). Anorexia and associated weight loss reduce body condition.

The CBC and chemistry panel findings reflect chronic disease and inflammation. Post-renal azotaemia can be present with obstructive masses. An elevation of alkaline phosphatase occurs in approximately 50% of cases, which is likely to be due to bone metastasis. Haematuria, pyuria, bacteriuria and atypical transitional cells can be found on urinalysis. Ultrasound-guided centesis of the prostate can provide cytologic evidence of malignancy, however malignant transitional cells appear similar to

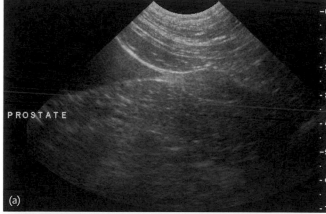

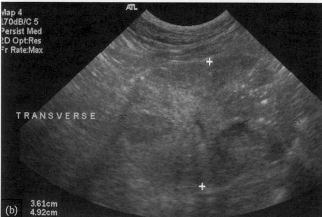

25.24 (a) Normal prostate of a neutered dog: homogeneous and small. (b) Prostatomegaly (between callipers) in a neutered dog with transitional cell carcinoma; the parenchyma is mottled, with calcification and mass effect.

reactive transitional cells, making biopsy of the prostate important (Figure 25.25). An open biopsy requires laparotomy or laparoscopy but is less likely to seed malignancy in the abdomen. Ultrasound-guided prostatic biopsy is a less invasive alternative; informed client consent is advised.

Thoracic radiographs are indicated to screen for pulmonary metastasis. Lumbar spinal radiographs can show vertebral metastasis. Mineralization in the enlarged prostate and sublumbar lymphadenopathy are suggestive of a malignant disease.

Abdominal ultrasonography is the most useful diagnostic tool, permitting evaluation of the prostatic parenchyma, regional lymph nodes, extension into the urinary bladder, urethral obstruction and the presence of hydroureter and hydronephrosis. Focal or multifocal hyperechoic prostatic parenchyma with asymmetry and irregular capsule outline and mineralization are common findings. Cavitary regions of necrosis and haemorrhage can be present. Sublumbar lymphadenopathy can be marked (Figures 25.26–25.29).

Definitive diagnosis requires histopathological examination of affected tissues and this can help to differentiate between TCC and ACA or other malignancies. Tissue samples are usually obtained by surgical biopsy. If the mass extends into the urinary bladder, cystoscopic biopsy is possible. Transabdominal ultrasound-guided biopsy is straightforward, but TCC are very exfoliative and seed readily, making the procedure risky for iatrogenic spread.

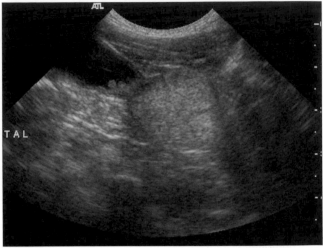

25.27 Sagittal ultrasound image of a prostatic transitional cell carcinoma. Note extension into the neck of the urinary bladder. The prostatic parenchyma retains striations, suggestive of benign prostatic hyperplasia.

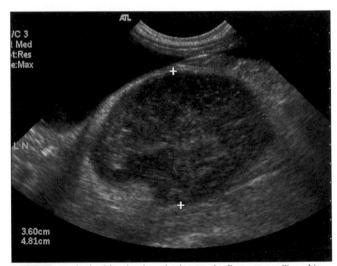

25.28 Marked sublumbar lymphadenopathy (between callipers) in a 10-year-old neutered Samoyed causing compression of the urethra.

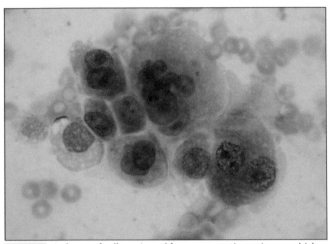

25.25 A cluster of cells aspirated from a prostatic carcinoma which exhibit criteria of malignancy: anisocytosis, anisokaryosis, multinucleated cells with prominent nucleoli, increased nuclear to cytoplasmic ratio and multiple nucleoli.

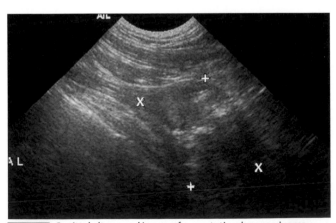

25.26 Sagittal ultrasound image of a prostatic adenocarcinoma (between callipers). Note the mineralization evident in the parenchyma.

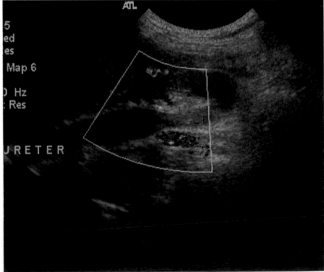

25.29 Sagittal ultrasound image of hydroureter resulting from extension of prostatic neoplasia into the trigonal region of the urinary bladder (colour-flow image).

Therapy

Poor quality of life is common with prostatic neoplasia; most dogs are euthanased within 2 months of the diagnosis. Castration has little benefit. Prostatectomy could be considered with local, intracapsular disease, but is associated with incontinence. Palliative radiation can relieve the clinical signs for some time. Urethral stenting can relieve urethral obstruction but can be associated with urinary incontinence and stent dislodgement. The use of non-steroidal anti-inflammatory drugs (NSAIDs) is associated with prolonged survival in dogs with prostatic carcinomas. Concurrent use of gastric protectants is advised. Oral analgesics that can be combined with NSAIDs can be helpful in controlling pain. Stool softeners are indicated if tenesmus is present. Intravenous bisphosphonates such as pamidronate can help with relief of the pain from skeletal metastases.

Chemotherapy can result in partial, short-term clinical responses. Agents used include mitoxantrone, vinblastine, carboplatin, gemcitabine and cisplatin (TCC) and carboplatin, cisplatin, doxorubicin and gemcitabine (ACA). The NSAID piroxicam, in combination with mitoxantrone, carboplatin or gemcitabine, improves success rates. Consultation with a veterinary oncologist is advised.

References and further reading

Barsanti JA (1992) Diagnosis and medical therapy of prostatic disorders. In: *Urologic Surgery of the Dog and Cat*, ed. EA Stone and JA Barsanti, pp.215–226. Lea & Febiger, Philadelphia

Barsanti JA and Finco DR (1995) Canine prostatic diseases. In: *Textbook of Veterinary Internal Medicine, 4th edn*, ed. S Ettinger and E Feldman, pp. 1662–1685. Elsevier Saunders, Philadelphia

Bjurström L (1992) Long-term study of aerobic bacteria in the genital tract in stud dogs. *American Journal of Veterinary Research* **53**, 670–673

Cohen SM, Taber KH and Malatesta PF (1991) Magnetic resonance imaging of the efficacy of specific inhibition of 5alpha-reductase in canine spontaneous benign prostatic hyperplasia. *Magnetic Resonance in Medicine* **21**, 55–70

Davidson AP and Baker TW (2009) Reproductive ultrasound of the dog and tom. *Topics in Companion Animal Medicine* **24**, 64–70

Grieco V, Riccardi E and Greppi GF (2008) Canine testicular tumors: a study on 232 dogs. *Journal of Comparative Pathology* **138**, 86–89

Mutsaers AJ, Widmer WR and Knapp DW (2003) Canine transitional cell carcinoma. *Journal of Veterinary Internal Medicine* **17**, 136–144

Peters MAJ (2000) Aging, testicular tumours and the pituitary–testis axis in dogs. *Journal of Endocrinology* **166**, 153–161

Pettersson A (2007) Age at surgery for undescended testis and risk of testicular cancer. *New England Journal of Medicine* **356**, 1835–1841

Purswell BJ, Parker NA and Forrester SD (2000) Prostatic diseases in dogs: A review. *Veterinary Medicine* **95**, 315–321

Rijsselaere T (2005) New techniques for the assessment of canine semen quality: a review. *Theriogenology* **64**, 706–719

Root Kustritz M (2005) Relationship between inflammatory cytology of canine seminal fluid and significant aerobic bacterial, anaerobic bacterial or *Mycoplasma* cultures of canine seminal fluid: 95 cases (1987–2000). *Theriogenology* **64**, 1333–1339

Sirinarumitr K, Johnston SD and Kustritz MR (2001) Effects of finasteride on size of the prostate gland and semen quality in dogs with benign prostatic hypertrophy. *Journal of the American Veterinary Medical Association* **218**, 1275–1280

Smith J (2008) Canine prostatic disease: A review of anatomy, pathology, diagnosis, and treatment. *Theriogenology* **70**, 375–383

Ström-Holst B (2003) Characterization of the bacterial population of the genital tract of adult cats. *American Journal of Veterinary Research* **64**, 963–968

Withrow SJ and Vail DM (2007) *Withrow and MacEwen's Small Animal Clinical Oncology, 4th edn*, pp.649–657. Saunders Elsevier, St. Louis

Chapter 26

Medical management of urolithiasis

Jodi L. Westropp and Jody Lulich

Urolithiasis is a general term referring to the causes and effects of stones anywhere in the urinary tract. Urolithiasis should not be viewed conceptually as a single disease with a single cause but rather as a sequela of multiple interacting underlying abnormalities. Thus, the syndrome of urolithiasis may be defined as the occurrence of familial, congenital or acquired pathophysiological factors that, in combination, progressively increase the risk of precipitation of excretory metabolites in urine to form stones (i.e. uroliths).

Many factors contribute to urolith formation and can vary with mineral composition; some of these factors are known and some are unknown. Risk factors known to influence urolith formation can be intrinsic, such as the animal's breed or genetic make-up, sex, age, congenital anomalies of the urinary tract or inherent disorders of metabolism (acid–base, water and nutrients), or extrinsic factors such as the animal's diet, environment, stress and acquired diseases (e.g. urinary tract infection, hypercalcaemia). Each factor may play a limited or significant role in the development and prevention of different types of uroliths. Nonetheless, recognition and control of lithogenic risk factors should minimize urolith formation and recurrence.

Diagnostic imaging for cystoliths

The indication for evaluating a dog or cat for urolithiasis is primarily based on urinary tract signs such as pollakiuria, stranguria or haematuria, or a combination of these, which suggests the possibility of cystoliths. In this clinical situation, medical imaging provides an accurate and sensitive method of confirming disease (see Chapter 7). The authors of an *in vitro* study concluded that ultrasonography was more sensitive than survey and contrast cystography for detection of cystoliths (Weichselbaum *et al.*, 1999). Moreover, the operator and patient are not exposed to ionizing radiation. However, if ultrasonography becomes the sole method of urolith detection, several important diagnostic features of uroliths would be overlooked, the most important being the radiopacity of the urolith, which aids in identification of urolith type. For example, struvite and calcium oxalate (CaOx), the two most common uroliths in cats and dogs, are radiodense, while urate and cystine are comparatively less radiodense or undetectable when

utilizing plain radiography. Furthermore, size may be more accurately predicted by radiography, and uroliths in the urethra of the male dog may be more easily detected via radiography (Byl *et al.*, 2010). This information is clinically relevant when developing surgical and minimally invasive strategies for urolith removal.

Diagnostic imaging for nephrolithiasis and ureterolithiasis

Clinical signs of nephrolithiasis and ureterolithiasis are variable and will depend on the presence or absence of ureteral obstruction and renal disease. In one study, upper tract urolithiasis was detected in 47% of cats with chronic kidney disease (CKD) (Ross *et al.*, 2007). Therefore, it is important to perform imaging studies in all cats with azotaemia. The sensitivity of survey abdominal radiography for the diagnosis of ureterolithiasis in cats is 81% (Kyles *et al.*, 2005). CaOx-containing ureteral calculi are the most common uroliths identified in the upper tract of cats (Cannon *et al.*, 2007) and are most readily identified in the retroperitoneal area on the lateral radiographic projection; however, visibility on lateral radiographs alone can lead to difficulty in determining which ureter is involved or whether one or both ureters are affected. Therefore, abdominal ultrasonography is recommended for cats suspected of having ureteroliths; it has a sensitivity for detecting a urolith of 77% (Kyles *et al.*, 2005). Although this is lower than the sensitivity of plain radiography, ultrasonography can help delineate which ureter is obstructed and the severity of hydronephrosis and hydroureter, if present (Figures 26.1 and 26.2). A combination of survey radiography and ultrasonography has a sensitivity of 90% for the diagnosis of ureterolithiasis, so it is the preferred approach.

In subacute ureteral obstructions, ureteral and pelvic dilatation may not be present, but this does not exclude the diagnosis of a ureteral obstruction. Additional imaging modalities, such as antegrade pyelography and computed tomography (CT) may be indicated to identify calculi that are not apparent on survey radiography or ultrasonograms, although many veterinary surgeons (veterinarians) feel these diagnostics do not provide additional information that will alter the therapeutic plan. Researchers evaluating imaging techniques in humans (Argüelles *et al.*,

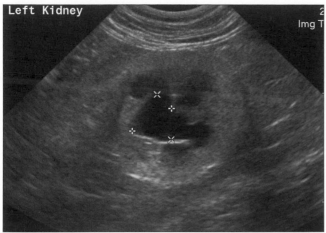

26.1 Ultrasonographic sagittal view of the left kidney of a 3-year-old neutered male Domestic Shorthaired Cat. The left kidney has moderate hydronephrosis and diverticular distension. There is a small focus of mineralization within each renal papilla and moderate dilatation of the left ureter was also present. This cat was treated conservatively with medical management due to the absence of azotaemia.

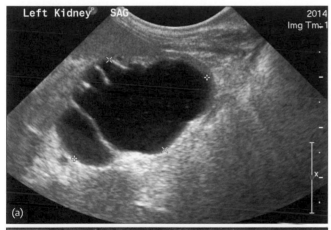

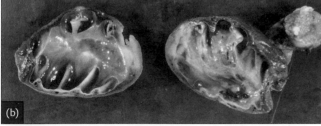

26.2 Ultrasonographic sagittal view of the left kidney of a 10-year-old neutered female Pomeranian presented for anorexia, fever and lethargy. (a) Marked hydronephrosis of the left kidney was noted, with only a thin (2.3 mm) mantel of parenchymal tissue remaining. The renal pelvis contained urine with suspended particulate material; pyelonephritis was suspected. (b) The kidney was subsequently removed because of suspected sepsis and a 5 mm urolith was confirmed in the left ureter approximately 2.6 cm distal to the pelvis. It was composed of 100% calcium oxalate. The dog recovered with appropriate antimicrobial therapy and supportive care.

2013) reported that CT scanning, using the bone window, provided the greatest *in vitro* accuracy from which actual stone measurements could be estimated; however, the craniocaudal diameter was overestimated. Furthermore, using the soft tissue window overestimated stone size. An abstract reported that CT (unenhanced or contrast enhanced) did not significantly improve the diagnostic performance for detection of ureteral obstruction in cats (Carr *et al.*, 2012).

Dissolution protocol for struvite urolithiasis

Struvite urolithiasis in cats and dogs is often amenable to medical dissolution. The authors consider dissolution more compassionate and an effective alternative to surgery. However, in animals with urolith-induced urinary tract obstruction surgical removal is the treatment of choice. In dogs, 70–80% of struvite uroliths occur in bitches. Although struvite uroliths are found most often in the bladder, they can be noted in the kidneys and ureters of dogs (Low *et al.*, 2010). They are usually larger than CaOx and often smooth in shape (Figure 26.3). Virtually all canine struvite calculi are infection induced, usually by *Staphylococcus pseudintermedius* or, less commonly, by *Proteus mirabilis*. These bacteria typically have the ability to hydrolyse urea to form ammonia and carbon dioxide. This reaction increases the urine pH and makes ammonium ions available to form magnesium ammonium phosphate crystals. When dissolving infection-induced struvite uroliths, the current recommendations are to provide antimicrobial therapy for the duration of the dissolution protocol. Ideally, the antimicrobial chosen should be based on susceptibility testing. Penicillins are usually an effective empirical antimicrobial choice, pending susceptibility results.

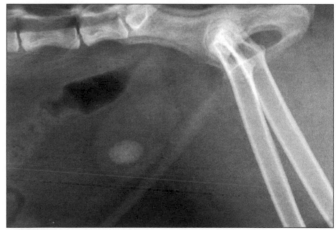

26.3 Survey radiograph of a 7-year-old Domestic Longhaired Cat illustrating a solitary radiodense stone. The stone dissolved completely in 4 weeks with a struvitolytic therapeutic food.

Occasionally, urine can be oversaturated with the minerals that comprise struvite, promoting stone formation in the absence of an infection. In fact, sterile struvite uroliths are the most common struvite stone in cats. In cats, struvite urolithiasis usually occurs as single larger cystic calculus (Figure 26.4). These uroliths are also amenable to dietary dissolution (Houston *et al.*, 2011; Lulich *et al.*, 2013). Three diets have been reported to be effective for dissolution of struvite uroliths in cats and two are marketed for dogs (Figure 26.5).

Because calculolysis usually occurs within 1 month in the cat (and can occur as quickly as 8–10 days), abdominal radiographs should be evaluated 2 weeks after the animal has fully adjusted to the dissolution protocol. Studies are currently underway to evaluate a dissolution protocol for dogs with struvite urolithiasis, but this protocol seems reasonable for dogs as well. If the urolith(s) appear(s) smaller, the urine is dilute (specific gravity <1.016) and the pH appropriate (<6.5), the dissolution protocol should be continued and the patient re-examined

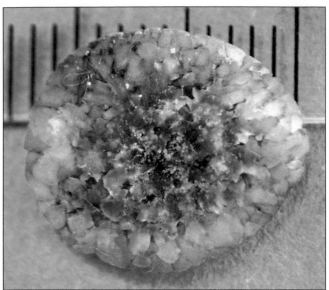

26.4 Stone removed from an 8-year-old European Shorthaired Cat and submitted for quantitative mineral analysis. The stone was composed of 100% magnesium ammonium phosphate. (Scale divisions shown on the ruler are millimeters.)

- Hill's® Prescription Diet® s/d® Feline (dry and canned)
- Hill's® Prescription Diet® c/d® Multicare/Feline Urinary Tract Health (dry and canned; reduced calorie also available)
- Royal Canin Veterinary Diet® Feline Urinary S/O (dry and canned; moderate calorie also available)
- Hill's® Prescription Diet® s/d® Canine (canned)
- Royal Canin Veterinary Diet® Canine Urinary S/O (dry and canned)

26.5 Commercial diets reported to be effective for struvite dissolution in cats and dogs.

in 3–4 weeks. If the urolith is not smaller with dietary intervention, the owner should be questioned regarding compliance. If compliance was good then the stone probably contains minerals other than struvite; in dogs, struvite uroliths can be layered with apatite (calcium phosphate), which may prevent complete dissolution.

Contraindications to attempting dissolution for suspected struvite urolithiasis include urethroliths or ureteroliths that are causing obstruction, or the patient's clinical signs being severe enough to warrant immediate stone removal. Furthermore, if the patient has a large cystolith that occupies most of the urinary bladder, dissolution is unlikely to be successful. The lower urinary tract signs associated with struvite urolithiasis can often be controlled with analgesics such as tramadol or non-steroidal anti-inflammatory drugs combined with dietary therapy; clinical signs should resolve within the first 24–28 hours.

Preventing recurrence of struvite urolithiasis in dogs should be aimed at preventing urinary tract infections (UTIs) because most dogs form infection-induced struvite stones. A search for underlying comorbidities (e.g. conformational abnormalities, obesity) should be initiated and the condition corrected, if possible. In cats, a diet should be fed that is high in moisture to decrease the urine concentration of mineral precursors that form struvite. This diet should produce a urinary pH that is acidified (<6.8), which is under the relative supersaturation threshold for struvite. Abdominal radiographs (including the entire urinary tract) should be performed periodically (every 2–3 months initially, then less often as the disease is managed) to assess for new urolith formation. If recurrent stones are detected when they are small, voiding urohydropropulsion may be an option for stone removal.

Calcium oxalate urolithiasis

Calcium oxalate (CaOx) is the most common urolith submitted to several stone laboratories from dogs and approximately equal in submission to struvite when evaluating data from cats. Although such stones are most often removed from the bladder, upper tract CaOx urolithiasis has been reported more frequently, especially in cats (Cannon *et al.*, 2007; Low *et al.*, 2010; Palm and Westropp, 2011). The mechanism of pathogenesis of CaOx stone formation in small animals is largely unknown, but several risk factors have been associated with CaOx formation. CaOx occurs slightly more often in males than in females and generally occurs in middle-aged cats and dogs. Diet can influence CaOx formation in some animals; low dietary potassium and calcium, decreased fluid intake and highly acidified urine are considered to be risk factors for CaOx urolithiasis in the cat and dog (Lekcharoensuk *et al.*, 2001; Trinchieri, 2013). Calcium should not be severely restricted in patients with a history of CaOx urolithiasis because dietary restriction of calcium causes hyperoxaluria and a potential for progressive loss of bone mineral component. Furthermore, oxalate absorption in the gut is dependent on the amount of dietary calcium consumed (Trinchieri, 2013). High protein diets could be a risk factor and the source of protein may be important to consider (e.g. hydroxyproline) as it is a precursor to oxalate. Some authors have also indicated that overweight and obese cats have a higher prevalence of urinary disease (defined as acute cystitis, feline urological syndrome, infection and urolithiasis) compared with those reported to be normal or underweight (Lund *et al.*, 2005). The association between obesity and CaOx urolithiasis in small animals has not been well investigated.

Once the urolith has been removed and identified as CaOx, strategies to prevent CaOx urolith recurrence may be used (Figure 26.6). It is important to address all patient-related factors and comorbidities that may be present in order to manage all of the patient's (and client's) needs appropriately. All dogs and cats with CaOx uroliths should have their serum calcium evaluated; if it is elevated, appropriate diagnostics should be pursued to investigate the cause of the hypercalcaemia.

In human medicine, evidence suggests that additional water consumption reduces urine saturation, the chemical driving force for urolith formation, by reducing the concentration of lithogenic precursors in urine (Borghi *et al.*, 1999; Lotan *et al.*, 2013); a similar approach seems prudent in animals. In addition to decreasing urine specific gravity (USG), increased water intake is likely to be associated with increased voiding frequency. Frequent voiding reduces crystal retention time, which theoretically should minimize urolith formation and growth.

Feeding canned formulations is one way to increase dietary moisture intake. In support of this recommendation, short-term studies (i.e. 12–19 days) in normal dogs and cats showed that foods containing high quantities of water (73% moisture) significantly reduced the relative supersaturation (RSS) for CaOx when compared with dry formulations (6.3% moisture) (Buckley *et al.*, 2011). Feeding canned rather than dry foods increases total water excretion, as does adding water to dry food (for dogs). When feeding dry foods, clients will need to add at least 2–3 cups of water per cup of dry food to attain adequate moisture content. This should be done gradually to allow the dog to adjust and to minimize food aversion.

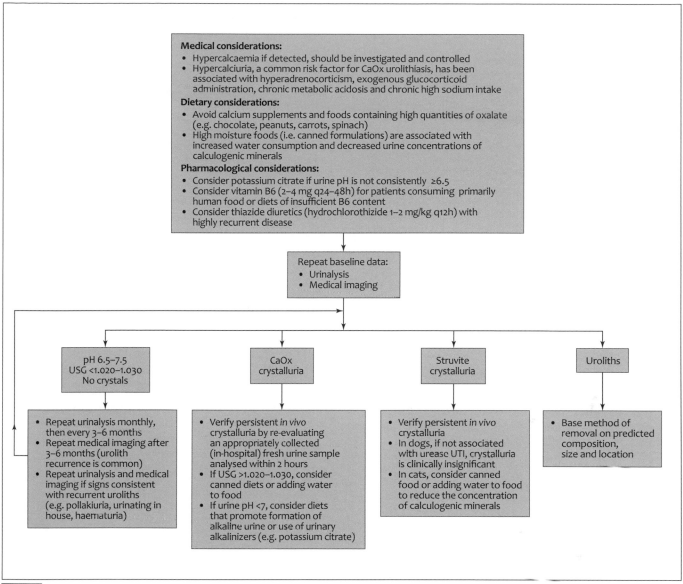

Medical considerations:
- Hypercalcaemia if detected, should be investigated and controlled
- Hypercalciuria, a common risk factor for CaOx urolithiasis, has been associated with hyperadrenocorticism, exogenous glucocorticoid administration, chronic metabolic acidosis and chronic high sodium intake

Dietary considerations:
- Avoid calcium supplements and foods containing high quantities of oxalate (e.g. chocolate, peanuts, carrots, spinach)
- High moisture foods (i.e. canned formulations) are associated with increased water consumption and decreased urine concentrations of calculogenic minerals

Pharmacological considerations:
- Consider potassium citrate if urine pH is not consistently ≥6.5
- Consider vitamin B6 (2–4 mg q24–48h) for patients consuming primarily human food or diets of insufficient B6 content
- Consider thiazide diuretics (hydrochlorothizide 1–2 mg/kg q12h) with highly recurrent disease

Repeat baseline data:
- Urinalysis
- Medical imaging

pH 6.5–7.5 USG <1.020–1.030 No crystals
- Repeat urinalysis monthly, then every 3–6 months
- Repeat medical imaging after 3–6 months (urolith recurrence is common)
- Repeat urinalysis and medical imaging if signs consistent with recurrent uroliths (e.g. pollakiuria, urinating in house, haematuria)

CaOx crystalluria
- Verify persistent *in vivo* crystalluria by re-evaluating an appropriately collected (in-hospital) fresh urine sample analysed within 2 hours
- If USG >1.020–1.030, consider canned diets or adding water to food
- If urine pH <7, consider diets that promote formation of alkaline urine or use of urinary alkalinizers (e.g. potassium citrate)

Struvite crystalluria
- Verify persistent *in vivo* crystalluria
- In dogs, if not associated with urease UTI, crystalluria is clinically insignificant
- In cats, consider canned food or adding water to food to reduce the concentration of calculogenic minerals

Uroliths
- Base method of removal on predicted composition, size and location

26.6 Algorithm for the prevention of recurrence of calcium oxalate (CaOx) uroliths. USG = urine specific gravity; UTI = urinary tract infection.

If owners cannot or will not feed canned food, the desired USG is not being met by providing additional water, and there is concern over urolith recurrence, the clinician may consider the addition of sodium chloride to the diet or feeding a diet that is higher in sodium chloride to try to prevent CaOx recurrence. In healthy dogs consuming foods that were considered higher in sodium (3 g/1000 kcal), CaOx RSS was decreased after 36 days (Stevenson et al., 2003). Longer term studies have not been performed. Absolute urinary calcium excretion increased, although the urine calcium concentration did not change, owing to the increased urine volume in healthy dogs consuming foods higher in sodium chloride. A study evaluating a higher-sodium diet (2.5 g/Mcal as fed) fed to older (mean age 10.4 years) cats had no adverse effects on renal function or blood pressure; however, the mean USG was only significantly lower at the 3-month time interval (over a 24-month study) compared with that of cats consuming a lower-sodium diet (mean USG: 1.034 versus 1.043). Cats in both groups had a mean USG of approximately

1.033 when assessed at 24 months (Reynolds et al., 2013). Adding dietary salt is contraindicated if the animal has concurrent kidney disease, hypertension or cardiovascular disease. It is also important that animals consuming higher salt diets have unrestricted access to water.

If dietary therapy fails to control CaOx urolith recurrence, hydrochlorothiazide (2 mg/kg orally q12h in dogs; 1 mg orally q12h in cats) can be administered, because this drug may decrease urinary calcium excretion and RSS for CaOx (Lulich et al., 2001; Hezel et al., 2007). Serum calcium concentration should be evaluated shortly after starting this drug to ensure that hypercalcaemia does not occur. Although there are no studies of the efficacy of hydrochlorothiazide in cats with CaOx uroliths, reports in healthy cats have suggested that this dose is well tolerated and reduces the RSS for CaOx. Additionally, potassium citrate may be helpful because the citrate can complex with calcium, thereby decreasing urinary concentrations of calcium oxalate. Potassium citrate will also alkalinize the urine.

Medical management of ureterolithiasis

Ureterolithiasis is more of a concern in cats than in dogs, and studies have suggested an increase in the frequency of ureterolithiasis in this species (Palm and Westropp, 2011). The clinical signs associated with ureterolithiasis are variable and are often related to the rate at which ureteral obstruction develops; cats and dogs with acute obstruction and rapid renal capsular distension show more pain than those with more insidious obstructions. Non-specific signs can include decreased appetite, weight loss, lethargy and hiding; haematuria (macroscopic or microscopic) also appears to be a common, but non-specific, clinical finding in animals with ureterolithiasis. However, upper tract uroliths can also be identified as incidental findings when imaging is performed for other indications. Depending on the degree of renal compromise, either pre-existing before obstruction or secondary to obstruction, many animals may also have clinical signs as a result of azotaemia.

If nephroliths are present but not distorting the renal parenchyma, removal is not advised and the animal should be monitored for progression (e.g. worsening azotaemia, increasing hydronephrosis). Likewise, if ureteroliths are diagnosed in animals without azotaemia or ureteral distension, the dog or cat can be monitored for progression. In these cases, a high-moisture diet (e.g. canned food) that is marketed for CaOx prevention is usually recommended. If evidence of kidney disease (International Renal Interest Society (IRIS) CKD Stage 2 or greater) is present, most urologists recommend using a diet reduced in phosphorus and protein that is formulated for kidney disease.

If ureteral dilatation is mild and the animal is stable, conservative medical management may be considered. Although there are no studies to evaluate the efficacy of any of the treatments mentioned, most veterinary urologists agree that expulsive therapy (see below) may play a role in the management of this disease in stable patients. Suggested therapies include intravenous fluid diuresis with administration of the diuretic mannitol, with or without other drug therapies. Drugs that have anecdotally been used for pets with ureterolithiasis include alpha-adrenoceptor antagonists such as phenoxybenzamine and prazosin. Tamsulosin, another alpha antagonist used in human patients, has also been anecdotally administered to cats for this disease. These drugs may help relax the ureter and allow passage of the stone into the bladder; response rates are variable. The tricyclic antidepressant amitriptyline has also been used because it may help inhibit smooth muscle contractions. Analgesics such as buprenorphine should also be used. During conservative management it is crucial to evaluate the stability of the patient and fluid status critically. Overhydration can occur, and fluid therapy should be discontinued if the animal's weight has increased and urine output is considered oliguric. Animals should be monitored by serial measurements of serum creatinine and blood urea nitrogen concentrations, because these are often the most reliable indicators that the obstruction has improved or progressed.

If ureteral dilatation progresses or obstruction persists, interventional therapy such as ureteral surgery, a ureteral stent or subcutaneous ureteral bypass placement should be considered, with the goal of preserving and restoring lost kidney function.

Urate urolithiasis

Dalmatians have a well described alteration in purine metabolism that leads to the excretion of uric acid in the urine rather than excretion of the more soluble metabolic endproduct, allantoin. All Dalmatians excrete relatively high amounts of uric acid (400–600 mg of uric acid per day, as compared with 10–60 mg per day in non-Dalmatian dogs); however, not all Dalmatians form urate uroliths. The prevalence of the clinical disease in male Dalmatians ranges from 26 to 34%, which is higher than that observed in bitches, probably due to anatomical differences between the sexes (Bartges et al., 1999). Genetic studies have identified the SLC2A9 transporter as the cause of the change in uric acid handling by Dalmatians, by positional cloning using an interbreed backcross (Bannasch et al., 2008; see also Chapter 14). Dogs of other unrelated breeds (including English Bulldogs, Black Russian Terriers and Australian Shepherds) have also been identified to be homozygous for the same mutation in SLC2A9 (Bannasch et al., 2008). For a list of other predisposed breeds and information on DNA testing to help owners and breeders identify affected and carrier dogs, please see the following website: www.vgl.ucdavis.edu/services/Hyperuricosuria.php.

Prevention strategies suggested for the management of urate uroliths in dogs with genetic hyperuricosuria include low-protein diets, bicarbonate supplementation, xanthine oxidase inhibitors and increased water intake (Case et al., 1993). Strategies for urate prevention in hyperuricosuric breeds are listed in Figure 26.7. Dietary purine restriction can be accomplished by feeding a low-protein diet (e.g. Hills Prescription Diet u/d® Canine Non-struvite urinary tract health), or diets that have higher protein but are restricted in purines (e.g. Royal Canin® Veterinary Diet Urinary U/C™ Low Purine Dry Dog Food). Vegetarian diets have also been anecdotally suggested for management of this disease.

If urate-containing calculi are found in dogs without the genetic predisposition, an investigation for a portovascular anomaly, such as a portosystemic shunt (PSS) or portal venous hypoplasia (PVH), and other causes of hepatic disorders should be pursued. Dogs with underlying liver disorders are likely to be predisposed to urate urolith formation due to the hyperammonuria and hyperuricosuria that result from the reduced ability of the liver to convert ammonia to urea and uric acid to allantoin. Correction of the vascular disorder should be addressed, if possible, to help prevent urate urolith recurrence. In dogs with inoperable PSS, or those with PVH, diets marketed for kidney disease or liver disease may be fed to help decrease the urinary ammonium urate and help control any signs of hepatic encephalopathy. If a portovascular anomaly cannot be documented, DNA testing for the hyperuricosuric genetic abnormality should be considered.

Much less is known about the pathophysiology of feline urate urolithiasis. In younger cats, or those with clinical signs and/or clinicopathological changes suggestive of a PSS (e.g. persistent ptyalism, neurological signs, microcytosis, elevated liver enzymes), further diagnostics such as abdominal ultrasonography and/or a technetium scan should be considered. The mean age of cats with urate uroliths is approximately 4–7 years; Siamese and Egyptian Mau cats have been reported to be over-represented (Albasan et al., 2009; Dear et al., 2011).

Management for dogs with genetic hyperuricosuria involves feeding a diet that is high in moisture and restricted in protein, such as those marketed for kidney disease. Anecdotally, a commercially available hydrolysed soy protein diet has been fed to affected cats in the hope of providing an adequate protein intake with low purine

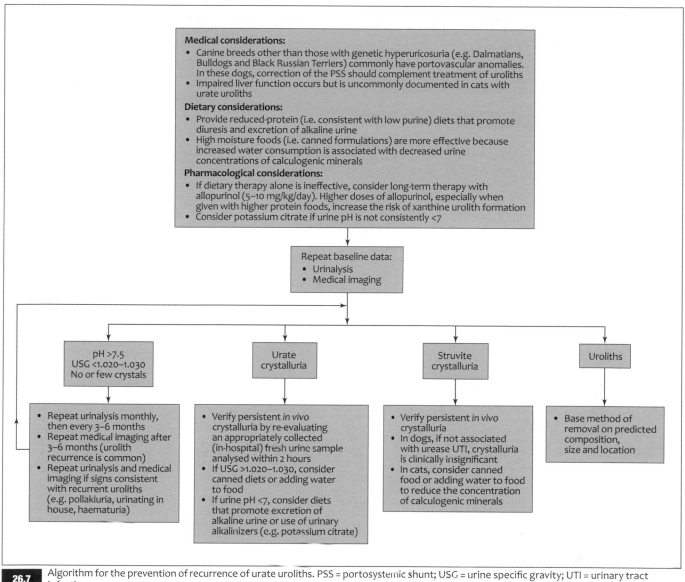

Medical considerations:
- Canine breeds other than those with genetic hyperuricosuria (e.g. Dalmatians, Bulldogs and Black Russian Terriers) commonly have portovascular anomalies. In these dogs, correction of the PSS should complement treatment of uroliths
- Impaired liver function occurs but is uncommonly documented in cats with urate uroliths

Dietary considerations:
- Provide reduced-protein (i.e. consistent with low purine) diets that promote diuresis and excretion of alkaline urine
- High moisture foods (i.e. canned formulations) are more effective because increased water consumption is associated with decreased urine concentrations of calculogenic minerals

Pharmacological considerations:
- If dietary therapy alone is ineffective, consider long-term therapy with allopurinol (5–10 mg/kg/day). Higher doses of allopurinol, especially when given with higher protein foods, increase the risk of xanthine urolith formation
- Consider potassium citrate if urine pH is not consistently <7

Repeat baseline data:
- Urinalysis
- Medical imaging

pH >7.5 USG <1.020–1.030 No or few crystals
- Repeat urinalysis monthly, then every 3–6 months
- Repeat medical imaging after 3–6 months (urolith recurrence is common)
- Repeat urinalysis and medical imaging if signs consistent with recurrent uroliths (e.g. pollakiuria, urinating in house, haematuria)

Urate crystalluria
- Verify persistent in vivo crystalluria by re-evaluating an appropriately collected (in-hospital) fresh urine sample analysed within 2 hours
- If USG >1.020–1.030, consider canned diets or adding water to food
- If urine pH <7, consider diets that promote excretion of alkaline urine or use of urinary alkalinizers (e.g. potassium citrate)

Struvite crystalluria
- Verify persistent in vivo crystalluria
- In dogs, if not associated with urease UTI, crystalluria is clinically insignificant
- In cats, consider canned food or adding water to food to reduce the concentration of calculogenic minerals

Uroliths
- Base method of removal on predicted composition, size and location

26.7 Algorithm for the prevention of recurrence of urate uroliths. PSS = portosystemic shunt; USG = urine specific gravity; UTI = urinary tract infection.

content (Royal Canin® Feline Hypoallergenic Hydrolyzed Adult HP). To the authors' knowledge, however, no controlled dietary trials in cats with urate uroliths have been performed. Periodic imaging using ultrasonography (because urate can be difficult to see on plain radiography) is also important to monitor for recurrence. Correction of an underlying liver disorder (such as PVH) is important for management in those patients where it has been documented.

Cystine urolithiasis

Cystine urolithiasis is much more common in dogs than in cats. Cystinuria in dogs results from a mutation in one of two genes: *SLC3A1* (type I-A, autosomal recessive inheritance; type II-A, autosomal dominant inheritance) and *SLC7A9* (type II-B; autosomal dominant inheritance). These genes encode subunits required for the dibasic amino acid transporter system that enables cysteine reabsorption from the glomerular filtrate (Brons *et al.*, 2013). Furthermore, an androgen-dependent type III cystinuria has been reported in entire male dogs of several breeds. A mutation

in the *SLC3A1* gene has also been reported in the cat (Mizukami *et al.*, 2015).

Cystine uroliths have been reported more often in younger male dogs and recurrence rates can be high. Dietary management includes feeding a diet high in moisture and low in protein (e.g. Hill's Prescription Diet u/d®, Royal Canin® Veterinary Diet Urinary U/C™), or feeding a vegetarian diet. Cystine is more soluble in alkaline urine and the recommended dietary therapy should result in a urine pH >6.5–7.0. If the optimal urinary pH is not achieved in this manner, potassium citrate (starting dose of 50–75 mg/kg q12h) can be added to alkalinize the urine, because citrate salts serve as a source of bicarbonate. The drug tiopronin (Thiola®, 2-mercaptopropionylglycine (2-MPG); 15–20 mg/kg orally q12h) can also be administered to help prevent (Hoppe and Denneberg, 2001) (or possibly dissolve) cystine stones; however, this sulphydryl compound can be cost prohibitive and limited in its availability. Therefore, veterinary surgeons may need to rely on compounding pharmacies to provide this medication. When using this drug, gastrointestinal and haematological adverse effects can occur. Dogs and cats should be monitored with appropriate imaging studies to evaluate the effectiveness of the therapeutic approach.

References and further reading

Albasan H, Osborne CA, Lulich JP *et al.* (2009) Rate and frequency of recurrence of uroliths after an initial ammonium urate, calcium oxalate, or struvite urolith in cats. *Journal of the American Medical Association* **235(12)**, 1450–1455

Argüelles SE, Aguilar García J, Lozano-Blasco JM *et al.* (2013) Lithiasis size estimation variability depending on image technical methodology. *Urolithiasis* **41(6)**, 517–522

Bannasch D, Safra N, Young A *et al.* (2008) Mutations in the *SLC2A9* gene cause hyperuricosuria and hyperuricemia in the dog. *PLoS Genetics* **4(11)**, e1000246

Bartges JW, Osborne CA, Lulich JP *et al.* (1999) Canine urate urolithiasis. Etiopathogenesis, diagnosis, and management. *Veterinary Clinics of North America: Small Animal Practice* **29(1)**, 161–191

Borghi L, Meschi T, Schianchi T *et al.* (1999) Urine volume: stone risk factor and preventive measure. *Nephron* **81(Suppl 1)**, 31–37

Brons AK, Henthorn PS, Raj K *et al.* (2013) *SLC3A1* and *SLC7A9* mutations in autosomal recessive or dominant canine cystinuria: a new classification system. *Journal of Veterinary Internal Medicine* **27(6)**, 1400–1408

Buckley CM, Hawthorne A, Colyer A and Stevenson AE (2011) Effect of dietary water intake on urinary output, specific gravity and relative supersaturation for calcium oxalate and struvite in the cat. *British Journal of Nutrition* **106(Suppl 1)**, S128–S130

Byl KM, Kruger JM, Kinns J *et al.* (2010) *In vitro* comparison of plain radiography, double-contrast cystography, ultrasonography, and computed tomography for estimation of cystolith size. *American Journal of Veterinary Research* **71**, 374–380

Cannon AB, Westropp JL, Ruby AL and Kass PH (2007) Evaluation of trends in urolith composition in cats: 5,230 cases (1985–2004). *Journal of the American Veterinary Medical Association* **231**, 570–576

Carr A, Wisner ER, Westropp JL and Mayhew PD (2012) Feline ureterolithiasis and ureteral obstruction: utility of computed tomography and ultrasound in clinical decision making. *Veterinary Radiology and Ultrasound* **53**, 680

Case LC, Ling GV, Ruby AL *et al.* (1993) Urolithiasis in Dalmatians: 275 cases (1981–1990). *Journal of the American Veterinary Medical Association* **203(1)**, 90–100

Dear JD, Shiraki R, Ruby AL and Westropp JL (2011) Feline urate urolithiasis: a retrospective study of 159 cases. *Journal of Feline Medicine and Surgery* **13(10)**, 725–732

Hezel A, Bartges JW, Kirk CA *et al.* (2007) Influence of hydrochlorothiazide on urinary calcium oxalate relative supersaturation in health young adult female domestic shorthaired cats. *Veterinary Therapeutics* **8(4)**, 247–254

Hoppe A and Denneberg T (2001) Cystinuria in the dog: clinical studies during 14 years of medical treatment. *Journal of Veterinary Internal Medicine* **15(4)**, 361–367

Houston DM, Moore AE, Favrin MG and Hoff B (2004) Canine urolithiasis: a look at over 16000 urolith submissions to the Canadian Veterinary Urolith Centre from February 1998 to April 2003. *Canadian Veterinary Journal* **45(3)**, 225–230

Houston DM, Weese HE, Evason MD, Biourge V and van Hoek I (2011) A diet with a struvite relative supersaturation less than 1 is effective in dissolving struvite stones *in vivo. British Journal of Nutrition* **Suppl 1**, S90–S92

Kyles AE, Hardie EM, Wooden BG *et al.* (2005) Clinical, clinicopathologic, radiographic, and ultrasonographic abnormalities in cats with ureteral calculi: 163 cases (1984–2002). *Journal of the American Veterinary Medical Association* **226**, 932–936

Lekcharoensuk C, Osborne CA and Lulich JP (2001) Epidemiologic study of risk factors for lower urinary tract diseases in cats. *Journal of the American Veterinary Medical Association* **218(9)**, 1429–1435

Lotan Y, Buendia Jiménez I, Lenoir-Wijnkoop I *et al.* (2013) Increased water intake as a prevention strategy for recurrent urolithiasis: major impact of compliance on cost-effectiveness. *Journal of Urology* **189(3)**, 935–939

Low WW, Uhl JM, Kass PH, Ruby AL and Westropp JL (2010) Evaluation of trends in urolith composition and characteristics of dogs with urolithiasis: 25,4999 cases (1985–2006). *Journal of the American Veterinary Medical Association* **236(2)**, 193–200

Lulich JP, Kruger JM, Macleay JM *et al.* (2013) Efficacy of two commercially available, low-magnesium, urine-acidifying dry foods for the dissolution of struvite uroliths in cats. *Journal of the American Veterinary Medical Association* **243(8)**, 1147–1153

Lulich JP, Osborne CA, Lekcharoensuk C, Kirk CA and Allen TA (2001) Effects of hydrochlorothiazide and diet in dogs with calcium oxalate urolithiasis. *Journal of the American Veterinary Medical Association* **218(10)**, 1583–1586

Lund EM, Armstrong J, Kirk CA and Klausner JS (2005) Prevalence and risk factors for obesity in adult cats from private US veterinary practices. *International Journal of Applied Research in Veterinary Medicine* **3(2)**, 88–96

Mizukami K, Raj K and Giger U (2015) Feline cystinuria caused by a missense mutation in the *SLC3A1* gene. *Journal of Veterinary Internal Medicine* **29(1)**, 120–125

Palm C and Westropp J (2011) Cats and calcium oxalate: strategies for managing lower and upper tract stone disease. *Journal of Feline Medicine and Surgery* **13(9)**, 651–660

Reynolds BS, Chetboul V, Nguyen P *et al.* (2013) Effects of dietary salt intake on renal function: a 2-year study in healthy aged cats. *Journal of Veterinary Internal Medicine* **27(3)**, 507–515

Ross SJ, Osbourne CA, Lekcharoensuk C, Koehler LA and Polzin DJ (2007) A case-control study of the effects of nephrolithiasis in cats with chronic kidney disease. *Journal of the American Veterinary Medicine Association* **230**, 1854–1859

Stevenson AE, Hynds WK and Markwell PJ (2003) Effect of dietary moisture and sodium content on urine composition and calcium oxalate relative supersaturation in healthy Miniature Schnauzers and Labrador Retrievers. *Research in Veterinary Science* **74(2)**, 145–151

Trinchieri A (2013) Diet and renal stone formation. *Minerva Medica* **104(1)**, 41–54

Weichselbaum RC, Feeney DA, Jessen CR *et al.* (1999) Urocystolith detection: comparison of survey, contrast radiographic and ultrasonographic techniques in an *in vitro* bladder phantom. *Veterinary Radiology and Ultrasound* **40**, 386–400

Chapter 27

Non-medical management of urolithiasis

William T. N. Culp and Carrie A. Palm

Urolithiasis is a relatively common syndrome affecting canine and feline patients and both medical and non-medical treatment options are regularly employed. The use of non-medical therapies in the treatment of urolithiasis is dependent on the clinical scenario (e.g. obstructive *versus* non-obstructive disease), the type of stone(s) present and their location within the urinary tract. The focus of this chapter will be on the non-medical techniques utilized for the treatment of urolithiasis in dogs and cats, as this field has undergone significant advancement over the last decade. Medical options are discussed in Chapter 26.

Nephrolithiasis

Nephrotomy

In the authors' practice, the number of nephrotomies and nephrostomy tube placements for the treatment of nephrolithiasis and ureterolithiasis has decreased because of the development of other treatment options with less morbidity; however, indications for these procedures may exist on a very limited basis. In some cases, nephrotomies to remove large nephroliths can be considered if recurrent urinary tract infections (UTIs) are documented that are refractory to medical management or the stone is large enough to obstruct the flow of urine.

The effect of performing bisection nephrotomies in normal dogs has been described (Gahring *et al.*, 1977). To perform the bisection nephrotomy, an incision was made on the convex surface of the kidney to divide the kidney into dorsal and ventral segments. This technique resulted in a 20–40% decrease in glomerular filtration rate (GFR) at 6 weeks post-nephrotomy.

Because of concerns about renal dysfunction after nephrotomy, a different technique utilizing the intersegmental blood supply as a guide for incision was developed in humans. This technique was also evaluated in normal dogs, and no significant difference in GFR was noted 7 days after surgery when comparing an intersegmental incision with a bisection nephrotomy (Stone *et al.*, 2002).

In two separate studies in cats (Bolliger *et al.*, 2005; King *et al.*, 2006), minimal long-term renal dysfunction was noted after bisection nephrotomy. It has also been reported (Bolliger *et al.*, 2005) that a modest relative reduction in single kidney GFR was observed in a kidney that had had a nephrotomy compared with a non-operated kidney. While these studies demonstrate that nephrotomy may be performed without major untoward effects in normal dogs and cats, the impact on diseased kidneys is unknown, and the reparative potential is likely to be compromised in those cases.

Nephrolithotomy/nephrolithotripsy

Nephrolithotomy and nephrolithotripsy involve the placement of a sheath into the renal pelvis through the renal cortex and parenchyma. In nephrolithotomy cases, the stones are removed directly through the sheath, whereas in nephrolithotripsy cases the stones are first fragmented into smaller pieces via holmium:YAG (yttrium, aluminium, garnet) laser lithotripsy and then removed through the sheath. In human medicine, these procedures are performed percutaneously through very small skin incisions (generally about 1 cm), and placement of the sheath is performed with ultrasound and fluoroscopic guidance. In dogs and cats, percutaneous placement of sheaths within the renal pelvis for nephrolithotomy or nephrolithotripsy has been difficult to perform, but some success has been achieved when these procedures are performed through a coeliotomy approach (Berent, 2014). Although a coeliotomy is not minimally invasive, the use of nephrolithotomy and nephrolithotripsy techniques prevents the massive trauma to normal renal tissue that occurs with traditional nephrotomy.

Nephrostomy tubes

Nephrostomy tubes can be placed temporarily to allow drainage of urine from the renal pelvis. Nephrostomy tubes are generally considered when patients are unstable (e.g. azotaemic, hyperkalaemic), and nephrostomy tube placement can stabilize a patient before a permanent treatment option is performed. The traditional surgical placement of these tubes involves a full coeliotomy and exposure of the kidneys with tunnelling of the tubes through the body wall to allow for external drainage. These tubes can be difficult to maintain and inadvertent removal is a common complication.

In the authors' clinic, percutaneous placement of nephrostomy tubes utilizing fluoroscopic and ultrasound guidance is preferred over open placement. To perform this procedure, the cat or dog is placed in lateral recumbency on the non-affected side. A stab incision is made in the skin overlying the kidney, and ultrasonography is utilized to guide placement of an 18 G over-the-needle catheter into the renal pelvis. Once the catheter is positioned, the needle is removed, and a 0.035-inch hydrophilic guide wire is introduced into the catheter and curled in the renal pelvis. The catheter is removed, and a locking-loop nephrostomy tube can be placed over the guide wire into the renal pelvis. The locking-loop nephrostomy tube is then locked to resist removal from the renal pelvis, and the tube is secured to the skin. While this technique can be quick and minimally invasive, the patient must still be anaethetized. Given this and the financial considerations, many veterinary surgeons (veterinarians) and owners choose definitive treatment initially, rather than temporary nephrostomy tube placement. Nonetheless, temporary tube placement may be the appropriate treatment for selected cases that are deemed unstable.

Extracorporeal shockwave therapy

Extracorporeal shockwave lithotripsy (ESWL) can be utilized to fragment nephroliths, typically requiring that the resultant fragments pass down the ureter. This procedure has demonstrated efficacy in dogs; however, the procedure is not generally recommended for cats (Adams *et al.*, 2005). It has been reported, in an *in vitro* study evaluating the impact of ESWL, that the ureteroliths fragmented poorly in cats compared with dogs, and the authors speculated that clinical application would probably result in unacceptable renal injury (Adams *et al.*, 2005). Placement of ureteral stents may be considered in conjunction with ESWL to help prevent ureteral obstruction due to the passing stone fragments.

Ureteronephrectomy

Ureteronephrectomy is not often recommended for urinary tract diseases involving the kidneys and ureters, but may be considered in selected cases. The decision to remove a kidney is not one that should be taken lightly and, when possible, other treatment options should be considered, especially if functional renal parenchyma is still present in the affected kidney. If ureteral or renal pelvic obstruction has resulted in severe hydronephrosis and minimal to no functional renal parenchyma is present, and secondary complications such as renal abscessation or compression from the space-occupying effects of an obstructed kidney have occurred, surgical removal should be considered. If that decision is made, it is critical for the attending clinician to consider the current and future function of the contralateral kidney. Ureteronephrectomy via a coeliotomy is a relatively straightforward procedure, and the outcome associated with the surgery is generally considered excellent. If the decision is made to pursue ureteronephrectomy, the kidney and ureter should be removed completely to prevent secondary complications that can occur, such as pyoureter or recurrent or persistent UTI.

Ureteronephrectomy is also being performed more regularly by laparoscopy in certain cases. A recent study described the technique in 12 cases (nine clinical), and laparoscopic ureteronephrectomy was determined to be a viable option (Mayhew *et al.*, 2013). In two cases, conversion to an open procedure was necessary owing to a severe hydroureter in one and retroperitoneal haemorrhage in the second. At the authors' clinic, laparoscopic ureteronephrectomy is the treatment of choice, whenever feasible.

Ureterolithiasis

Ureterotomy/ureterectomy/ureteroneocystostomy

Ureteral obstruction is a complex condition that affects both dogs and cats. Ureteral obstruction in dogs and cats with severe azotaemia is generally diagnosed relatively quickly, but diagnosis of ureteral obstruction can be more difficult in a non-azotaemic patient. In these cases, the animal may present with nonspecific clinical signs, such as inappetence and lethargy, or the obstruction may be found incidentally during evaluation for another problem. The decision to pursue treatment can be more difficult in patients that show minimal or no outward clinical signs, but a basic understanding of the physiology of ureteral obstruction, as well as treatment options and outcomes, will allow the attending clinician to provide as much information as possible to clients so they can make informed decisions regarding their pet's care.

Several diagnostic tests should be performed during evaluation of a patient with a ureteral obstruction. Bloodwork, with particular attention paid to renal values, will allow the veterinary surgeon to evaluate the patient fully and to determine how quickly intervention is re-quired. It is important to recognize that even with non-azotaemic ureteral obstruction, damage to the renal parenchyma is occurring while obstruction is present, so treatment to alleviate the obstruction should be pursued as soon as possible. Concurrent UTI may be present, and it is critical for a urinalysis and urine culture to be performed in all affected patients. Abdominal ultrasonography is typically the most useful test for diagnosis of ureteral obstruction. Ultrasonographic changes seen with ureteral obstruction are often obvious (e.g. significant dilatation of the urinary collecting system); however, in early obstruction changes may not be clear, requiring a clinician to put the entire clinical picture together to make a diagnosis. The lack of an obvious obstructing lesion within the ureter does not exclude ureteral obstruction. Abdominal radiographs can identify radiopaque ureteral and kidney stones (e.g. calcium oxalate, struvite); more advanced imaging with computed tomography is not typically indicated.

Historically, ureterotomy has been recommended for treatment of obstructive ureteral stones in veterinary medicine, and in some practices is still commonly utilized for treatment of single obstructive ureteral stones. One study suggested that most cases of proximal ureteral obstruction were treated by ureterotomy whereas most cases of distal ureteral obstruction were treated by partial ureterectomy or ureteroneocystostomy (Kyles *et al.*, 2005b). However, cases of ureteral obstruction are often not straightforward; some stones may not be noted on imaging studies. Furthermore, some dogs and cats may have multiple stones, an accumulation of crystals, strictures, or scarring and inflammation from previous ureteral passage of stones, making diagnosis and management difficult. In addition, stones may not be luminal, but embedded in the ureteral mucosa, making removal difficult. The extremely small size of the ureter, especially in cats, and its retroperitoneal position make surgery technically challenging and can be associated with complications. The ureteral diameter of a normal cat ureter is approximately 0.4 mm, and in dogs it can range from 5 to 15 mm. Some ureteral surgery requires specialized equipment such as microscopy, surgical loupes and instrumentation designed to hold and manipulate the ureter and small suture material.

Reports of treatment of obstructive ureteral disease are uncommon, but a small number of studies have evaluated outcomes of ureterotomy in cats treated for obstructive ureteral calculi (Kyles *et al.*, 2005a; 2005b). The postoperative complication rate in one series of cats was 31%, with urine leakage and persistent ureteral obstruction being the most common complications reported, occurring in 16% and 6% of cases, respectively (Kyles *et al.*, 2005b). Reported mortality rates have been as high as 18% (Kyles *et al.*, 2005b).

Ureteral stent placement

In the past several years, the placement of ureteral stents has revolutionized the treatment of ureteral obstruction in veterinary medicine, especially in cats (Figure 27.1).

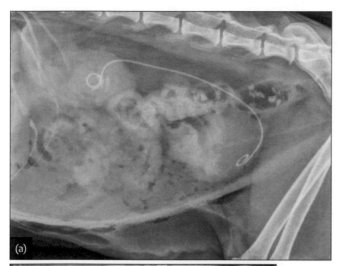

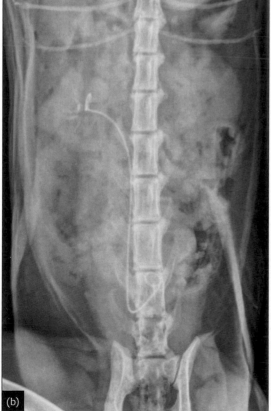

27.1 A ureteral stent has been placed in this 10-year-old neutered male Domestic Shorthaired Cat with a right ureteral obstruction. (a) Lateral radiograph and (b) ventrodorsal radiograph.

Ureteral stenting involves the placement of a double pigtail stent that is anchored within both the renal pelvis and the bladder. Ureteral stents can be placed surgically, percutaneously or cystoscopically. Stents allow passage of urine from the kidney into the bladder, initially through the stent and then, over time, by flow around the stent as passive ureteral dilatation develops (Lennon *et al.*, 1997). Stents may also be used to prevent stricture formation following surgery of the ureter or ureterovesicular junction (Auge and Preminger, 2002). Critical evaluation of the use of ureteral stents in companion animals is underway, but the use of ureteral stents in humans is well established (Auge and Preminger, 2002).

Ureteral stenting for benign disease in dogs and cats is being performed more regularly (Zaid *et al.*, 2011; Nicoli *et al.*, 2012; Horowitz *et al.*, 2013; Manassero *et al.*, 2013; Berent *et al.*, 2014). In most feline cases, ureteral stents are placed surgically and access to the ureter may be antegrade (through the kidney) or retrograde (from the ureteral orifice). In bitches, many stents can be placed with cystoscopic guidance; this is also possible in male dogs, although the author prefers to use perineal access.

Subcutaneous ureteral bypass

The subcutaneous ureteral bypass (SUB™) system was developed as an alternative to ureteral stent placement for ureteral obstruction. With this technique, urine passes through an artificial surgically placed system and, as the name suggests, the endogenous ureter is completely bypassed and does not need to be patent. The current subcutaneous ureteral bypass system employed most commonly in veterinary medicine involves the placement of nephrostomy and cystostomy tubes that sit subcutaneously, and are typically connected at a subcutaneous access port (Figure 27.2); this port allows the subcutaneous ureteral bypass system system to be flushed easily if needed.

Subcutaneous ureteral bypass is currently performed via coeliotomy in dogs and cats. An 18 G over-the-needle catheter is introduced into the renal pelvis, generally from the caudal pole, and a guide wire is introduced into the renal pelvis through the catheter. The catheter is removed, and the locking-loop nephrostomy tube is placed over the guide wire into the renal pelvis. A cystostomy tube is then placed in the bladder through a stab incision. Both tubes are secured to the respective organs and then connected via a port or male-to-male adapter. The system is secured subcutaneously.

Subcutaneous ureteral bypass has been described experimentally in dogs and clinically in cats in separate studies (Horowitz *et al.*, 2013; Steinhaus *et al.*, 2015). Subcutaneous ureteral bypass is the newest of the renal decompression techniques described for cats and dogs, and early results are promising. In one study, a subcutaneous ureteral bypass system was utilized to relieve ureteral obstructions in cats with both circumcaval and non-circumcaval ureters; the majority of the cases were noted to have ureterolithiasis (Steinhaus *et al.*, 2015). The long-term outcome in those cases was good, and it was reported the subcutaneous ureteral bypass system device did not obstruct as often as ureteral stents did (Steinhaus *et al.*, 2015). While these newer techniques for treatment of ureteral obstruction in veterinary patients are not without complications, and critical evaluation is still underway, initial results are promising and in the authors' experience they have greatly improved patient outcomes.

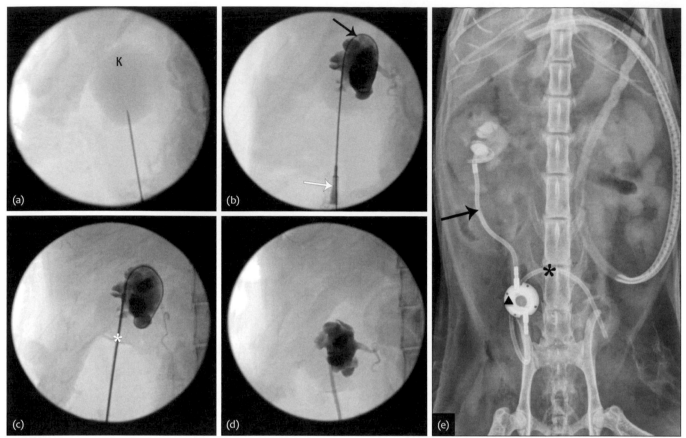

27.2 Placement of a subcutaneous ureteral bypass (SUB™) device in a 12-year-old neutered female Domestic Longhaired Cat with a right ureteral obstruction. Fluoroscopic images: (a) An 18 G over-the-needle catheter is being inserted from the caudal pole of the kidney (K) and directed into the renal pelvis. (b) The needle has been removed and a 0.035-inch guide wire (black arrow) has been introduced into the renal pelvis through the over-the-needle catheter (white arrow). (c) The over-the-needle catheter has been removed, and a nephrostomy tube (*) has been introduced over the guide wire into the renal pelvis. (d) The guide wire has been removed, and the nephrostomy tube is now locked within the renal pelvis. (e) A postoperative ventrodorsal radiograph immediately after placement. The nephrostomy tube (arrowed), cystostomy tube (*) and connecting subcutaneous port (triangle) can all be seen in this image.

Cystolithiasis

Cystotomy

Cystotomy is probably the most common urinary tract procedure performed in companion animals, and the performance of a cystotomy via a coeliotomy has been described extensively. Over the last several years, several novel minimally invasive techniques for removal of cystic calculi have been developed and described in veterinary patients. Recently, three less invasive techniques for cystotomy have been reported. A laparoscopic-assisted cystoscopy technique was described by Rawlings et al. in 2003. With this technique, two ports are placed, one for the camera and one for grasping the bladder. After the bladder has been grasped, stay sutures are placed in the bladder to secure it in a fixed position. A small cystotomy can then be performed and the cystoscope can be introduced into the bladder to assist in stone removal and to allow better visualization of the bladder and urethral mucosa (Rawlings et al., 2003). A more recent study (Pinel et al., 2013) made modifications to the originally described technique, including establishment of a temporary cystopexy, retrograde hydropropulsion and the use of a laparoscope as opposed to a cystoscope. Both of these less invasive techniques have been shown to be safe and effective for the removal of cystoliths and to allow visualization of the bladder and urethral mucosa (Rawlings et al., 2003; Pinel et al., 2013). Percutaneous

cystolithotomy was also reported recently and involves the placement of a port in the bladder after it has been exteriorized (Runge et al., 2011). Stones can be flushed from the urethra via the port site or grasped with forceps and baskets (Runge et al., 2011). With any of these techniques, it is critical that the clinician ensures removal of the entire stone burden, with careful intraprocedural evaluation and postoperative imaging.

Laser lithotripsy

Holmium:YAG laser lithotripsy has been utilized in companion animals for minimally invasive removal of cystic and urethral calculi. With this intracoporeal technique, a cystoscope is used to visualize the calculus within the urethra or bladder and a laser fibre is then passed through the working channel of the cystoscope so that the fibre comes in contact with the calculus. Laser energy is then applied to the calculus, resulting in photothermal fragmentation of the stone. Fragments are then removed by a combination of basket retrieval and voiding urohydropropulsion (Figure 27.3). Successful completion of lithotripsy requires that the patient be of adequate size for passage of a cystoscope with a working channel that will accommodate the laser fibre, and that all stone fragments can be removed or voided through the urethra. This necessitates that fragments are small enough and that intraprocedural haemorrhage, inflammation and swelling do

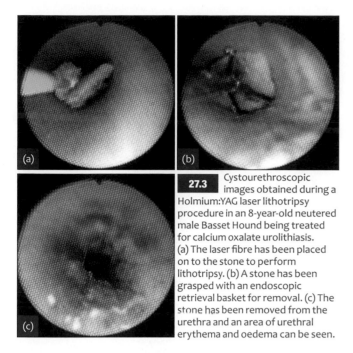

27.3 Cystourethroscopic images obtained during a Holmium:YAG laser lithotripsy procedure in an 8-year-old neutered male Basset Hound being treated for calcium oxalate urolithiasis. (a) The laser fibre has been placed on to the stone to perform lithotripsy. (b) A stone has been grasped with an endoscopic retrieval basket for removal. (c) The stone has been removed from the urethra and an area of urethral erythema and oedema can be seen.

not preclude complete removal. Staged procedures may be necessary in some cases. Case selection, based on stone size and number, patient size and sex, and comorbidities such as urethral stricture that might preclude passage of instrumentation or removal of fragments, is critical to maximize success.

At the authors' institution, laser lithotripsy is reserved for cases with a small to moderate stone burden. In cases of urethral obstruction, when a concurrent large stone burden is present in the bladder, retrograde hydropropulsion is attempted so that all stones can efficiently be removed via one of the cystotomy techniques discussed above. In rare cases where retropulsion is not successful, lithotripsy is recommended so that urethrotomy can be avoided. In male dogs, owing to the poor visibility achieved in the bladder with flexible cystoscopes and the difficulty in atraumatically removing a large volume of fragments through the male urethra, lithotripsy is typically only recommended for treatment of urethral stones. Careful attention should be paid to ensure that the entire stone burden is gone; this includes post-procedural imaging.

There are limited numbers of studies that have evaluated the use of laser lithotripsy in dogs. One study evaluating 100 dogs undergoing laser lithotripsy for treatment of urethral and cystic calculi reported an 82% rate of complete stone removal (Lulich et al., 2009). Complete removal of calculi was reported to be effective in males and females; however, it was more likely for complete removal of all calculi to be achieved in bitches (Lulich et al., 2009). Similarly, a separate study identified sex (females) as a predictor of success (Grant et al., 2008). In that study, lithotripsy in male dogs was reported to be technically more difficult to perform, required longer treatment times, and was less successful overall, when compared with bitches (Grant et al., 2008). Additionally, smaller bodyweight, large stone burden and increasing stone size increased the time required to perform lithotripsy (Grant et al., 2008). In a study comparing laser lithotripsy with cystotomy, lithotripsy was found to be a safe and effective treatment option in the removal of cystic and urethral calculi with no significant differences in resources or complications when compared with cystotomy; hospitalization time was significantly shorter for lithotripsy cases. (Bevan et al., 2009).

Voiding urohydropropulsion

Small bladder stones can be removed by voiding urohydropropulsion (VUH). To perform VUH, it is critical that the patient is given a general anaesthetic. A urinary catheter is passed through the urethra into the bladder, and the bladder is infused with sterile saline until it is moderately distended; excessive distension could lead to bladder wall mucosal haemorrhage and, less commonly, to bladder rupture. The urethral catheter is then removed while the urethral orifice is held closed to prevent the outflow of the infused saline. The patient is placed in a vertical position so the stones can fall into the bladder trigone. The bladder is expressed manually and the contents collected. During manual bladder expression, firm pressure should be applied; however, the attending clinician must monitor for development of urethral obstruction caused by passing fragments. Patients selected for VUH should have small stone burdens that will fit through the urethra. While the authors have performed VUH on large-breed dogs, smaller dogs (<20–25 kg) are more easily manipulated during voiding. The authors do not recommend VUH for male cats because of the small urethral size and the risk of urethral obstruction from resulting blood clots.

Urethrolithiasis

Urethral catheterization/cystostomy tube placement

Urethral obstruction is a common presenting complaint in veterinary clinics, in both dogs and cats. Many techniques have been developed to assist in urethral catheterization, allowing urine expulsion, although this procedure remains extremely challenging in some instances. Advances in instrumentation and the availability of this instrumentation have improved clinicians' ability to accomplish urethral catheterization on a regular basis. The use of hydrophilic guide wires (0.035-inch in dogs and 0.018-inch in cats) can provide assistance and can facilitate placement of a urethral catheter. These guide wires can usually be inserted retrograde into the urethral lumen, which then provides access for open-ended catheters to be placed over the guide wires.

Antegrade placement of a guide wire can be considered when retrograde placement has been unsuccessful. A urethral catheter can then be placed over the guide wire. To place a urethral catheter over a guide wire placed in antegrade fashion, the patient is placed in dorsal recumbency (dogs and cats) or lateral recumbency (generally cats). A region over the bladder is clipped and prepared using aseptic technique. In dogs, an 18 G over-the-needle catheter is introduced into the bladder near the apex; this allows introduction of a 0.035-inch guide wire. In cats, a 22 G over-the-needle catheter can be used and an 0.018-inch guide wire is recommended. The guide wire is then passed (using fluoroscopic guidance) from the bladder into the urethra; the dilatation of the urethra that is often seen proximal to the obstruction can assist in passage of the wire. Given that urethral tears often occur secondary to traumatic retrograde urethral catheterization attempts, guide wires often pass successfully when placed antegrade, and will not get caught in the torn mucosal flaps. Once guide wire access has been achieved out of the urethra, a urinary catheter can be passed over the guide wire into the urinary bladder in a retrograde-fashion. The chances of catheter placement are increased because through-and-through guide wire access allows for improved passage. A study evaluated this technique in nine cats with urethral obstructions secondary to iatrogenic urethral tears (6/9), urethral calculi (1/9), urethral ulceration (1/9) and urethral stricture (1/9) (Holmes *et al.*, 2012). The technique was determined to be a useful minimally invasive option for rapid placement of a urethral catheter.

Urethral stricture and subsequent urethral obstruction are major complications that can develop after urethrolithiasis or urethral catheterization. Treatment options for opening of the stricture include ballooning and stenting (or a combination of the two). To bypass a urethral stricture, a guide wire is passed retrograde or antegrade into the urinary bladder. A balloon (high pressure, low volume) can be introduced over the guide wire into the region of the stricture. The balloon can be inflated to cause dilation of the stricture and increase the luminal diameter in that region. If the lesion has been previously ballooned or there is a reason to decrease the overall number of procedures in that particular patient (e.g. patient morbidity or owner's wishes), then a stent can be immediately placed. If ballooning alone is attempted, it is likely that several sessions will be necessary. For benign urethral strictures, a covered urethral stent is recommended to prevent ingrowth of scar tissue.

If a patient needs to be stabilized prior to more definitive surgery or a minimally invasive treatment option, percutaneous drainage tube placement under fluoroscopic image guidance can be performed. Similar to antegrade urethral catheterization, an over-the-needle catheter is placed intra-abdominally or into the bladder, depending on whether peritoneal cavity or bladder drainage is required. After initial catheter placement, a guide wire is introduced into the cavity and the over-the-needle catheter is removed. A locking-loop pigtail catheter can be advanced over the guide wire and, as the guide wire is removed, the catheter pigtail should be locked to prevent inadvertent removal.

Urethrotomy/urethrostomy

With the success of retrograde hydropropulsion and laser lithotripsy, the use of urethrotomy to remove urethral stones is extremely rare. Urethrotomies can be performed in any location along the urethra, and closure of the site is generally recommended although healing by second intention has been described. In cases of serial or chronic urethrolithiasis that have failed medical management, permanent urethrostomies can be performed. The goal of the urethrostomy is to create an opening that is larger than the natural urethral orifice to allow easier passage of small stones; it is considered in patients with recurrent stone formation and urethral obstruction despite appropriate medical management. While these procedures decrease the risk of urethral obstruction, it can still occur. Prescrotal or scrotal and perineal urethrostomies are most commonly performed in dogs and cats, respectively.

When creating permanent urethrostomies, appropriate surgical technique is essential. Urethral stricture can occur at the surgical site, and other complications such as UTI have also been documented (McLoughlin, 2011). However, the outcome with these procedures is generally considered good.

References and further reading

Adams LG, Williams JC, Mcateer JA *et al.* (2005) *In vitro* evaluation of canine and feline calcium oxalate urolith fragility via shock wave lithotripsy. *American Journal of Veterinary Research* **66**, 1651–1654

Auge BK and Preminger GM (2002) Ureteral stents and their use in endourology. *Current Opinion in Urology* **12**, 217–222

Berent AC (2014) New techniques on the horizon: interventional radiology and interventional endoscopy of the urinary tract ('endourology'). *Journal of Feline Medicine and Surgery* **16**, 51–65

Berent AC, Weisse CW, Todd K and Bagley DH (2014) Technical and clinical outcomes of ureteral stenting in cats with benign ureteral obstruction: 69 cases (2006–2010). *Journal of the American Veterinary Medical Association* **244**, 559–576

Bevan JM, Lulich JP, Albasan H and Osborne CA (2009) Comparison of laser lithotripsy and cystotomy for the management of dogs with urolithiasis. *Journal of the American Veterinary Medical Association* **234**, 1286–1294

Bolliger C, Walshaw R, Kruger JM *et al.* (2005) Evaluation of the effects of nephrotomy on renal function in clinically normal cats. *American Journal of Veterinary Research* **66**, 1400–1407

Gahring DR, Crowe DT, Powers TE *et al.* (1977) Comparative renal function studies of nephrotomy closure with and without sutures in dogs. *Journal of the American Veterinary Medical Association* **171**, 537–541

Grant DC, Werre SR and Gevedon ML (2008) Holmium:YAG laser lithotripsy for urolithiasis in dogs. *Journal of Veterinary Internal Medicine* **22**, 534–539

Holmes ES, Weisse C and Berent AC (2012) Use of fluoroscopically guided percutaneous antegrade urethral catheterization for the treatment of urethral obstruction in male cats: 9 cases (2000–2009). *Journal of the American Veterinary Medical Association* **241**, 603–607

Horowitz C, Berent A, Weisse C, Langston C and Bagley D (2013) Predictors of outcome for cats with ureteral obstructions after interventional management using ureteral stents or a subcutaneous ureteral bypass device. *Journal of Feline Medicine and Surgery* **15**, 1052–1062

King MD, Waldron DR, Barber DL *et al.* (2006) Effect of nephrotomy on renal function and morphology in normal cats. *Veterinary Surgery* **35**, 749–758

Kyles AE, Hardie EM, Wooden BG *et al.* (2005a) Clinical, clinicopathologic, radiographic, and ultrasonographic abnormalities in cats with ureteral calculi: 163 cases (1984–2002). *Journal of the American Veterinary Medical Association* **226**, 932–936

Kyles AE, Hardie EM, Wooden BG *et al.* (2005b) Management and outcome of cats with ureteral calculi: 153 cases (1984–2002). *Journal of the American Veterinary Medical Association* **226**, 937–944

Lennon GM, Thornhill JA, Grainger R, Mcdermott TE and Butler MR (1997) Double pigtail ureteric stent *versus* percutaneous nephrostomy: effects on stone transit and ureteric motility. *European Urology* **31**, 24–29

Lulich JP, Berent AC, Adams LG, Westropp JL, Bartges JW and Osborne CA (2016) ACVIM Small Animal Consensus Recommendations on the Treatment and Prevention of Uroliths in Dogs and Cats. *Journal of Veterinary Internal Medicine* **30(5)**, 1564–1574

Lulich JP, Osborne CA, Albasan H, Monga M and Bevan JM (2009) Efficacy and safety of laser lithotripsy in fragmentation of urocystoliths and urethroliths for removal in dogs. *Journal of the American Veterinary Medical Association* **234**, 1279–1285

Manassero M, Decambron A, Viateau V *et al.* (2013) Indwelling double pigtail ureteral stent combined or not with surgery for feline ureterolithiasis: complications and outcome in 15 cases. *Journal of Feline Medicine and Surgery* **16**, 623–630

Mayhew PD, Mehler SJ, Mayhew KN, Steffey MA and Culp WT (2013) Experimental and clinical evaluation of transperitoneal laparoscopic ureteronephrectomy in dogs. *Veterinary Surgery* **42**, 565–571

McLoughlin MA (2011) Complications of lower urinary tract surgery in small animals. *Veterinary Clinics of North America: Small Animal Practice* **41**, 889–913

Nicoli S, Morello E, Martano M, Pisoni L and Buracco P (2012) Double-J ureteral stenting in nine cats with ureteral obstruction. *Veterinary Journal* **194**, 60–65

Pinel CB, Monnet E and Reems MR (2013) Laparoscopic-assisted cystotomy for urolith removal in dogs and cats – 23 cases. *Canadian Veterinary Journal* **54**, 36–41

Rawlings CA, Mahaffey MB, Barsanti JA and Canalis C (2003) Use of laparoscopic-assisted cystoscopy for removal of urinary calculi in dogs. *Journal of the American Veterinary Medical Association* **222**, 759–761

Runge JJ, Berent AC, Mayhew PD and Weisse C (2011) Transvesicular percutaneous cystolithotomy for the retrieval of cystic and urethral calculi in dogs and cats: 27 cases (2006–2008). *Journal of the American Veterinary Medical Association* **239**, 344–349

Steinhaus J, Berent AC, Weisse C *et al.* (2015) Clinical presentation and outcome of cats with circumcaval ureters associated with a ureteral obstruction. *Journal of Veterinary Internal Medicine* **29**, 63–70

Stone EA, Robertson JL and Metcalf MR (2002) The effect of nephrotomy on renal function and morphology in dogs. *Veterinary Surgery* **31**, 391–397

Zaid MS, Berent AC, Weisse C and Caceres A (2011) Feline ureteral strictures: 10 cases (2007–2009). *Journal of Veterinary Internal Medicine* **25**, 222–229

Chapter 28

Management of non-obstructive idiopathic/interstitial cystitis in cats

Tony Buffington and Dennis J. Chew

Lower urinary tract signs (LUTS) are common in pet cats. These signs include increased frequency of urination, stranguria, haematuria, vocalizing during urination and periuria (urinating in the house outside of the cat's litter container). These signs have a variety of causes (Osborne *et al.*, 1996). Urinary incontinence without urgency is not common in cats.

The terms FUS (feline urological syndrome) and FLUTD (feline lower urinary tract disease) were coined in the 1970s and 1980s to describe cats with LUTS; unfortunately, these terms have come to mean a specific disorder to some, rather than the possibility of several distinct diagnoses. The terms feline idiopathic and interstitial cystitis were first used in the 1990s to describe cats with LUTS in which urolithiasis, bacterial urinary infection, anatomical abnormalities and neoplasia had been excluded. A better term might have been chronic idiopathic LUTS, because the term cystitis (or any term referable to the lower urinary tract (LUT)) tended to over-focus attention on this organ at the expense of a more broad-based investigation during the history and physical examination. Feline interstitial cystitis (FIC) was defined as a chronic condition, whereas idiopathic cystitis can be acute or chronic. For the purposes of this chapter the authors have used the abbreviation FIC interchangeably for interstitial cystitis and chronic idiopathic cystitis.

Results of studies over the past two decades suggest that FIC can result when a 'sensitive individual' is exposed to a 'provocative environment'. Sensitive individuals are cats with more vulnerability (genetic, environmental) than resilience factors, which can sensitize the central stress response system (SRS) to threats. A provocative environment is one in which the animal's perception of threat exceeds its perception of control ('stress'), which can result in chronic activation of the SRS (Figure 28.1).

FIC seems to result from complex interactions between the bladder, nervous system, adrenal glands, husbandry practices and the environment in which the cat lives. Additionally, housing and stress have been associated with a number of other common disorders of cats, including behavioural problems, type 2 diabetes, dental disease, hyperthyroidism, obesity, separation anxiety disorder and urolithiasis, suggesting that sensitive individuals and provocative environments may be more common than previously thought. This research has led to the hypothesis that FIC may be one example of a 'Pandora syndrome' in

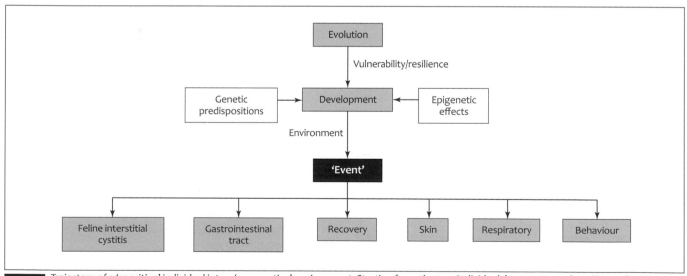

28.1 Trajectory of a 'sensitive' individual into a 'provocative' environment. Starting from the top, individuals' genes are sculpted by evolution and received from both parents, resulting in individual genetic predispositions. Which genes are read can then be determined by environmentally influenced epigenetic modulation of gene expression, in some cases resulting in individuals that are unusually sensitive to their surroundings. Most individuals are exposed to threatening 'events' during life, such as injury, infection or assault, and recover uneventfully. In sensitized individuals, however, the event may unmask the underlying susceptibility, and result in a variety of chronic disease problems. (Adapted from Kirkengen and Ulvestad, 2007)

cats, comparable with the 'central sensitivity syndromes' of interstitial cystitis, irritable bowel syndrome, fibromyalgia, panic disorder, etc. described in humans. The term 'Pandora syndrome' is proposed to describe cats with chronic recurrent LUTS in the presence of comorbid disorders (e.g. behavioural, dermatological, endocrine, gastrointestinal) until a more biologically appropriate term is identified (Buffington, 2011; Buffington *et al.*, 2014).

Diagnosis

Signalment

LUTS occur in both male and female cats, although middle-aged neutered males and females may be at increased risk compared with their intact counterparts. An affected cat typically is 1–10 years of age (peak risk 2–6 years), spends all or nearly all of its time living indoors with humans, is expected to eliminate in a litter container, and eats 75–100% dry food. Obesity and a variety of other comorbid conditions have been associated with FIC. Owners sometimes note that affected cats are unusually nervous, fearful, defensively aggressive, hypervigilant, or even excessively attached to their owner(s) compared with healthy cats. Cats with access to the outdoors can still be affected, especially if the cat perceives the outdoor environment to be threatening.

History and clinical signs

Cats can be presented for an initial occurrence of LUTS and may not return for care owing to an (often presumed) improvement in the condition, or can return with recurrent LUTS. Both sexes appear to be affected equally. Although cats with LUTS can be obstructed or not when presented, urethral obstruction is far more common in male cats than in queens, with no difference reported between intact and castrated males. In addition to potential genetic and early adverse life events, other factors associated with an increased risk of FIC have been reported, including excessive bodyweight, decreased activity, multi-cat households, indoor housing and a variety of environmental stressors such as conflict with another cat in the household.

Some of the most common causes of LUTS are presented in Figure 28.2; some 30 distinct causes have been described. When presented with a cat with LUTS, determining whether one is seeing the cat's initial *versus* a recurrent episode and what other health problems the cat may have permits judicious utilization of resources by choosing appropriate diagnostic tests to allow individually tailored treatment recommendations. Documenting the frequency and severity of the LUTS is important because this information can be used to assess improvement following treatment.

A detailed environmental history can help the clinician to identify likely causes even at an initial presentation, because perception of threat in the cat's surroundings can result in periuria even in otherwise healthy cats (Stella *et al.*, 2011). A standardized questionnaire for indoor-housed cats with instructions for use is available to obtain a detailed survey regarding food and water, litter container management, environmental considerations, resting opportunities, movement and social contact (Buffington, 2014). Client responses to these questions can facilitate conversations with the client, and can be helpful when prescribing environmental modifications (described later). A detailed history often reveals stressors in the cat or owner's life that may contribute to creating or perpetuating clinical signs.

Physical examination

A thorough physical examination of cats with LUTS permits evaluation of the presence or absence of abnormalities in all body systems. Careful examination of cats with FIC may reveal variable combinations of dysfunction of the gastrointestinal tract, skin, lungs, heart, as well as obesity and behavioural abnormalities. The bladder is usually small during active bouts of cystitis, but careful abdominal palpation may reveal stones or wall thickening and/or elicit pain. Cats with FIC sometimes also 'barber' the hair on their caudal ventral abdomen and inner thighs, possibly a manifestation of referred pain (Figure 28.3). Whether or not cats with LUTS from other causes also do this has not been reported, to the author's knowledge, and should be investigated.

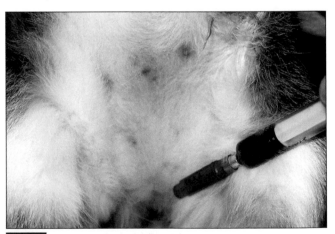

28.3 'Barbered' abdomen of a cat with feline interstitial cystitis.

How many diagnostics to pursue and when to pursue them

Figure 28.4 provides a list of differential diagnoses for many of the possible causes of LUTS in cats. Some combination of history, physical examination, urinalysis, quantitative urinalysis and imaging with radiography, ultrasonography or cystoscopy usually allows a diagnosis of inclusion or exclusion to be established.

In cats <10 years of age when first presented

- 55–70% have FIC
- 10–20% have urolithiasis, most commonly either calcium oxalate or struvite
- About 10% have a structural abnormality such as urachal diverticulum or urethral stricture
- About 10% have what appears to be a behavioural disorder
- Fewer than 2% of cases in the United States have a bacterial urinary tract infection
- Fewer than 1% have bladder or urethral neoplasia
- Very rare causes include cyclophosphamide (Cytoxan) treatment and parasitic cystitis associated with *Capillaria felis*

In cats ≥ 10 years of age when first presented

- About 5% have FIC
- More than half have a bacterial urinary tract infection, either alone or in association with urolithiasis. Many of these cats have chronic kidney disease and submaximally concentrated urine

28.2 Differential diagnoses for cats that present with lower urinary tract signs (LUTS), based on age group. FIC = feline interstitial cystitis.

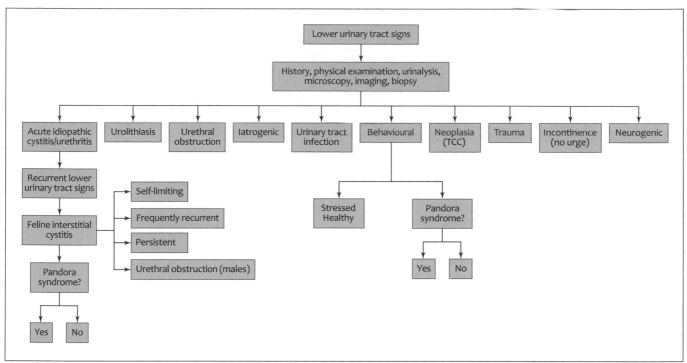

28.4 Some possible causes of lower urinary tract signs (LUTS) in cats after appropriate diagnostic evaluation. Imaging includes some combination of radiography, contrast urography, ultrasonography and/or uroendoscopy. Not all tests are appropriate for every cat, so diagnostic evaluations tailored to the individual cat are most likely to arrive at the correct diagnosis. TCC = transitional cell carcinoma.

An otherwise healthy young cat presented for a first episode of LUTS may not need diagnostic investigations beyond a complete history, physical examination and environmental assessment unless the clinical signs progress, or do not abate within a week. Clinical signs in many cats with FIC resolve during this time, only to recur within 6–12 months when environmental modification has not been successfully implemented; 52% recurred within 12 months in a recent study (Kruger et al., 2015). Clients can be offered a survey abdominal radiograph to exclude radiopaque urinary stones and urinalysis with aerobic bacterial urine culture to exclude the presence of a polyuric condition or bacterial urinary tract infection (UTI), respectively. A presumptive diagnosis of FIC consists of **exclusion** of urolithiasis, UTI and neoplasia, as well as **inclusion** of a compatible history, physical examination, environmental assessment and results from laboratory testing and imaging as described below.

Urinary tract imaging

Urinary tract imaging is appropriate for all cats with recurrent LUTS. Survey radiographs can identify radiodense calculi such as calcium oxalate or struvite, ≥2–3 mm in size. Advanced imaging should be pursued for cats with multiple recurrences or persistence of clinical signs if survey radiographs were normal, to exclude radiolucent calculi and anatomical defects.

Contrast cystourethrography is normal in about 85% of cats with FIC, but occasionally reveals focal or diffuse thickening of the bladder wall, permeation of contrast agent into the bladder wall or abdomen, and filling defects in the contrast pool (blood clots and cellular debris). Positive-contrast urethrography of male cats occasionally reveals the presence of a focal urethral stricture. Symmetrical annular urethral strictures are very difficult to diagnose, and proper filling of the bladder with contrast agent is important to help delineate these abnormalities. Positive-contrast

urethrography is important to perform in male cats that have undergone previous instrumentation both with urethral catheters and now have recurrence of LUTS, to evaluate urethral diameter and to exclude the presence of a urinary catheter remnant and urethral trauma.

Ultrasonography provides a less invasive method of imaging than contrast urethrocystography. Bladder wall thickness can be measured readily if the bladder is adequately distended with urine (overestimation of bladder wall thickness commonly occurs when there is inadequate distension with urine). Ultrasonography can document the presence of bladder calculi regardless of their radiodensity. Discrimination between urinary debris that settles to dependent bladder locations, urinary 'sand' and small stones is difficult and frustrating even for experienced sonographers; small stones may not 'shadow' and sometimes debris that piles up appears to shadow. Ultrasonography of affected and normal cats sometimes reveals hyperechogenic acoustic interfaces of suspended particles. The identity of these echogenic particles remains to be determined, but they do not appear to be crystals. In one study, 36 of 40 normal cats were described to have suspended echogenic particles within urine in the bladder, none of which was gravitating or exhibited distal acoustic shadowing, reverberation or twinkle artefact. Gravitating particles are more likely to be crystalline. The clinical relevance of these particles has also not yet been determined and they probably do not contribute to LUTS. The proximal urethra can be examined with ultrasonography, but this is not a good method to image the urethra, because most of the urethra cannot be examined using this modality (Sislak et al., 2014).

Uroendoscopy (cystoscopy), while no longer used to diagnose FIC, can be very useful for identifying or excluding the presence of other abnormalities of the LUT (e.g. strictures, small stones, urachal diverticuli, neoplasia, foreign body). Cystoscopy is available at some referral centres, especially for queens that can accommodate a rigid paediatric cystoscope. Urethroscopy of male cats is possible with the use of very small fibrescopes, but this instrumentation is not widely available (see Chapter 8).

Laboratory evaluation

Normal results of complete blood count (CBC) and routine serum biochemistry are found in cats with FIC. Thyroxine (T4) concentrations and serology for feline leukaemia virus (FeLV) and feline immunodeficiency virus (FIV) should be analysed, because hyperthyroidism or infection with FeLV or FIV also can result in LUTS.

Urinalysis: Urinalysis findings (Lund *et al.*, 2013) are neither sensitive nor specific for FIC. The classical findings of haematuria and proteinuria wax and wane between days, and even within the same day (Westropp *et al.*, 2006). Additionally, it is impossible to know with certainty that red cells and protein in the urine did not enter the sample during collection by cystocentesis when urine is collected by this method. The classical positive finding is 'haemorrhagic inflammation', a preponderance of red blood cells with few neutrophils in the urine sediment.

Crystals are often not present when fresh urine is evaluated. When crystals are observed, they are usually present in low numbers. Refrigeration can cause the appearance of crystals *ex vivo*, so it is physiologically normal to observe a few crystals in urinary sediment, especially when the urine is highly concentrated, and more so in samples stored under refrigeration until analysis. Moreover, the presence or absence of crystals has no known diagnostic or pathophysiological impact on non-obstructive FIC; struvite or calcium oxalate crystals do not appear to damage healthy urothelium (Khan *et al.*, 1984; Cohen *et al.*, 1991) but are more likely to adhere to injured tissue. The likely sequence of events is that sterile inflammation occurs first, plasma proteins exude into the urine, urinary pH increases, and then struvite crystals precipitate as a secondary event.

The urine specific gravity (USG) of healthy cats should be greater than 1.035 (Rishniw and Bicalho, 2015). Consumption of diets with higher moisture content was associated with a slightly lower USG, but only in queens. It was found that 25% of queens fed largely or exclusively canned diets had a USG of <1.035 and 50% had a USG of >1.040, whereas 75% of male cats fed similar diets had a USG of >1.040, and only 6% had a USG of <1.035. The authors could not explain the reason for the selective effect of sex and diet type on USG.

Current evidence suggests that the pH of the urine is not involved in the pathophysiology or management of cats with FIC. Most cats in North America consume foods that tend to acidify the urine. A neutral urine pH in cats affected with FIC at the time of evaluation does not necessarily reflect a failure of the diet to acidify the urine. The pH of the urine depends on a complex interaction of factors other than diet, including (transportation) stress-induced acute respiratory alkalosis, the presence of urease-producing bacterial UTI, and the amount of plasma proteins (pH approximately 7.4) leaked into urine as a consequence of the neurogenic inflammatory process.

Microbiology: Although microorganisms in the LUT have not been identified as a common cause of FIC or associated with chronic LUTS in the USA, one study from Norway of 134 cats with a variety of obstructive and non-obstructive causes of LUTS found a surprisingly high number of cats with quantitative bacteriuria, either alone or with variable combinations of crystals and uroliths (Eggertsdottir *et al.*, 2007). The percentages were much higher than those reported from other studies. Interpretation of these findings is complicated by the percentages of samples obtained from voided midstream (46%) or catheterized urine samples (21%) rather than by cystocentesis (21%; in 10% of cases the method of urine collection was not recorded). The authors speculated that the higher rate for discovery of UTI they observed might have resulted from differences between cases diagnosed at primary and tertiary care facilities, although geographical differences in the development of UTI cannot be excluded. Quantitative growth from midstream voided samples from healthy cats also can be substantial; one study found >10³ colony-forming units (cfu)/ml in cultures from 55% of males and 40% of females (Lees, 1984).

In the authors' experience, in both tertiary and primary care practice, quantitative culture reveals significant bacterial growth (>10³ cfu/ml) in only 1–2% of the samples of urine collected by cystocentesis from young cats with LUTS; special cultures for ureaplasma and mycoplasma are routinely negative. It may not be necessary to perform urine culture in cats <10 years of age with LUTS that have USG >1.040 and <5 white blood cells per high-power field (WBC/hpf) on urinary sediment. Urine culture is recommended for all cats with recurrent LUTS, USG <1.040, >5 WBC/hpf, azotaemia, previous perineal urethrostomy, or a history of urethral catheterization within the past 6 months.

Management

FIC is a chronic waxing and waning syndrome with no currently known cure. Despite this, statistically and clinically significant reductions in signs have been demonstrated in both clinical and laboratory studies using effective multi-modal environmental modification (MEMO) (Buffington *et al.*, 2006a; Westropp *et al.*, 2006; Stella *et al.*, 2011).

Realistic expectations for successful management of a cat with FIC depend on the specific cat, and the ability of the veterinary surgeon (veterinarian) and owner to identify, agree on and implement effective treatments and changes in husbandry practices. Although cats with severe chronic FIC may be more difficult to manage successfully than those provided earlier intervention, our experience with cats donated to our research programme with intractable FIC suggests that >95% of severely affected cats can recover in effectively enriched environments. Most cats can substantially improve, as perceived by their owners. Success ultimately is defined by the owner's perception of the cat using the litter container more often (fewer episodes of periuria), less macroscopic haematuria, fewer painful behaviours (stranguria, dysuria, howling, pain when picked up) and improved interactions with the owners. Though it is possible to have resolution of all the LUTS following treatment for long periods, many owners still perceive success when only partial improvement is achieved. The American Association of Feline Practitioners (AAFP) and the International Society of Feline Medicine (ISFM) recently published *Feline Environmental Needs Guidelines*, including a client brochure, based upon MEMO principles, which can be used to guide recommendations (Ellis *et al.*, 2013).

The authors offer stepwise tiers of MEMO based on evaluation of each particular situation (Figure 28.5); additional treatments may be added when effective implementation of first tier treatment recommendations fails to

Initial episode: 'watchful waiting' – spontaneous resolution of LUTS is common
• Analgesia • Provide client education about FIC and environmental modifications • Explain effective litter container management • Introduce unscented, clumping litter as appropriate • Provide a ventilated accessible secluded location for the litter container • Clean the litter container at least once daily • Clean up and eliminate 'accident' urine odours
Signs recur
• Analgesia • Obtain a sample for urinalysis and abdominal radiography as indicated • Offer consistent diet • Consider increasing water intake • Emphasize incorporation of effective MEMO
Signs recur again
• Analgesia • Obtain a sample for urine culture and contrast radiography and ultrasonography as indicated • Consider introducing pheromones • Review MEMO efforts
Signs frequently recur or persist
• Analgesia • Consider referral for cystoscopy and repeat diagnostics as indicated • Consider use of amitriptyline and analgesia • Review MEMO efforts

28.5 Stepwise approach to the management of cats with feline interstitial cystitis (FIC). More diagnostics should be performed when lower urinary tract signs (LUTS) do not resolve within 7 days and when signs recur, to ensure that the diagnosis is truly compatible with FIC. MEMO = multimodal environmental modification.

resolve the LUTS. All cats affected with FIC (and urinary stone disease) are provided with the first tier of recommendations. The authors also explain how to clean up urine deposited outside the litter container, enhance the management of the litter container, provide pain relief, increase water intake and introduce MEMO. Analgesics and a mild dose of tranquilizers (e.g. acepromazine) are often prescribed for cats severely affected with FIC during an acute episode or flare in LUTS. Subsequent tiers of treatment may include more advanced MEMO measures, and possibly pharmacological therapy.

Treatment of a first episode or an infrequent acute flare

Resolution of LUTS occurs in most cats within a week, often without treatment. Clinical signs persisting longer than 7 days are beyond the point of spontaneous resolution for most cats, so specific recommendations for further diagnostics and treatment are justified at that time.

Analgesia

The best approach to analgesia for bladder pain (visceral) has yet to be determined. Butorphanol has been used, but its effects are less long-lived or potent than those of buprenorphine (Steagall *et al.*, 2014). Sustained release formulations of buprenorphine have recently become available that can provide up to 72 hours of therapeutic drug levels for pain relief following a single injection. Fentanyl patches have been used in rare cases in which bladder pain was assessed as severe. Anecdotal reports of the usefulness of non-steroidal anti-inflammatory drugs (NSAIDs), especially

meloxicam and ketoprofen, abound, but no studies of safety or effectiveness are available for review. Some specialists have prescribed piroxicam for use on alternate days, but there are no controlled clinical trials of its effectiveness or safety. NSAIDs are not commonly used for treatment of interstitial cystitis in humans. NSAIDs that are authorized for use in cats list indications for pre-emptive pain management, usually as a single treatment before anaesthesia and surgery. Chronic use of NSAIDs in cats can be dangerous owing to the possibility for development of acute kidney injury, especially should the cat become dehydrated for any reason at the time of NSAID administration (see Chapter 20). The US Food and Drug Administration (FDA) recently required the following statement to be added to the label for meloxicam use in cats: 'Repeated use of meloxicam in cats has been associated with acute renal failure and death. Do not administer additional injectable or oral meloxicam to cats. See Contraindications, Warnings, and Precautions for detailed information.' Robenacoxib, a long-acting NSAID, has recently become available for use in cats; its effectiveness for cats with FIC has yet to be reported, to the authors' knowledge. Other analgesics such as gabapentin have been used without clinical evidence as to their efficacy.

The authors currently treat acute episodes or flares of LUTS in cats with FIC with oral buprenorphine at 10–20 µg/kg q6–12h for 7 days. This analgesic regimen is most often combined with acepromazine (0.25 mg/cat i.m. or 2.5 mg orally q8h) for 2–4 days as part of the standard approach to care. As with other analgesics, effectiveness of such treatment has not been demonstrated in controlled trials, so it is only the authors' clinical impression that it provides relief to affected cats in practice. Whether provision of analgesia for acute episodes impacts development of future episodes is not known.

Cleaning soiled areas

It is important to clean all areas of the house soiled by urine so that other cats in the household do not start urinating in these places, and so the affected cat does not continue to urinate these areas (Herron, 2010). Enzymatic cleaners are the most effective approaches to reduce and prevent the return of urine odour. Injector kits are available to inject enzymes into padding beneath carpets to break down urine, but removing urine that has seeped into these spaces can be difficult or impossible. Though it is tempting to use chemical deodorizers, these products render enzyme treatments useless. Products with strong odours also lessen the effects of feline facial pheromones should they be chosen for use at the same time, thereby reducing their effectiveness. In situations with extensive urine soiling, it may not be possible to neutralize urine in the carpet, so removing the carpet and underlying pad may be the only solution. After treatment, aluminium foil, sticky tape or citrus fragranced deodorants may be applied to the cleaned area to reduce the risk of cats using these areas again. As with any environmental modification strategy, one must be sure that efforts to make a resource aversive are matched by provision of a preferable alternative, from the cat's point of view.

Multimodal environmental modification – Tier 1

The overarching premise of MEMO is that some cats suffer adverse consequences of indoor housing, especially when forced to spend nearly all of their time indoors in association with people and other animals in confined spaces. Ethological and behavioural studies demonstrate that captivity activates the SRS in some cats. The cat's environment can be barren and monotonous, threatening, or chaotic, any of which can activate the SRS (Figure 28.6).

Effective MEMO can reduce the activity of the SRS and decrease the severity and frequency of LUTS and signs of comorbid disorders in cats with FIC (Buffington, 2011). MEMO consists of owner education about cats in general, their cat's disease, optimal food, water and litter container management, modification of the environment to reduce perceived threats, and working with owners in multi-cat households to reduce inter-cat conflict. The individual cat's preferences are determined for food and feeding, water and watering, litter container and litter substrates, space, and interactions with humans and other animals. In multi-cat households, increasing the number and locations of resources can decrease competition for food and water and opportunities for elimination that might contribute to LUTS. MEMO is intended to provide activities that are natural and enjoyable to the cat. Especially sensitive cats may perceive any change in routine, feeding schedule, owner work schedule, addition or removal of humans or pets from the household, and the owner's emotions, as threatening. Therefore, changes in the environment of a sensitive cat should be kept to a minimum, made gradually and tailored for each individual cat according to the needs and limitations of each cat, owner and household.

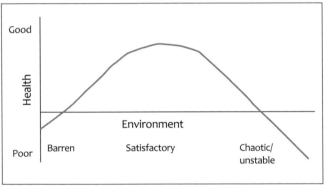

28.6 Quadratic relationship between environmental quality and health. Cats with feline interstitial cystitis (and those with Pandora syndrome) appear to tolerate a narrower range of environmental conditions than do healthy cats. For example, they may be more threatened by other cats, their owners, or features of their environment that would not adversely affect an otherwise healthy cat. (Reproduced from Buffington et al., 2014 with permission from the Journal of Feline Medicine and Surgery)

Asserting the authority to confine an animal implies the responsibility to provide an effectively enriched environment. Owners of cats and their veterinary surgeons have an obligation to maximize the quality of the cat's living experience. Prolonged housing in unenriched environments may not cause FIC, but it can contribute to its development and maintenance by unmasking the tendency of a particular cat to develop LUTS in response to external risk factors. The goal of MEMO is to provide environmental modifications that decrease the frequency of activation of the SRS and provide the cat sufficient perception of control of its environment to permit it to live below its clinical threshold for sickness behaviours or clinical signs of disease.

Effective MEMO in most cases obviates the need for drug administration, which can be threatening to cats and stressful for both cats and owners. In both clinical observational (Buffington et al., 2006b) and laboratory studies

(Stella et al., 2011), approximately 90% of cats with FIC had dramatic reductions in clinical signs when implementing only MEMO therapy for the initial episode (see Figure 28.5).

Most of the authors' experience has been with implementation of MEMO for cats with relatively severe FIC. The concepts advocated here seem likely to benefit cats with a first episode of LUTS (in fact, the authors' advocate them for all confined cats).

How is environmental enrichment provided for cats that live extensively indoors? Understanding some basic concepts regarding cat behaviour/husbandry is important in the development of indoor housing strategies that minimize perception of threat for a particular cat. Although not asocial, cats appear to have evolved as solitary hunters of small prey in relatively large spaces. Unlike dogs and humans, cats are not group hunters. In the wild, cats eat small meals (birds, rodents, insects) and hunt whenever prey is available. Indoor housing seriously reduces the area available for hunting and roaming activities, no prey are provided and cats are expected to adapt to the rhythmic activities of humans with which they share space, and many times also to live with dogs. The average household with cats in the USA has more than two cats. Living with other cats in confinement can be inherently stressful for some cats, and owners or veterinary surgeons may not recognize conflict and stress in these situations.

Cats that perceive chronic threat activate the SRS, which can adversely affect both the physiology and the behaviour of cats. Activation of the SRS in an individual cat can result from problematic interactions between cats, between cats and humans, between cats and their environments, and variable combinations of these. Identification and quantification of feline stressors can be quite difficult, but strategies for stress reduction are important if successful outcomes in reduction of severity or duration of clinical signs of FIC are to be achieved.

Owner education:
General: Some clients have not had much experience with cats, and so may not understand their basic husbandry needs. In such cases there are a variety of resources that can be recommended; these are listed at the end of the chapter. Access to the internet when discussing which resource options to provide to the cat permits one to perform an image search for the resource (food puzzle, climbing structure, scratching device, etc.) to show clients the range of possibilities, and to let them choose the ones they believe will be most appropriate in their situation. This also creates some level of investment in the MEMO process on the part of the client, which can facilitate the therapeutic relationship.

Litter container management: Cats prefer clean safe litter containers; nothing should discourage the cat from using the litter container. For cats confined indoors, the number of litter containers that are provided and their locations are important management issues. The general rule for the number of available litter containers is to have one more than the number of cats in the household, out of sight of all the others. The litter containers need to be easily and safely accessible to the cats. Placing litter containers in different locations (and on different levels in multi-level houses) is recommended to the extent possible, so that ample toileting opportunities are provided. Placing litter containers in quiet, convenient locations that provide an escape route if necessary for the cat also improves conditions for normal elimination behaviours by preventing other cats from blocking access to the elimination area.

The litter container should be scooped twice daily, and a full litter exchange performed weekly for sensitive cats that might be deterred from litter container use by less frequent cleaning. The value of providing enough litter containers that are frequently cleaned cannot be over-emphasized. However, cleaning of litter containers with detergents that leave a strong or citrus odour can discourage some cats from willingly entering the litter container.

The nature of the container and the substrate(s) preferred (or avoided) are also important considerations, and individual cat preferences vary. Consequently, it may take a while to find the best container and substrate for a specific cat. In general, the container needs to be large enough to accommodate the cat completely. A recent study showed that cats generally preferred larger litter containers than are often provided (Guy et al., 2014).

Covered litter containers can be tricky, in that some cats prefer the privacy, but owners often do not clean these containers often enough to prevent accumulation of elimination and odours. Unscented clumping litter is recommended; some litter scents deter use of the container by some cats, and use of clumping litter has been associated with improved use of the litter container by cats in some settings.

Trials with different litter substrates may reveal preferences for one type over another. Having two litter containers next to each other with different substrates in each is one way to determine which litter may be preferred – multiple tests may be required before a substrate is identified that the affected cat really seems to enjoy. If urine and faeces are not well covered in the litter container, it is likely that the cat does not want to paw the litter to cover the excrement. Well-covered faeces and urine spots usually mean that the cat is willing to use that particular litter. The AAFP and ISFM recently published Guidelines for Diagnosing and Solving House-Soiling Behavior in Cats, including a client brochure, that contains more complete discussions of types of litter container, litter and management techniques (Carney et al., 2014).

Water intake: Dilution of the urine towards a target USG of 1.025 has been proposed to reduce the risk of recurrence of signs in cats with FIC (Westropp and Buffington, 2010). A recent study reported USG measurements of >1.035 in most apparently healthy cats presenting to first-opinion practices (Rishniw and Bicalho, 2015). They found that USG decreased with increasing feeding of canned food in queens but not in male cats, and that most cats still had USGs of >1.040 regardless of the moisture content of the diet(s) consumed. After consumption of a dry therapeutic diet for 6 months, USG measurements from cats with FIC were 1.051 ± 0.012 and had not changed significantly from entry to the study, whereas cats with FIC fed a commercial therapeutic canned diet had a USG of 1.039 ± 0.018, which was significantly lower than the group receiving the dried diet and from their baseline USG. LUTS recurred in two of 18 cats fed the canned diet, and 11 of 28 cats fed the dry diet (p <0.05). One cat in the dry diet group in which clinical signs recurred had a urinary tract infection at re-evaluation. The analysis of the dataset after exclusion of this cat revealed a lack of statistical significance (p = 0.11). Additionally, both laboratory and clinical studies that did not focus on dilution of the urine have reported large reductions in recurrence of signs in cats with FIC, so any salutary effect of urine dilution appears to be modest.

Although increased water intake has not been demonstrated to be beneficial in general, it is unlikely to be detrimental and may be helpful in some cases. To ensure adequate water intake, the cat's preferences can be investigated. Considerations can include water freshness, taste and movement (still or running), depth of water, type of bowl, flavouring and location. All may need to be modified until the individual cat's preferences are determined. Water fountains, dripping taps, flavoured water (meat, fish or clam juice) and bottled water (especially if in areas with heavily mineralized or chlorinated tap water) may increase water intake in some cats. Some cats will drink more water when the water bowl is filled to the top several times a day – other cats prefer to find water in obscure places. Two studies of running water fountains showed that some cats increased water intake, but that this did not lower the USG. Despite no change for the average cat, some cats do show a preference for running water and increase their water intake when provided with fountains.

Nutrition: Some diets are marketed for feeding to cats with FIC. Attributes of these foods include increases in water content to reduce USG and changes in the amounts of minerals, sodium chloride, omega-3 fatty acids, antioxidants, tryptophan and alpha-casozepine. Unfortunately, no results of independently conducted properly randomized controlled trials of any of the diets currently sold for cats with FIC are available in the peer-reviewed scientific literature.

A recently published study compared a test diet designed to differ from the control diet in large part by its increased content of antioxidants and omega-3 oil (Kruger et al., 2015). Cats with FIC fed the test diet had a recurrence rate comparable with that recorded in other studies (Kruger et al., 2003; Gunn-Moore and Shenoy, 2004; Buffington et al., 2006b; Chew et al., 2009; Stella et al., 2011), whereas those fed the control diet had more frequent recurrences. Tryptophan, an essential amino acid, has been added to some diets, based on the idea that it may increase central serotonin concentrations, which might then exert an anxiolytic effect. Most studies of tryptophan's effects on mood are acute feeding studies, with very little, if any, evidence of long-term effects (Soh and Walter, 2011). Moreover, dietary tryptophan may not exert this effect on serotonin in cats (Trulson, 1985) and, even if it did, one would still need to demonstrate that this led to the desired clinical outcome in the target population with a particular diet, because other dietary constituents influence tryptophan availability. An open-label industry-funded study of a diet supplemented with alpha-casozepine and tryptophan fed to 10 cats with FIC was recently reported (Meyer and Beěvářová, 2016). The study lasted only 8 weeks and had no comparator diet group. Additionally MEMO was prescribed at the same time so any beneficial effects of the diet to reduce LUTS can not be separated from the effects of MEMO.

Recommending a diet change seems most reasonable when either the owner or the cat does not like the diet currently fed. Some owners and cats prefer dry foods, and may object to a forced transition to canned foods, particularly when they are of no demonstrable therapeutic value. Attempts to alter the urine to minimize crystalluria are not indicated; no evidence supports the notion that the common types of crystal in cat urine damage the urothelium, or worsen LUTS in non-obstructive forms of FIC. Perhaps more important is maintaining the consistency, composition and constancy of the diet that is fed. Consistency refers to the water content of the food, composition refers to the nutrient content of the diet being fed and constancy refers to minimizing changes in the diet that is being fed. For example, if a change in diet is deemed advisable (constancy), it should be first be the client's, and then the cat's, choice to switch to the new diet by offering the new food at mealtime next to the usual food in a separate container so the cat can express its preference. If the cat chooses the new food, the old food can be removed. To the authors' knowledge no nutrient or ingredient has been demonstrated to exacerbate or alleviate LUTS in cats with FIC.

Another aspect of the nutritional care of cats with FIC includes feeding management. Cats generally prefer to eat individually in a quiet location where they will not be startled by other animals, sudden movement or activity of an air duct or appliance that may begin operation unexpectedly. Natural cat feeding behaviour also includes predatory activities such as stalking and pouncing. These may be simulated by hiding small amounts of food around the house, or by putting food in a 'puzzle' feeding device, from which the cat has to extract individual pieces or move to release the food pieces, if such interventions appeal to the cat. Opportunities to express species-typical prey behaviours are commonly used in captive felids to provide enrichment (Shepherdson *et al.*, 1993; Damasceno and Genaro, 2014; Ruskell *et al.*, 2015) and, although not yet carefully studied in domestic cats, it appears to benefit some cats with FIC and related disorders (e.g. obesity) as well (Dantas *et al.*, 2016).

Conflict: Conflict among cats commonly is present when multiple cats are housed indoors together and health problems are present. Conflict among cats can develop because of threats to a cat's perception of its overall status or rank in the home, from other animals in the home, or from outside cats. The goal is to reduce conflict to a more manageable level for the cats involved.

Signs of open conflict are easy to recognize. The signs of silent conflict can be so subtle they are easily missed. Threatened cats may attempt to circumvent agonistic encounters by avoiding other cats, by decreasing their activity, or both. Threatened cats often spend increasingly large amounts of time away from the family, staying in areas of the house that others do not use, or they attempt to interact with family members only when the assertive cat is elsewhere. Although either the assertive or threatened cat can exhibit conflict-related urine marking, in our experience FIC usually occurs in the threatened cat.

A common cause of conflict between indoor-housed cats appears to be competition for resources. Cats may engage in open or silent conflict over space, food, water, litter containers, perches, sunny areas, safe places where the cat can watch its environment, or attention from people. Conflict can develop even when there is no obvious limitation to access to resources. Open conflict seems most likely to occur when a new cat is introduced into the house.

Treatment for conflict between indoor cats involves providing a separate set of resources for each cat, preferably in locations where the cats can use them without being seen by other cats. Neutering all of the cats may also reduce conflict. Trimming all nails may also be helpful. Whenever the cats involved in the conflict cannot be directly supervised, the threatened cat should be provided with a refuge in a separate protected space. Conflict between indoor-housed cats and outside cats can occur when a new cat enters the area around the house the affected cat lives in. To cats, windows are no protection from a threatening cat outside. If outside cats are the source of the problem, a variety of strategies are available to make the client's garden less desirable to them.

Toys/prey/play: Effective MEMO includes appropriate provision of resources and interactions with and for cats that simulate some of the activities they would encounter in the wild. Simulations of prey that include laser lights, lures and feathered fishing pole toys can be useful interactions for some cats. Cats often enjoy playing with toys, particularly those that are small, move, and mimic prey characteristics. Use of containers or toys that intermittently release food during play may provide actions to simulate hunting behaviour.

Identifying a cat's 'prey preference' allows one to buy or make toys that the cat will be more likely to play with. Prey preference can be identified by paying close attention to the cat's reaction to toys with specific qualities, such as those that resemble birds (feather toys), small animals (e.g. 'furry mice') or insects (laser pointers, pieces of dry food) presented one at a time or together. Expandable tunnels provide opportunities for cats to play by themselves and for hiding. Many cats also prefer novelty, so a variety of toys should be provided, and rotated or replaced regularly to sustain their interest.

Play activities with the owners may decrease stress in a cat's life if the owners are not the source of the stress in the first place. Some cats seem to prefer to be petted and groomed, whereas others may prefer play interactions with owners. Cats also can be trained to perform behaviours ('tricks'); cats respond much better to praise than to force, and seem to be more amenable to learning if the behaviour is shaped before feeding.

Space: Cats generally prefer more space than the average house or apartment provides. Cats interact with both the physical structures and other animals, including humans, in their environment. The physical environment should include opportunities for scratching (both horizontal and vertical may be necessary), climbing, hiding and resting undisturbed. Some cats seem to prefer to monitor their surroundings from elevated vantage points, so climbing frames, hammocks, platforms, raised walkways, shelves or window seats may appeal to them. The addition of elevated spaces such as shelves, 'kitty condos', cardboard boxes, beds or crates may provide enough space to reduce conflict in multi-cat households to a tolerable level and to provide increased stimulation to housed cats in general. Playing a radio to habituate cats to sudden changes in sound and human voices has also been recommended. Videotapes to provide visual stimulation from possible prey are available and seem to be captivating for some cats.

Pheromonotherapy: Synthetic feline facial pheromones are marketed to reduce urine marking or spraying behaviours in cats (e.g. Feliway®). Natural pheromones from the head and cheeks are rubbed by cats on to objects in their environment as a means of communicating familiarity and noting them as non-threatening. By so doing they exert a calming effect on the cat. These pheromones reduce the vigilance of the cat so that the cat's need to mark or spray its territory is reduced. Since vigilance of cats is maintained largely by activity of the sympathetic nervous system, it is possible that use of these pheromones contributes to decreased adrenergic outflow from the brainstem in some cats. If so, they could be useful for treatment of FIC in cats, although a systematic review has questioned their efficacy (Frank *et al.*, 2010). There appears to be a salutary effect of these pheromones in some cats, and the authors continue to prescribe their use. In some cases, the authors prefer use of the electric room diffuser form that continually disperses the pheromone over the manual pump spray formulation. One or more diffusers should be placed in rooms where the cat may be the most stressed – near windows and doors, soiled furniture and/or the litter container. The authors recommend the use of pheromonotherapy for cats with FIC after (or during) implementation of MEMO when it has been found to be insufficient to control signs.

Frequent recurrence or persistence of signs
Further environmental enrichment

If initial implementation of MEMO does not adequately reduce the signs of FIC, the clinician must go back and review what the client did and did not implement. Alternative attempts at enrichment can be suggested for those that were not initially implemented, and additional enrichments may be considered at this time.

Increased access to the outdoors can be helpful in the management of some cats as long as it does not increase the risk of morbidity and mortality following infectious diseases, trauma or becoming prey for outdoor predators. In some locales, increased exposure to the outdoors may be contraindicated if the density of cats or other threats in the area is particularly high.

A dramatic improvement occurs in some cats that are allowed at least a few hours of outdoor activities daily. Partial access to the outdoors can be attempted in contained yards or with the use of enclosures on patios or special fences designed to keep pet cats inside and prevent access of other outside cats. An Internet search for images of 'cat enclosures' yields hundreds of options.

Drugs

Drug therapy is not attempted until analgesics have been administered and level-1 environmental enrichment implemented without adequate resolution of clinical signs (including low-grade persistent signs, or frequent recurrence of clinical signs).

Tricyclic analgesics/antidepressants: Tricyclic analgesics/ antidepressants (TCA) can exert powerful effects that decrease clinical signs in cats with FIC, even in the absence of changes in cystoscopic appearance (Chew *et al.*, 1998). Although many different mechanisms could account for a salutary effect of TCA, none has been proven in a setting of natural disease in cats.

Two studies have found no benefit from the use of TCA to treat acute bouts of FIC (Kraijer *et al.*, 2003; Kruger *et al.*, 2003); abrupt cessation of TCA administration after 7 days increased the severity of clinical signs and frequency of recurrence in one study (Kruger *et al.*, 2003). In one open-ended non-placebo-controlled study, prescription of amitriptyline was associated with resolution of clinical signs in 60% of cats with severe FIC for 1 year during administration of 10 mg orally q24h at the owner's bedtime. Despite the decrease in clinical signs, no improvement in the cystoscopic appearance of the bladder mucosa was observed (Chew *et al.*, 1998)

The authors consider use of TCA only when other treatments described above have not been helpful. Cats often have markedly decreased clinical signs of FIC during such treatment with amitriptyline, the TCA with which the authors have had the most experience. Despite the improvement in clinical signs, the behaviour of these cats is different and is associated with weight gain and poor grooming. If the situation is desperate for the owner and the clinical signs

severe, the authors recommend starting with 10 mg amitriptyline q24h. If there is less urgency for immediate improvement, they will usually start with 5 mg q24h and either decrease or increase the dose to an eventual 2.5–12.5 mg total daily dose of amitriptyline. Sometimes TCA is prescribed while environmental enrichment is being implemented. If environmental enrichment is successful in reducing the cat's perceived stress, it may be possible to taper the dose of TCA gradually and in some instances to stop this form of medication.

Owing to possible effects on liver enzymes or function during administration of TCA, the authors recommend a serum biochemical panel prior to starting the drug and again at 1, 3 and 6 months during treatment. A CBC is also recommended to ensure no adverse effects of chronic treatment are occurring (thrombocytopenia and neutropenia). TCA should be used cautiously if at all in cats with serious heart disease.

Treatment with the so-called behaviour modification class of drugs has the possibility of decreasing the activity of the sympathetic nervous system and could have benefits for cats with FIC. Fluoxetine, clomipramine and pheromonotherapy may assist in managing urine spraying beyond placebo-based interventions (Mills *et al.*, 2011), but no clinical trials of their efficacy in cats with FIC have been published, to the authors' knowledge.

Glycosaminoglycans: Given that urinary glycosaminoglycans (GAG) excretion in cats affected with FIC appeared to be decreased, compared with that of healthy cats, GAG administration has been tested. Studies to date have shown no benefit of oral glucosamine (Gunn-Moore and Shenoy, 2004) or pentosan polysulphate (PPS) supplementation by mouth (Chew *et al.*, 2009) or by subcutaneous injection (Wallius and Tidholm, 2009) over that of placebo in cats with FIC (or humans with interstitial cystitis (Nickel *et al.*, 2015)).

Antimicrobials: Bacterial urinary infections are exceedingly uncommon in cats less than 10 years of age, and therefore it is very unlikely that antimicrobials have a role in the treatment of most LUT conditions in cats. An exception would be in male cats that have previously undergone perineal urethrostomy or those that have been instrumented with urinary catheters within the previous 6 months. Much greater risk for a true bacterial UTI exists in these cats, as well as in cats with submaximally concentrated urine (USG <1.035), because this may suggest an underlying disease that predisposes to UTI.

Prognosis for successful treatment of FIC

The prognosis for diseases affected by environmental factors may depend on parameters of the patient, the housing situation and the client. Patient factors include the animal's genetic predisposition and prior individual experience, the duration of the problem, the frequency of occurrences and, for inappropriate urination, the number of areas and different types of surface soiled. Housing factors include the number of cats in the household, the number of affected cats, the advisability of allowing limited outdoor access and the feasibility of rearranging the environment. Client factors include the owners' ability to identify modifiable causes, the strength of their bond to affected cats, their willingness to pay for treatment, the amount of time available to devote to solving the problem and the willingness to accept and use adjunctive medications as indicated.

The prognosis for successful treatment of FIC will vary with the degree of empowerment attained by the owners. Empowerment of the owner with knowledge, resources and encouragement allows reduction of external modifiable risk factors in some cats.

Conclusions

Converging evidence from a variety of studies suggests that FIC in some cats is more likely to be a disorder affecting the bladder than a primary bladder disorder; this led to the 'Pandora syndrome' hypothesis (Buffington, 2011). Cats with FIC have variably severe involvement of the SRS, and are exposed to a range of environmental stimuli. Given the current state of our knowledge, we have limited capacity to treat the internal factors, and therefore have focused on modification of external factors pending development of strategies to modulate the activity or output of the SRS.

Although many indoor-housed cats appear to accommodate to a wide range of surroundings, the neuroendocrine abnormalities in the cats we treat with FIC do not seem to permit them the adaptive capacity of healthy cats. Clinicians should thus focus on external factors in environments that appear adequate for healthy cats to accommodate disease-induced limitations of cats with FIC. Moreover, because external factors have been shown to unmask susceptibility to many common chronic diseases in cats, the authors recommend effective environmental enrichment as preventive health care for all cats, just as they recommend appropriate vaccination and provision of satisfactory nutrition.

Selected client education resources

An internet search for 'cat care' returns a large number of options from around the world that can be reviewed and shared with clients as appropriate.

The American Association of Feline Practitioners
www.catvets.com/guidelines/client-brochures

Cornell Feline Health Center
www.vet.cornell.edu/FHC

From the Cat's Point of View
www.perfectpaws.com/bookpreview/cpvpreview2.html

The Indoor Pet Initiative
https://indoorpet.osu.edu/cats

International Cat Care
www.icatcare.org:8080/advice

References and further reading

Buffington CA (2011) Idiopathic cystitis in domestic cats – beyond the lower urinary tract. *Journal of Veterinary Internal Medicine* **25**, 784–796

Buffington CA (2014) *Household Resource Checklist*. The Indoor Pet Initiative. Available at: indoorpet.osu.edu/assets/documents/Fillable-Household-Resource-Checklist_06-03-14.pdf

Buffington CA, Westropp JL and Chew DJ (2014) From FUS to Pandora syndrome. *Journal of Feline Medicine and Surgery* **16**, 385–394

Buffington CA, Westropp JL, Chew DJ and Bolus RR (2006a) Clinical evaluation of multimodal environmental modification (MEMO) in the management of cats with idiopathic cystitis. *Journal of Feline Medicine and Surgery* **8**, 261–268

Buffington CA, Westropp JL, Chew DJ and Bolus RR (2006b) Clinical evaluation of multimodal environmental modification (MEMO) in the management of cats with idiopathic cystitis. *Journal of Feline Medicine and Surgery* **8**, 261–268

Carney HC, Sadek TP, Curtis TM *et al.* (2014) AAFP and ISFM guidelines for diagnosing and solving house-soiling behavior in cats. *Journal of Feline Medicine and Surgery* **16**, 579–598

Chew DJ, Bartges JW, Adams LG, Kruger JM and Buffington CAT (2009) Randomized, placebo-controlled clinical trial of pentosan polysulfate sodium for treatment of feline interstitial (idiopathic) cystitis. *ACVIM Forum 2009, Montreal, Quebec*

Chew DJ, Buffington CAT, Kendall MS, Dibartola SP and Woodworth BE (1998) Amitriptyline treatment for idiopathic cystitis in cats (15 cases, 1994–1996). *Journal of the American Veterinary Medical Association* **213**, 1282–1286

Cohen SM, Cano M, Earl RA, Carson SD and Garland EM (1991) A proposed role for silicates and protein in the proliferative effects of saccharin on the male rat urothelium. *Carcinogenesis* **12**, 1551–1555

Damasceno J and Genaro G (2014) Dynamics of the access of captive domestic cats to a feed environmental enrichment item. *Applied Animal Behaviour Science* **151**, 67–74

Dantas LM, Delgado MM, Johnson I and Buffington T (2016) Food puzzles for cats: feeding for physical and emotional well being. *Journal of Feline Medicine and Surgery* **18**, 723–732

Eggertsdottir AV, Lund HS, Krontveit R and Sorum H (2007) Bacteriuria in cats with feline lower urinary tract disease: a clinical study of 134 cases in Norway. *Journal of Feline Medicine and Surgery* **9**, 458–465

Ellis SL, Rodan I, Carney HC *et al.* (2013) AAFP and ISFM feline environmental needs guidelines. *Journal of Feline Medicine and Surgery* **15**, 219–230

Frank D, Beauchamp G and Palestrini C (2010) Systematic review of the use of pheromones for treatment of undesirable behavior in cats and dogs. *Journal of the American Veterinary Medical Association* **236**, 1308–1316

Gunn-Moore DA and Shenoy CM (2004) Oral glucosamine and the management of feline idiopathic cystitis. *Journal of Feline Medicine and Surgery* **6**, 219–225

Guy NC, Hopson M and Vanderstichel R (2014) Litterbox size preference in domestic cats (*Felis catus*). *Journal of Veterinary Behavior: Clinical Applications and Research* **9**, 78–82

Herron ME (2010) Advances in understanding and treatment of feline inappropriate elimination. *Topics in Companion Animal Medicine* **25**, 195–202

Khan SR, Cockrell CA, Finlayson B and Hackett RL (1984) Crystal retention by injured urothelium of the rat urinary bladder. *Journal of Urology* **132**, 153–157

Kirkengen AL and Ulvestad E (2007) Heavy burdens and complex disease – an integrated perspective. *The Journal of the Norwegian Medical Association* **127**, 3228–3231

Kraijer M, Fink-Gremmels J and Nickel RF (2003) The short-term clinical efficacy of amitriptyline in the management of idiopathic feline lower urinary tract disease: a controlled clinical study. *Journal of Feline Medicine and Surgery* **5**, 191–196

Kruger JM, Conway TS, Kaneene JB *et al.* (2003) Randomized controlled trial of the efficacy of short-term amitriptyline administration for treatment of acute, nonobstructive, idiopathic lower urinary tract disease in cats. *Journal of the American Veterinary Medical Association* **222**, 749–758

Kruger JM, Lulich JP, MacLeay J *et al.* (2015) Comparison of foods with differing nutritional profiles for long-term management of acute nonobstructive idiopathic cystitis in cats. *Journal of the American Veterinary Medical Association* **247**, 508–517

Lees GE (1984) Epidemiology of naturally occurring feline bacterial urinary tract infections. *Veterinary Clinics of North America: Small Animal Practice* **14**, 471–479

Lund HS, Krontveit RI, Halvorsen I and Eggertsdottir AV (2013) Evaluation of urinalyses from untreated adult cats with lower urinary tract disease and healthy control cats: predictive abilities and clinical relevance. *Journal of Feline Medicine and Surgery* **15**, 1086–1097

Markwell PJ, Buffington CAT, Chew DJ *et al.* (1999) Clinical evaluation of commercially available urinary acidification diets in the management of idiopathic cystitis in cats. *Journal of the American Veterinary Medical Association* **214**, 361–365

Meyer HP and Bečvářová I (2016) Effects of a urinary food supplemented with milk protein hydrolysate and L-tryptophan on feline idiopathic cystitis–results of a case series in 10 cats. *International Journal of Applied Research in Veterinary Medicine* **14**, 59–65

Mills DS, Redgate SE and Landsberg GM (2011) A meta-analysis of studies of treatments for feline urine spraying. *PLoS One* **6**, e18448

Nickel JC, Herschorn S, Whitmore KE *et al.* (2015) Pentosan polysulfate sodium for treatment of interstitial cystitis/bladder pain syndrome: insights from a randomized, double-blind, placebo-controlled study. *Journal of Urology* **193**, 857–862

Osborne CA, Lulich JP, Thumchai R *et al.* (1996) Feline urolithiasis. Etiology and pathophysiology. *Veterinary Clinics of North America: Small Animal Practice* **26**, 217–232

Rishniw M and Bicalho R (2015) Factors affecting urine specific gravity in apparently healthy cats presenting to first-opinion practice for routine evaluation. *Journal of Feline Medicine and Surgery* **17**, 329–337

Ruskell AD, Meiers ST, Jenkins SE and Santymire RM (2015) Effect of bungee-carcass enrichment on behavior and fecal glucocorticoid metabolites in two species of zoo-housed felids. *Zoo Biology* **34**, 170–177

Shepherdson DJ, Carlstead K, Mellen JD and Seidensticker J (1993) The influence of food presentation on the behavior of small cats in confined environments. *Zoo Biology* **12**, 203–216

Sislak MD, Spaulding KA, Zoran DL, Bauer JE and Thompson A (2014) Ultrasonographic characteristics of lipiduria in clinically normal cats. *Veterinary Radiology and Ultrasound* **55**, 195–201

Soh NL and Walter G (2011) Tryptophan and depression: can diet alone be the answer? *Acta Neuropsychiatrica* **23**, 3–11

Steagall PV, Monteiro-Steagall BP and Taylor PM (2014) A review of the studies using buprenorphine in cats. *Journal of Veterinary Internal Medicine* **28**, 762–770

Stella JL, Lord LK and Buffington CA (2011) Sickness behaviors in response to unusual external events in healthy cats and cats with feline interstitial cystitis. *Journal of the American Veterinary Medical Association* **238**, 67–73

Trulson ME (1985) Dietary tryptophan does not alter the function of brain serotonin neurons. *Life Sciences* **37**, 1067–1072

Wallius BM and Tidholm AE (2009) Use of pentosan polysulphate in cats with idiopathic, non-obstructive lower urinary tract disease: a double-blind, randomised, placebo-controlled trial. *Journal of Feline Medicine and Surgery* **11**, 409–412

Westropp JL and Buffington CAT (2010) Lower urinary tract disorders in cats. In: *Textbook of Veterinary Internal Medicine, 7th edn*, ed. SJ Ettinger and EC Feldman. Elsevier-Saunders, St. Louis

Westropp JL, Kass PH and Buffington CA (2006) Evaluation of the effects of stress in cats with idiopathic cystitis. *American Journal of Veterinary Research* **67**, 731–736

Chapter 29

Urinary tract infections

Joe Bartges and Shelly Olin

Urinary tract infections (UTIs) develop when a temporary or permanent breach in host defence mechanisms allows virulent microbes to adhere, multiply and persist within the urinary tract. UTIs are most commonly caused by bacteria, although fungi and viruses may infect the urinary tract. UTIs may involve more than one anatomical location; the infection should be categorized as upper urinary tract (kidneys and ureters) or lower urinary tract (bladder, urethra, prostate or vagina). Determining which anatomical sites are infected is necessary when prescribing the type and duration of antimicrobial treatment, determining whether additional treatments are necessary (e.g. neutering male dogs with prostatitis) and future monitoring. Bacteriuria may or may not result in a clinical UTI.

Aetiopathogenesis of UTIs

Host defences

Although the urinary tract communicates with the microbe-ladened external environment, most of the urinary tract is sterile, and local defences are present throughout the tract to resist infection. Mechanisms of host resistance to UTIs (Figure 29.1) are typically divided into natural inherent resistance factors and acquired or induced resistance factors activated by bacteriuria or UTI.

- **Normal micturition**
  - Adequate urine volume
  - Frequent voiding
  - Complete voiding
  - Urinary continence
- **Anatomical structures**
  - Urethral high-pressure zones
  - Surface characteristics of urothelium
  - Urethral peristalsis
  - Prostatic secretions (antibacterial fraction and immunoglobulins)
  - Length of urethra
  - Ureterovesical flap valves
  - Ureteral peristalsis
  - Glomerular mesangial cells (?)
  - Extensive renal blood supply and flow
- **Mucosal defence barriers**
  - Antibody production
  - Surface layer of glycosaminoglycans
  - Intrinsic mucosal antimicrobial properties
  - Exfoliation of urothelial cells

29.1 Natural and acquired host defences of the urinary tract. (continues)

- **Mucosal defence barriers** *continued*
  - Bacterial interference by commensal microbes of distal urogenital tract
  - Mucosal innate immunity: Toll-like receptors, etc.
- **Antimicrobial properties of urine**
  - Extremely high or low urine pH
  - Hyperosmolality
  - High concentration of urea
  - Organic acids
  - Low molecular weight carbohydrates
  - Tamm–Horsfall mucoproteins
  - Host defence peptides (e.g. defensins)
- **Systemic immunocompetence**
  - Cell-mediated immunity
  - Humoral-mediated immunity

29.1 (continued) Natural and acquired host defences of the urinary tract.

UTI causative organisms

Most UTIs result from ascending migration of pathogens from the distal urogenital tract into the normally sterile proximal urethra, bladder and/or upper urinary tract. The external genitalia and distal urethra of dogs are not sterile environments; the resident population of bacteria may inhibit adherence or multiplication of uropathogens, but may themselves also become uropathogens if host defences are altered (Figure 29.2).

- *Escherichia coli*
  - Certain O (somatic) antigens
    - Outer polysaccharide portion of bacterial envelope
    - Indirect marker of virulence (human studies)
  - Certain K (capsular) antigens
    - Capsule surrounds bacterium
    - May inhibit phagocytosis and complement-mediated bactericidal activity
    - Increased resistance to inflammation favours persistence of bacteria in tissue
  - Adhesive fimbriae (pili)
    - Proteinaceous filamentous organelles that protrude from the surface of the bacterium
    - Specific types of fimbriae (p-fimbriae) enhance the ability of a bacterium to remain adherent to uroepithelium despite cleansing action of urinary system
  - Haemolysin
    - Increases amount of free iron available for bacterial growth
    - May cause tissue damage

29.2 Selected factors that may enhance the virulence (uropathogenicity) of bacteria causing urinary tract infections. (continues)

- ***Escherichia coli** (continued)*
  - Aerobactin
    - Iron-binding protein
    - Facilitates bacterial growth
  - R-plasmids
    - Promote resistance to antimicrobial agents
  - Resistance to serum bactericidal activity
  - Rapid replication in urine
- ***Proteus** spp., **Staphylococcus** spp. and some **Klebsiella** spp.*
  - Adherence factors
  - Urease activity
    - Bacterial enzyme that hydrolyses urea to ammonia
    - Ammonia directly injures uroepithelium
    - Urease promotes production of magnesium ammonium phosphate uroliths, which serve as niduses for infection
  - R-plasmids
- ***Pseudomonas** spp.*
  - Heavy mucoid polysaccharide capsule
    - Prevents antibody adherence
  - R-plasmids

29.2 (continued) Selected factors that may enhance the virulence (uropathogenicity) of bacteria causing urinary tract infections.

Bacterial isolates

A single bacterial pathogen is isolated from approximately 75% of infections, 20% of UTIs are caused by two species, and approximately 5% are caused by three species. The bacteria that most commonly cause UTIs are similar in dogs and cats. *Escherichia coli* is most common (Figure 29.3), followed by Gram-positive cocci, and then various others including *Proteus* spp., *Klebsiella* spp., *Pasteurella* spp., *Pseudomonas* spp., *Corynebacterium* spp. and several other rarely reported genera. *Mycoplasma* spp. are isolated from the urine of dogs with clinical signs of lower urinary tract infection in less than 5% of samples; whether or not *Mycoplasma* spp. are associated with urinary tract disease in cats is controversial. Cats may be infected with a unique strain of *Staphylococcus*, *S. felis*, and commercial phenotypic identification systems may not differentiate between *S. felis* and other coagulase-negative *Staphylococcus* spp. Litster *et al.* (2007) found that *S. felis* was the third most common isolate, based on 16S ribosomal (r) DNA sequencing, suggesting that *S. felis* is the most common staphylococcal species causing UTI in cats.

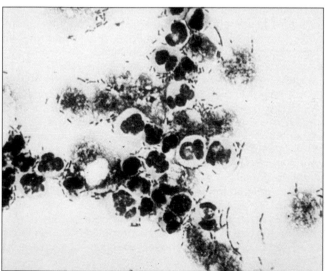

29.3 Rods (*Escherichia coli*) and white blood cells in modified Wright's stained urine sediment from a dog with bacterial cystitis.

Fungal isolates

Fungal UTI is uncommon. As with bacterial UTI, fungal UTI occurs when there is a temporary or permanent breach in local or systemic immunity of the lower urinary tract. Funguria may be due to primary infections of the lower urinary tract or secondary to shedding of fungal elements into the urine in animals with systemic infections. Primary fungal UTI is most commonly due to *Candida* spp., commensal inhabitants of the genital mucosa, upper respiratory tract and gastrointestinal tract. *C. albicans* is the most commonly identified species, followed by *C. glabrata* and *C. tropicalis*. Other ubiquitous fungi may also occasionally cause primary fungal UTI, including *Aspergillus* spp., *Blastomyces* spp. (Figure 29.4) and *Cryptococcus* spp.

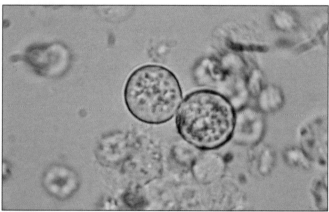

29.4 *Blastomyces* spp. organisms observed on microscopic examination of urine sediment from a 2-year-old neutered male Dobermann with lower urinary tract signs.

Viral isolates

Viral-induced diseases, especially of the upper urinary tract, are increasingly recognized in humans. However, it can be difficult to determine cause-and-effect relationships because virus-induced disease may occur in the absence of detectable replicating virus. Several viruses have been associated with canine and feline urinary disease, but causality has yet to be determined (Figure 29.5).

Species	Upper urinary tract disease	Lower urinary tract disease
Dog	• Canine adenovirus type I • Canine herpesvirus	• Not applicable
Cat	• Feline coronavirus • Feline immunodeficiency virus • Feline leukaemia virus • Feline foamy (syncytium-forming) virus	• Feline calicivirus • Bovine herpesvirus-4 • Feline foamy (syncytium-forming) virus

29.5 Viruses associated with urinary tract disease in dogs and cats. (Data from Kruger *et al.*, 2011)

Diagnosis

Dogs and cats with microburia may or may not have clinical signs. Clinical signs associated with UTI are variable and depend on the virulence and number of uropathogens, the presence or absence of concurrent diseases of the urinary tract, the immune system's response to infection, the duration of infection and the site(s) of infection (Figure 29.6). Various combinations of pollakiuria, stranguria, dysuria, haematuria and inappropriate

Parameter	Lower urinary tract infection	Upper urinary tract infection	Acute prostatitis or prostatic abscessation	Chronic prostatitis
History	• Dysuria, stranguria, pollakiuria • Urge incontinence • Signs of abnormal detrusor reflex (overflow incontinence, large residual volume) • Gross haematuria at end of micturition • Cloudy urine with abnormal odour • Recent catheterization or cystotomy	• Polyuria, polydipsia • ± Signs of systemic infection • ± Kidney disease	• Urethral discharge independent of micturition • Signs of systemic infection • ± Reluctance to urinate or defecate	• Recurrent urinary tract infections • Urethral discharge independent of urination • ± Dysuria, stranguria
Physical examination findings	• Small, painful, thickened bladder • Palpable masses in urethra or bladder • Flaccid bladder wall, large residual volume • Abnormal micturition reflex • ± Palpation of uroliths • May be normal	• ± Detectable abnormalities • ± Fever and other signs of systemic infection • ± Abdominal, flank (renal) pain • Kidney(s) normal or increased in size	• ± Fever and other signs of systemic infection • ± Painful prostate and/or painful abdomen • ± Prostatomegaly or asymmetrical prostate	• Often no detectable abnormalities • ± Prostatomegaly or asymmetrical prostate
Laboratory findings	• *Complete blood count (CBC)*: Normal • *Urinalysis*: Pyuria, haematuria, proteinuria, bacteriuria • *Urine culture*: Significant bacteriuria	• *CBC*: ± Leucocytosis • *Urinalysis*: Pyuria, haematuria, proteinuria, bacteriuria, white blood cell or granular casts • Impaired urine concentration • ± Azotaemia and other findings of kidney disease	• *CBC*: ± Leucocytosis • *Urinalysis*: Pyuria, haematuria, proteinuria, bacteriuria • *Prostate or prostatic fluid cytology*: Inflammation and infection	• *CBC*: Normal • *Urinalysis*: Pyuria, haematuria, proteinuria, bacteriuria
Diagnostic imaging findings	• Normal kidneys • Structural abnormalities of lower urinary tract • ± Urocystoliths and/or urethroliths • ± Thickening of bladder wall and irregularity of mucosa • ± Emphysematous cystitis	• Renomegaly • ± Abnormal kidney shape • ± Nephroliths, ureteroliths • ± Dilated renal pelves, dilated pelvic diverticulae • ± Evidence of outflow obstruction	• ± Indistinct cranial border of prostate • ± Prostatomegaly • ± Prostatic cysts • ± Reflux of contrast medium into prostate	• ± Prostatomegaly • ± Prostatic cysts • ± Prostatic mineralization

29.6 Abnormalities that help localize urinary tract infections.

urination may occur with lower UTIs. Animals with upper UTIs may have abdominal pain localized to one or both kidneys, micro- or macroscopic haematuria, polyuria, or clinical signs due to septicaemia or kidney disease. If the UTI is associated with a predisposing condition (e.g. diabetes mellitus, hyperadrenocorticism or bladder neoplasia), clinical signs associated with that condition may predominate. Urinary incontinence may be noted in patients with lower UTIs, presumably due to inflammation-induced detrusor hyperreflexivity and/or urethritis. However, patients with urinary incontinence prior to the time of infection may have ectopic ureters, urethral sphincter mechanism incompetence or overflow incontinence due to neurological disease, all of which predispose to the development of bacterial UTI.

Physical examination abnormalities directly due to the presence of a UTI are rare. Occasionally, mucopurulent discharge from the external genitalia may be noted, particularly in bitches. Nevertheless, all animals with suspected or confirmed UTIs should have thorough examinations of the external genitalia in order to identify potential predisposing causes of infection. Bitches with anatomical abnormalities of the vulva, severe perivulvar dermatitis or vaginal stenosis may be at increased risk for the development of UTI, and digital vaginal examinations should be performed in patients with recurrent infections. Male cats with perineal urethrostomies also have an increased risk of UTI.

Urinalysis

A complete urinalysis (i.e. urine specific gravity determination, dipstick analysis and urine sediment examination) is part of the minimum database. Cystocentesis is the gold standard for collecting urine when evaluating a dog or cat for UTI, because this minimizes the likelihood of contamination of the urine sample by distal urethral or genital flora. If infectious prostatitis or vaginitis is suspected, these anatomical areas should be evaluated using alternative techniques (see Chapter 25 for evaluation of the patient with prostatitis).

Urine specific gravity is variable in dogs or cats with urinary tract infection; inappropriately dilute urine usually occurs when infection involves the upper urinary tract or there is an associated disease that has affected urine concentrating ability. Dipstick analysis often, but not always, reveals haematuria and proteinuria. Leucocyte esterase (white blood cells (WBCs)) and nitrite (bacteria) dipstick test pads are not reliable in dogs and cats. Nitrites are produced by several human bacterial uropathogens, but bacterial strains isolated from veterinary patients result in frequent false-negative results. Leucocyte test strips detect human granulocyte esterase protein activity; in dogs, this dipstick pad has low sensitivity, whereas in cats it has very low specificity.

Urine sediment examination is more useful for detection of infection than dipstick analysis. The presence of a significant number of WBCs (>0–5 per high-power field (hpf)) on urine sediment examination suggests inflammation, particularly when associated with haematuria and proteinuria. Detection of significant microburia with pyuria indicates active inflammation associated with an infection, if clinical signs are present. Bacteria and fungi may be difficult to identify in dilute urine, making diagnosis of UTI by sediment examination problematic; also, UTIs may often be present without concurrent inflammation when host defences are compromised by systemic diseases (e.g. hyperadrenocorticism, feline leukaemia virus infection).

The sensitivity for detection of rod-shaped bacteria in unstained urine sediment preparations is good when >10,000 bacteria/ml are present. Cocci are more difficult to detect in urine sediment, and typically >100,000 bacteria/ml are required for consistent detection. Although detection of bacteria on urine sediment examination strongly suggests bacterial UTI, this finding should be verified by urine culture if clinically indicated. The sensitivity and specificity for detection of bacterial UTI in dog or cat urine by examination of unstained urine sediment are 82.4% and 76.4%, respectively. False positives are often due to misidentification of fat globules or other urine debris as bacteria, and false negatives may be due to the number of bacteria being too low to be identified. The diagnostic accuracy of UTI diagnosis by urine sediment examination is increased by staining sediment with Gram's stain or new methylene blue; nevertheless, urine culture is the gold standard for diagnosis of UTI.

Urine culture

Aerobic bacterial urine culture is the gold standard for diagnosis of bacterial UTI. A diagnosis of UTI based solely on clinical signs or urinalysis findings of haematuria and/or urinary tract inflammation may result in misdiagnosis, does not allow precise identification of the infecting organism or determination of sensitivity to various antimicrobials, and therefore possibly leads to inadequate or inappropriate treatment. Under some circumstances, antimicrobial therapy may be considered without first obtaining the results of urine culture; however, samples for urine culture should be collected before antimicrobial therapy is started. If antimicrobial therapy has occurred, it should be discontinued for 3–5 days prior to collection of urine for urine culture, to minimize *in vitro* inhibition of microbial growth.

Following collection of urine, samples should be preserved and transported so as to avoid bacterial contamination, proliferation or death. Urine specimens for aerobic bacterial culture should be stored and transported in sealed, sterilized containers, and processing should begin as soon as possible. A variety of sterile containers can be used which do not contain preservatives or inhibitors; these are suitable only when samples are immediately transported and processed by microbiology laboratories, because they will not prevent bacterial proliferation (thus falsely increasing the number of colony-forming units (cfu) per millilitre of urine) or eventual death (and thus may result in false-negative results). Bacterial counts may double every 20–45 minutes at room temperature. Multiplication or destruction of bacteria may occur within 1 hour of collection. When these standard transport containers are used and laboratory processing is delayed by more than 30 minutes, urine specimens should be refrigerated at 4°C. Refrigerated samples should be plated within 8–12 hours of collection.

If samples cannot be processed immediately for urine culture, several alternatives are available. In-clinic urine culture kits allow immediate processing of urine and may also decrease the cost to owners by allowing veterinary surgeons (veterinarians) to select only positive samples for species identification and sensitivity testing by outside laboratories. Blood agar and MacConkey's agar plates may also be inoculated and incubated for 24–48 hours. A calibrated bacteriological loop or a microlitre mechanical pipette that delivers exactly 0.01 or 0.001 ml of urine to the culture plates should be used to estimate cfu/ml, and urine should be streaked over the plates using conventional methods. Blood agar supports the growth of most aerobic bacterial uropathogens, and MacConkey's agar provides morphological information that aids in the identification of bacteria and prevents 'swarming' of *Proteus* spp. Plates are incubated or placed under an incandescent light. Prior to obtaining in-clinic cultures, the clinician should ascertain whether the plates could be submitted to their reference laboratory for identification and determination of antimicrobial sensitivities. If no growth occurs after 48–72 hours, the plates may be discarded. If in-clinic cultures are performed, appropriate laboratory facilities, proper equipment and biosafety level 2 containment and waste management, in addition to appropriately trained personnel, should be in place.

Commercially available urine culture collection tubes containing preservative, which may or may not be combined with refrigeration, may be used to preserve specimens for up to 72 hours before processing occurs. The advantage of these preservative tubes is that they allow delay in the submission of samples for urine culture until results of other diagnostic tests, such as urinalysis, become available. Inoculation of urine into 'enrichment' media (such as thioglycollate) may allow detection of low numbers of bacteria; this is most useful when urine culture during antimicrobial therapy cannot be avoided.

A quantitative urine culture includes isolation and identification of the infecting organism and determination of the number of bacteria (i.e. cfu per unit volume; cfu/ml). Quantitation allows interpretation of the significance of bacteria present in a urine sample. The presence of bacteria, even in low numbers, in urine collected aseptically by cystocentesis indicates a UTI. Although urine obtained from most dogs without a UTI by any method is usually sterile or contains <10,000 cfu/ml, counts of 100,000 cfu/ml or higher nevertheless occur with sufficient frequency to make collection of urine by midstream voiding or manual expression unsatisfactory in most cases.

Treatment

Antimicrobial drugs are the cornerstone of treatment for bacterial UTIs. The antimicrobial agent selected should be: easy to administer; associated with few, if any, adverse effects; inexpensive; able to attain urine concentrations (and tissue concentrations in the event of kidney or prostatic infection) that exceed the minimum inhibitory concentration (MIC) for the uropathogen by at least fourfold; and unlikely to affect the animal's resident gastrointestinal flora adversely. In most cases the antimicrobial agent chosen should be based on susceptibility testing of the uropathogen.

Determining whether an infection is uncomplicated or complicated is essential to guide the diagnostic and therapeutic plan. A simple uncomplicated UTI occurs sporadically in an otherwise healthy animal with a normal structural and functional urinary tract. In contrast, infections are complicated if there is: involvement of the upper urinary tract and/or prostate; an underlying comorbidity that alters the structure or function of the urinary tract, such as an endocrinopathy or chronic kidney disease (CKD); or recurrent infection. Recurrent infections are further categorized as relapsing, refractory/persistent, reinfection, or superinfection (Figure 29.7). Most cats with bacterial UTI have complicated infections. Additional laboratory testing and imaging studies are often required for complicated infections (Figure 29.8). Duration of treatment and monitoring of patients depends on what type of UTI is present (Figure 29.9).

Term	Definition	Underlying aetiology
Uncomplicated UTI	• Healthy individual, normal urinary tract anatomy and function	• Sporadic infection

Complicated UTI Comorbidity	• Disease that alters the structure or function of the urinary tract
	• Relevant comorbidity can predispose to persistent or recurrent infection
		• Endocrinopathies:
		  • Diabetes mellitus
		  • Hyperadrenocorticism
		  • Hyperthyroidism
		• Chronic kidney disease
		• Urinary or reproductive tract anatomical abnormality
		• Immunosuppression
		• Neurogenic bladder
		• Pregnancy

Recurrent infection (relapsing)	• Recurrence within weeks to months of a successfully treated infection
	• Sterile bladder during treatment
	• Same organism
		• Failure to eradicate pathogen
		• Deep-seated niche:
		  • Pyelonephritis
		  • Prostatitis
		  • Bladder submucosa
		  • Stone
		  • Bladder neoplasia

Refractory/persistent infection	• Persistently positive culture with original pathogen despite *in vitro* antimicrobial susceptibility • No elimination of bacteriuria during or after treatment	• Rare • Failure of host defences • Structural abnormality • Patient/client incompliance • Abnormal metabolism/excretion of antimicrobial

Reinfection	• Recurrence with different organism
	• Variable time course after previous infection
		• Poor systemic immune function:
		  • Endocrinopathy
		  • Immunosuppression
		• Loss of urine antimicrobial properties:
		  • Glucosuria
		  • Dilute urine
		• Anatomical abnormality
		• Physiological predisposition:
		  • Neurogenic bladder
		  • Urinary incontinence

Superinfection	• Infection with different pathogen during treatment for the original infection	• Cystotomy tube • Indwelling urinary catheter • Neoplasia

29.7 Uncomplicated and complicated urinary tract infections (UTIs).

• Urinalysis
• Urine culture (ideally, cystocentesis sample)
• Complete blood count
• Chemistry profile with electrolytes
• Digital rectal examination
• Feline leukaemia virus/feline immunodeficiency virus (cats)
• Thyroid testing:
  • Cats: total thyroxine (T4)
• Adrenal testing:
  • Low-dose dexamethasone suppression test
  • Adrenocorticotrophic hormone stimulation test
• Abdominal radiography
• Abdominal ultrasonography
• Contrast radiography:
  • Excretory urography
  • Contrast cystourethrography
  • Double-contrast cystography
  • Contrast vaginourethrography
• Prostatic wash/aspirate

29.8 Extended diagnostic testing for complicated urinary tract infections (UTIs).

Bacterial UTI
Uncomplicated (simple) UTI

Antimicrobial drugs are the cornerstone of treatment for UTI. In most cases, the antimicrobial agent chosen should be based on susceptibility testing of the uropathogen. Overuse and misuse of antimicrobial drugs may result in the emergence of resistant organisms, a situation that has implications for successful treatment of infections in the patient as well as overall veterinary and human health.

Patients with uncomplicated UTI and those with clinical signs severe enough to merit therapy prior to the results of urine culture and sensitivity testing should receive a broad-spectrum antimicrobial that has excellent urine penetration. Suggested first-line antimicrobials for uncomplicated UTIs include amoxicillin, cefalexin and trimethoprim/sulfamethoxazole (Figure 29.10). The use of potentiated beta-lactams (e.g. amoxicillin/clavulanic acid), fluoroquinolones, or extended release cefalexin (e.g. cefovecin) is inappropriate for most uncomplicated UTIs, and should be reserved for complicated or resistant infections (Figure 29.11).

Infection	Treatment duration	Monitoring urine culture
Uncomplicated bacterial UTI	7–14 days	5–7 days after discontinuation of antimicrobials
Complicated bacterial UTI	Minimum 3–6 weeks	1 week into therapy; before therapy discontinuation; 5–7 days after discontinuation of antimicrobial; 1 month and 2 months post-treatment
Asymptomatic bacteriuria	Treatment not recommended unless high risk of ascending or systemic infection	If clinical signs develop
Fungal UTI	Minimum 6–8 weeks	As above for complicated bacterial UTI

29.9 Treatment duration and monitoring for urinary tract infections (UTIs).

Infection	First-line drug options
Uncomplicated UTI	Amoxicillin, trimethoprim/sulphonamide
Complicated UTI	Guided by culture and susceptibility testing, but consider amoxicillin or trimethoprim/sulphonamide initially
Subclinical bacteriuria	Antimicrobial therapy not recommended unless high risk for ascending infection; if so, treat as for complicated UTI
Pyelonephritis	Start with a fluoroquinolone, with reassessment based on culture and susceptibility testing
Prostatitis	Trimethoprim/sulphonamide, enrofloxacin, chloramphenicol

29.10 Summary of first-line antimicrobial options for bacterial urinary tract infections (UTIs) in the dog and cat.

Drug	Dose	Comments
Amikacin	Dogs: 15–30 mg/kg i.v., i.m., s.c. q24h Cats: 10–14 mg/kg i.v., i.m., s.c. q24h	Not recommended for routine use but may be useful for treatment of multidrug-resistant organisms. Potentially nephrotoxic. Avoid in animals with renal insufficiency
Amoxicillin	11–15 mg/kg orally q8h or 22 mg/kg orally q12h	Good first-line option for UTIs. Excreted in urine predominantly in active form if normal renal function is present. Ineffective against beta-lactamase-producing bacteria
Amoxicillin/clavulanate	12.5–25 mg/kg orally q8h (dose based on combination of amoxicillin + clavulanate)	Not established whether there is any advantage over amoxicillin alone
Ampicillin	Not recommended	Not recommended because of poor oral bioavailability. Amoxicillin is preferred
Cefadroxil, cefalexin	12–25 mg/kg orally q12h	Enterococci are resistant. Resistance may be common in Enterobacteriaceae in some regions
Cefovecin	8 mg/kg single s.c. injection. Can be repeated once after 7–14 days	Should only be used in situations where oral treatment is problematic. Enterococci are resistant. Pharmacokinetic data are available to support the use in dogs and cats, with a duration of 14 days (dogs) and 21 days (cats). The long duration of excretion in the urine makes it difficult to interpret post-treatment culture results
Cefpodoxime proxetil	5–10 mg/kg orally q24h	Enterococci are resistant
Ceftiofur	2 mg/kg s.c. q12–24h	Approved for treatment of UTIs in dogs in some regions. Enterococci are resistant
Chloramphenicol	Dogs: 40–50 mg/kg orally q8h Cats: 12.5–20 mg/kg orally q12h or 50 mg total dose orally q12h	Reserved for multidrug-resistant infections with few other options. Myelosuppression can occur, particularly with long-term therapy. Avoid contact by humans because of rare idiosyncratic aplastic anaemia
Ciprofloxacin	30 mg/kg orally q24h	Sometimes used because of lower cost than enrofloxacin. Lower and more variable oral bioavailability than enrofloxacin, marbofloxacin and orbifloxacin. Difficult to justify over approved fluoroquinolones. Dosing recommendations are empirical
Doxycycline	3–5 mg/kg orally q12h	Highly metabolized and excreted through intestinal tract, so urine levels may be low. Not recommended for routine use
Enrofloxacin	Dogs: 10–20 mg/kg orally q24h Cats: 5 mg/kg orally q24h	Excreted in urine predominantly in active form. Reserve for documented resistant UTIs but good first-line choice for pyelonephritis (dogs 20 mg/kg orally q24h). Limited efficacy against enterococci. Associated with risk of retinopathy in cats. Do not exceed 5 mg/kg/day of enrofloxacin in cats
Imipenem/cilastatin	5 mg/kg i.v., i.m. q6–8h	Reserve for treatment of multidrug-resistant infections, particularly those caused by Enterobacteriaceae or *Pseudomonas aeruginosa*. Recommend consultation with a urinary or infectious disease veterinary specialist or veterinary pharmacologist prior to use
Marbofloxacin	2.7–5.5 mg/kg orally q24h	Excreted in urine predominantly in active form. Reserve for documented resistant UTIs but good first-line choice for pyelonephritis. Limited efficacy against enterococci
Meropenem	8.5 mg/kg s.c. q12h or i.v. q8h	Reserve for treatment of multidrug-resistant infections, particularly those caused by Enterobacteriaceae or *Pseudomonas aeruginosa*. Recommend consultation with a urinary or infectious disease veterinary specialist or veterinary pharmacologist prior to use
Nitrofurantoin	4.4–5 mg/kg orally q8h	Good second-line option for simple uncomplicated UTI, particularly when multidrug-resistant pathogens are involved. Contraindicated for pyelonephritis owing to lack of tissue penetration
Orbifloxacin	Tablets: 2.5–7.5 mg/kg orally q24h; oral suspension: 7.5 mg/kg orally q24h (cats) or 2.5–7.5 mg/kg orally q24h (dogs)	Excreted in urine predominantly in active form
Pradofloxacin	Dogs: 3 mg/kg orally q24h[a] Cats: 5 mg/kg orally q24h[a]	May cause bone marrow suppression resulting in severe thrombocytopenia and neutropenia in dogs
Trimethoprim/sulfadiazine	15 mg/kg orally q12h Note: dosing is based on total trimethoprim + sulfadiazine concentration	Good first-line option. Concerns regarding idiosyncratic and immune-mediated adverse effects in some patients, especially with prolonged therapy. If prolonged (>7 days) therapy is anticipated, baseline Schirmer's tear testing is recommended (dogs), with periodic re-evaluation and owner monitoring for ocular discharge. Avoid in dogs that may be sensitive to potential adverse effects such as keratoconjunctivitis sicca, hepatopathy, hypersensitivity and skin eruptions

29.11 Antimicrobial treatment options for urinary tract infection (UTI) in dogs and cats.
([a] Dose extrapolated from Lees, 2013)

Empirical antimicrobial therapy: Treatment of uncomplicated bacterial UTIs of acute onset may be undertaken without antimicrobial susceptibility testing, provided the dog or cat has not been administered antimicrobial agents within the previous 4 to 6 weeks; and the UTI is an initial or infrequent occurrence. In such situations, the antimicrobial should be chosen for its known urine-penetrating properties and with understanding of the bacterial species that most commonly cause UTI in dogs and cats. Identification of bacteria on urine sediment examination, particularly if Gram's staining is performed, increases the likelihood of empirically choosing an appropriate antimicrobial. For example, *Escherichia coli*, a Gram-negative rod, is the most common cause of bacterial UTI in dogs and cats, and is usually associated with aciduria. Conversely, *Staphylococcus* spp. are Gram-positive cocci commonly associated with alkaluria because they produce urease, which metabolizes urea to ammonia, resulting in an alkaline urine pH.

Short duration antimicrobial therapy: In human medicine, short duration antimicrobial therapy, commonly trimethoprim/sulfamethoxazole or a fluoroquinolone, has become the standard treatment for acute uncomplicated bacterial cystitis in women. The recommendations are antimicrobial specific because not all antimicrobials have comparable efficacy when given as only a 3-day treatment. Benefits of shorter therapy include better compliance, lower cost and decreased adverse effects. The goal of treatment is to decrease the bacterial load enough to control clinical signs, with the immune system eliminating remaining organisms. Westropp *et al.* (2012) and Clare *et al.* (2014) evaluated short duration treatment in dogs with uncomplicated bacterial UTI. The first study compared 3-day high-dose enrofloxacin (*n* = 35, 20 mg/kg orally q24h) to standard doses of amoxicillin/clavulanic acid (*n* = 33, 13.75–20 mg/kg orally q12h). Clinical and microbiological cure was evaluated 7 days after antimicrobial discontinuation, and short-term high-dose treatment was not inferior to standard treatment. The second study was double blinded and compared 3-day trimethoprim/sulfamethoxazole (*n* = 20, 15 mg/kg orally q12h) plus 7-day placebo to 10 days of cefalexin (*n* = 18, 20 mg/kg orally q12h). There was no significant difference in the short-term (4 days post-treatment) and long-term (30 days post-treatment) clinical and microbiological cure rates between the treatment groups. Clinical cure at 30 days was 50–65% and microbiological cure was 20–44%. Additional studies are needed to determine the appropriate treatment duration for uncomplicated bacterial UTI.

Combination therapy: If multiple bacteria are isolated, the relative importance of each must be assessed on the basis of quantification and suspected pathogenicity. Ideally, an antimicrobial effective against all pathogens is selected. If this is not possible then combination therapy with multiple antimicrobials may be considered. Assuming that there is no evidence of pyelonephritis or increased risk of ascending infection, targeting antimicrobial therapy against the pathogen with most clinical relevance is reasonable. For example, anecdotally, resolution of *Enterococcus* spp. infection is often possible after treatment of concurrent infection.

Complicated UTI

Sexually intact dogs, most cats, and animals with identifiable predisposing causes for UTI (e.g. chronic kidney disease, hyperadrenocorticism, diabetes mellitus) should be considered to have complicated UTIs (see Figures 29.8, 29.9 and 29.10). Likewise, patients with infections of the upper urinary tract (pyelonephritis) are considered to have complicated UTIs, because penetration of antimicrobials into the kidneys is less than into the urine in many cases, and the complications associated with unsuccessful treatment are much more severe than with uncomplicated lower UTIs. Treatment with antimicrobials for longer than the routine 10–14 days is usually indicated, particularly for pyelonephritis and prostatitis, with treatment courses usually continuing for 4–6 weeks. The duration of treatment in animals with other comorbidities has not been studied; longer-duration therapy may or may not be necessary. The urine dipstick and sediment should be re-evaluated in the first week of treatment for response to therapy and also before discontinuation of therapy. Intact male dogs with UTIs should be assumed to have prostatic infection, and thus when choosing antimicrobial therapy consideration must be given to which drugs adequately penetrate the blood–prostate barrier (see Chapter 25). Cats are often considered to have complicated UTIs because infections in this species are much more commonly associated with systemic disease.

Catheter-associated UTI

There is no evidence to support routine urine culture or culture of the urinary catheter tip following removal in patients without clinical signs; such cultures do not predict the development of catheter-associated infection. In contrast, urine culture is always indicated for a patient with clinical signs of UTI, fever of undetermined origin or abnormal urine cytology (i.e. haematuria, pyuria). If the patient develops new clinical signs or fever after a urinary catheter has been placed, ideally the urine catheter should be removed and a cystocentesis performed to provide a sample for culture once the bladder fills. Alternatively, the original urinary catheter is replaced and a urine sample is collected through the second catheter. It is less ideal to sample the urine through the original catheter and a sample from the collection bag should never be used.

Asymptomatic bacteriuria

Asymptomatic bacteriuria (AB) is a common and often benign finding in healthy women. Risk factors include pregnancy, diabetes mellitus, spinal cord injury, indwelling urinary catheter and being an elderly nursing home resident. Women with AB have more frequent symptomatic episodes, but antimicrobial treatment does not decrease the number of episodes. A benefit of treatment has not been found with clinical trials in humans, whereas potential complications include adverse drug reactions and the development of antimicrobial resistance. The prevalence of AB in healthy dogs and cats is low (2–9%). Animals with underlying comorbidities, such as hyperthyroidism, diabetes mellitus or CKD, or recurrent infection, have increased prevalence of AB, up to 30% and 50% respectively. There are no prospective studies comparing clinical outcome in veterinary patients with or without antimicrobial treatment for AB. Wan *et al.* (2014) found that, of dogs with AB, 50% had transient colonization and 50% had persistent bacteriuria over a 3-month period; no dog developed clinical signs at any time. Similar to general recommendations in humans, treatment is not recommended for AB unless there is a high risk of ascending or systemic infection (e.g. immunocompromised patients, CKD).

Fungal UTI

Diagnosis of fungal UTI most commonly occurs by identification of fungal elements during routine or concentrated urine sediment examination. Fungal culture and sensitivity are ideal prior to treatment, especially in cases other than *Candida albicans*, which tend to be more resistant.

Viral UTI

Routine diagnostic tests, including urinalysis and light microscopy, cannot identify viruses or virus-induced disease. Virus isolation is the gold standard for diagnosis, but this technique is expensive, time-consuming and requires live replicating virus. Diagnostic polymerase chain reaction (PCR) assays are rapid and sensitive, but methods to optimize nucleic acid preparation are essential because the nucleic acids are easily degraded in urine.

Resistance

The emergence of multidrug-resistant bacteria is concerning and has important implications for both the patient and public health. There are trends towards increasing resistance in both faecal and environmental reservoirs. In addition to acquiring resistance genes via plasmids, there are other bacterial strategies for persistence within the urinary tract. For example, uropathogenic *Escherichia coli* can invade and persist within the superficial bladder wall epithelial cells. These bacteria may remain dormant for a period of time, followed by recrudescence.

Biofilms

Some bacteria have the capacity for biofilm formation, which facilitates colonization. A biofilm is composed of organisms adhered together by a self-produced polysaccharide matrix. It has been suggested that the bacteria within the biofilm become sessile; they are protected from the immune system and antimicrobials, and are inherently resistant to shear forces of removal. In humans, bacteria with the capacity to produce biofilms have been associated with AB. Biofilms are also implicated in the development of catheter-associated UTI.

Strategies to prevent catheter-associated biofilms include using materials that are less amenable to biofilm formation and coatings or surface modifications that decrease biofilm formation. For example, silicone catheters are preferred over latex because scanning electron microscope imaging reveals that latex surfaces are more irregular and promote microbial adherence. An example of an agent used for catheter coating is the antiseptic chlorhexidine. In a veterinary prospective study by Segev *et al.* (2013), ($n = 26$ dogs) evaluating biofilm formation on indwelling urinary catheters, a sustained-release varnish on chlorhexidine-coated urinary catheters statistically decreased biofilm formation. There is an array of other catheter coatings and modifications to decrease bacterial adherence and biofilm formation that have primarily been studied in a research setting, including silver coating, nanoparticles, iontophoresis, antimicrobials, urease and other enzyme inhibitors, liposomes and bacteriophages. Other novel strategies include quorum sensing inhibitors and vibroacoustic stimulation (Figure 29.12). A detailed discussion of comparison is beyond the scope of this article and the reader is referred elsewhere. Some oral antimicrobials, in particular combination therapy with clarithromycin, have shown promise *in vitro* for anti-biofilm activity. For example, *P. aeruginosa* biofilm was eliminated by a synergistic combination of clarithromycin and ciprofloxacin. Likewise, combination therapy of clarithromycin with fosfomycin was more effective than either treatment alone in reducing *Staphylococcus pseudintermedius* biofilm. *In vivo* studies are needed for further evaluation of the efficacy of these therapies.

Fungal resistance

Infections that fail to respond completely to fluconazole should be recultured and antifungal sensitivity testing performed. Some susceptible isolates may respond to intravesicular administration of 1% clotrimazole or amphotericin B. Urinary alkalinization has also been historically proposed as adjunctive therapy in patients with fungal UTI, because increased urine pH may inhibit fungal growth. However, this is not currently favoured for treatment of fungal UTI in humans, and is of questionable efficacy in veterinary patients.

Strategy	Definition	Mechanism of action
Silver coating	Catheter coating	Bactericidal activity of silver ion inhibits enzymatic pathways and disrupts the cell wall
Nanoparticles	Nanometre-sized particles that attach to and penetrate bacterial cells	Disrupt cell membranes via lipid peroxidation and interacting with DNA
Iontophoresis	Application of an electrical field with low intensity direct current	Bioelectric effect enhances antimicrobial efficacy against bacteria within biofilms
Urease and other enzyme inhibitors	For example, acetohydroxamic acid, fluorofamide, N-acetyl-D-glucosamine-1-phosphate acetyltransferase inhibitors	*In vitro*, reduce encrustation and alter biofilm integrity
Liposomes	Act as carriers for hydrophobic and hydrophilic drugs	Increase drug half-life, decrease adverse effects, protect drug from environment
Bacteriophages	Viruses that selectively infect bacteria	Bacteriophages rapidly divide within bacteria and lyse bacterial cells. Bacteria can develop resistance
Quorum-sensing inhibitors	Quorum sensing describes a system of molecular signalling (i.e. auto-inducers) that controls population density and gene expression necessary for bacteria to develop the biofilm phenotype	For example, *Delisea pulchra* algae produce a molecule that inhibits auto-inducer signalling
Vibroacoustic stimulation	Low acoustic waves form a vibrating coat along the catheter surface	Inhibit bacterial adhesion and quorum-sensing electrical gradients

29.12 Strategies to prevent biofilm formation.

Prophylaxis

Pulse antimicrobial therapy

There are no good studies evaluating pulse (intermittent) or chronic low dose prophylactic antimicrobial therapy in animals with frequent reinfections, but anecdotally some animals may benefit. Careful patient selection is required and the impact of promoting antimicrobial resistance should be considered. Before prophylactic treatment is undertaken, urine culture and susceptibility testing should be done to ensure that the bacterial UTI has been eradicated. For long-term prophylaxis, a drug that is excreted in high concentrations in urine and is unlikely to cause adverse effects is selected. Often a fluoroquinolone, cephalosporin or a beta-lactam antimicrobial is chosen. The antimicrobial agent is administered at approximately one third of the therapeutic daily dose immediately after the patient has voided, at a time when the drug and its metabolites will be retained in the urinary tract for 6–8 hours (typically at night). The drug is given for a minimum of 6 months. Urine samples, preferably collected by cystocentesis (not by catheterization because this may induce bacterial UTI), are collected every 4–8 weeks for urinalysis and quantitative urine culture. If the sample is free of infection then prophylactic treatment is continued. If bacterial UTI is identified, active (breakthrough) infection is treated as a complicated bacterial UTI prior to returning to a prophylactic strategy. If a breakthrough bacterial UTI does not occur after 6 months of prophylactic antimicrobial therapy, treatment may be discontinued and the patient should be monitored for reinfection.

D-Mannose

D-Mannose is used to prevent recurrent UTI, but there are no studies of clinical efficacy in veterinary patients. The D-mannose sugar competitively binds to mannose fimbriae on certain *E. coli* strains, thereby inhibiting adhesion to the uroepithelium. There are few data available for other bacteria that may express mannose fimbriae. An extrapolated anecdotal dose for dogs is ¼ teaspoon per 20 pounds (9 kg) bodyweight three times daily.

Methenamine

Methenamine salt is a urinary antiseptic that is converted to bacteriostatic formaldehyde in an acidic environment (urine pH <5.5). There is controversy in human medicine as to whether methenamine prevents UTI, although there is some evidence that it may be effective for short-term prophylaxis. It is unknown whether the two salts described in the literature, hippurate and mandelate, are equally effective; the mandelate salt is difficult to find. There is limited veterinary literature on the use of methenamine in small animals, although there is a theoretical benefit. Studies of safety, efficacy and appropriate dosing are lacking. Commonly recommended doses are 10–20 mg/kg orally q12h (dog) and 250 mg/cat orally q12h. Gastrointestinal upset and dysuria are the most commonly reported adverse events; methenamine is poorly tolerated by feline patients. Methenamine should not be used in cases of kidney disease. Concurrent use of a urinary acidifier, such as DL-methionine, is usually required for maximal effect.

Cranberry

Proanthocyanidin, the 'active ingredient' in cranberry, alters the genotypic or phenotypic expression of fimbriae, which subsequently inhibits *E. coli* adherence to human bladder and vaginal epithelial cells. Studies in humans reveal inconsistent efficacy for prevention of UTIs. However, in a meta-analysis (n = 1049), human patients supplemented with cranberry products had fewer UTIs over a 12-month period compared with placebo. There are few veterinary studies in healthy dogs and no feline studies. Additionally, quality and potency are variable among over-the-counter products; ideally each formulation would be tested in the species of interest. The Consensus of the Antimicrobial Guidelines Working Group of the International Society for Companion Animal Infectious Diseases is that there is insufficient evidence to support the use of cranberry extract to prevent recurrent UTIs in dogs and cats.

Local therapy

Local infusions with antimicrobials, antiseptics and dimethylsulphoxide (DMSO) can be irritating and are not retained within the urinary bladder. Anecdotally, instillation of dilute chlorhexidine (1:100, 0.02%) and/or EDTA-tromethamine (EDTA-tris) via cystotomy tube may decrease the incidence of bacterial UTI. In a small study on humans, bladder irrigation with dilute 0.02% chlorhexidine significantly decreased postoperative bacteriuria, although it did not eliminate pre-existing infection, and did not appear to damage the bladder mucosa. It has been postulated that EDTA-tris has synergistic effects with systemic antimicrobials as well as local chlorhexidine irrigation. Proposed mechanisms included divalent ion binding causing alteration of bacterial DNA synthesis, cell wall permeability and ribosomal stability. Additionally, *in vitro* studies suggest that the presence of EDTA-tris reduces the minimum inhibitory concentration of various antimicrobial drugs. In a small study by Farca *et al.* (1997), (n =17 dogs, n = 4 with chronic cystitis), daily local infusion via sterile urinary catheter (25 ml EDTA at 37°C) for 7 days was well tolerated and dogs had negative urine cultures up to 180 days post treatment. Additional studies are needed to determine the short- and long-term effects of EDTA-tris therapy.

Complications of UTIs

UTIs may be associated with several complications. Repeated UTI and subsequent antimicrobial therapy may result in multidrug resistance. Bacterial organisms that produce urease, an enzyme that metabolizes urinary urea resulting in formation of magnesium ammonium phosphate hexahydrate (struvite) uroliths, include *Staphylococcus* spp., *Enterococcus* spp., *Proteus* spp. and *Corynebacterium urealyticum*. Deep-seated tissue infections may occur, resulting in polypoid cystitis, emphysematous cystitis, pyelonephritis and prostatitis. Polypoid cystitis lesions are niduses of deep-seated bacterial infection, and should be treated as complicated UTIs. In some cases long-term antimicrobial therapy may result in successful resolution of lesions. However, partial cystectomy results in more rapid resolution of clinical signs, is likely to be associated with improved rates for long-term resolution of infection, and allows shorter antimicrobial treatment courses.

Emphysematous cystitis refers to accumulation of air within the bladder wall and lumen, secondary to infection with glucose-fermenting bacteria. Most cases are due to *Escherichia coli* infection, but *Proteus* spp., *Clostridum* spp. and *Aerobacter aerogenes* have also been reported. Emphysematous cystitis most commonly develops in dogs and cats with diabetes mellitus because of the high concentration of fermentable substrate. Treatment of emphysematous cystitis should be as described for complicated UTI; if glucosuria is present then appropriate treatment should be initiated for the underlying cause.

Although no systematic reviews of pyelonephritis in dogs or cats have been performed, animals with systemically compromised immunity (e.g. hyperadrenocorticism, diabetes mellitus), dogs or cats with CKD, and patients with any cause of vesicoureteral reflux may be predisposed to development of pyelonephritis. Chronic pyelonephritis is probably underdiagnosed as a cause of chronic kidney disease in dogs and cats, and should be especially considered in patients with previously stable CKD that have unexpected worsening of azotaemia (i.e. 'acute-on-chronic' renal failure).

Prostatic abscessation is a sequel to prostatitis and is characterized by accumulations of purulent fluid within the prostatic tissue. Clinical signs are variable and dependent upon the size and extent of the abscess, as well as systemic involvement. Prostatic abscesses are generally easily identified with ultrasonography, and the goal of therapy is to provide drainage either through ultrasound-guided percutaneous drainage or surgery. Surgical options include partial prostatectomy and prostate ometalization. Further information on prostatitis can be found in Chapter 25.

References and further reading

Ball A, Carr T, Gillespie W et al. (1987) Bladder irrigation with chlorhexidine for the prevention of urinary infection after transurethral operations: a prospective controlled study. Journal of Urology 138, 491–494

Barsanti J (2012) Genitourinary infections. In: Infectious Diseases of the Dog and Cat, 4th edn, ed. CE Greene, pp.1013–1031. Elsevier Saunders, St. Louis

Bartges D and Blanco L (2001) Bacterial urinary tract infections in cats. Compendium Standard Care 3, 1–5

Clare S, Hartmann F, Jooss M et al. (2014) Short- and long-term cure rates of short-duration trimethoprim-sulfamethoxazole treatment in female dogs with uncomplicated bacterial cystitis. Journal of Veterinary Internal Medicine 28, 818–826

Farca A, Piromalli G, Maffei F et al. (1997) Potentiating effect of EDTA-tris on the activity of antibiotics against resistant bacteria associated with otitis, dermatitis and cystitis. Journal of Small Animal Practice 38, 243–245

Forward ZA, Legendre AM and Khalsa HD (2002) Use of intermittent bladder infusion with clotrimazole for treatment of candiduria in a dog. Journal of the American Veterinary Medical Association 220, 1496–1498

Kranjčec B, Papeš D and Altarac S (2014) D-mannose powder for prophylaxis of recurrent urinary tract infections in women: a randomized clinical trial. World Journal of Urology 32, 79–84

Kruger JM, Osborne CA, Wise AG et al. (2011) Urinary tract infections – viruses. In: Nephrology and Urology of Small Animals, ed. JW Bartges and DJ Polzin, pp.725–733. Blackwell Publishing Ltd, Ames

Lees P (2013) Pharmacokinetics, pharmacodynamics and therapeutics of pradofloxacin in the dog and cat. Journal of Veterinary Pharmacology and Therapeutics 36, 209–221

Litster A, Moss SM, Honnery M et al. (2007) Prevalence of bacterial species in cats with clinical signs of lower urinary tract disease: recognition of Staphylococcus felis as a possible feline urinary tract pathogen. Veterinary Microbiology 121, 182–188

Litster A, Thompson M, Moss S et al. (2011) Feline bacterial urinary tract infections: An update on an evolving clinical problem. Veterinary Journal 187, 18–22

Pressler BM. Urinary tract infections – fungal. In: Nephrology and Urology of Small Animals, ed. JW Bartges and DJ Polzin, pp.717–724. Blackwell Publishing Ltd, Ames

Segev G, Bankirer T, Steinberg D et al. (2013) Evaluation of urinary catheters coated with sustained-release varnish of chlorhexidine in mitigating biofilm formation on urinary catheters in dogs. Journal of Veterinary Internal Medicine 27, 39–46

Wan SY, Hartmann FA, Jooss MK et al. (2014) Prevalence and clinical outcome of subclinical bacteriuria in female dogs. Journal of the American Veterinary Medical Association 245, 106–112

Weese JS, Blondeau JM, Boothe D et al. (2011) Antimicrobial use guidelines for treatment of urinary tract disease in dogs and cats: antimicrobial guidelines working group of the international society for companion animal infectious diseases. Veterinary Medicine International 263768, doi: 10.4061/2011/263768, http://www.hindawi.com/journals/vmi/2011/263768/

Westropp J, Sykes J, Irom S et al. (2012) Evaluation of the efficacy and safety of high dose short duration enrofloxacin treatment regimen for uncomplicated urinary tract infections in dogs. Journal of Veterinary Internal Medicine 26, 506–512

Chapter 30

Medical and surgical management of urinary incontinence

Allyson Berent and Philipp Mayhew

Micturition is the physiological process of storage and voiding of urine. Disorders of micturition interfere with these normal processes and can often lead to urinary incontinence or the inability to voluntarily control the flow of urine through the urethra. This chapter focuses on the medical, endoscopic and surgical management of urinary incontinence in small animal veterinary patients. The reader is referred to Chapter 3 for more details on lower urinary tract anatomy and micturition physiology, and to Chapter 9 for the diagnostic approach to the incontinent patient.

Aetiology of urinary incontinence

Urinary incontinence is most commonly seen in female dogs, but has certainly been recognized in both male dogs and male and female cats. There are various causes of urinary incontinence, which are listed in Figure 30.1. When there is an abnormality in either the structure or function of the urine storage phase of micturition, dogs can present with urinary incontinence. The reasons for this include:

- Failure of the urethra to appropriately close during urine storage (urethral sphincter mechanism incompetence, USMI)
- An anatomical abnormality of the ureteral termination (ureteral ectopia), urinary bladder shape and/or size, or shape, size and/or length of the urethra
- Urinary bladder dysfunction (failure of the urinary bladder to accommodate urine during the storage phase due to size, location, strength or neuromuscular function).

Epidemiology and pathophysiology
Urethral sphincter mechanism incompetence

A 'weak' urethra (decreased urethral closure pressure) is the most common cause of urinary incontinence in dogs and is mainly reported in neutered female dogs, although it can occur in entire dogs as well. This form of urinary incontinence is referred to as USMI, previously known as 'hormone-responsive incontinence'. Approximately 5–20% of female dogs are reported to develop USMI an average of 3 years after neutering, with larger breed dogs (>20 kg) being at higher risk (31% versus 9.3%). USMI is particularly common in certain breeds of dog, including

Cause	Examples	Other associated conditions
Urethral sphincter mechanism incompetence – acquired	Not applicable	Short, wide urethra Intrapelvic bladder
Urethral sphincter mechanism incompetence – congenital	Not applicable	Short, wide urethra
Ectopic ureter	Intramural or extramural	Urethral sphincter mechanism incompetence Short, wide urethra Hypoplastic bladder Persistent paramesonephric remnant
Vaginal defects	Persistent parasmesonephric remnant Vaginal septum Dual vaginas	Ectopic ureters
Prostatic disease	Prostatitis Prostatic neoplasia Benign prostatic hyperplasia	Haematuria Pollakiuria Prostatomegaly
Urinary storage dysfunction	Detrusor–urethral dyssynergia Overactive bladder	Large, overdistended bladder (detrusor–urethral dyssynergia) Small, empty bladder (overactive bladder)
Miscellaneous	Overflow incontinence Feline leukaemia virus-associated incontinence	Large, soft bladder with minimal tone

30.1 Causes of urinary incontinence.

Newfoundlands, Golden Retrievers, Labrador Retrievers, Old English Sheepdogs, Rottweilers, Dobermanns, Weimeraners, Boxers, Irish Setters and various other pure and mixed breeds. There is controversy regarding the timing of neutering and the effect of developing urinary incontinence. Most recommendations to date encourage neutering after 3 months of age, but before the first season (although recommendations vary).

The apparent beneficial effect of oestrogen on USMI has been investigated and is considered to be related to an oestrogen-induced increase in expression of alpha-1 adrenoreceptors on the urethral smooth muscle and sensitivity to alpha adrenergic agents in female dogs. Clinical responses to exogenous oestrogen therapy is mixed in female dogs with a poor response seen in male dogs and male and female cats.

Investigation into the role of follicle-stimulating hormone (FSH) and luteinizing hormone (LH) in incontinent female dogs found little relationship between concentrations of these hormones and maximal urethral closure pressure. There is a beneficial effect seen with the treatment of a gonadotrophin-releasing hormone (GnRH) analogue in some female dogs, and this effect is hypothesized to be independent of measurable urethral pressures (Reichler et al., 2006b).

The underlying cause of USMI is not known, as there are various factors that may contribute to urinary incontinence, including increasing age, decreased urethral alpha adrenoceptor responsiveness, short urethral length or wide width, abnormal bladder neck or urethral position (sitting caudally within the pelvis), obesity and vestibulovaginal septal defects. Decreased urethral closure pressures have been reported in dogs with USMI. It is important to realize that some female dogs that are continent also have low maximal urethral closure pressure on urethral pressure profiles (see Chapter 9) following ovariectomy or ovariohysterectomy, suggesting that numerous factors may result in urinary incontinence. Neutering has been found to result in a significantly higher percentage of collagen than smooth muscle in the urethral wall, which is speculated to affect urethral closure pressure. In addition, there have been some anatomical differences described in the urinary tract of incontinent female dogs compared with continent female dogs, but these are often subtle.

The most significant anatomical factor associated with continence in female dogs is the location of the bladder neck. In a study of 57 incontinent and 42 continent female dogs, an intrapelvic bladder location was found in 54 of the 57 incontinent dogs and only 7 of the 42 continent dogs (Holt, 1985c), suggesting a strong association of USMI and bladder neck location, resulting in a shortened urethral length. There is controversy as to whether it is the abdominal location of the bladder neck and urethra providing increased intra-abdominal pressure for improved continence or the shorter urethral functional length associated with an intrapelvic bladder location.

In male dogs, intrapelvic bladder location was also seen with incontinence, although this was not found to be associated with a shorter urethral length. Castration was shown to be a risk factor for incontinence in the same study (Power et al., 1998) likely associated with a smaller prostate gland and a more intrapelvic bladder location.

In cats, acquired USMI is uncommonly reported and most cases are considered congenital anomalies. Clinical signs are usually severe. Most cats have concurrent anatomical abnormalities, with urethral hypoplasia being the most common. Vaginal aplasia was present in 8 of the 9 cats in one study (Holt and Gibbs, 1992) and the uterine horns were found to enter the dorsal aspect of the bladder in the majority of cases.

Ectopic ureters

Ectopic ureters are the result of dysembryogenesis of the metanephric duct system. This congenital anomaly can be of one or both ureters and is typically associated with the ureteral orifice being located distal to the bladder neck. This can be in the urethra, vagina, uterus or vestibule in female dogs or anywhere along the urethra in male dogs. Intravesicular ectopic ureters are typically documented as ureteral openings within the urinary bladder proximal to the trigone, but enter in an abnormal location or are an abnormal shape. This finding can be associated with little clinical relevance but in one study it was found, at times, to be associated with some degree of hydronephrosis (North et al., 2010).

Extravesicular ectopic ureters are most commonly found in female cats, with a female:male ratio of 20:1; 43% of reported cases were seen in females in one series (Holt and Gibbs, 1992). Although ectopic ureters have been reported in both pure and mixed breed dogs, it seems to occur with greater frequency in the Labrador and Golden Retriever, Siberian Husky, terrier breeds, Newfoundland and Poodle (miniature and toy).

Intramural ectopic ureters enter the bladder neck in the normal position, fail to open into the bladder lumen, tunnel beyond the normal ureteral orifice position within the submucosa and exit distally at variable locations within the urogenital tract. Over 99% of ectopic ureters are considered intramural, with 100% of 175 ectopic ureters in one study found to be intramural (Holt, 1995). In another study, 32% of dogs had multiple openings of the intramural ureter (Cannizzo et al., 2003) so care should be taken to investigate the entire lower urinary tract. Extramural ectopic ureters do not tunnel within the normal ureteral trajectory but bypass the bladder and trigone and enter the urogenital tract distally (Figure 30.2). This is rarely reported in dogs and is more commonly seen in cats.

Male dogs with ectopic ureters may present for evaluation of severe 'megaureter' and hydronephrosis (see Figure 30.8). In the author's [AB] practice this has been seen most commonly in young to middle-aged Labrador Retrievers. These ectopic ureters are typically associated with a very narrow intramural tunnel. This has also been seen in the author's [AB] practice in a small number of female dogs. Ureteral orifice stenosis associated with ectopic ureters in young male dogs should be a differential diagnosis for megaureter to the level of the urinary bladder. This condition is often not associated with urinary incontinence. Laser ablation (see below) can be an effective therapy for both ectopic ureters and ureteral stenosis.

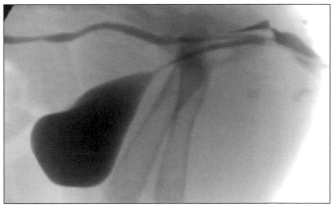

30.2 Fluoroscopic image of a female dog taken during a retrograde vaginovestibulogram showing an extramural ectopic ureter.
(Courtesy of Dr Carrie Palm and Dr Bill Culp)

In >90% of cases ureteral ectopia is associated with multiple anomalies of the urinary tract, including urinary tract infections (64–85%), renal agenesis (4.8%), hydroureter (50%), hydronephrosis (50%), short urethra, intrapelvic bladder (20–40%), hypoplastic bladder (16%) and persistent paramesonephric remnants/vaginal septum or dual vagina (93%).

The history of urinary incontinence can usually be traced to the time of weaning, although male dogs often present later in life (median 3 years old). Male dogs tend to have a very narrow ureteral orifice with a very thick intramural tunnel. This results in a ureteral outflow tract obstruction and is most commonly (85% of cases) associated with moderate to severe hydroureter and hydronephrosis. At least half of the male dogs with ectopic ureters seen at the author's [AB] practice are not incontinent. The reason the ectopic ureters are initially diagnosed is due to the severe hydronephrosis and hydroureter seen on abdominal ultrasonography. In the author's [AB] experience, this condition is typically seen in Labrador Retrievers although it has also been reported in a small group of Entlebucher dogs (North et al., 2010).

USMI and other voiding dysfunctions have been reported in 89% of female dogs with concurrent ectopic ureters evaluated by urodynamic studies (Lane et al., 1995). Dogs that remained incontinent following surgical correction of ureteral ectopia had a significantly lower maximal urethral pressure (MUP) and maximal urethral closure pressure (MUCP) preoperatively compared with those dogs that were continent postoperatively. It has been suggested that dogs with a MUCP <19 cmH$_2$O have an increased risk of postoperative incontinence (Lane et al., 1995). Care needs to be taken in interpretation of the clinical utility of urethral pressure profiles, as dogs with abnormal profiles can still ultimately become continent, whilst those with more normal profiles can remain incontinent. Furthermore, the urethral pressure profiles should be standardized for anaesthetic drugs and depth when making comparisons between various studies. In male dogs, it has been hypothesized that the longer functional urethral length may help to maintain continence, regardless of the displaced ureteral orifice, and is likely to be the reason male dogs with ureteral ectopia are often continent at the time of diagnosis, or go undiagnosed.

Urinary bladder dysfunction

Involuntary contractions of the bladder detrusor muscle when it contains only a small volume of urine results in the condition characterized as 'overactive bladder (OAB) syndrome'. In dogs, the terms detrusor hyperactivity or instability are also used, depending on the origin of the contraction. Evidence of OAB syndrome can be seen on urodynamic studies by performing a cystometrogram.

One study found that >30% of incontinent dogs had poor bladder storage function, over half of which also had poor urethral closure pressure. This may be associated with increased collagen deposition in the bladder in neutered female dogs. In addition, in juvenile dogs and cats with congenital incontinence (for example, ectopic ureters, hypoplastic bladder, hypoplastic urethra, USMI), bladder storage dysfunction associated with low compliance is also suspected based on urodynamic studies. When dogs are suspected of having OAB syndrome as well as USMI, they are often referred to as having 'mixed urinary incontinence'.

Miscellaneous causes

Several other less common causes of incontinence occur in dogs and cats. Prostatic disease has been hypothesized to interfere with the normal functioning of the urethral sphincter mechanism. For further information on the diagnostic approach to urinary incontinence in entire male dogs, see Chapter 9. Studies in dogs following total prostatectomy for prostatic disease revealed postoperative urinary incontinence in the majority of cases, whilst continence was maintained following the procedure in dogs without pre-existing prostatic disease.

Detrusor–urethral dyssynergia (DUD) is a complex condition that is rarely reported in veterinary patients, but is likely to be underestimated. This condition is considered a functional anomaly where contraction of the detrusor muscle and relaxation of the urethral sphincter are uncoordinated, resulting in inappropriate micturition, typically leading to urinary retention and possibly overflow incontinence.

Mass lesions associated with inflammatory or neoplastic disease can be occasional causes of urinary incontinence in dogs and this is presumably due to interference with the normal functioning of the urethral sphincter mechanism. Dogs presenting with transitional cell carcinoma of the bladder or urethral wall can also be incontinent. It is unclear whether this is overflow incontinence secondary to partial urethral obstruction or neurogenic incontinence from the inflammation associated with the tumour.

Diagnostic approach to urinary incontinence

The diagnostic approach to evaluating a dog or cat with urinary incontinence should involve a thorough history, physical examination, continence scoring, a minimum database including urinalysis and urine culture, and various diagnostic imaging studies (e.g. abdominal radiography, ultrasonography of the urinary tract). Cystoscopy may also be clinically indicated (see Chapter 8). The diagnostic approach to the incontinent patient is detailed in Chapter 9.

Continence scoring

A continence score should be obtained (Figure 30.3). The authors use a scoring system which uses a 10 point scale, where:

1 Animal does not posture to urinate and there is constant dribbling of urine and leaking at rest and at play.
2.5 Animal has the ability to produce a stream of urine but there is a large volume of leakage between urinations and at rest.
5 Animal has the ability to produce a good stream and void a large volume of urine but there is a small amount of dribbling seen between urinations and a large volume of leakage at rest.
7.5 Animal only leaks urine when at rest and not between urinations.
9 Animal leaks urine 1–2 times per week (not daily) and evidence of urine leaking found only on the hair around the vulva or penis.
10 Animal shows no urine leaking at all.

Continence evaluation sheet

Age of spay:...

Age when dog acquired:...

Is urine? (circle one):

    Bloody: Y   N   (if Y: sometimes   always   infrequent)

    Odorous: Y   N   (if Y: sometimes   always   infrequent)

Straining to urinate: Y N   Passes full stream of urine: Y N   Postures to urinate frequently: Y N

Duration of signs:..

Onset of clinical signs (acute *versus* chronic):...

Progression of signs *versus* static:...

Continence score: (0 always leaks – 10 never leaks):

1...2.5...5.0..7.5...................................10

1.0:   always leaks, never able to produce a puddle of urine

2.5:   can posture and urinate but leaks more volume than produces during urination

5.0:   postures and urinates normally but leaks when laying down and when walking around

7.5:   only leaks when laying down and does not leak when walking around

9.0:   only leaks a few times a week

10.0: never leaks urine

Urinary tract infections (Y/N):..

Treatments/responses:...

Anatomic abnormalities (vulva, vagina):..

Concurrent medical conditions:...

Previous diagnostics performed (results):...

Previous medical therapy and doses (response: partial/none):...

....

Additional comments:..

....

30.3   Continence evaluation sheet.

Treatment strategies for urinary incontinence

Pharmacological management

A formulary for the pharmacological management of the various forms of urinary incontinence is given in Figure 30.4. A large proportion (approaching 90%) of dogs with USMI respond to medical management, and many dogs with ureteral ectopia have concurrent USMI that requires medical intervention following successful relocation of the ureterovesicular junction into the urinary bladder.

Alpha adrenergic agonists

The most frequently used class of drugs in dogs are the alpha adrenergic agonists (sympathomimetics) including phenylpropanolamine and pseudoephedrine. These drugs increase contraction of the smooth muscle of mainly the bladder neck and proximal urethra. Urodynamic studies have shown that phenylpropanolamine increases MUP and MUCP. Various reports have demonstrated continence rates in incontinent female dogs ranging between 75 and 90% after phenylpropanolamine therapy (Richter and Ling, 1985; White and Pomeroy, 1989; Bacon *et al.*, 2002; Scott *et al.*, 2002; Noël *et al.*, 2010). Some dogs are documented to become less responsive to phenylpropanolamine with prolonged administration, suggesting desensitization of the alpha adrenoceptors over time. Possible side effects of phenylpropanolamine include anxiety, restlessness, tachycardia and hypertension, all of which are typically minor in otherwise healthy dogs. Response in male dogs to phenylpropanolamine for USMI treatment appears to be less predictable. In one study, only about a third of male dogs were continent after treatment with phenylpropanolamine and in another smaller study over 85% were responsive (Aaron *et al.*, 1996; Power *et al.*, 1998). Little information exists on the effectiveness of phenylpropanolamine in feline USMI, but it is typically considered minimally effective. Ephedrine and pseudoephedrine are mixed-acting sympathomimetic drugs and have lower efficacy, and potentially more side effects, than phenylpropanolamine. Ephedrine was shown to have a complete response in 74% of female dogs and some improvement in most of the other dogs (Arnold *et al.*, 1989a).

Drug class	Dosage	Indications	Contraindications	Side effects
Alpha adrenergic agonists				
Phenylpropanolamine	1.0–1.5 mg/kg orally q8–12h	USMI in female dogs ± male dogs ± cats	Renal insufficiency; hypertension; allergic reaction to the drug; glaucoma; enlarged prostate; hyperthyroidism; diabetes mellitus; heart disease; pregnancy or breeding	Anxiety; restlessness; loss of appetite; weakness; hypertension; seizures; tachycardia; difficulty urinating
Ephedrine	Dogs: 1.2 mg/kg orally q8–12h Cats: 2–4 mg/kg orally q8–12h			
Pseudoephedrine	Dogs <25 kg: 15 mg/dog orally q8h Dogs >25 kg: 30 mg/dog orally q8h			
Oestrogen analogues				
Diethylstilbestrol	0.1–0.3 mg/kg/day (up to 1 mg/dog) orally for 7–10 days then 1 mg/dog/week	Oestrogen-responsive incontinence	Pregnancy; history of polyuria and polydipsia	Vomiting; polydipsia; polyuria; swollen vulva; oestrus; lethargy; diarrhoea; pyometra; feminization Rare: blood dyscrasia with an ultimate fatal aplastic anaemia
Estriol	1–2 mg once daily and then titrate to lowest effective dose daily or every 2–3 days			
Stilbestrol	0.04–0.06 mg/dog orally q24h for 7 days, reduced weekly to 0.01–0.02 mg/dog/day			
Testosterone analogues				
Methyltestosterone	0.5 mg/kg orally q24h	Male dogs with suspected USMI	Entire; history of prostatic neoplasia; aggressive behaviour	
Testosterone propionate	2.2 mg/kg i.m. every 2–3 days			
Testosterone cypionate	2.2 mg/kg i.m. every 30–60 days			
Gonadotrophin-releasing hormone (GnRH) analogues				
Leuprolide acetate	11.25 mg i.m. every 3 months[a]	USMI in spayed female dogs	Entire; pregnant; lactating	Pain at injection site; dyspnoea; lethargy; tachyphylaxis
Antimuscarinic and spasmalytic agents				
Oxybutynin (antispasmodic of detrusor muscle and smooth muscle of the small and large bowel)	Dogs: 0.2 mg/kg orally q8–12h with 1.25–3.75 mg (total dose) orally q8–12h Cats: 0.5–1.25 mg (total dose) orally q8–12h	Detrusor hyperreflexia; overactive bladder	Gastrointestinal obstruction; urine retention; intestinal atony; glaucoma; cardiac disease; hyperthyroidism; prostatic disease; colitis; obstructive uropathy	Diarrhoea; constipation; urinary retention; hypersalivation; sedation; anorexia; tachycardia; dry eyes/mouth; weakness; mydriasis
Alpha-1 adrenergic blockers				
Tamsulosin	Dogs: 0.1–0.2 mg/10 kg/day orally	Urethral relaxation; DUD	Hypotension; urethral incontinence; renal insufficiency; *MDR1* mutation	Hypotension; syncope; lethargy; dizziness; gastrointestinal distress
Prazosin	Dogs: 1 mg/15 kg orally q12h Cats: 0.25 mg orally q12h			
Alpha-1 and -2 adrenergic blockers				
Phenoxybenzamine	0.25 mg/kg orally q12–24h	Urethral relaxation; DUD	Hypotension; urethral incontinence; renal insufficiency; glaucoma	Hypotension; miosis; increased intraocular pressure; nasal congestion; gastrointestinal upset; weakness
Tricyclic antidepressants				
Imipramine	5–15 mg (total dose) orally q12h	USMI	Seizure disorders	Seizures; sedation; dry mouth; constipation
Other drugs				
Diazepam	0.2–0.5 mg/kg orally q8h	DUD	Use of other benzodiazepines; liver disease	Sedation
Dantrolene	1–5 mg/kg orally q8–12h	DUD	Can cause hepatotoxicity; use with caution in patients with cardiac dysfunction; monitor body temperature and liver chemistry	Weakness; sedation; dizziness; headache; gastrointestinal upset
Gabapentin	5–10 mg/kg orally q12h to 10–20 mg/kg orally q8h	DUD; overactive bladder	Avoid human oral solution as it contains xylitol; lower dosage in renal insufficiency; withdrawal can be seen if abruptly discontinued	Sedation; ataxia

30.4 Pharmacological treatment of incontinence. [a] This is an extrapolated dose from the literature but there are no reported acceptable doses available for dogs and cats to date. DUD = detrusor–urethral dyssynergia; USMI = urethral sphincter mechanism incompetence.

Oestrogen therapy

Oestrogen therapy is also commonly administered to dogs for the treatment of USMI due to the association between neutering, loss of endogenous oestrogen production and the development of USMI. Exogenous oestrogen therapy has few reported side effects, including pyometra, bone marrow suppression, vulvar swelling, metrorrhagia and attractiveness of males. Anecdotally, the longer acting formulation, diethylstilbestrol, has been reported to cause a dose-dependent potential for bone marrow suppression, although this is not something that has been seen to date in the author's [AB] practice at dosages used to treat USMI. Oestrogens are contraindicated in entire female patients with congenital USMI, which is the case for most female cats and some young female dogs, as it can result in negative feedback on the pituitary axis. Oestrogens are thought to upregulate both the expression and sensitivity of alpha adrenoceptors, creating a synergistic effect and potentially allowing dose reductions of both drugs over time. Newer oestrogen analogues are available that are shorter acting and equally effective (e.g. oral estriol).

Several oestrogen preparations are available, including diethylstilbestrol, stilbestrol and estriol. Reports in the literature on the use of oestrogen therapy suggest ranges in the response, which are typically between 60 and 90%. The largest study showed a 61% continence rate at 42 days post-treatment with a further 22% showing improvement (Mandigers and Nell, 2001). No dog in the study had evidence of bone marrow suppression.

Overall, it is considered that alpha adrenergic agonists are more effective for the treatment of USMI in female dogs compared with oestrogen therapy. Male dogs generally have a poor response to treatment with oestrogen, with one study showing that none of the eight dogs treated was continent following therapy (Aaron et al., 1996). The use of testosterone in neutered male dogs has also been reported with typically poor results, although the use of methyltestosterone in a small group of male dogs has been used with some success in the author's [AB] practice. Little information is available regarding the use of oestrogens in cats, although their use has been discouraged.

Gonadotrophin-releasing hormone analogues

GnRH analogues (e.g. leuprolide acetate) have been reported for the treatment of USMI in neutered female dogs. The rapid rise in plasma FSH and LH that occurs after neutering has been hypothesized to be involved in the pathogenesis of USMI in female dogs (Reichler et al., 2006ab); however, treatment with leuprolide acetate did not increase the MUCP on urethral pressure profilometry, regardless of the decrease in FSH and LH levels following therapy. Nonetheless, a clinical response to therapy has been noted with one study reporting a 63% complete continence rate with its use (Reichler et al., 2006ab). In the absence of evidence of a direct effect of GnRH on urethral closure pressure, the authors hypothesize that the effect may be mediated through an increased bladder storage volume, as shown by cystometric studies.

Tricyclic antidepressants

Tricyclic antidepressants, such as imipramine, have been used for the treatment of USMI, OAB and mixed urinary incontinence with limited success. Imipramine has antimuscarinic and sympathomimetic effects, as well as sedative properties (Acierno and Labato, 2006). This can increase concentrations of serotonin and noradrenaline (norepinephrine) at the synaptic level in the central nervous system. This medication facilitates urine storage by decreasing bladder contractility and increasing outlet resistance through alpha adrenergic effects on the bladder neck and an antispasmodic effect on the detrusor muscle.

Detrusor–urethral dyssynergia

Medical management for DUD can be challenging as the diagnosis is difficult to confirm and the underlying cause is often unknown. DUD is often associated with urine retention. Patients with DUD most often present for stranguria (a poor 'water pick' type of urine stream). If incontinence occurs at rest, in the presence of a large, overdistended bladder, this is more consistent with overflow incontinence, which can be associated with DUD. If DUD is suspected then sympathetic or somatic dyssynergia may be present. In these cases, specific drug therapy to reduce smooth muscle tone (e.g. prazosin, tamsulosin, phenoxybenzamine) or striated muscle external sphincter pressure (dantrolene, diazepam) could be administered to the patient.

The author [AB] has also had some anecdotal success using tramadol and gabapentin for the treatment of DUD. This success was likely related to the effect on any component of detrusor overactivity associated with DUD. The modulation of bladder receptor and/or spinal cord neuronal activity is a possible mechanism that helps to control involuntary detrusor contractions. Gabapentin acts on the afferent pathways and may help to improve clinical signs if the condition is neurogenic in origin. If it is not possible to clinically distinguish which part of the sphincter mechanism is most affected, it is usually recommended to initiate a therapeutic trial with a sympatholytic drug in the first instance. An alpha adrenergic agonist (e.g. phenylpropanolamine) should never be used in cases where stranguria and urine retention are present. In addition, some veterinary surgeons (veterinarians) administer bethanecol (a parasympathomimetic) to patients with DUD, which in the author's [AB] experience often exacerbates the condition and should not be used unless the urethral outflow obstruction is resolved. Overall, the literature would suggest a poor prognosis for medical success with pharmacological management, but the author [AB] has seen dramatic improvements with tailored medical combinations.

In the authors' experience, when pharmacological therapy fails, the alternative options are:

- To consider temporarily stenting various parts of the intrapelvic and then penile urethra with a temporary catheter
- Endoscopic botulinum-A toxin injections (see below) into the muscle of the urethra
- Self-expanding metallic stent placement if the location can be determined
- For intractable urethral obstructions due to DUD, the author [AB] will often place a temporary cystostomy tube while various medications are tried.

Overactive bladder

Detrusor hyperactivity or OAB is associated with excessive, spastic elimination, typically associated with a good stream of urine but significant urgency to urinate. Underlying causes for cystitis should be ruled out first (e.g. bacterial cystitis, urolithiasis, cystic neoplasia). If incontinence occurs with an empty bladder, it is typically due to abnormal detrusor contractions during the storage phase.

For OAB, anticholinergic drugs such as oxybutynin are most commonly used. This can be combined with alpha adrenergic agonists if needed. Owners should be aware of the potential for gastrointestinal upset with the administration of anticholinergic medications. In addition, the use of medications to control OAB, such as gabapentin, have been tried with moderate anecdotal success.

Endoscopic-assisted management
Urethral sphincter mechanism incompetence

Various injectable bulking agents have been used in women for more than 80 years for the treatment of stress incontinence (similar to USMI in dogs) and over the past 15 years this technique has been adapted for use in veterinary medicine. This is typically reserved for dogs that have failed medical management for USMI or are intolerant of the side effects associated with the drugs used to treat USMI. The reason for using bulking agents is to decrease the diameter of the internal urethral wall in such a way that allows coaptation of the urethral mucosa and narrowing of the lumen, creating increased resistance to urine outflow. These agents also increase stretch in the urethral muscle fibres, which may allow the muscle to close more effectively. The success of this procedure is often user dependent, so appropriate training is needed.

Various agents have been used, including bovine cross-linked collagen, polytetrafluoroethylene paste, calcium hydroxylapetite, polydimethylsiloxane (PDMS-Macroplastique®), autologous fat and carbon-coated zirconium beads (Durasphere®). At this time only calcium hydroxylapetite (Coaptite®), carbon-coated beads (Durasphere), polydimethylsiloxane (PDMS-Macroplastique®) and a newly available cross-linked bovine collagen material (ReGain™) are commercially available. Glutaraldehyde cross-linked bovine collagen (Contigen®) was the most commonly used bulking agent in dogs and humans, but has since been taken off the market for the treatment of USMI in the United States.

Injections are performed using cystoscopic guidance (Figure 30.5). Routine cystoscopy is performed to exclude other anatomical anomalies such as ectopic ureters, persistent paramesonephric remnants, ureteral troughs and a short/wide urethra. Once the ureteral openings are identified in their normal anatomical position, the operator identifies the proper location to inject the bulking agent; typically approximately 2–3 cm caudal to the trigone at a point where the normal urethral lumen has maximal coaptation and is the most narrow. The bulking agent is provided in a syringe and a long, flexible injection needle is required that fits easily through the working channel of the rigid cystoscope.

Once the ideal location within the urethra is identified, the needle is exteriorized from the proximal tip of the cystoscope. It is very important to stay parallel to the urethral lumen and this requires utilizing the 30 degree cystoscope to align each bleb appropriately. Once the needle is nearly parallel with the mucosal lumen, the tip is gently pierced through the urethral mucosa, remaining fairly superficial so that the muscularis is not entered and the material is only injected in the submucosa. If the material is injected too deep, then the blebs will not form towards the lumen of the urethra, but instead will be outside the lumen in the muscle or periurethral tissue. This will then not contribute to any coaptation. Once the bevel of the needle is inserted in the tissue, the cystoscope should remain very stable and an assistant can inject the material in 0.1 ml

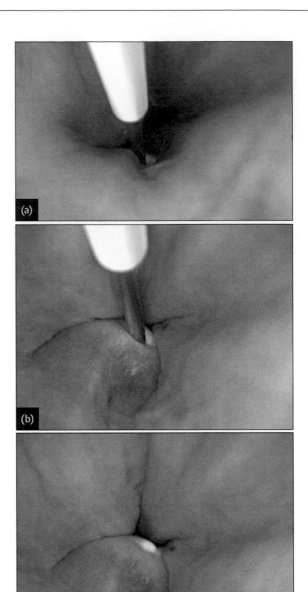

30.5 Endoscopic images taken during the injection of bulking agents in a female dog with USMI in dorsal recumbency. (a) The injection needle is passed through the working channel of the endoscope and pierces the urethral mucosa. (b) Infusion of the bulking material into the submucosal layer, creating a bleb. (c) After the bleb is formed, the needle is removed and the urethral lumen begins to coaptate.

increments until an appropriate sized bleb is seen. It is recommended that 3–4 blebs are made at the 2, 6 and 10 (or 3, 6, 9 and 12) o'clock position. The goal is to have all of the blebs coaptate in the lumen of the urethra so that it appears almost closed, but can be expressed. It is the author's [AB] impression that injecting two rows of blebs improves the continence rate and duration of effect, and does not increase the complication rate. It is not unusual for a small amount of bleeding to occur after removing the needle, but this typically resolves within a few minutes. After delivering each bleb, the author [AB] leaves the needle in place without any further injection of material for 10–15 seconds to allow a blood clot to form prior to removing the needle.

The main complication seen with bulking agent injections is temporary urethral outflow tract obstruction, which is rare and short-lived. This will resolve within 24 hours of urethral catheterization if absolutely needed. A bulking agent should never be injected in the face of an active urinary tract infection; therefore, an aerobic bacterial urine culture should be performed prior to the procedure. If results are positive, treatment with appropriate antimicrobials for at least 3 days prior to the procedure is warranted. The authors also typically treat the patient with antimicrobials for 3 days following the procedure and analgesia is administered on an as needed basis (similar to that used for routine cystoscopy). Patients can be discharged the same day as the procedure. Response rates with bulking agents are variable and range from 3 months to longer than 3 years, depending on the material used (Arnold *et al.*, 1996; Barth *et al.*, 2005; Bartges and Callens, 2011; Byron *et al.*, 2011).

Ectopic ureters

Cystoscopic-guided laser ablation for ectopic ureters (CLA-EU) provides a minimally invasive alternative to surgery in both male and female dogs with intramural ectopic ureters. This procedure enables simultaneous diagnosis and therapeutic intervention, and may also avoid some of the complications associated with open surgical techniques (see below). Utilizing the combination of cystoscopy and fluoroscopy, each ureteral orifice can be directly visualized, other urinary anomalies can be assessed (vaginal septal remnants, hypoplastic bladder, intrapelvic bladder, hydroureter and hydronephrosis) and the differentiation of intramural *versus* extramural tunnelling can be made. Once the diagnosis of an intramural ectopic ureter is confirmed with cystoscopy and fluoroscopy, the laser can be used to ablate the medial ectopic ureteral wall and reposition the opening cranial to the bladder trigone.

Only an experienced endoscopist, comfortable using a diode or Holmium:YAG (yttrium, aluminium, garnet) laser and performing cystoscopy, should attempt this procedure (Figure 30.6). The most substantial risk is not appreciating an extramural ureter and accidentally cutting it with the laser. This is considered a contraindication to the laser procedure, making concurrent fluoroscopy recommended (Figure 30.7). Other risks include urethral perforation during cystoscopy and development of a proliferative reaction along the laser tract (known as a 'delayed laser reaction'). Both of these complications are very rare in the authors' experience (seen in <3% of cases). This is typically an outpatient procedure.

In a study evaluating 30 female dogs (48 ectopic ureters) following CLA-EU, 47% were completely continent at a median follow-up of 2.7 years (Berent *et al.*, 2012). The addition of medical management (approximately 20% response), transurethral bulking agent injections (approximately 30% response) and the placement of a hydraulic occluder (approximately 80–90% response) improved the overall urinary continence rate to 77%. Another study (Curraro *et al.*, 2013) retrospectively reported an additional 18 female cases using a similar technique and similar results were obtained. The procedure has also been reported in four male dogs, all of which were continent following laser ablation (Berent *et al.*, 2008); since this time more than 20 dogs have been treated and the continence rate is approximately 85%. Nearly 85–90% of male dogs have evidence of hydroureter and/or hydronephrosis on screening ultrasonography and not all male dogs are incontinent, despite the presence of ectopic ureters. This ureteral and renal pelvis dilatation is associated with ureteral orifice stenosis (Figure 30.8); the ureteral opening is typically ectopic.

Dogs with a history of ectopic ureters should be routinely monitored throughout their lives as they are at an increased risk for the development of recurrent urinary tract infections (Berent *et al.*, 2012), of which haematuria and pyuria might be subtle, or the only sign may be increased urinary incontinence that may be responsive to antimicrobial therapy. Furthermore, the urinary tract infection may be associated with an increased urine odour and/or pollakiuria. Positive urine cultures were identified in >80% of female dogs prior to CLA and 35% post-CLA. Antimicrobial therapy should be implemented if clinically indicated.

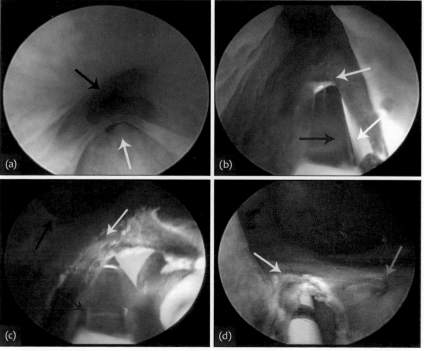

30.6 Endoscopic images of a female dog taken during cystoscopic-guided laser ablation of a right intramural ectopic ureter. The dog is in dorsal recumbency. (a) Urethral lumen (black arrow) showing the intramural ectopic ureteral opening in the mid-urethra (yellow arrow). (b) A urethral catheter (white arrow) and a laser fibre (red arrow) have been inserted into the lumen of the ectopic ureter (yellow arrow) prior to laser ablation. (c) Laser ablation being performed. The ureteral tissue (yellow arrow) is being cut with the laser (red arrow) towards the urethral lumen and trigone (black arrow). (d) The trigone of the bladder following laser ablation showing the new ureteral opening (yellow arrow) and the left normal ureteral opening (blue arrow).

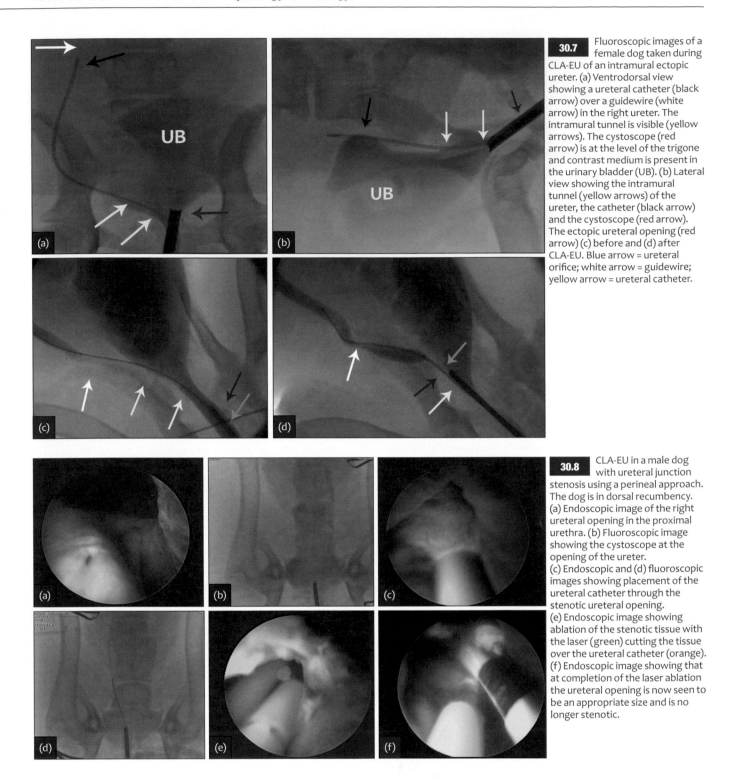

30.7 Fluoroscopic images of a female dog taken during CLA-EU of an intramural ectopic ureter. (a) Ventrodorsal view showing a ureteral catheter (black arrow) over a guidewire (white arrow) in the right ureter. The intramural tunnel is visible (yellow arrows). The cystoscope (red arrow) is at the level of the trigone and contrast medium is present in the urinary bladder (UB). (b) Lateral view showing the intramural tunnel (yellow arrows) of the ureter, the catheter (black arrow) and the cystoscope (red arrow). The ectopic ureteral opening (red arrow) (c) before and (d) after CLA-EU. Blue arrow = ureteral orifice; white arrow = guidewire; yellow arrow = ureteral catheter.

30.8 CLA-EU in a male dog with ureteral junction stenosis using a perineal approach. The dog is in dorsal recumbency. (a) Endoscopic image of the right ureteral opening in the proximal urethra. (b) Fluoroscopic image showing the cystoscope at the opening of the ureter. (c) Endoscopic and (d) fluoroscopic images showing placement of the ureteral catheter through the stenotic ureteral opening. (e) Endoscopic image showing ablation of the stenotic tissue with the laser (green) cutting the tissue over the ureteral catheter (orange). (f) Endoscopic image showing that at completion of the laser ablation the ureteral opening is now seen to be an appropriate size and is no longer stenotic.

Vestibulovaginal remnants

Dogs affected by vestibulovaginal remnants, including persistent paramesonephric remnant (PPMR), vaginal septum and dual vaginas, are suggested to display various signs such as natural breeding difficulties, persistent urinary incontinence, vaginal pooling of urine, chronic recurrent urinary tract infections, dysuria, vaginitis, dystocia and vulvar dermatitis. In a recent study (Burdick *et al.*, 2013), endoscopic laser ablation of vestibulovaginal septal remnants (ELA-VR) was shown to improve continence scores and decrease urinary tract infections in dogs; however, the small number of dogs without multiple concurrent malformations precluded the significance of resolving these lesions. As the current implications of these malformations remain unknown, having a non-invasive and effective treatment option such as endoscopic-guided laser ablation is ideal when the alternative is surgical vaginectomy.

The procedure is undertaken using a cystoscope and either a diode or Holmium:YAG laser (Figure 30.9). Each malformation is classified as either a PPMR (<1 cm), vaginal septum (>1 cm) or dual vagina (entire vagina to the cervix). The malformation is ablated using the laser from the caudal aspect to the most cranial aspect, until the vagina is one open tube. This is also an outpatient procedure. In 30 dogs in which this procedure was performed and the patients were re-evaluated 6 weeks later, no dog had reformation of their vestibulovaginal septal remnant (Burdick *et al.*, 2013).

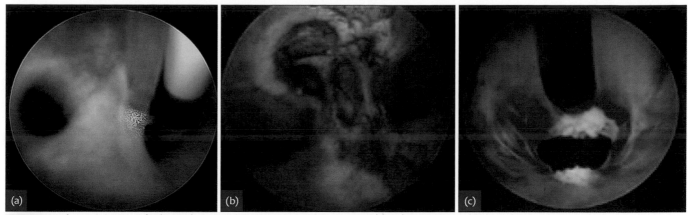

30.9 Endoscopic images of a dog with a persistent paramesonephric remnant (PPMR) during laser ablation of the remnant. The dog is in dorsal recumbency. (a) Laser fibre at the band of tissue with a catheter is one compartment of the vagina. (b) Charring of the tissue during laser ablation. (c) An open vaginal opening following laser ablation.

Detrusor–urethral dyssynergia and overactive bladder

Idiopathic DUD is a rare (but may be underdiagnosed) condition, commonly seen in middle-aged, large-breed male dogs (see above). It is typically a diagnosis by exclusion (see Chapter 9). In one retrospective study the prognosis was considered grave as only 1 of the 22 dogs responded to medical management and the others were euthanased (Diaz Espineira *et al.*, 1998). A more recent study described using self-expanding metallic urethral stents in dogs with DUD with moderate success in a small number of dogs (Hill *et al.*, 2014) (Figure 30.10).

OAB, also rarely diagnosed in dogs, is seen more commonly in young, large-breed dogs and can be associated with behavioural problems. It can be managed medically with drugs such as oxybutynin, but when refractory can be incredibly frustrating for the owner. In human medicine, DUD is also considered very rare, but OAB is quite common. In a recent report, botulinum-A toxin was found to be successful as a therapy for various voiding disorders such as DUD and OAB (Leippold *et al.*, 2003). Botulinum toxin is produced by *Clostridium botulinum* and is a neurotoxin that acts as a presynaptic neuromuscular blocking agent, resulting in muscle weakness for up to several months when injected intramuscularly. In the human literature, external urethral sphincter pressure, voiding pressure and post-void residual volume was

decreased after injection into the external urethral sphincter, lasting 2–9 months (Leippold *et al.*, 2003). For humans with OAB, injections of botulinum-A toxin into the detrusor muscle for relaxation has been associated with excellent results, improving incontinence. This has been performed for DUD in the author's [AB] practice in one dog when medical management failed. The botulinum-A toxin was injected intramuscularly into the urethra under cystoscopic guidance. This was successful for approximately 8 weeks until the effect subsided.

Surgical management
Urethral sphincter mechanism incompetence

Surgical treatment of USMI in dogs and cats is indicated when medical treatment has failed and a variety of techniques have been described for achieving continence is these cases. The principal aims of surgical procedures that use native tissues to treat USMI are either to relocate the bladder neck and proximal urethra into the abdomen to expose them to increases in intra-abdominal pressure or to increase the resistance to urine outflow in the urethra by direct pressure or constriction. The literature would suggest that male dogs do not respond as well as females to these surgical approaches to USMI. Hydraulic occluders (see Figure 30.11), a device that provides a potentially dynamic and titratable degree of compression to the mid-urethra of female dogs and the proximal or mid-urethra in male dogs, have been introduced in recent years. Early evidence suggests that they are well tolerated and provide a superior degree of continence control compared with other standard surgical approaches, can be used in both dogs and cats, but may be associated with severe complications (Currao *et al.*, 2013; Reeves *et al.*, 2013; Wilson *et al.*, 2015). However, there are currently no studies that have critically compared outcomes and complication rates of implantable occlusion devices and the techniques that use native tissues only.

Techniques for female dogs:
Colposuspension: The therapeutic hypothesis behind colposuspension is that by increasing pressure transmission to the proximal urethra and bladder neck, continence will be re-established. This is achieved by cranial traction on the bladder to re-establish it in an intra-abdominal position. The bladder is anchored in this new location by placing mattress sutures through the prepubic tendon and subsequently through the lateral aspect of the muscular

30.10 Fluroroscopic image of a urethral stent in the proximal urethra of a male dog that has DUD.

wall of the vagina. Initial studies reporting the results of colposuspension were encouraging. In a large cohort of 150 dogs, resolution of incontinence was seen in 53% of cases and a further 37% were significantly improved long-term (Holt, 1990b). However, the durability of the effect has been contradicted by studies showing that initial improvements are not sustained in many animals, with only 14% being completely continent 1 year after surgery without medication (Rawlings *et al.*, 2001). However, when colposuspension and medical management were combined, 81% of dogs were considered either completely continent or greatly improved (Rawlings *et al.*, 2001). Complications of colposuspension are uncommon with dysuria occurring in 6% of cases in one study (Holt, 1990b).

Urethropexy and cystourethropexy: Urethropexy aims to create a similar effect to colposuspension by moving the bladder and urethra cranially into an intra-abdominal position but does so by placement of sutures directly into the urethral wall (rather than creating a vaginal sling around the urethra as is the case with colposuspension). It has been suggested that as well as repositioning the bladder and urethra, urethropexy might also work by directly increasing urethral resistance at the level where the sutures are applied. In one study, an appreciable 'kink' was consistently seen on postoperative retrograde vaginourethrograms and a palpable increase in pressure during postoperative passage of a urethral catheter in many dogs was appreciated (Martinoli *et al.*, 2014). In a study of 10 female dogs treated by cystourethropexy, only two were continent postoperatively with surgery alone, and four were continent at 3–12 months postoperatively when treated with surgery and medical management (Massat *et al.*, 1993). In a subsequent report of a cohort of 100 dogs undergoing urethropexy, continence was restored in 56% of patients postoperatively and 83% were deemed to be improved by surgery for a mean of 22 months (White, 2001). However, similarly to colposuspension, the effect may not be durable in a proportion of dogs with only 48% being described as having an 'excellent' outcome >3 years postoperatively. Complications reported with these techniques are related to excessive constriction of urinary outflow. In one study, 21% of dogs had postoperative complications consisting of increased frequency of micturition in 14% of dogs, dysuria in 6% of cases and anuria in 3% of cases (White, 2001). In the three dogs that became anuric postoperatively, a second procedure was performed to release the overly tight sutures and allow urination to resume.

Colposuspension in combination with urethropexy: Recently, a report of a combined approach in female dogs with USMI involving placement of both urethropexy and colposuspension sutures has been described (Martinoli *et al.*, 2014). The authors suggest that this technique might provide improvement in results by repositioning the bladder and proximal urethra within the abdominal cavity, as well as exerting a constrictive effect on the proximal urethra to increase urethral resistance. Of the 30 dogs undergoing the procedure, 70% were judged to be completely continent with a further 26% experiencing only occasional incontinence. The effect appeared to be more durable compared with reports of either technique performed in isolation, with the results reported at a median follow-up time of 39.5 months.

Urethral sling procedures: Several procedures that involve the creation of a sling around the proximal to mid-urethra without necessarily changing the position of the bladder or urethra have been reported in small numbers of dogs, but have not gained widespread use. One technique involves creation of a sling from two rectangular seromuscular pedicle flaps that are elevated from the ventral bladder trigone area and passed around the bladder neck and sutured together dorsally. This technique was not very effective. Another modification of the sling technique used a polyester ribbon passed through the obturator foramina, around the urethra and secured ventral to the pelvis with a titanium clip. Postoperative stranguria was seen in 23% of cases and two dogs developed fistulation associated with the ribbon 2 and 3 years postoperatively (Nickel *et al.*, 1998). Continence was achieved in 65% of cases, with or without concurrent medication. A more promising, less invasive, approach was reported in seven dogs and consists of a modification of a technique used in women for stress incontinence (Claeys *et al.*, 2010). Performed through a median episiotomy incision, the authors used polypropylene tape to create a urethral sling, which was reported to restore continence to six of the seven dogs with USMI. The effect was durable in the six dogs with a median follow-up time of 11.3 months.

Hydraulic occluders: Artificial hydraulic urethral occluders have been used for refractory incontinence in human medicine since the early 1970s. The placement of a hydraulic occluder was first reported in four dogs in 2009. These devices are inflatable silicone occluders that are placed around the proximal urethra and attached to a subcutaneously placed vascular access port (Figure 30.11). The use of a custom designed veterinary device was tested

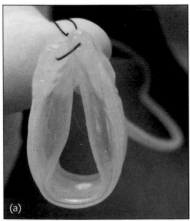
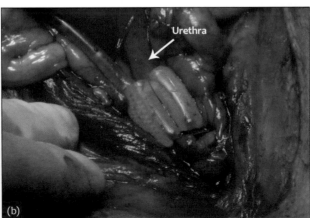
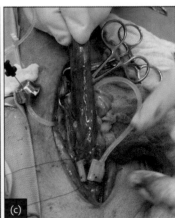

30.11 Hydraulic occluder placement in a female dog with USMI. (a) The silicone ring prior to implantation into the patient with permanent suture material placed through the islets of the device. (b) The occluder is placed around the lumen of the urethra, approximately 1.5 cm caudal to the trigone. (c) The ring is placed around the proximal urethra and the tubing exiting the body wall is attached to the access port. Note the black Huber needle being used to flush the device with saline.

urodynamically in six canine cadavers and inflation of the device to 25% and 50% resulted in an increase in the MUCP and cystourethral leak point pressure. In a recent report of 18 dogs with refractory urinary incontinence that failed ectopic ureter surgery/CLA-EU, medical management and/or bulking agent injection, an overall continence rate of 67% was achieved and when client compliance was attained, the continence score was 92% for a median of 32 months (Currao *et al.*, 2013). The development of a urethral stricture around the hydraulic occluder, resulting in a complete urethral obstruction was reported to occur in 8–17% of dogs and this should be considered prior to device placement. If this occurs, removal of the device has been shown to improve the clinical signs. In another study (Reeves *et al.*, 2013) evaluating the placement of a hydraulic occluder in 27 dogs (24 female dogs and 3 male dogs), a urethral obstruction developed in 7% of dogs with a follow-up time of 12.5 months. The majority of patients did not have a prior ectopic ureter.

Techniques for male dogs:

Vas deferentopexy: Vas deferentopexy seeks to emulate the effects of colposuspension in male dogs. The vas deferens is surgically advanced in a cranial direction, leading to cranial movement of the urethra. Traction is maintained until the prostate gland is seen to move approximately 1 cm cranially. The deferentopexy is then performed by pulling the vas deferens though two muscular tunnels created in the right and left rectus sheath. If not already neutered, dogs must be castrated prior to undergoing vas deferentopexy. The technique has been performed in seven dogs, five of which had intrapelvic bladders preoperatively. The bladders of all seven dogs were located intra-abdominally postoperatively. Clinically, three of the seven dogs were continent following surgery and a further three were improved but only continent with medical therapy in a follow-up time ranging from 12 to 49 months (Holt *et al.*, 2005). No other major complications were recorded. A laparoscopic approach to the technique has also been described in the literature. Long-term outcomes have not been reported in a large cohort of dogs treated with this technique.

Prostatopexy: This technique avoids the need for neutering that is required with vas deferentopexy. Prostatopexy aims to move the bladder neck and proximal urethra into an intra-abdominal position. It involves the placement of two non-absorbable monofilament sutures through the pre-pubic tendon and through the ventral and caudal prostatic capsule approximately 1 cm from the urethra on either side after cranial traction has been placed on the bladder. As an association between neutering and USMI has been made in male dogs, maintenance of dogs in an intact state may be beneficial in these cases. In one clinical report of prostatopexy in male dogs with USMI, only one of the nine dogs in the study was cured, although four were significantly improved for a mean of 2.5 years (Holt *et al.*, 2005).

Techniques for female cats:

The pathophysiology of USMI in cats appears to differ from that in dogs, making the use of the above mentioned techniques inappropriate in many cases. Anatomical abnormalities of the feline lower urogenital tract are often present, including severe urethral and vaginal hypoplasia, with bladder hypoplasia occurring less commonly.

Bladder neck reconstruction: This technique involves the creation of a longer urethra aimed at increasing the potential resistance to urine outflow. Two techniques have been

described and involve either resection of the caudoventral bladder to a point close to the ureterovesicular junctions or the creation of bladder flaps to augment urethral length. It has been suggested that cats with bladder hypoplasia might be better treated using the flap reconstruction technique, whereas cats with normal sized bladders may be adequately treated with the bladder neck resection technique. Of eight cats treated with one of these two techniques, three became continent, four were significantly improved, and one experienced postoperative dysuria (Holt, 1993).

Ectopic ureters

Management of ectopic ureters can either be performed through an open celiotomy approach or by CLA-EU (see above). The aims of surgery are to restore continence, prevent ongoing urinary tract infection or pyelonephritis and to prevent progression of, or reverse, hydroureter and hydronephrosis. Surgical options for ectopic ureters involve either removal of the ectopic ureter along with the affected kidney (ureteronephrectomy), reimplantation of the ureter into the bladder wall (ureteroneocystostomy) or creation of a new opening into the bladder (neoureterostomy). Unfortunately, no single surgical technique has been shown to be successful in controlling urinary incontinence in all cases, although when used in combination with medical management, endoscopic augmentation and/or other surgical procedures, many dogs can have continence restored to an extent where quality of life for the pet and owner are deemed good to excellent. Postoperative continence rates in female dogs treated by neoureterostomy or ureteroneocystostomy vary from 22–58%. The prognosis in male dogs appears to be more favourable with neoureterostomy, ureteroneocystostomy or ureteronephrectomy, rendering 82% of dogs continent in one study (Anders *et al.*, 2012).

Ureteronephrectomy: This procedure should only be considered in dogs when end-stage renal damage is present unilaterally and contralateral kidney function is judged to be adequate. Standard techniques for ureteronephrectomy have been described and are usually performed via an open celiotomy approach. This technique is rarely necessary.

Neoureterostomy: This technique is performed for intramural ectopic ureters, which are present in the vast majority of canine and feline cases. A new ureteral opening in the bladder is created and the remaining intramural tunnel is either sutured closed or removed in its entirety (sometimes termed trigonal reconstruction) (Figure 30.12). The key to neoureterostomy is recognition of the ectopic ureteral wall within the bladder mucosa, which is variably challenging. Once located, it is incised parallel to the longitudinal axis of the ureter at the level of the bladder trigone. The edges of the ureteral incision are sutured to the bladder mucosa to create a new ureteral stoma using a fine synthetic absorbable monofilament suture material (1–1.5 metric, 5/0–4/0 USP) in a simple interrupted pattern. The distal urethral segment can either be double ligated or completely excised. A continuation of the cystotomy incision into a proximal urethrotomy will be required to excise the distal segment in most patients and in some cases a pubic symphisiotomy may be required if access to the entirety of the distal segment is desired. The value of distal segment resection remains controversial with one study unable to demonstrate differences

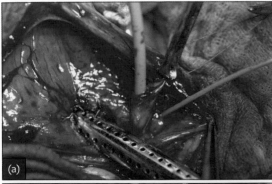

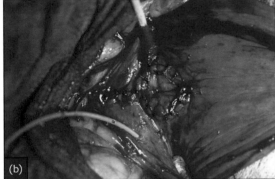

30.12 Neoureterostomy in a female dog with unilateral ureteral ectopia and severe hydroureter. (a) A neoureterostomy has been created (the Poole suction tip is located in the stoma). The more distal intramural tunnel (large red rubber catheter) has been partially dissected prior to excision. The smaller red rubber catheter is positioned in the contralateral normally positioned ureterovesicular junction. (b) After excision of the intramural ectopic ureteral segment, the mucosa has been sutured in a simple interrupted fashion to re-establish continuity of the bladder mucosa and the site of the neoureterostomy can be clearly seen.

in postoperative continence between dogs that had the distal segment simply ligated or completely resected (Mayhew *et al.*, 2006).

Ureteroneocystostomy: Extramural ectopic ureters are very rare in dogs and cats and are usually treated with ureteroneocystostomy (ureteral reimplantation). A variety of techniques have been described, but in all cases the distal end of the ectopic ureter is initially identified and ligated as close to its termination as possible. In dogs, a submucosal tunnel technique and a transverse pull-through technique have been described (Figure 30.13). Complications following ureteroneocystostomy include postoperative hydroureter

and hydronephrosis or stricture at the site of the new ureterovesicular junction, which has been reported in up to 25% of cases after this procedure. In cats, ureteroneocystostomy is a microsurgical technique due to the tiny dimensions of the feline ureter. Extravesicular and intravesicular techniques have been described in cats, with the former seemingly having some advantages.

Conclusion

Overall, urinary incontinence presents a major frustration to owners and veterinary surgeons, but with the appropriate diagnostic tests to define the underlying aetiology and tailored treatment regimens, the chance of dramatic improvement is possible in the majority of cases. As more options become available, greater success for managing the various causes of urinary incontinence is being reported.

References and further reading

Aaron A, Eggleton K, Power C *et al.* (1996) Urethral sphincter mechanism incompetence in male dogs: a retrospective analysis of 54 cases. *Veterinary Record* **139**, 542–546

Acierno MJ and Labato MA (2006) Canine incontinence. *Compendium on Continuing Education for the Practicing Veterinarian* **28**, 591–598

Adams WM and DiBartola SP (1983) Radiographic and clinical features of pelvic bladder in the dog. *Journal of the American Veterinary Medical Association* **182**, 1212–1217

Adin CA, Farese JP, Cross AR *et al.* (2004) Urodynamic effects of a percutaneously controlled static hydraulic urethral sphincter in canine cadavers. *American Journal of Veterinary Research* **65**, 283–288

Anders KJ, McLoughlin MA, Samii VF *et al.* (2012) Ectopic ureters in male dogs: review of 16 clinical cases (1999–2007). *Journal of the American Animal Hospital Association* **48(6)**, 390–398

Angioletti A, De Francessco I, Vergottini M *et al.* (2004) Urinary incontinence after spaying in the bitch: incidence and oestrogen therapy. *Veterinary Research Communications* **28**, 153–155

Arnold S, Arnold P, Hubler M *et al.* (1989a) Urinary incontinence in spayed bitches: prevalence and breed predisposition. *Schweizer Archiv fur Tierheilkunde* **131**, 259–263

Arnold S, Hubler M, Lott-Stolz G *et al.* (1996) Treatment of urinary incontinence in bitches by endoscopic injection of glutaraldehyde cross-linked collagen. *Journal of Small Animal Practice* **37**, 163–168

Arnold S, Jäger P, DiBartola SP *et al.* (1989) Treatment of urinary incontinence in dogs by endoscopic injection of Teflon. *Journal of the American Veterinary Medical Association* **195**, 1369–1374

Awad SA and Downie JW (1976) Relative contributions of smooth and striated muscles to the canine urethral pressure profile. *British Journal of Urology* **48**, 347–354

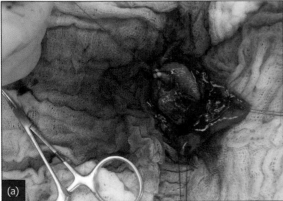

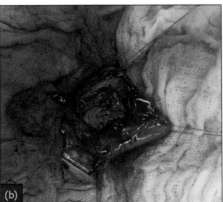

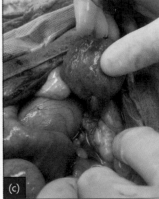

30.13 Ureteroneocystostomy in a dog with extramural ectopic ureters. (a) The distal aspect of the ureter has been ligated and sectioned and is being pulled through a tunnel created in the dorsal aspect of the bladder wall in preparation for ureteroneocystostomy. (b) The completed ureteroneocystostomy has been completed by placement of fine gauge absorbable sutures in a simple interrupted pattern to appose ureteral to bladder mucosa. (c) The completed ureteroneocystostomy can be seen from the external surface of the bladder after closure of the cystotomy incision

Bacon NJ, Oni O and White RAS (2002) Treatment of urethral sphincter mechanism incompetence in 11 bitches with a sustained-release formulation of phenylpropanolamine hydrochloride. *Veterinary Record* **151**, 373–376

Barsanti JA and Downey R (1984) Urinary incontinence in cats. *Journal of the American Animal Hospital Association* **20**, 979–982

Bartges JW and Callens A (2011) Polydimethylsiloxane urethral bulking agent (PDMS UBA) injection for treatment of female canine urinary incontinence – preliminary results. *Journal of Veterinary Internal Medicine* **25**, 748–749

Barth A, Reichler IM, Hubler M *et al.* (2005) Evaluation of long-term effects of endoscopic injection of collagen into the urethral submucosa for treatment of urethral sphincter incompetence in female dogs: 40 cases (1993–2000). *Journal of the American Veterinary Medical Association* **226**, 73–76

Barthez PY, Smeak DD, Wisner ER *et al.* (2000) Ureteral obstruction after ureteroneocystostomy in dogs assessed by technetium TC 99m die-thylenetriamine pentaacetic acid scintigraphy. *Veterinary Surgery* **29**, 499–506

Basinger RR, Rawlings CA, Barsanti JA *et al.* (1987) Urodynamic alterations after prostatectomy in dogs without clinical prostatic disease. *Veterinary Surgery* **16**, 405–410

Basinger RR, Rawlings CA, Barsanti JA *et al.* (1989) Urodynamic alterations associated with clinical prostatic diseases and prostatic surgery in 23 dogs. *Journal of the American Animal Hospital Association* **25**, 385–392

Berent AC, Mayhew PD and Porat-Mosenco Y (2008) Use of cystoscopic-guided laser ablation for treatment of intramural ureteral ectopia in male dogs: four cases (2006–2007). *Journal of the American Veterinary Medical Association* **232**, 1026–1034

Berent AC, Weisse C and Mayhew PD (2012) Evaluation of cystoscopic-guided laser ablation of intramural ectopic ureters in female dogs. *Journal of the American Veterinary Medical Association* **240**, 716–725

Burdick S, Berent AC and Weisse C (2013) Endoscopic-guided laser ablation of vestibulovaginal septal remnants in dogs: 36 cases (2007–2011). *Journal of the American Veterinary Medical Association* **244(8)**, 944–949

Byron JK, Chew DJ and McLoughlin MA (2009) Urinary incontinence: treatment with injectable bulking agents. In: *Current Veterinary Therapy XIV*, ed. JD Bonagura and DC Twedt, pp. 960–964. Saunders Elsevier, St. Louis

Byron JK, Chew DJ and McLoughlin ML (2011) Retrospective evaluation of urethral bovine cross-linked collagen implantation for treatment of urinary incontinence in female dogs. *Journal of Veterinary Internal Medicine* **25**, 980–984

Cannizzo KL, McLoughlin MA, Chew DJ *et al.* (2001) Uroendoscopy. *Veterinary Clinics of North America: Small Animal Practice* **31**, 789–807

Cannizzo KL, McLoughlin MA, Mattoon JS *et al.* (2003) Evaluation of transurethral cystoscopy and excretory urography for diagnosis of ectopic ureters in female dogs: 25 cases (1992–2000). *Journal of the American Veterinary Medical Association* **223**, 475–481

Claeys S, de Leval J and Hamaide A (2010) Transobturator vaginal tape inside out for treatment of urethral sphincter mechanism incompetence: preliminary results in 7 female dogs. *Veterinary Surgery* **39(8)**, 669–679

Creed KE (1983) Effect of hormones on urethral sensitivity to phenylephrine in normal and incontinent dogs. *Research in Veterinary Science* **34**, 177–181

Cullen WC, Fletcher TF and Bradley WE (1981) Histology of the canine urethra I. Morphometry of the female urethra. *Anatomical Record* **199**, 177–186

Cullen WC, Fletcher TF and Bradley WE (1983) Morphometry of the female feline urethra. *The Journal of Urology* **129**, 190–192

Cullen WC, Fletcher TF and Bradley WE (1983) Morphometry of the male feline pelvic urethra. *The Journal of Urology* **129**, 186–189

Currao R, Berent AC and Weisse C (2013) Use of a percutaneously controlled urethral hydraulic occluder for treatment of refractory urinary incontinence in 18 female dogs. *Veterinary Surgery* **42(4)**, 440–447

Diaz Espineira MM, Viehoff FW and Nickel RF (1998) Idiopathic detrusor-urethral dyssynergia in dogs: a retrospective analysis of 22 cases. *Journal of Small Animal Practice* **39**, 264–270

Forsee KM, Davis GJ, Mouat EE *et al.* (2013) Evaluation of the prevalence of urinary incontinence in spayed female dogs: 566 cases (2003–2008). *Journal of the American Veterinary Medical Association* **242(7)**, 959–962

Frenier SL, Knowlen GG, Speth RC *et al.* (1992) Urethral pressure response to alpha-adrenergic agonist and antagonist drugs in anesthetized healthy male cats. *American Journal of Veterinary Research* **53**, 1161–1165

Gookin JL and Bunch SE (1996a) Detrusor-striated sphincter dyssynergia in a dog. *Journal of Veterinary Internal Medicine* **10**, 339–344

Gregory CR (1984) Electromyographic and urethral pressure profilometry: clinical application in male cats. *Veterinary Clinics of North America: Small Animal Practice* **14**, 567–574

Gregory SP, Holt PE, Parkinson TJ *et al.* (1999) Vaginal position and length in the bitch: relationship to spaying and urinary incontinence. *Journal of Small Animal Practice* **40**, 180–184

Hardie EM, Stone EA, Spaulding KA *et al.* (1990) Subtotal canine prostatectomy with the neodymium:yttrium-aluminum-garnet laser. *Veterinary Surgery* **19**, 348–355

Hill TL, Berent AC and Weisse CW (2014) Evaluation of urethral stent placement for benign urethral obstructions in dogs. *Journal of Veterinary Internal Medicine* **28**, 1384–1390

Holt PE (1985a) Urinary incontinence in the bitch due to sphincter mechanism incompetence: prevalence in referred dogs and retrospective analysis of sixty cases. *Journal of Small Animal Practice* **26**, 181–190

Holt PE (1985b) Urinary incontinence in the bitch due to sphincter mechanism incompetence: surgical treatment. *Journal of Small Animal Practice* **26**, 237–246

Holt PE (1985c) Importance of urethral length, bladder neck position and vestibulovaginal stenosis in sphincter mechanism incompetence in the incontinent bitch. *Research in Veterinary Science* **39**, 364–372

Holt PE (1990a) Urinary incontinence in dogs and cats. *Veterinary Record* **127**, 347–350

Holt PE (1990b) Long-term evaluation of colposuspension in the treatment of urinary incontinence due to incompetence of the urethral sphincter mechanism in the bitch. *Veterinary Record* **127**, 537–542

Holt PE (1993) Surgical management of congenital urethral sphincter mechanism incompetence in eight female cats and a bitch. *Veterinary Surgery* **22**, 98–104

Holt PE (1995) Feline urinary incontinence. In: *Current Veterinary Therapy XII*, ed. J Bonagura and RW Kirk, pp. 1018–1021. WB Saunders, Philadelphia

Holt PE, Coe RJ and Hotston Moore A (2005) Prostatopexy as a treatment for urethral sphincter mechanism incompetence in male dogs. *Journal of Small Animal Practice* **46**, 567–570

Holt PE and Gibbs C (1992) Congenital urinary incontinence in cats: a review of 19 cases. *Veterinary Record* **130**, 437–442

Holt PE and Hotston Moore A (1995) Canine ureteral ectopia: an analysis of 175 cases and comparison of surgical treatments. *Veterinary Record* **136**, 345–349

Holt PE and Stone EA (1997) Colposuspension for urinary incontinence. In: *Current Techniques in Small Animal Surgery, 4th edn*, ed. MJ Bojrab, pp. 455–459. Williams and Wilkins, Baltimore

Holt PE and Thrusfield MV (1993) Association in bitches between breed, size, neutering and docking, and acquired urinary incontinence due to incompetence of the urethral sphincter mechanism. *Veterinary Record* **133**, 177–180

Kershen RT, Dmochowski RR and Appell RA (2002) Beyond collagen: injectable therapies for the treatment of female stress urinary incontinence in the new millennium. *Urologic Clinics of North America* **29**, 559–574

Lane IF, Lappin MR and Seim HB (1995) Evaluation of results of preoperative urodynamic measurements in nine dogs with ectopic ureters. *Journal of the American Veterinary Medical Association* **206**, 1348–1357

Lane IF and Westropp JL (2009) Urinary incontinence and micturition disorders: pharmacologic management. In: *Current Veterinary Therapy XIV*, ed. JD Bonagura and DC Twedt, pp. 955–959. Saunders Elsevier, St. Louis

Leippold T, Reitz A and Schurch B (2003) Botulinum toxin as a new therapy option for voiding disorders: current state of the art. *European Urology* **44**, 165–174

Lose G (2001) Urethral pressure measurement: problems and clinical value. *Scandinavian Journal of Urology and Nephrology (Supplement)* **207**, 61–66

Mandigers PJJ and Nell T (2001) Treatment of bitches with acquired urinary incontinence with oestriol. *Veterinary Record* **149**, 764–767

Martinoli S, Nelissen P and White R (2014) The outcome of combined urethropexy and colposuspension for management of bitches with urinary incontinence associated with urethral sphincter mechanism incompetence. *Veterinary Surgery* **43(1)**, 52–57

Massat BJ, Gregory CR, Ling GV *et al.* (1993) Cystourethropexy to correct refractory urinary incontinence due to urethral sphincter mechanism incompetence. *Veterinary Surgery* **22**, 260–269

Mayhew PD, Lee KCL, Gregory SP *et al.* (2006) Comparison of two surgical techniques for management of intramural ureteral ectopia in dogs: 36 cases (1994–2004). *Journal of the American Veterinary Medical Association* **229**, 389–393

McLoughlin MA and Chew DJ (2000) Diagnosis and surgical management of ectopic ureters. *Clinical Techniques in Small Animal Practice* **15**, 17–24

Mehl ML, Kyles AE, Pollard R *et al.* (2005) Comparison of 3 techniques for ureteroneocystostomy in cats. *Veterinary Surgery* **34**, 114–119

Meler E, Berent AC, Weisse C *et al.* (2014) Treatment of congenital ureterovesicular junction stenosis using laser ablation in dogs: 10 cases (2010–2013) *American College of Veterinary Internal Medicine, Nashville* [Abstract]

Miodrag A, Castleden CM and Vallance TR (1988) Sex hormones and the female urinary tract. *Drugs* **36**, 491–504

Muir P, Goldsmid SE and Bellenger CR (1994) Management of urinary incontinence in five bitches with incompetence of the urethral sphincter mechanism by colposuspension and a modified sling urethroplasty. *Veterinary Record* **134**, 38–41

Nickel RF, Wiegand U and Van den Brom WE (1998) Evaluation of a transpelvic sling procedure with and without colposuspension for treatment of female dogs with refractory urethral sphincter mechanism incompetence. *Veterinary Surgery* **27**, 94–104

Noël S, Cambier C, Baert K *et al.* (2010) Combined pharmacokinetic and urodynamic study of the effects of oral administration of phenylpropanolamine in female Beagle dogs. *The Veterinary Journal* **184**, 201–207

Norris AM, Laing EJ, Valli VE *et al.* (1992) Canine bladder and urethral tumors: a retrospective study of 115 cases (1980–1985). *Journal of Veterinary Internal Medicine* **6**, 145–153

North C, Kruger JM, Venta PJ, Miller JM, Rosenstein DS *et al.* (2010) Congenital ureteral ectopia in continent and incontinent-related Entlebucher Mountain Dogs: 13 cases (2006–2009). *Journal of Veterinary Internal Medicine* **24(5)**, 1055–1062

Power SC, Eggleton KE, Aaron AJ *et al.* (1998) Urethral sphincter mechanism incompetence in the male dog: importance of bladder neck position, proximal urethral length and castration. *Journal of Small Animal Practice* **39**, 69–72

Rawlings CA, Barsanti JA, Mahaffey MB *et al.* (2001) Evaluation of colposuspension for treatment of incontinence in spayed female dogs. *Journal of the American Veterinary Medical Association* **219**, 770–775

Reeves L, Adin C, McLoughlin M *et al.* (2013) Outcome after placement of an artificial urethral sphincter in 27 dogs. *Veterinary Surgery* **42(1)**, 12–18

Reichler IM, Barth A, Piche CA *et al.* (2006a) Urodynamic parameters and plasma LF/FSH in spayed Beagle bitches before and 8 weeks after GnRH depot analogue treatment. *Theriogenology* **66**, 2127–2136

Reichler IM, Jochle W, Piche CA *et al.* (2006b) Effect of a long acting GnRH analogue or placebo on plasma LH/FSH, urethral pressure profiles and clinical signs of urinary incontinence due to sphincter mechanism incontinence in bitches. *Theriogenology* **66**, 1227–1236

Reichler IM, Pfeiffer E, Piche A *et al.* (2004) Changes in plasma gonadotropin concentrations and urethral closure pressure in the bitch during the 12 months following ovariectomy. *Theriogenology* **62**, 1391–1402

Richter KP and Ling GV (1985) Clinical response and urethral pressure profile changes after phenylpropanolamine in dogs with primary sphincter incompetence. *Journal of the American Veterinary Medical Association* **187**, 605–611

Rose SA, Adin CA, Ellison GW *et al.* (2009) Long-term efficacy of a percutaneously adjustable hydraulic urethral sphincter for treatment of urinary incontinence in four dogs. *Veterinary Surgery* **38**, 747–753

Salomon JF, Cotard JP and Viguier E (2002) Management of urethral sphincter mechanism incompetence in a male dog with laparoscopic-guided deferentopexy. *Journal of Small Animal Practice* **43**, 501–505

Scott L, Leedy M, Bernay F *et al.* (2002) Evaluation of phenylpropanolamine in the treatment of urethral sphincter mechanism incompetence in the bitch. *Journal of Small Animal Practice* **43**, 493–496

Smith AL, Radlinkay MG and Rawlings CA (2010) Cystoscopic diagnosis and treatment of ectopic ureters in female dogs: 16 cases (2005–2008). *Journal of the American Veterinary Medical Association* **237**, 191–195

Thrusfield MV (1985) Association between urinary incontinence and spaying in bitches. *Veterinary Record* **116**, 695

Thrusfield MV, Holt PE and Muirhead RH (1998) Acquired urinary incontinence in bitches: its incidence and relationship to neutering practices. *Journal of Small Animal Practice* **39**, 559–566

van Kerrebroeck P, ter Meulen F, Farrelly E *et al.* (2003) Treatment of stress urinary incontinence: recent developments in the role of urethral injection. *Urological Research* **30**, 356–362

Weber UT, Arnold A, Hubler M *et al.* (1997) Surgical treatment of male dogs with urinary incontinence due to urethral sphincter mechanism incompetence. *Veterinary Surgery* **26**, 51–56

Wilson K, Berent AC and Weisse C (2016) Use of a percutaneously controlled hydraulic urethral occluder for the treatment of urinary incontinence in 3 cats. *Journal of the American Veterinary Medical Association* **248**, 544–551

White RAS and Pomeroy CJ (1989) Phenylpropanolamine: an a-adrenergic agent for the management of urinary incontinence in the bitch associated with urethral sphincter mechanism incompetence. *Veterinary Record* **125**, 478–480

White RN (2001) Urethropexy for the management of urethral sphincter mechanism incompetence in the bitch. *Journal of Small Animal Practice* **42**, 481–486

Conversion tables

Haematology

Parameter	SI unit	Conversion factor	Conventional unit
Red blood cell count	10^{12}/l	1	10^6/µl
Haemoglobin	g/l	0.1	g/dl
MCH	pg/cell	1	pg/cell
MCHC	g/l	0.1	g/dl
MCV	fl	1	µm³
Platelet count	10^9/l	1	10^3/µl
White blood cell count	10^9/l	1	10^3/µl

Biochemistry

Parameter	SI unit	Conversion factor	Conventional unit
Alanine transferase	IU/l	1	IU/l
Albumin	g/l	0.1	g/dl
Aldosterone	pmol/l	0.36	pg/ml
Alkaline phosphatase	IU/l	1	IU/l
Antiduirectic hormone	pmol/l	1.084	pg/ml
Aspartate transaminase	IU/l	1	IU/l
Bilirubin	µmol/l	0.0584	mg/dl
BUN	mmol/l	2.8	mg/dl
Calcitriol	pmol/l	0.417	pg/ml
Calcium	mmol/l	4	mg/dl
Carbon dioxide (total)	mmol/l	1	mEq/l
Cholesterol	mmol/l	38.61	mg/dl
Chloride	mmol/l	1	mEq/l
Cortisol	nmol/l	0.362	ng/ml
Creatine kinase	IU/l	1	IU/l
Creatinine	µmol/l	0.0113	mg/dl
Erythropoietin	IU/l	1	mIU/l
Glucose	mmol/l	18.02	mg/dl
Insulin	pmol/l	0.1394	µIU/ml
Iron	µmol/l	5.587	µg/dl
Magnesium	mmol/l	2.4	mg/dl
Parathyroid hormone	pmol/l	9.4	pg/ml
Phosphorus	mmol/l	3.1	mg/dl
Potassium	mmol/l	1	mEq/l
Sodium	mmol/l	1	mEq/l
Total protein	g/l	0.1	g/dl
Thyroxine (T4) (free)	pmol/l	0.0775	ng/dl
Thyroxine (T4) (total)	nmol/l	0.0775	µg/dl
Tri-iodothyronine (T3)	nmol/l	65.1	ng/dl
Triglycerides	mmol/l	88.5	mg/dl

Index

Page numbers in *italics* indicate figures